Bayesian Thinking in Biostatistics

CHAPMAN & HALL/CRC
Texts in Statistical Science Series

Joseph K. Blitzstein, *Harvard University, USA*
Julian J. Faraway, *University of Bath, UK*
Martin Tanner, *Northwestern University, USA*
Jim Zidek, *University of British Columbia, Canada*

Recently Published Titles

Practical Multivariate Analysis, Sixth Edition
Abdelmonem Afifi, Susanne May, Robin A. Donatello, and Virginia A. Clark

Time Series: A First Course with Bootstrap Starter
Tucker S. McElroy and Dimitris N. Politis

Probability and Bayesian Modeling
Jim Albert and Jingchen Hu

Surrogates
Gaussian Process Modeling, Design, and Optimization for the Applied Sciences
Robert B. Gramacy

Statistical Analysis of Financial Data
With Examples in R
James Gentle

Statistical Rethinking
A Bayesian Course with Examples in R and STAN, Second Edition
Richard McElreath

Statistical Machine Learning
A Model-Based Approach
Richard Golden

Randomization, Bootstrap and Monte Carlo Methods in Biology
Fourth Edition
Bryan F. J. Manly, Jorje A. Navarro Alberto

Principles of Uncertainty, Second Edition
Joseph B. Kadane

Beyond Multiple Linear Regression
Applied Generalized Linear Models and Multilevel Models in R
Paul Roback, Julie Legler

Bayesian Thinking in Biostatistics
Gary L. Rosner, Purushottam W. Laud, and Wesley O. Johnson

Modern Data Science with R, Second Edition
Benjamin S. Baumer, Daniel T. Kaplan, and Nicholas J. Horton

Probability and Statistical Inference
From Basic Principles to Advanced Models
Miltiadis Mavrakakis and Jeremy Penzer

For more information about this series, please visit: https://www.crcpress.com/Chapman--Hall-CRC-Texts-in-Statistical-Science/book-series/CHTEXSTASCI

Bayesian Thinking in Biostatistics

by
Gary L. Rosner
Purushottam W. Laud
Wesley O. Johnson

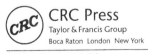

CRC Press
Taylor & Francis Group
Boca Raton London New York

CRC Press is an imprint of the
Taylor & Francis Group, an **informa** business

A CHAPMAN & HALL BOOK

First edition published 2021
by CRC Press
6000 Broken Sound Parkway NW, Suite 300, Boca Raton, FL 33487-2742

and by CRC Press
2 Park Square, Milton Park, Abingdon, Oxon, OX14 4RN

© 2021 Taylor & Francis Group, LLC

CRC Press is an imprint of Taylor & Francis Group, LLC

Library of Congress Cataloging-in-Publication Data

Names: Rosner, Gary L., author. | Laud, Purushottam, 1948- author. | Johnson, Wesley O., author.
Title: Bayesian thinking in biostatistics / Gary L. Rosner, Purushottam W. Laud, Wesley O. Johnson.
Description: First edition. | Boca Raton : CRC Press, 2021. | Includes bibliographical references and index.
Identifiers: LCCN 2020049870 (print) | LCCN 2020049871 (ebook) | ISBN 9781439800089 (hardcover) | ISBN 9781439800102 (ebook)
Subjects: LCSH: Biometry--Methodology. | Bayesian statistical decision theory.
Classification: LCC QH323.5 .R68 2021 (print) | LCC QH323.5 (ebook) | DDC
570.1/5195--dc23
LC record available at https://lccn.loc.gov/2020049870
LC ebook record available at https://lccn.loc.gov/2020049871

ISBN: 978-1-4398-0008-9 (hbk)

To my wife, Naomi, and my children, Joshua and Molly, for their support, understanding, patience, and, most of all, love. GLR

To Kaye and the boys – Raj, Kavi, Sanjiv and Filip – who have believed since its conception that this project would come to fruition. PWL

To my friend and mentor, Seymour Geisser. I miss him very much. WOJ

Contents

Preface

How could they see anything but the shadows if they were never allowed to move their heads? (Plato, The allegory of the cave, *The Republic*, Book VII)

Why an introductory book on Bayesian biostatistics?

Bayesian statistical methods have found increased use and acceptance in biomedical research. More and more clinical trials are including Bayesian considerations in their designs. Interim analyses based on posterior or predictive probabilities have appeared in protocols for clinical studies sponsored by the largest pharmaceutical companies and at internationally renowned academic medical centers. Governmental regulatory agencies, such as the U.S. Food and Drug Administration and the European Medicines Agency, are becoming more open to considering clinical trials with Bayesian designs. In our roles as biostatisticians at active academic medical centers, we have used Bayesian methods in our collaborations. We receive frequent requests for information about Bayesian methods from our colleagues in other disciplines. We teach courses on Bayesian methods, focusing on biostatistical applications, and our students come from many different departments. Given this widespread interest—especially from our colleagues in disciplines outside of statistics—we felt the time is right for an introductory textbook that reviews Bayesian inference from the standpoint of someone whose interest is biostatistical but whose background is not. Aside from providing a summary of the concepts and theory of Bayesian inference, information that one can find in many available texts, we also discuss methods that biomedical investigators would want to use for their research. We cover Bayesian methods for analyzing time-to-event data (i.e., survival analysis), clinical trial design, longitudinal data analysis, and diagnostic tests.

Another factor that has contributed to broader use of Bayesian methods in biostatistics is the availability of computer programs to carry out the necessary computations. The stand-alone packages WinBUGS (and its current incarnation OpenBUGS), JAGS, and Stan, as well as packages and functions written for the statistical computing environment R, have put the ability to carry out rather sophisticated and complex data analyses in the hands of more people than ever before. The availability of these tools provides the opportunity to promote the use of Bayesian biostatistical methods to a wider audience. In the book and an accompanying website, we provide programs in the BUGS language, with variants for JAGS and Stan, that one can use or adapt for one's own research.

The topics we cover are the applications we see most often in our respective institutions. We are not able to cover each topic as thoroughly as we might like, since one could expand each method-focused chapter into a book. (In fact, books are available that focus on each chapter's topic.) We have, however, endeavored to cover the elements that we consider to be the more important or useful aspects of each topic and provide the necessary background to allow further study if the reader wishes. We have ended each chapter with a section called "Recap and Readings" in which we provide references to books or research papers that contain further details or development of methods we discuss in the chapter.

What this book tries to accomplish

As mentioned above, we wrote this book for use by scientists and researchers who may not have extensive background in mathematics and statistics. Although we do include some of the mathematics, anyone with an understanding of basic calculus will be able to appreciate the underlying theory. Furthermore, we explain in words the concepts that underlie complicated methods. The goal is to give the scientist the ability to think about and use statistical models effectively in the context of the data available for analysis, as well as other information that may inform that analysis. In doing so, the analysis can focus on questions raised by the science, not restrictions imposed by the statistical method.

We describe the basics of Bayesian inference and explain many ways in which one may apply this statistical approach to carry out inference in one's research. We describe models based on assumptions of particularly convenient distributions, such as the binomial, Gaussian (or normal) distributions, as do many standard textbooks. Unlike several other textbooks, however, we emphasize the availability of information with which one can form informed prior distributions. We feel strongly that one should put some thought into prior distributions instead of immediately using standard reference or so-called "non-informative" prior distributions. In many biomedical settings, we statisticians and our subject-matter collaborators know enough to be able to say that certain outcomes are highly unlikely (e.g., living 200 years after suffering a myocardial infarction at age 65) or even impossible. The prior distribution is, after all, part of the statistical model. In our view, an advantage of the Bayesian approach is that it forces each member of the study team to think carefully about assumptions, including the assumptions that underlie statistical models.

We go beyond standard statistical models in the book. We introduce a few Bayesian nonparametric methods and illustrate their uses in data analysis. Bayesian nonparametric models provide a flexible and less restrictive approach to inference. These statistical models place uncertainty on the underlying probability distributions in the inferential model. This extra uncertainty relaxes one of the most ubiquitous assumptions in statistics, namely, that random continuous quantities follow normal distributions. Aside from removing the distributional assumption of normality, the extra flexibility also carries over into characterizing relationships between outcomes and covariates not as, say, linear but as mixtures of linear regressions. This freedom from more rigid modeling assumptions allows for exploration and a touchstone against which to assess parametric assumptions and particular models. Each of us has applied Bayesian nonparametric models in our research and written on its application in complex problems. The availability of DPPackage in R and approximations via other software packages make these flexible inferential approaches available for use by many researchers who are not skilled at writing their own computer programs. We illustrate these methods in the book.

As it is natural in the Bayesian approach, we emphasize estimation of biomedically relevant quantities and assessment of the uncertainty in this estimation. This is in contrast to an emphasis on hypothesis formulation and testing that appears in most standard textbooks in biostatistics.

How to navigate and learn from the book

The first chapter introduces the components that are necessary for carrying out Bayesian inference and presents some biomedical example studies that we analyze in later sections of the book. In particular, this chapter presents our understanding and vision of what statistical inference in science is all about. This philosophy underlies Bayesian thinking. Chapter 2 presents the fundamentals of Bayesian inference. Chapter 3 illustrates Bayesian inference with some basic statistical models. Chapter 4 reviews computational methods for carrying out Bayesian inference, emphasizing Markov chain Monte Carlo methods and software to implement these computational approaches. Comparing populations is common in biostatistics, and Chapter 5 contains many models for such analyses. Chapter 6 covers the important topic of prior distributions, including prior elicitation and implementation via Markov chain Monte Carlo. Linear regression from a Bayesian perspective is covered in Chapter 7, and regression models for dichotomous outcomes are covered in Chapter 8. Several other regression models are given in Chapter 9. Once one has fit a model or models, one has to decide which of several competing models appears to fit the best and also assess how well the model actually fits the data. We cover this important topic in Chapter 10. Many biostatistical analyses concern time-to-event data, and Chapters 11 and 12 cover this topic from a Bayesian perspective. We provide a brief review of Bayesian approaches to designing clinical trials in Chapter 13. Hierarchical models and longitudinal data are the subjects of Chapter 14. We present some basic models for evaluating diagnostic tests in Chapter 15.

There are also three appendices that provide some reference or background material. Appendix A reviews elementary probability theory that forms the basis of statistical inference. We include several probability distributions in the book, and Appendix B contains a table of these distributions' densities and key characteristics. Since computation is critical for modern Bayesian data analysis, Appendix C contains brief descriptions of several software tools that one can use in one's own research when one analyzes data. Readers will likely find several of the more general packages useful when doing the exercises at the end of each chapter.

We recommend that one read Chapters 1–6 in order before choosing topics from the remaining chapters. The choice of topics, chapters to cover, and the order could depend on available time, instructor or student interest, and other courses the student or reader may take as part of a degree program. One possibility is to include linear and binary regression (Chapters 7 and 8), followed by model criticism and choice (Chapter 10).

Another choice could be to include survival analysis (Chapters 11 and 12), along with some discussion of clinical trials (Chapter 13). There are many combinations that will fill a good semester of Bayesian biostatistics.

Sections with an asterisk (*) in their title involve more difficult probability calculus that some readers may prefer to skip on first reading. Later chapters and sections not marked with * will not require the material in these sections. The * sections will be beneficial for those who wish to have a deeper understanding of the Bayesian approach to statistics and the underlying theory, but they are not necessary in order to practice it.

Web material

The book has a dedicated website that provides example programs written for use with WinBUGS (or OpenBUGS), JAGS, and Stan, along with data, at https://github.com/BTB-RLJ. We will post corrections we learn about on this site, as well as any addenda to the material already in the book. We hope this website will be dynamic and allow us to expand the models and discussion relating to Bayesian inference in biostatistics, as we receive comments and suggestions from readers, students, and teachers.

What this book does not do and where you can find that information

As we stated earlier, we cannot in this introductory book cover all application areas of Bayesian inference in biostatistics. Additionally, the field is dynamic and a rapidly expanding area of research, with new models arising all the time to address new subject-matter research questions and sources of biomedical data. Although we provide citations and references in each chapter, we will now provide a small list of references that some readers may wish to consult alongside or after reading this book.

A general introduction to Bayesian thinking that does not use any calculus is given in the book by Donald Berry [36]. The books by Gelman et al. [133] and Carlin and Louis [63] provide a general but modern (i.e., computational) presentation of the Bayesian approach to inference. Christensen et al. [79] cover some (but not all) of the same methods that we present in this book. A very good source of interesting examples is *The BUGS Book* by Lunn et al. (2012) [232]. Another good source for examples is McElreath (2020) [241]. Kadane (2011) [196] presents the theoretical foundations underlying Bayesian statistical models, including decision theory.

Acknowledgments

We wish to thank our teachers and colleagues for their inspiration and guidance. We also thank our students for always helping us learn new things or gain a new understanding of methods and theory. Many people have helped us along the way in writing this book. We thank Yushu Shi and Jacob Fiksel for their programming help. We have made use of materials in the book *Bayesian Ideas and Data Analysis: An Introduction for Scientists and Statisticians* [79] in the writing of this book. We appreciate the authors' efforts that have in turn helped us in our efforts. We also wish to express our appreciation for David Grubbs of Chapman & Hall/CRC for his patience and guidance throughout the process. Last, but definitely not least, we thank our families for their never ending support.

Chapter 1

Scientific Data Analysis

Bayesian statistical methods follow a well-defined set of principles and rely on the mathematics of probabilities. These principles require a focus on a model for the data to be analyzed and on the information available about the model in sources extraneous to these data. The method combines this information with the information in the data, and then proceeds to make scientific conclusions with *quantified* certainty. Typically, the certainty of conclusions is captured in clear probability statements and in predictions for future data. Such post-data statements consist of what is termed "inference." Essentially, this is the culmination of taking the external-to-data knowledge about a biomedical mechanism and its outcome, learning from the collected data, and arriving at an updated state of knowledge.

As an example, suppose data will be collected to study the extent of the rotational acceleration involved in injuries leading to a concussion diagnosis during high school football games. The gathering of such data would involve helmets equipped with sophisticated measuring devices [154]. The resulting data may be regarded as repeated measurements, in units of radians per second squared, corresponding to each concussion event. Describing the data via statistical summary measures (e.g., means and standard deviations) and via graphical displays (e.g., histograms and boxplots) is an important first step in the analysis. However, as there will be variation in these numbers from one event to another, it is also very useful next to think of the mechanism by which data similar to those collected could arise. This thought process is called modeling the data, the model specifying a probabilistic mechanism that might have generated the data. Methods of Bayesian statistics emphasize the model-based approach to data analysis. As an initial step, we could think of the rotational acceleration data as arising from a normal distribution, and without any probabilistic distinction from one event to another. Now, the data-generating normal distribution has some mean and standard deviation. These two unknown quantities, in turn, are represented by probability distributions assigned to their possible values. Such distributions for unknowns are to characterize mathematically any possible external information available from sources (perhaps laboratory data in animal models, historical reports) distinct from the data to be collected. Bayesian inference then represents data-incorporated knowledge about the unknowns, combining the data and the outside-data information. This knowledge is characterized by probability statements that include estimates and uncertainty about the estimates, as well as used to predict future data.

In this chapter, after a description of our approach, we introduce some examples and then give brief general presentations of the pieces needed for Bayesian analysis.

1.1 Philosophy

We motivate the book with a general philosophy of data analysis that will be illustrated in the next section, with details to follow in the remainder of the book:

- that a primary role of statistics in science and society is to provide appropriate tools for addressing *scientific* questions;

- that appropriate statistical analysis of data involves a collaborative effort between subject-matter scientists and statisticians;

- that it is both appropriate and necessary to incorporate the scientist's expertise into making decisions related to the data;

- that foundational issues matter in statistics;

- that prediction is of fundamental importance.

To achieve these aims, we have adopted a Bayesian approach. Bayesian statistical analysis is based on the premise that all uncertainty should be modeled using probabilities and that statistical inferences should be logical conclusions based on the laws of probability.

The field of statistics has long embraced the concept of probability models for data. Such models typically involve parameters that are presumed to be related to characteristics of the sampled populations. These parameters can range from few in number with simple interpretations to an uncountable number. Parameters can never be known with absolute certainty unless we sample the entire population. Moreover, parameters may not have physical interpretations since, inevitably, models rarely are precisely true. Models are, we hope, useful approximations to some truth that can provide good predictions. Nonetheless, statistical inquiry has focused more on the estimation of parameters than on prediction.

As we already indicated, given a statistical model for the data, the Bayesian approach mandates an additional probability model for all unknown parameters in the data model. Our approach is to model this uncertainty about the parameters using scientific expert information, or what we will term knowledge-based information. This information must be obtained independently of the data being analyzed. One way to guarantee that scientific input about model parameters is independent of the data is to acquire that information before the data have been collected. However this is often unrealistic except in situations such as a well-planned clinical trial. Our experience is that it is generally possible to obtain independent information from sources such as existing literature or colleagues of the scientists who collected the current data. We also discuss the formation of so-called "reference" or "flat" priors, when there is an absence of knowledge-based information. There is an art to the formation of probability distributions that incorporate available scientific knowledge, and the lack of it.

1.2 Examples

We now provide a glimpse into the types of data that we analyze later in the book to illustrate concepts and methods in Bayesian analysis. In later chapters, we will elaborate on some of these examples, and introduce additional examples as more advanced models are considered.

Example 1.1. Dr. Jeffrey Whittle designed and conducted a study of hypertension in members of U.S. veterans' organizations such as the Veterans of Foreign Wars (VFW) and the American Legion. Blood pressure (systolic and diastolic), height and weight were measured at baseline, and after 6 and 12 months. Blood pressure is measured in millimeters of mercury (mm Hg), height in inches and weight in pounds. These measurements were a part of a randomized trial [353] to compare two different methods of educating and encouraging hypertensive veterans to achieve better control of this condition. One method recruited and trained leaders from the organizations' posts (or local chapters) who then educated and encouraged their peers. The other method consisted of seminars given by health professionals at the posts. Data on the 405 participants are in the data file named VetBP.csv. We will refer to this example and the data set with the name **VetBP**.

Example 1.2. In a study of breast cancer survivors, Dr. Tina Yen and colleagues considered possible risk factors for lymphedema, a condition caused by a blockage of lymph vessels that drain fluids from body tissues. Lymphedema results in arm swelling, possibly leading to decreased functioning, skin breakdown and chronic infections if untreated. The reported article [356] uses data on women 65 to 89 years of age collected from telephone surveys, Medicare claims, and state cancer registries. The measured variables include patient demographics such as age and race, tumor characteristics such as size and grade, and treatment variables such as type of surgery, number of lymph nodes examined and receipt of radiation, chemo and hormonal therapy. Data for 1,307 patients are included in the file named LE.csv. We will refer to this example and its data with the name **LE**.

Example 1.3. Mild traumatic brain injury (MTBI) is a term currently used by the scientific community studying what is commonly known as concussion. It is caused by a rapid linear or rotational acceleration of the head, typically caused by a blunt impact. McCrea [237] gives an excellent overview of the field. As an example, we will focus on the data that led to a threshold for predicting MTBI [363] and refer to this example and its data with the name **MTBI**.

Example 1.4. Patients brought to a trauma center after severe injuries often face heavy odds against short-term survival. Dr. Turner Osler, a trauma surgeon and former head of the Burn Unit at the University of New Mexico Trauma Center, was interested in studying which factors are associated with such odds. In particular, he targeted measurements routinely available from trauma center records: injury severity score, revised trauma score, age, and whether the injury is blunt or penetrating. Analysis resulting from Dr. Osler's data is discussed in [24]. We refer to these data and this example with the name **Trauma**.

Example 1.5. Falls in the elderly are quite common and can have serious consequences. Unintentional falls cause approximately 2 million injuries requiring care in emergency departments per year among Americans over the age of 65. Many falls lead to fractures and hospital admissions for trauma. Each year, 16,000 deaths are attributed to complications from such falls. For the state of Wisconsin, summary data of yearly emergency department visits are available at the website www.dhs.wisconsin.gov/wish. Accompanying analysis of a multi-county intervention was led by Dr. Peter Layde and reported in [153] We will refer to this example and its data with the name **Falls**.

Example 1.6. To study biomechanical aspects of various severe brain injuries caused by motor vehicle crashes as well as penetrating objects, computer simulation is a major tool. Such simulation requires good measurements of the material properties of the brain tissue, such as the coefficient value in a stress–strain relationship. For this purpose, animal tissue is harvested after sacrifice, stored and later used in laboratory measurements. Dr. Yoganandan's laboratory conducted a study [362] to determine if the temperature at which the tissue is stored affects the coefficient measurement obtained. Stress and strain measurements were made at the same lab temperature on two groups of specimens of tissue, one group preserved ice-cold and the other at $37°C$. The file named Brain.csv contains these data. We will refer to this example and its data with the name **Brain**.

Example 1.7. Dr. Ann Nattinger and her research team conducted a longitudinal survey of women over 65 who had incident breast cancer in 2003 [247]. There were four waves of this survey, following the patients for 5 years beyond surgery. The file BRCAsurvey.csv contains data on all 3,083 patients. The variables in the data set include survival information (five-year survival as a yes/no outcome, and time of death if applicable), age at surgery, type of surgery (breast conserving or mastectomy), some tumor characteristics such as size and grade, an index of comorbidity (the variable named `nci`), case volume measures for the patient's surgeon and hospital, and others. We will refer to this example and its data with the name **BRCAsurvey**.

Example 1.8. This example illustrates the analysis of *time-to-event data*, data about how long it takes for something to happen. How long until a drug kicks in? How long does a person with a fatal disease survive? Bedrick, Christensen, and Johnson [25] consider data on 45 cows that naturally aborted their fetuses prematurely. It is of interest to dairy managers to determine whether cows infected with *Neospora caninum* typically abort later than uninfected cows; 19 of the 45 cows were infected. The times to abortion in the uninfected group are 60, 74, 37, 45, 75, 40, 50, 50, 146, 70, 50, 84, 60, 149, 50, 90, 259, 40, 90, 101, 70, 90, 254, 130, 80, and 40 days. For the infected group the times are 50, 130, 100, 130, 50, 140, 129, 76, 138, 69, 70, 144, 70, 130, 70, 150, 251, 110, and 120 days. One way to answer the study question is to compute a summary statistic, such as the mean or median, for each group of cows and decide if the difference between these group-specific summary measures is reasonably close to zero. How close to zero one considers to be reasonably close to zero will determine the inference about the association between infection with *Neospora caninum* and a cow's time to abortion. We will refer to this example as **DairyCattle**.

Example 1.9. Our next example is another illustration of *time-to-event data*. The Cancer and Leukemia Group B (CALGB) conducted a randomized clinical trial to compare the benefits of different dose intense regimens of a three-drug combination to treat non-metastatic breast cancer. Benefit in this study referred to living longer without the breast cancer recurring, sometimes called disease-free survival (DFS). The study, CALGB 8541 [59], randomized over 1,500 women to one of three treatment regimens.

The analysis of time-to-event data is often complicated by the fact that one does not get to see when the event occurs in all study participants. That is, some patients are alive and free of breast cancer at the time of analysis. If the recurrence occurs in these patients, it occurs in the future, but we do not know when in the future. This complicating factor is called *censoring*. Some people buy a refrigerator because their previous one broke. Those people know how long their refrigerator survived. But many people replace their refrigerator before it breaks, so the data on how long it would last are censored. All they know is that it was still running when it was replaced. Censoring is discussed more extensively in Chapter 11.

Since there are known patient or disease characteristics that may affect DFS beyond any treatment effect, the analyst may want to account for potential differences in the distribution of these prognostic characteristics across the treatment groups. Regression methods allow one to adjust for any differences in characteristics, and we will illustrate these methods in Chapter 12 in the context of the analysis of time-to-event data.

These breast cancer study data, contained in the file CALGB8541.csv, also appeared in [37]. We will refer to this example and its data with the name **CALGB8541**. CALGB also conducted other studies, some of which we will describe and use as examples in later chapters.

1.3 Essential Ingredients for Bayesian Analysis

In science, one carries out experiments to learn about the world around us. In this book we focus on biological sciences, but many, if not most, of the concepts we present apply more broadly. Scientists ask questions and design studies to obtain answers. Why do certain people get cancer? Why do some patients respond to drug A while other patients do not? Will intervention X reduce the risk of heart disease? When analyzing data from a study, it is conceptually useful to step back from the data at hand and consider the question (or questions) the study data are supposed to answer. Ask, for example, what was known about this question when the investigators designed the study, and why the study's investigators designed the study as they did. What was the state of knowledge prior to the analysis of these data? Thinking about the state of knowledge and the goals of the study helps us understand the ingredients of Bayesian data analysis and how the data analyst combines them.

Consider the **VetBP** blood pressure study, for example. The study planned to recruit members from veterans' organizations and measure their systolic and diastolic blood pressure at recruitment. Although the full study had many other goals, let us focus only on this baseline measurement for the moment. As a simple goal, consider quantifying the mean and variation of blood pressure in the population from which the study subjects were selected.

Here then is a list of ingredients we need, described in a little more detail in this section, and elaborated throughout the book:

- the *observable* measurements and the *process* of collecting these observables;

- the *unobservables or unknowns* of scientific interest;

- the *probability mechanism or model* that will generate the data;

- the state of *pre-data or outside-data* knowledge about the unknowns;

- the *mathematical formulation* (or a learning mechanism) by which the data will add to this knowledge;

- the resulting *post-data or data-informed* knowledge.

1.3.1 Observables and Design for Their Collection

It is good to begin with the definition of measurements that are to be made during data collection. In the **VetBP** study the central measurement was the blood pressure, both systolic (SBP) and diastolic (DBP) in millimeters of mercury. It is also important to consider the design for subject recruitment for the study. Veterans' organizations in the Milwaukee area were contacted with participation requests and visited upon invitation, subsequently enrolling individuals with their written consent. Here the observables are blood pressure measurements on individuals from the population of veterans known to these organizations in the area and accessible via these organizations.

1.3.2 Unknowns of Scientific Interest

In scientific inquiry, study objectives often focus on learning about interesting unknowns such as the probability of surviving at least 5 years after a cancer diagnosis (Example 1.9, **CALGB8541**); the effect of treatment on the risk of lymphedema among breast cancer survivors (Example 1.2, **LE**); or the effect of injury severity, revised trauma score, age, and type of injury on the probability of death while being treated for trauma in an emergency department (Example 1.4, **Trauma**). Typical unknowns of scientific interest are summary measures, such as the mean, median, or standard deviation, of the *population* from which the individuals in the study were recruited.

A typical statistical model may also include unknowns that, by themselves, are not of particular scientific interest but that nonetheless are useful in specifying a model that fits the data well. It will often be the case that some functions of model parameters are of scientific interest. This will be a recurring theme throughout the book. Knowledge about these unknowns is updated by using the collected data.

Several quantities relating to the veteran population were of interest to Dr. Whittle, the study's principal investigator (Example 1.1, **VetBP**). These quantities include the population mean SBP and DBP, standard deviations of these in the population, SBP and DBP ranges that describe the middle 50% of the population and, most importantly, the percentage of the veteran population with SBP greater than 140 mm Hg or DBP greater than 90 mm Hg. Of even greater interest is the effect of treatment on reducing both types of BP.

1.3.3 Probability Models and Model Parameters

We begin with the simplest models that characterize the generation of a study's data; we introduce numerous additional models in subsequent chapters.

By regarding participants in Dr. Whittle's study as a random sample from the population, we can consider blood pressure (BP) measurements on individuals to be interchangeable, with no characteristics distinguishing one subject from the next. The model assumes a distributional form for the BP measurements, starting with the assumption of a normal distribution, which must be checked. We may also consider the possibility of a log-normal distribution, namely, that the logarithms of the BP measurements are normally distributed. We would want to compare normal and log-normal models to see which is preferable. Model parameters are typically means and variances of familiar or interpretable measurements; in the case of a log-normal model, it is not the mean on the log scale that is of primary scientific interest, but rather the mean or median on the scale of the original data measured in millimeters of mercury.

1.3.4 External Knowledge (or Prior) Distribution

Bayesian inference requires one to quantify one's current state of knowledge about the unknowns prior to (or apart from) collecting the current data. For illustration, consider the case where a study is to be performed to assess the effect of taking statins in order to lower BP. On the web we found a reference to a meta-analysis of a number of studies that examined this question [310]. We only focus on one piece of their study, which involved 12 studies of patients whose SBP at the beginning of the study exceeded 130 mm Hg. Patients were randomly assigned to either a placebo or to a particular statin regimen, and estimates of the differences in average SBP were obtained for each study. The (overall, meta-analysis-based) estimated reduction in average SBP was 4 mm Hg with a 95% confidence interval for the difference in means of $(-5.8, -2.2)$. Here we consider a hypothetical situation where a new study is to be performed with a new type of statin that is cheaper than those used in the above studies, and which is hoped (or expected) to improve on the reduction in mean SBP.

The actual improvement is of course unknown. There are approaches that can be taken to specify a prior distribution on the unknown difference in means. A conservative approach would virtually ignore the above information and place a uniform distribution on a very wide interval, say $(-35, 35)$, to reflect prior uncertainty for the difference in average SBP. In this case, we would be saying that we were 100% certain that the reduction could be no more than 35 mm Hg and that it would be possible that new average difference could be an increase in average SBP up to 35 mm Hg. A somewhat less conservative approach would place a $N(0, 15^2)$ distribution on the difference in mean SBPs. The normal prior would convey that we were about 97.5% certain that the improvement would be at most 30 and similarly that there was a 97.5% chance that the new statin could increase average SBP up to 30 mm Hg. The most likely improvements would be closer to zero than to 30 and similarly if the new statin worked against lowering SBP.

These two priors would be considered to be quite diffuse relative to the information from the above study. A physician with lots of experience with statins may pick a less diffuse prior that also allows for less probability that the statin would increase mean SBP relative to the placebo. For example, they may have good reason to believe that it is impossible to drop average SBP by more than 10 mm Hg and that, if the new statin did increase mean SBP relative to the placebo, it would be unlikely to be more than 3 mm Hg. In this case a uniform prior on the interval $(-10, 5)$ might be sensible, or a comparable $N(-1, 3^2)$ prior.

Alternatively, the same physician may prefer to take account of the above information from the meta-analysis. Note that the width of the confidence interval is only 3.6. So we could imagine a prior that was centered on -4 and that still allowed for the new statin to be worse than placebo, say a uniform distribution on $(-10, 2)$, or a $N(-4, 3^2)$ distribution, to reflect substantive prior information from these studies.

In addition to the above possible specifications, we would need a prior specification for the average SBP among individuals who were taking the placebo. Focusing on mean SBP, it would be very safe to say that the mean SBP in this population is likely greater than 120 mm Hg and less than 200 mm Hg, keeping in mind that the population under study consists of individuals with SBP > 130. We emphasize that this range is for the possible values of the *mean* and *not* for *individual blood pressure values* in the population. We could represent the pre-data knowledge about the unknown population mean for this population with a $N(160, 20^2)$ distribution or a uniform distribution on $(120, 200)$. The range of likely values for the mean SBP is expected to be different in a different type of patient population.

In Chapter 6, we address in more detail how to turn a range of likely values into a distribution. We also consider the possibility of not having external information in Chapter 6.

The rest of the book expands on these essential concepts of Bayesian inference and presents the mathematical tools needed for Bayesian analysis in biostatistics, such as probability models for data and knowledge distributions for unknowns.

1.4   Recap and Readings

In this chapter, we addressed general notions of statistical and scientific inference, putting in perspective how Bayesian analysis weaves these together. We then gave a brief listing of what ingredients are essential for Bayesian analysis. We also presented a few motivating examples of statistics at work in the biomedical sciences. Many other excellent textbooks present Bayesian thinking as applied to data analysis. Examples include the books by Carlin and Louis [63], Gelman et al. [133], Christensen et al. [79], Robert [271] and Hoff [166].

We did not discuss one topic often presented early by many authors: the so-called subjectivity of Bayesian methods that requires a prior distribution. Chapter 6 covers some ground in this area, while an accessible discussion can be found in a pair of articles by Berger and Goldstein [30, 146].

Chapter 2

Fundamentals I: Bayes' Theorem, Knowledge Distributions, Prediction

In this chapter we introduce the principles and basic tools of Bayesian statistical inference. In particular, we consider an approach to statistical inference that leads to making probability statements about unknown quantities of interest or events, for example the occurrence of a disease such as cancer (yes/no) in a particular patient, or the event of surviving at least 5 years after diagnosis with stage 3 breast cancer.

We begin with an elementary form of Bayes' theorem. Bayes' theorem follows from the mathematical definition of conditional probability, which we also discuss. This elementary form of Bayes' theorem describes how to handle unknown quantities that are dichotomous (two categories) or polychotomous (multiple categories). For example, we may sample individuals and test them for an infection, in which case there is a simple yes/no or 1/0 dichotomous outcome, or we may observe in addition, for individuals who are infected, whether they are in an early or late stage of infection, in which case the outcome is trichotomous. We provide illustrations of basic probability concepts that illustrate these probability rules before proceeding to discuss probability models for unknowns of interest, for example, the proportion of HIV infections among blood donors or the proportion of a population with uncontrolled hypertension.

Next is a discussion by example of how to transform scientific knowledge about population characteristics of interest into probability models that describe and characterize that knowledge. Then we introduce and discuss the concepts of continuous and discrete random variables (RVs). Random variables are numerical outcomes associated with studies or events that are not precisely predictable. A continuous outcome in theory has a continuum of possible values, while a discrete outcome has a finite or countably infinite number of possible values. An example of the former case might involve a study where systolic blood pressure (SBP) values were collected from a population with an interest in the reduction in average SBP when using a new treatment regimen compared with a standard treatment. In the latter case, we may be observing cancer counts over time with an ultimate goal of studying and comparing cancer rates under differing circumstances. A binary response coded as 0/1 is a special case of a discrete RV.

A more general Bayes' theorem is presented in conjunction with the concept of a *likelihood function*. The likelihood function encapsulates the information in the data while scientific knowledge about population characteristics is encapsulated in the form of a so-called prior probability distribution. These are combined using

Bayes' theorem to produce the ultimate Bayesian inference, the so-called posterior distribution. It is then shown how the posterior distribution is used to make specific statistical inferences for objects of interest.

The chapter concludes with an introduction to the important problem of prediction and an introduction to Bayesian computation.

2.1 Elementary Bayes' Theorem: Simple but Fundamental Probability Computations

The mathematical basis for combining data and external knowledge to arrive at an updated state of knowledge is provided by Bayes' theorem. Our initial discussion below is somewhat removed from Dr. Whittle's BP study in order to introduce the ideas in simpler situations. The theorem addresses conditional probabilities, which we introduce first.

A systematic development of probability is an extensive undertaking. Here we take the pragmatic view that the reader has had previous exposure to probability and views it in terms of long-run relative frequencies (e.g., the home team wins 54% of professional baseball games) or a degree of certainty (e.g., the probability of precipitation in my city tomorrow is 80%).

Regardless, it is important to recognize that the probability of an event can depend on knowledge of whether or not another related event has occurred. For example, suppose we roll two six-sided dice sequentially. We focus on the probability that the sum is 6. With 36 equally likely possible outcomes, and 5 of these—$(1,5), (2,4), (3,3), (4,2), (5,1)$—resulting in a sum of 6, we can write $P(\text{sum equals } 6) = 5/36$.

Now suppose we are told that the first die shows a number less than 4. So we know that one of the 18 possible outcomes, $\{(j,1), (j,2), (j,3), (j,4), (j,5), (j,6) : j = 1, 2, 3\}$, occurred. How does this affect the 5/36 probability? We see that there are three outcomes that result in a 6 that are also outcomes that result in the first toss being less than 4. We are now seeking the *conditional probability* that the sum equals 6 *given* the first die shows a number less than 4. Intuitively, this should be $3/18 = 1/6$. The definition of the conditional probability of A given that an event B has occurred is

$$P(A \mid B) = \frac{P(A \cap B)}{P(B)}, \tag{2.1}$$

where $\cap$ means "and," and $P(B)$ must be greater than zero. One can explain this formula as meaning the proportion of the probability of B that is associated with A. For the two events above, $A \cap B$ is represented by the outcomes $(1,5), (2,4), (3,3)$ and thus has probability 3/36, and the conditioning event B has probability 18/36 = 1/2. Thus the desired conditional probability is $(3/36)/(18/36) = 1/6$. Knowing B increased slightly the probability of A from 5/36 to $1/6 = 6/36$. Knowledge of some other events can have a dramatic impact. Consider, for example, $C =$ "first die shows a number greater than 5." Then $P(A \mid C) = 0$.

Observe that A and B are not generally interchangeable in that $P(A \mid B)$ may not equal $P(B \mid A)$. Indeed, a moment's reflection reveals that these two probabilities usually have entirely different meanings. Yet, this is a common point of confusion. For example, nearly 46% of smokers are women but only about 18% of women smoke. An overwhelming majority of race car drivers are men but only a small fraction of men are race car drivers! And in our dice throwing example, $P(B \mid A) = 3/5$ while $P(A \mid B) = 1/6$.

Bayes' theorem provides the link that enables proper reversal of conditioning. In its simplest form, we have the following version for two events.

Bayes' Theorem for Two Events. Let A and B be two events with $P(A) > 0$. Then

$$P(B \mid A) = \frac{P(A \mid B)P(B)}{P(A)} = \frac{P(A \mid B)P(B)}{P(A \mid B)P(B) + P(A \mid B^c)P(B^c)} \tag{2.2}$$

where the superscript c stands for complement (i.e., "not").

The right-hand side of this equation follows from the definition of conditional probability as a ratio, and the denominator follows from the law of total probability (see Appendix A). Notice that this reversal of conditioning requires $P(B)$ and $P(A \mid B^c)$ in addition to $P(A \mid B)$.

Example 2.1. Diagnostic testing for diseases is seldom perfect. It is thus useful to know the probability that an individual has the disease after the testing result is available. Experiments evaluating a new diagnostic test typically enroll a fixed number of individuals with the disease and a fixed number without the disease and apply the diagnostic test to both groups. These experiments tell us directly what the chance of a positive (or negative) test result is given that the person has the disease (or does not have the disease). We want to know, however, what the probability is that a person with a positive test result has the disease.

Let $T+$ and $T-$ denote the events that a person tests positive and negative, respectively. Similarly define $D+$ and $D-$ as true disease status. For a person testing positive, we are interested in $P(D+ \mid T+)$. To calculate this we need: (i) $P(D+)$, the unconditional or marginal probability of disease in the population (or *prevalence*, i.e., the probability of disease without regard to test outcome); (ii) $P(T+ \mid D+)$, the probability that an individual with the disease tests positive; and (iii) $P(T+ \mid D-)$, the probability that an individual without the disease tests positive. In Chapter 15 we define these probabilities in more detail. Here we point out that Bayes' theorem allows us to carry out the necessary calculations if appropriate probabilities are available.

Example 2.2. Nattinger et al. [246] constructed an algorithm that inspects billing records of patients in the Medicare system in the U.S. to determine incident cases of breast cancer. By using records of patients with known incident breast cancer as well as cancer-free controls (as determined by the carefully constructed and highly regarded SEER-Medicare linked registry [289]), they estimated that the algorithm detects a true case with probability 0.80 and falsely declares a non-case as a case of incident breast cancer with probability 0.0005. Taking the overall cancer incidence in this population to be 0.005, we calculate the chance that an algorithm-declared case is indeed an incident breast cancer case. Using the notation $A+$ for algorithm positive, $A-$ for algorithm negative, $D+$ for true case, $D-$ for true non-case, we compute $P(D+ \mid A+)$. The form of Bayes' theorem in equation (2.2) gives

$$
\begin{aligned}
P(D+ \mid A+) &= \frac{P(A+ \mid D+)P(D+)}{P(A+ \mid D+)P(D+) + P(A+ \mid D-)P(D-)} \\
&= \frac{0.80 \times 0.005}{0.80 \times 0.005 + 0.0005 \times (1 - 0.005)} \\
&= \frac{0.004}{0.004 + 0.0004975} = \frac{0.004}{0.0045030} \doteq 0.89,
\end{aligned}
$$

where $\doteq$ means "is approximately equal to."

We now introduce a second, and more commonly stated, form of Bayes' theorem. This is an extension of the above form, replacing the pair of complementary events B and B^c by a general partition consisting of mutually exclusive events $B_1, \ldots, B_k$ that constitute all possibilities. In other words, we mean a collection of non-overlapping (or disjoint or mutually exclusive) events that cover all possibilities (i.e., the entire event space). In this case, again using the definition of conditional probability and the law of total probability, we have the following result.

Bayes' Theorem for an Event-Space Partition. Let $B_1, \ldots, B_k$ be a finite partition of an event space Ω, that is, $B_1 \cup \cdots \cup B_k = \Omega$ and $B_i \cap B_j = \phi$, $1 \le i < j \le k$. Let A be an event in Ω with $P(A) > 0$. Then

$$
P(B_i \mid A) = \frac{P(A \mid B_i)P(B_i)}{P(A \mid B_1)P(B_1) + \cdots + P(A \mid B_k)P(B_k)}, \quad i = 1, \ldots, k. \qquad (2.3)
$$

Notice that this equation allows us to compute the conditional probabilities of all k events in the partition, all conditioned on the same event A. The formula requires the unconditional probabilities of all partitioning events. In addition, we need the conditional probability of A given each partitioning event. Although at first sight this appears to be more demanding than equation (2.2), it turns out that working with general partitions gives more freedom in terms of model specification. The theorem will be further generalized for this purpose, ultimately conditioning on the data from a scientific experiment, analogous to conditioning on the event A in this simpler setting. This will be made precise shortly.

Example 2.3. Returning to Example 2.2, Nattinger et al. [246] observe that the algorithm's performance varies for the following four groups of the target population of women enrolled in Medicare:

D_1+ : women with first breast cancer in the incidence year;

D_2+ : women with prevalent breast cancer (i.e., incident in a prior year);

D_3+ : women with incident or prevalent cancer other than breast cancer;

$D-$: women who have never had any cancer.

Observe that the four events constitute a partition of the set of possible outcomes. Recall that $A+$ denotes that the algorithm indicates incident cancer. So now we are interested to know which cancer category is more likely when the algorithm detects cancer, namely, we calculate $P(D_i+ \mid A+)$ for a randomly chosen woman from the population. Notice, however, that $D+$ from the previous example and D_1+ are the same event.

Based on data from the SEER registries [288], the authors give the following unconditional probabilities for the partitioning events: $P(D_1+) = 0.005$, $P(D_2+) = 0.03$, $P(D_3+) = 0.07$, $P(D-) = 0.895$. They also quantify the performance of the algorithm as $P(A+ \mid D_1+) = 0.80$, $P(A+ \mid D_2+) = 0.0065$, $P(A+ \mid D_3+) = 0.0007$, $P(A+ \mid D-) = 0.0003$. This leads to

$$
\begin{aligned}
P(D_1+ \mid A+) &= \frac{P(A+ \mid D_1+)P(D_1+)}{P(A+ \mid D_1+)P(D_1+) + \cdots + P(A+ \mid D-)P(D-)} \\
&= \frac{0.80 \times 0.005}{0.80 \times 0.005 + 0.0065 \times 0.03 + 0.0007 \times 0.07 + 0.0003 \times 0.895} \\
&= \frac{0.0040055}{0.0040055 + 0.0001950 + 0.0000490 + 0.0002685} \\
&= \frac{0.0040055}{0.004518} \doteq 0.89.
\end{aligned}
$$

Similarly, $P(D_2+ \mid A+) = 0.0432$, $P(D_3+ \mid A+) = 0.0108$, $P(D- \mid A+) = 1 - 0.8866 - 0.0432 - 0.0108 = 0.0594$. So the algorithm is clearly most likely to detect incident breast cancer, as we already knew since $P(D+ \mid A+) = P(D_1+ \mid A+)$.

Finally, we observe that $P(D- \mid A-) = 0.895\,(1 - 0.003)/(1 - 0.004518) = 0.8964 \doteq P(D-)$. So we have an example where the events $D-$ and $A-$ are, for practical purposes, independent. Knowing that the algorithm says "no cancer" for a particular individual gives us very little additional information beyond the "prior" belief that there is no cancer.

Data-Informed Knowledge (or Posterior) Distribution. To illustrate how information from data can update our knowledge about unknowns, we continue to look at Example 2.3. If a Medicare-enrolled woman over 65 is chosen at random, our (pre-data) knowledge about her breast cancer status, $(D_1+, D_2+, D_3+, D-)$, is represented by a probability distribution with respective event probabilities $(0.005, 0.03, 0.07, 0.895)$.

Next consider the information contained in the billing records of the randomly chosen woman. If it results in the algorithm declaring the woman positive or negative for incident breast cancer, calculations like those in Example 2.3 result in new, data-informed knowledge about her breast cancer status. We summarize this in Table 2.1.

TABLE 2.1: Knowledge distributions for breast cancer status

| Status | Conditioning (billing record) information | | |
	$P(D_*)$	$P(D_* \mid A+)$	$P(D_* \mid A-)$
D_1+: Incident breast cancer	0.0050	0.8866	0.0010
D_2+: Prevalent breast cancer	0.0300	0.0432	0.0300
D_3+ : Incident or prevalent other cancer	0.0700	0.0108	0.0703
$D-$: Cancer-free	0.895	0.0594	0.8987

Each column shows the knowledge distribution under different information-based scenarios about the randomly chosen woman. Most of the probabilities of incident breast cancer, and of being cancer-free, change dramatically with information. Of course, the algorithm was constructed precisely to achieve this ability to respond to different information about the patient.

2.2 Science and Knowledge about Uncertain Quantities

Fundamentally, the field of statistics is about using probability models to analyze data in the presence of variation or uncertainty. There are two major philosophical positions about the use of probability models. One is that probabilities are determined by the outside world. The other is that probabilities exist in people's heads. Historically, probability theory was developed to explain games of chance. For example, the physical structures involved in rolling dice, spinning roulette wheels, and dealing well-shuffled decks of cards suggest obvious probabilities for various outcomes.

The notion of probability as a belief is more subtle. For example, suppose that you are in my presence when I flip a coin. Prior to flipping the coin, the physical mechanism involved suggests probabilities of 0.5 for each of the outcomes, heads and tails. But now I have flipped the coin, looked at the result, but not told you the outcome. As long as you believe I am not cheating you, you would naturally continue to describe the probabilities for heads and tails as 0.5. But this probability is no longer the probability associated with the physical mechanism involved, because you and I have different probabilities. I know whether the coin is heads or tails, and your probability is simply describing your personal state of knowledge.

Bayesian statistics starts by using (*knowledge-based or prior*) probabilities to describe current states of knowledge. It then incorporates information through data collection. Updating the knowledge given the data, according to the rules of probability calculus, results in new (*posterior*) probabilities to describe your state of knowledge after combining the prior information with the data.

In Bayesian statistics, uncertainty and information are incorporated through the use of probability distributions, and conclusions obey the laws of probability theory.

Some form of prior information is always available. If our inferential goal is to estimate the mean SBP of American men, we all know that this average cannot exceed 200 mm Hg. The probability of death during trauma surgery for a 20-year-old with a small injury and good vital signs is not close to 1. Very conservatively, the probability of being transfused with HIV infected blood in the U.S. cannot possibly be above 5%. At a minimum, a prior distribution for a parameter θ can easily exclude values that are simply unrealistic, and it seems silly to ignore such information. Our goal is not to find the "perfect" knowledge distribution but rather to incorporate salient features of available scientific knowledge into the data analysis. As such, we need to examine whether other reasonable prior distributions lead to substantively similar posterior conclusions.

Example 2.4. Gastwirth, Johnson, and Reneau [122] studied the prevalence of HIV infection in the blood supply in the U.S. In the medical literature, they found an estimate of the proportion of infected blood donors at that time to be 0.0004. They used this information to construct a beta distribution ($Be(a, b)$) that had a mode of 0.0004. Their goal was to estimate the actual proportion of infected blood units after screening for HIV that would be available for transfusion; this proportion was expected to be much smaller than 0.0004 since test accuracies were reasonably high. Here we imagine the simpler goal of estimating prevalence of HIV among blood donors.

We suppose that an expert might posit a 95th percentile of 0.05. That is, the expert would be 95% certain that the prevalence among U.S. donors at that time, say θ, was less than 0.05. The expert's best estimate of that prevalence is 0.0004. One can approximately characterize this uncertainty with a $Be(1, 59)$ distribution, using a method that we describe later. We note that a one-sided 95% probability interval is $(0, 0.05)$, a two-sided 90% interval is $(0.00087, 0.05)$, the median is 0.012, and the mean is 0.017. Since the prior distribution is so skewed, we have very different values for the mean, median, and mode. The main purpose here was to provide a distribution that covers a plausible range of values. A somewhat reasonable alternative to this choice might be a $U(0, 0.1)$ distribution, if the expert was 100% certain that the proportion could not be above 0.1, a likely possibility given that their best estimate was 0.0004.

As we proceed through the book, we will perform what are called sensitivity analyses. For these analyses, we will start with an expert-knowledge-based prior and consider plausible alternatives to that prior. Applying the inferential tools we discuss throughout the book, we will obtain posterior inferences based on each prior (expert and alternative) to see what impact the choice of prior has on the corresponding inferences. The ideal situation is when there is minimal impact. When inferences are sensitive to the choice of prior, this must be reported in any analysis.

Example 2.5. A team of researchers plans to collect data to ascertain whether dieting or exercise is preferable for weight loss in men. We assume that men are randomly assigned at the beginning of the study to be either in the dieting group or the exercise group, and that all participants agree to only use the protocol presented to them by the scientists. Also assume that the data (i.e., weight loss) will be reasonably approximated for each group by normal distributions with different means. Let Δ be the difference in mean weight loss for the dieting group minus that for the exercise group.

Suppose that, based on real data from a previous experiment, the dieting group had lost more weight on average than the exercise group, and also suppose that the scientists involved with the current study are interested to see if the previous study results will hold up in their own study. If an estimated effect of $\hat{\Delta} = 5$ had been presented in the literature with a 95% interval of $(2, 8)$, that information can be used as the basis for specifying a prior distribution for the current study. It will generally be the case that one would specify a prior distribution that expresses additional uncertainty beyond that conveyed by an analysis of previous data. Alternatively, physicians might be asked to simply provide their *expert* best guess for θ and to specify an interval in which they are, say, at least 95% certain that Δ would lie.

In practice, we typically obtain expert information or knowledge about some characteristics in the population under study, obtaining as much information as is reasonable and convenient to elicit. We then incorporate this information into a suitable class of distributions in ways that will be described throughout the book. Such information must be collected independently of the current data.

Describing uncertainty with a prior distribution is a collaborative effort between scientist and statistician and should ultimately involve validation by the expert to be certain that the selected knowledge distribution is a reasonable approximation to the expert's actual information.

Example 2.6. Consider the weight loss study above with 95% interval for Δ of $(2, 8)$. If we use a normal distribution to model scientific information about Δ, say $\Delta \sim N(a, b^2)$, then the 95% interval around the mean must have endpoints of about $a \pm 2b$. We set the best guess for Δ to be $\Delta_0 = 5$, so $a = 5$. With $a + 2b = 8$, we obtain $b = 1.5$. The size of b is directly related to the width of the specified 95% interval. Note that this technique used the fact that $(2, 8)$ is centered around $\Delta_0 = 5$. If we wanted to add uncertainty, say by considering the wider interval $(1, 9)$ as a 95% interval, then we would get $b = 2$ since $5 + 4 = 9$ is two standard deviations above the mean.

As previously suggested, it is often difficult for experts to provide direct information on the parameters of statistical models because they are not comfortable with the parameterization. In such cases, we elicit information about quantities that are more familiar to the expert and use that information to induce a prior on the model parameters. Typically, experimenters would have some ideas about mean weight loss under specified protocols and could give a best guess and, perhaps, a wide probability interval for it. When considering a difference in means as above, the choice of 0 for the difference in means will often be a reasonable choice, unless one has good reason to expect that one treatment is superior to another. On the other hand, it is more difficult for experts to think directly about likely values for a standard deviation.

To address this question, we propose the following. Suppose that weight loss for a randomly selected individual under a particular treatment can be modeled with a $N(\mu, \sigma^2)$ distribution. How would we place a prior on σ? Since σ is not easy to think about, we could ask questions about the lower quartile of weight losses among the population of men that would use the given protocol for weight loss. This number has 75% of the values above it and 25% below. The lower quartile of a normal distribution is $\mu - 0.675\sigma$, so if our expert's experience suggested that the lower quartile was about -5, and that μ was about $\mu_0 = -2$, then a natural guess for σ is $\sigma_0 = (-2 + 5)/0.675 = 4.44$. For σ^2, we could pick a distribution that had a median or mode equal to the best guess, 4.44^2, and which was suitably diffuse. We discuss both diffuse and informative priors for σ in some detail later on.

Although parameters are often mere conveniences, frequently a parameter θ has some basis in physical reality. This was the case for our parameter Δ in the above example. Rather than describing where θ *exactly* is, the prior describes *beliefs* about where θ is. The probabilities specified by the physicians are their beliefs about θ. Different physicians, or groups of physicians, will have different knowledge bases and, therefore, different probabilities for θ. If they analyze the same data, they will continue to have different beliefs about θ until sufficient data are collected so that they reach a consensus. This consensus should occur unless one or more of them is unrealistically dogmatic. For example, when considering extrasensory perception (ESP), some people refuse to place any positive probability on the phenomenon's existence, so no amount of data will change their beliefs [337]. A nice feature of Bayesian statistics is that scientist–statistician collaborations require that preconceptions be openly asserted. So a prior of 10^{-40} that ESP exists pretty much says that there is no need to collect data.

2.3   More on Bayes' Theorem: Inference for Model Unknowns

In Section 2.1 we discussed knowledge-based probabilities for events followed by their updated versions, conditioned on a potentially informative event (data). We also discussed in Section 2.2 some issues related to specifying knowledge-based information for model parameters that are on a continuum. In biostatistics it is most common to observe numerical data in the form of variables that are either continuous or discrete. For example, for the **VetBP** data (Example 1.1) the information is a collection of blood pressure values that are treated as continuous outcomes.

On the other hand, for the **LE** data of Example 1.2, the outcome is discrete, since occurrence of lymphedema is coded as a 1 and non-occurrence is coded as a 0. This leads us to a discussion of random variables.

Random Variable. A random variable (RV), say X, is a numerical outcome associated with a randomly selected person or experiment. We use capital letters, generally towards the end of the Latin alphabet, to represent RVs. When X is observed, we denote the actual outcome by the corresponding lower-case letter, namely $X = x$. If X is SBP and is observed to be 120, we say $X = 120$ was observed, but the generic x is a useful notation. Not all RVs are observable, however.

Population parameters are fundamental to all of statistical modeling. Random effects also play an important role in statistical modeling, as we shall see later in the book (Chapter 14). Neither is observable, even after data collection. Such unknowable quantities are treated as RVs in Bayesian analysis, and thus the statistician specifies probability distributions for them, since all uncertainty is to be modeled with probability. In Example 2.3, a knowledge-based distribution was placed on the different breast cancer event probabilities that were then modified when conditioned on $A+$ or $A-$. Here again, distributions for model parameters (and random effects variables) are modified when distributions are conditioned on observed data. Typically, we use lower-case Greek letters(e.g., $\mu, \sigma, \lambda, \theta$) for these unobservable quantities. Corresponding upper-case Greek letters denote the space of possible values taken by the unknowable quantities. For example, Θ is the set of all possible values for θ.

In specifying a model for data to be collected, observable and unobservable quantities can be either discrete or continuous. Probability mass functions (pmfs) are used as descriptors for the behavior of discrete random variables, and probability density functions (pdfs) are used for continuous random variables (see Appendix A). In this book, we often blur the distinction and simply call these descriptors probability density functions for the random variables, regardless of whether continuous or discrete. We use the letter p to denote density functions, and we often write that "the distribution of X is $p(\cdot)$" or equivalently "$X \sim p(\cdot)$."

We denote conditional distributions (see Appendix A) in a way that is similar to conditional probabilities for events, namely, by using a vertical bar. For example, $X \mid \theta$ is read as "X given θ" and represents the random variable X when the conditioning variable takes the particular value θ. This notation will be used in the specification of a probability model for the data, X, given the model parameter(s) θ. For example, we could say $X \mid \theta \sim p(\cdot \mid \theta)$ where $p(\cdot \mid \theta)$ is the conditional density for the random variable X.

We write $p(x \mid \theta)$ and $X \mid \theta \sim p(\cdot \mid \theta)$ interchangeably. When we think of x as observed data on X, we will be very much interested in the (posterior) density $p(\theta \mid x)$. We present these notational conventions in Table 2.2.

With this notation in hand, we return to Bayes' theorem, now stated for random variables. This takes a similar form to that for events (as in Section 2.1), with the

TABLE 2.2: Notational conventions

Quantity	Letter/symbol	Examples
Observable RVs (will become data)	UC Latin, end of alphabet	X, Y, Z
Observed data	LC Latin, end of alphabet	x, y, z
Unknowable RV (parameter)	LC Greek	μ, σ, λ, θ
Parameter Space of Unknowable RV	UC Greek	Λ, Θ
pmf or pdf	$p(\cdot)$	$p(x)$
"Distributed as" or "has distribution"	$\sim$	$X \sim p(\cdot)$, $Y \sim p(\cdot)$
Conditional RV	Vertical bar $\mid$	$X \mid Y = y$ $\theta \mid y$, $Y \mid \theta$
Conditional distribution	$p(\cdot \mid \cdot)$	$p(y \mid x, \theta)$, $p(\theta \mid y)$

sum in the denominator replaced by an integral. Consider two random variables: an observable Y and an unobservable θ. Let $p(\theta)$ be the density for θ representing the external (or prior) knowledge about θ. A model for the observable specifies $p(y \mid \theta)$, a conditional probability density. We then have the following result.

Bayes' Theorem for Two Random Variables. Let Y and θ be two random variables. Then

$$p(\theta \mid y) = \frac{p(y \mid \theta)p(\theta)}{\int p(y \mid \theta)p(\theta)d\theta}, \quad \theta \in \Theta, \tag{2.4}$$

where the integral is over Θ, the entire space for θ. The equality follows from the definition of a conditional density, and the denominator is simply the marginal density for Y, $p(y)$, using the law of total probability.

To illustrate, suppose Y is the (binary) indicator[1] of heads on a coin flip and θ is the unknown probability of heads. Then the distribution of $Y \mid \theta$ is Bernoulli with parameter θ, that is, $p(y \mid \theta) = \theta^y(1 - \theta)^{(1-y)}$ (see Appendix B). We say that $Y \mid \theta \sim Ber(\theta)$. We might consider taking the prior distribution of θ to be uniform on $(0, 1)$, since θ is constrained to lie between 0 and 1. That is, we assign equal probability across the range of values θ may take. We can write $p(\theta) = 1$ for $\theta \in (0, 1)$, and apply Bayes' theorem to get

$$p(\theta \mid y) = \frac{\theta^y(1 - \theta)^{1-y}}{\int_0^1 \theta^y(1 - \theta)^{1-y}d\theta}.$$

---

[1]The indicator of an event equals 1 if the event happens, 0 if it does not.

If the coin shows heads, we have the update

$$p(\theta \mid y = 1) = \frac{\theta}{\int_0^1 \theta \, d\theta} = 2\theta,$$

while tails results in

$$p(\theta \mid y = 0) = \frac{1 - \theta}{\int_0^1 (1 - \theta) \, d\theta} = 2(1 - \theta).$$

Figure 2.1 shows how pre-data knowledge about the probability of heads is updated by data. Although the Bayes' theorem above is stated for two random variables, it is

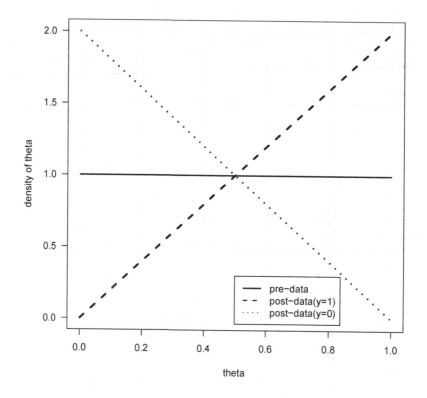

FIGURE 2.1: Bayesian knowledge updates after coin flip data.

quite general in that y and θ can be made up of many components or even collections of mathematical objects. Of course, specifying the density requires much care and can be quite intricate, depending on the structure of these objects. In general, it is useful to think of y as (possibly multivariate) data and θ as (a vector of) parameters (or unobservables). We can then state our next result.

Bayes' Theorem for Modeled Data. From here on, we allow for the generic parameter or unobservables $\boldsymbol{\theta} \in \boldsymbol{\Theta}$ to be a vector of, say, r elements, $(\theta_1, \ldots, \theta_r)$.

Most statistical models have more than one parameter, but when $r = 1$, this reduces to the single-parameter case. Bayesian inference for the parameter vector, $\boldsymbol{\theta}$, is just the joint posterior distribution. The joint posterior pdf is

$$p(\boldsymbol{\theta} \mid \boldsymbol{y}) = \frac{p(\boldsymbol{y} \mid \boldsymbol{\theta}) \, p(\boldsymbol{\theta})}{\int_{\Theta} p(\boldsymbol{y} \mid \boldsymbol{\theta}) \, p(\boldsymbol{\theta}) \, d\boldsymbol{\theta}} \tag{2.5}$$

where the integral is over the entire r-dimensional space, Θ, for the unobservables.

Using Bayes' Theorem for Inference. Equation (2.5) provides the density that contains post-data knowledge about unobservables or parameters. We now describe how it can be used explicitly for inference.

With multiple parameters, such as $\boldsymbol{\theta} = (\theta_1, \theta_2)$, we will usually be interested in some function of them, say $\gamma(\boldsymbol{\theta})$, as the primary scientific target of inference. For example, we might be interested in $\gamma_1 = \theta_1/\theta_2$ or $\gamma_2 = \theta_1 - \theta_2$, or $\gamma_3 = \theta_1$, or $\gamma_4 = P(\theta_1 > \theta_2)$, or in all four. Inferences for θ_i derive from the marginal posterior for θ_i. This is obtained by integrating the joint posterior with respect to all $r - 1$ elements of the Θ vector other than θ_i. For example, with $r = 2$, we obtain

$$p(\theta_1 \mid \boldsymbol{y}) = \int p(\theta_1, \theta_2 \mid \boldsymbol{y}) d\theta_2.$$

We remind the reader of our emphasis on the distinction between model parameters, $\boldsymbol{\theta}$, and parameters of scientific interest, say $\boldsymbol{\gamma} = \boldsymbol{\gamma}(\boldsymbol{\theta})$. There will often be more than one scientifically relevant parameter, so we would generally regard $\boldsymbol{\gamma}$ as a vector of parameters. In practice, however, we generally focus on a single parameter at a time. For the rest of this discussion, we consider a scalar γ. The Bayesian approach to inferences for γ is based solely on its posterior distribution, or equivalently $p(\gamma \mid \boldsymbol{y}) = p(\gamma(\boldsymbol{\theta}) \mid \boldsymbol{y})$.

In a calculus-based probability class, techniques are developed for finding the pdfs for functions of random variables. This can be hard work, however, and it is most often impossible to obtain an analytically tractable (nice) expression for $p(\boldsymbol{\theta} \mid \boldsymbol{y})$ or $p(\gamma \mid \boldsymbol{y})$. These issues are resolved by using Monte Carlo numerical techniques to approximate posterior distributions, regardless of the complexity. Numerical approximations are discussed in detail in Chapter 4. We give a preview illustration of their use later in this chapter, in Section 2.5.

Point inferences for γ provide a one-number summary of the (marginal) posterior, $p(\gamma \mid \boldsymbol{y})$. A natural choice to consider first is the posterior mean, $\tilde{\gamma}$,

$$\tilde{\gamma} \equiv E(\gamma \mid \boldsymbol{y}) = \int \gamma p(\gamma \mid \boldsymbol{y}) d\gamma.$$

But, as just indicated, the posterior for γ may not be analytically tractable. For the moment, suppose we know the joint posterior for $\boldsymbol{\theta}$. We can then obtain

$$\tilde{\gamma} = E(\gamma(\boldsymbol{\theta}) \mid \boldsymbol{y}) = \int \gamma(\boldsymbol{\theta}) p(\boldsymbol{\theta} \mid \boldsymbol{y}) d\boldsymbol{\theta}$$

from a convenient result in probability theory that avoids first obtaining $p(\gamma \mid \boldsymbol{y})$.

If the posterior for γ is skewed (has a long tail in one direction and a shorter tail in the other), the middle of the distribution is better represented by the median of the posterior, $\text{med}(\gamma \mid \boldsymbol{y})$, which is the value m that satisfies

$$\int_{-\infty}^{m} p(\gamma \mid \boldsymbol{y})d\gamma = 0.5 = \int_{m}^{\infty} p(\gamma \mid \boldsymbol{y})d\gamma.$$

Another quantity of interest is the mode of the posterior, which is the value, say $\hat{\gamma}$, that achieves the maximum $p(\gamma \mid \boldsymbol{y})$ over all possible γ. This is usually obtained by taking the derivative, $\frac{d}{d\gamma} \ln(p(\gamma \mid \boldsymbol{y}))$, setting it to zero, and solving for $\hat{\gamma}$.

We are also interested in a measure of how spread out or diffuse the posterior for γ is. The posterior variance is

$$\text{Var}(\gamma \mid \boldsymbol{y}) = \int (\gamma - \tilde{\gamma})^2 p(\gamma \mid \boldsymbol{y})d\gamma$$

and the posterior standard deviation, $\text{sd}(\gamma \mid \boldsymbol{y}) = \sqrt{\text{Var}(\gamma \mid \boldsymbol{y})}$.

Point estimates such as $\tilde{\gamma}$ and $\hat{\gamma}$ do not convey any quantitative uncertainty about the unknown. While the posterior standard deviation takes a step in quantifying uncertainty, we can be more direct by computing an interval with a specified high probability under the posterior density. In other words, intervals (l, u) for which $P(l < \gamma < u \mid \boldsymbol{y}) = 1 - \alpha$, where α is often chosen to be 0.05. If the posterior is symmetric about $\tilde{\gamma}$, then the mean, mode, and median are all the same. Moreover, the natural choice for l and u will be equidistant from $\tilde{\gamma}$ with $\alpha/2$ area under the posterior to the left of l and to the right of u. With a skewed posterior, there are other possible choices for intervals, but we will generally find intervals that have $\alpha/2$ area to the left of l, and $\alpha/2$ area to the right of u, so that there is $1 - \alpha$ area in between these values. Thus we have

$$\int_{l}^{u} p(\gamma \mid \boldsymbol{y})d\gamma = 1 - \alpha.$$

We may also be interested in one-sided versions, namely where $P(\gamma < u \mid \boldsymbol{y}) = 0.95$ or 0.99, etc.

Summary inferences for a Bayesian analysis generally involve presentation of a point estimate, a 95% interval estimate, and a posterior standard deviation. If the posterior is symmetric, then the mean should be presented; however, if it is skewed, then the median should be presented. These quantities, except for the posterior mode, are all obtained approximately using Monte Carlo methods, which are discussed in Chapter 4.

Bayes' Theorem in Proportionality Form. This helpful form avoids some unnecessary calculations when dealing with $p(\theta \mid \boldsymbol{y})$. To see this we first return to equation (2.5). Both sides of this equation should be seen as functions of θ only, as $\boldsymbol{y}$ represents observed numerical data that are regarded as fixed in any Bayesian analysis. Also observe that the denominator on the right-hand side is a definite integral and is free of $\boldsymbol{\theta}$. In other words, the denominator is a constant with respect to $\boldsymbol{\theta}$. In fact, it is the constant that makes the post-data density integrate to 1. Thus, the post-data density of $\boldsymbol{\theta}$ is determined up to a multiplicative constant by the numerator alone. Stated another way, this density is proportional to the numerator.

In addition, there are often multiplicative constants in $p(\boldsymbol{y} \mid \boldsymbol{\theta})$ and $p(\boldsymbol{\theta})$ as well. Observe that any such constants will cancel out in the ratio in equation (2.5), since this same term is in both the numerator and the denominator. Removing the multiplicative constant from $p(\boldsymbol{y} \mid \boldsymbol{\theta})$, we write

$$Lik(\boldsymbol{\theta}) \propto p(\boldsymbol{y} \mid \boldsymbol{\theta}).$$

This function of $\boldsymbol{\theta}$ is called the (Fisher) likelihood function. Thus with $\boldsymbol{y}$ representing observed data and $\boldsymbol{\theta}$ denoting the collection of unobservables, the data-informed knowledge distribution for $\boldsymbol{\theta}$ is determined by

$$p(\boldsymbol{\theta} \mid \boldsymbol{y}) \propto p(\boldsymbol{y} \mid \boldsymbol{\theta})\, p(\boldsymbol{\theta}) \propto Lik(\boldsymbol{\theta})\, p(\boldsymbol{\theta}), \tag{2.6}$$

where the proportionality constant is $\{\int_{\boldsymbol{\Theta}} Lik(\boldsymbol{\theta})\, p(\boldsymbol{\theta}) d\boldsymbol{\theta}\}^{-1}$, which is just the constant of integration that makes the joint posterior integrate to 1. The symbol $\propto$ is read as "is proportional to."

The main purpose of deriving expression (2.6) is to simplify calculations. This simplification occurs since we will often be able to recognize the name of the posterior density by simply knowing its functional form as a function of $\boldsymbol{\theta}$, making it unnecessary to keep track of constants. Also, keeping track of all of the constants can be quite tedious. In addition, even when we are not able to recognize the form, we will find in Chapter 4 that it is still not necessary to keep track of the constant of integration for reasons that will be discussed there.

Example 2.7. Using a small portion of the **VetBP** data of Example 1.1, we illustrate how one specifies a model for the data and an external knowledge distribution (or prior) for the unknowns in that model. Recall that Dr. Whittle's study recruited hypertensive veterans. Many with this condition are successful in controlling their hypertension through diet and medication while others are not. We focus here on one interesting unknown: the percentage of veterans who have uncontrolled hypertension. As a fraction, we denote this by $\theta =$ probability that a random veteran has uncontrolled hypertension.[2]

For now, we make no distinctions among individuals in the sample.[3] Consider data from 404 participants in the **VetBP** study. Let $\boldsymbol{y} = y_1, \ldots, y_{404}$, where y_i indicates whether or not the ith person in the study had uncontrolled hypertension. We assume that $Y_i \mid \theta \overset{iid}{\sim} Ber(\theta)$ for $i = 1, \ldots, 404$, where θ is the proportion of

---

[2]Dr. Whittle defined this as systolic blood pressure greater than 140 mm Hg or diastolic greater than 90 mm Hg, decreasing these cut-points by 10 mm Hg for diabetics.

[3]For simplicity at the outset, we disregard individual characteristics that may be related to the outcome, such as age and body mass index.

individuals in the population that have uncontrolled hypertension. We use *iid* to mean that these observations are independent and identically distributed, in this case conditional on the given value of θ. Because of this assumption, we have

$$p(\boldsymbol{y} \mid \theta) = \prod_{i=1}^{404} \theta^{y_i}(1-\theta)^{1-y_i} = \theta^S(1-\theta)^{404-S},$$

where $S = \sum_{i=1}^{404} y_i$ counts the number of individuals out of the 404 who have uncontrolled hypertension. It turns out that $S = 184$, so that $404 - S = 220$ for these data and $Lik(\theta) = \theta^{184}(1-\theta)^{220}$.

Now suppose, for the moment, that we want to act as though absolutely nothing is known about what θ might be for this population before data collection. Then a reasonable prior would be $p(\theta) = 1$ if $\theta \in (0,1)$ and 0 otherwise. We can also express this as $p(\theta) = I_{(0,1)}(\theta)$, where I is the indicator function. Alternatively, $\theta \sim U(0,1)$, which means that we believe all values of θ are equally plausible at the outset. Then using expression (2.6), we obtain

$$p(\theta \mid \boldsymbol{y}) \propto \theta^{184+1-1}(1-\theta)^{220+1-1},$$

which is the kernel of a $Be(185, 221)$ density function (see Appendix B), meaning that this is a beta pdf up to the constant of integration. Thus we have the very nice result that $\theta \mid \boldsymbol{y} \sim Be(185, 221)$. The prior and posterior pdfs are shown in Figure 2.2. It indicates that much information was gained about θ through the data.

Bayes' Theorem in Proportionality Form for an Event-Space Partition. Let $B_1, \ldots, B_k$ be a finite partition of an event space Ω. Let A be an event in Ω with $P(A) > 0$. Then

$$P(B_i \mid A) \propto P(A \mid B_i)P(B_i), \quad i = 1, \ldots, k, \tag{2.7}$$

where the proportionality constant is $\{\sum_{j=1}^{k} P(A \mid B_j)P(B_j)\}^{-1}$. Recall that the denominator in equation (2.3) is the normalizing constant that follows from the law of total probability. Its inverse is the constant of proportionality in expression (2.7). Let us see how this helps with calculations via the next example.

Example 2.8. We return to Example 2.3 and consider the observed event "the algorithm indicates that the randomly chosen woman has incident breast cancer." Conditioned on this event (data), we can calculate (posterior) probabilities for $(D_1+, D_2+, D_3+, D-)$. We show the calculations in Table 2.3.

The normalizing constant is the sum of the entries in the "product" column; it equals 0.004518. Dividing the products by this sum yields the last column. Notice that the procedure is to multiply the prior and the likelihood columns and normalize the resulting column of products by dividing each entry by the sum of the column. The final column would remain the same even if we multiplied each of the first two columns by distinct positive numbers. It is the relative size of the entries within each of the first two columns that is important in the calculation of the final column.

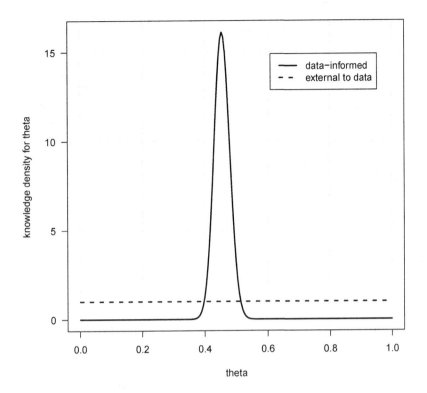

FIGURE 2.2: Prior and posterior distributions for fraction of uncontrolled hypertension among hypertensive veterans.

2.4 Prediction

Inference for unknowns in a model given the data leads naturally to prediction of quantities that involve future observations. Prediction is destined to play a major role in the future of biostatistics. Continuing with the **VetBP** data of Example 1.1, we extend Example 2.7 to prediction. Suppose we are planning a future study for which 100 veterans are to be recruited. We then ask the question (as did Dr. Whittle), how many of the 100 veterans to be sampled will have uncontrolled hypertension?

We tackle a simpler prediction problem first. Consider a single veteran in the future study. Let Z denote his or her status regarding uncontrolled hypertension, with $Z = 1$ if the veteran's hypertension is uncontrolled and 0 otherwise. Given the data from the 404 participants in the **VetBP** study, that is, given $\boldsymbol{y} = (y_1, \ldots, y_{404})$, where again y_i indicates whether or not the ith person in the study had uncontrolled hypertension, we wish to determine the predictive probability $P(Z = 1 \mid \boldsymbol{y})$. Using

TABLE 2.3: Posterior distribution given algorithm positive

Partition event	Prior prob. of part. event	Prob. of obs. data given part. event	Product	Post. prob. of part event
D_1+: Incident BC	0.0050	0.8011	0.0040055	0.8866
D_2+: Prevalent BC	0.0300	0.0065	0.0001950	0.0432
D_3+: Inc. or prev. other cancer	0.0700	0.0007	0.0000490	0.0108
$D-$: Cancer-free	0.8950	0.0003	0.0002685	0.0594

the law of total probability, we have

$$P(Z = z \mid \boldsymbol{y}) = \int_{\Theta} p(z, \theta \mid \boldsymbol{y}) d\theta = \int_{\Theta} p(z \mid \theta, \boldsymbol{y}) p(\theta \mid \boldsymbol{y}) d\theta.$$

The second equality follows from the fact that a joint pdf equals one of the marginals times a conditional (the multiplication rule for pdfs), for the same reason that the multiplication rule for events is $P(A \cap B) = P(B \mid A)P(A)$.

Now consider the first term in the integrand on the far right above. Assuming that past and future data are independent, conditional on θ, means that Z and $\boldsymbol{y}$ are independent when θ is regarded as fixed and known. Therefore, the conditioning on $\boldsymbol{y}$ in the first term in the integrand can be dropped. More formally, we write

$$P(Z = z \mid \theta, \boldsymbol{y}) = \frac{p(z, \theta, \boldsymbol{y})}{p(\theta, \boldsymbol{y})} = \frac{p(z, \boldsymbol{y} \mid \theta)p(\theta)}{p(\boldsymbol{y} \mid \theta)p(\theta)} = \frac{p(z \mid \theta)p(\boldsymbol{y} \mid \theta)}{p(\boldsymbol{y} \mid \theta)} = p(z \mid \theta),$$

which here is just $\theta^z (1 - \theta)^{1-z}$. As a consequence, in general we get

$$P(Z = z \mid \boldsymbol{y}) = \int_{\Theta} p(z \mid \theta) p(\theta \mid \boldsymbol{y}) d\theta. \tag{2.8}$$

From Example 2.7 we know that $\theta \mid \boldsymbol{y} \sim Be(185, 221)$. Substituting into equation (2.8) yields

$$
\begin{aligned}
P(Z = z \mid \boldsymbol{y}) &= \int_0^1 \{\theta^z (1 - \theta)^{1-z}\} \frac{\theta^{185-1}(1 - \theta)^{221-1}}{B(185, 221)} d\theta \\
&= \frac{1}{B(185, 221)} \int_0^1 \theta^{185+z-1}(1 - \theta)^{221+1-z-1} d\theta \\
&= \frac{B(185 + z, 222 - z)}{B(185, 221)} \\
&= \frac{\Gamma(185 + z)\Gamma(222 - z)}{\Gamma(407)} \frac{\Gamma(406)}{\Gamma(185)\Gamma(221)}, \quad z = 0, 1.
\end{aligned}
$$

In the equation, $B(a, b)$ is the beta function (not density) defined in terms of the gamma function, and equals $\Gamma(a)\Gamma(b)/\Gamma(a + b)$. It is the constant of integration for the $Be(a, b)$ distribution. The third equality above follows, since the integrand in the second equality is just the kernel of a $Be(185 + z, 221 + 1 - z)$ distribution. Then dividing the integrand in line 2 by $B(185 + z, 221 + 1 - z)$ results in an integral of 1. It remains to multiply by the same constant, which is what we see in line 3. For the predictive probability that $Z = 1$, the last expression takes the form

$$\frac{\Gamma(186)\Gamma(221)}{\Gamma(407)} \frac{\Gamma(406)}{\Gamma(185)\Gamma(221)} = \frac{185}{406} = 0.456$$

as $\Gamma(186) = 185 \times \Gamma(185)$ and $\Gamma(407) = 406 \times \Gamma(406)$ by the factorial property of the gamma function. A similar calculation results in $221/406$ for $Z = 0$. We could also get this last result by noting that $P(Z = 0 \mid \boldsymbol{y}) = 1 - P(Z = 1 \mid \boldsymbol{y})$.

Returning to the future study of 100 veterans, denote the future observations by $\mathbf{Z} = (Z_1, \ldots, Z_{100})$, the vector of unknown status values (uncontrolled hypertension or not) for all veterans in the future sample. The joint predictive density for $\mathbf{Z}$ can be obtained by the same argument that led to equation (2.8) above, simply replacing z with $\boldsymbol{z}$. The resulting joint predictive density is obtained below.

Joint Predictive Density. When future $\mathbf{Z}$ and data $\mathbf{Y}$ are conditionally independent given the unobservable θ, the joint predictive density is

$$P(\mathbf{Z} = \boldsymbol{z} \mid \boldsymbol{y}) = \int_{\Theta} p(\boldsymbol{z} \mid \theta)p(\theta \mid \boldsymbol{y})d\theta, \tag{2.9}$$

where boldface denotes a vector.

Example 2.9. For the future study of 100 veterans, we are interested in the distribution of $S_F = \sum_{i=1}^{100} Z_i$ given $\boldsymbol{y} = (y_1, \ldots, y_{404})$. Clearly, S_F is a function of $\mathbf{Z}$. Since we have conditional independence between S_F and $\mathbf{Y}$ given θ, equation (2.9) can be applied directly, that is, we have

$$P(S_F = s \mid \boldsymbol{y}) = \int_{\Theta} p(s \mid \theta)p(\theta \mid \boldsymbol{y})d\theta.$$

From elementary probability, we note that $S_F \mid \theta \sim Bin(100, \theta)$. We thus obtain

$$P(S_F = s \mid \boldsymbol{y}) = \int_0^1 \frac{100!}{s!(100 - s)!}\theta^s(1 - \theta)^{100-s} \frac{\theta^{185-1}(1 - \theta)^{221-1}}{B(185, 221)}d\theta,$$

$s = 0, \ldots, 100$. While it is straightforward to obtain an analytical result using the same technique used in the scalar case, it is somewhat ugly. Moreover, there is no actual necessity for having analytic formulas, as we now discuss.

In practice, most predictive distributions or densities turn out to be quite complex. Equation (2.9), for example, requires an integration over a possibly high-dimensional space, Θ. Fortunately, it is usually much easier to employ sampling-based Monte Carlo computation, which will be described briefly in the next section, and in detail in Chapter 4. Figure 2.3 gives precisely such a numerical approximation to the predictive density for the **VetBP** problem discussed above.

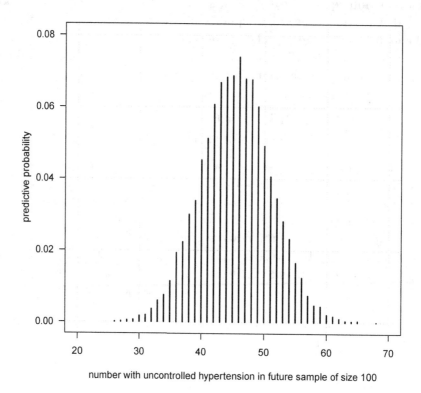

FIGURE 2.3: Predictive density.

Historical note. The predictive distribution defined in equation (2.8) goes back to at least the early to mid-1960s. We refer to Geisser (1971) [123], who was an ardent proponent of Bayesian prediction and who made a strong effort to clarify its utility as an important tool for making statistical inferences. Aitchison and Dunsmore (1975) [3] and Geisser (1993) [127] continued to make this case. More recently, at least since Gelman et al. (1995) [134], equation (2.8) has been termed the posterior predictive distribution. We will also introduce what has been termed the marginal predictive distribution (sometimes called the marginal likelihood of the observed data). This is obtained from equation (2.8) as $p(\boldsymbol{y}) = \int_{\Theta} p(\boldsymbol{y} \mid \theta)p(\theta)d\theta$, which has also more recently been termed the prior predictive distribution. We will, however, continue to use the original terminology.

2.5 Monte Carlo Approximation

Numerical approximations for Bayesian statistical inferences are presented in Chapter 4. It is these approximations that make the modern Bayesian inference so powerful in handling complex scientific problems. Here, we give a brief overview of what is coming for estimation and for prediction. We assume the background model for the data, $p(\boldsymbol{y} \mid \theta)$, the pre-data scientific input, $p(\theta)$, and a model for future data, $p(\boldsymbol{z} \mid \theta)$, where past and future are assumed to be independent given the parameters. We again assume the scientific estimation goal is for a parameter $\gamma = \gamma(\boldsymbol{\theta})$.

Suppose it is possible to sample vectors (using a computer algorithm), say $\{\boldsymbol{\theta}^{(1)}, \boldsymbol{\theta}^{(2)}, \ldots, \boldsymbol{\theta}^{(M)}\}$ for large M, from the posterior distribution $p(\boldsymbol{\theta} \mid \boldsymbol{y})$. Then, calculating the corresponding values for $\{\gamma^{(j)} \equiv \gamma(\boldsymbol{\theta}^{(j)}) : j = 1, \ldots, M\}$ results in a large sample from the (marginal) posterior of interest, $p(\gamma \mid \boldsymbol{y})$. This sample can be used to approximate the density of γ using a variety of techniques, including just smoothing a histogram of these samples. The posterior mean is approximated by $\hat{\gamma} = \sum_{j=1}^{M} \gamma^{(j)}/M$, the posterior standard deviation is approximated by $\sqrt{\sum_{j=1}^{M} (\gamma^{(j)} - \hat{\gamma})^2 / M}$, and quantiles of the posterior are obtained by ordering the $\gamma^{(j)}$ from smallest to largest. Of particular interest are the 0.025, 0.5, and 0.975 quantiles of this Monte Carlo sample. The sample median is a numerical approximation to the median of the underlying posterior distribution, and the 0.025 and 0.0975 sample quantiles give numerical approximations to (l, u), the posterior interval for the parameter of interest.

Sampling from the Predictive Distribution. Monte Carlo samples from $p(\boldsymbol{z} \mid \boldsymbol{y})$ can be obtained as follows. For each $\boldsymbol{\theta}^{(j)}$, sample

$$\mathbf{Z}^{(j)} \mid \boldsymbol{\theta}^{(j)} \sim p(\mathbf{Z} \mid \boldsymbol{\theta}^{(j)}),$$

independently for $j = 1, \ldots, M$. Under conditional independence, this amounts to sampling from the distribution with density $p(\boldsymbol{z} \mid \boldsymbol{\theta}^{(j)}, \boldsymbol{y})$, independently for all $j = 1, \ldots, M$, which results in a random sample from the predictive distribution with pdf $p(z \mid \boldsymbol{y})$. One then uses either the mean or the median of this distribution as a point estimate, depending on whether or not it is skewed. One can also take quantiles of this distribution to obtain prediction intervals. Monte Carlo samples of functions of $\mathbf{Z}$, such as S_F in Example 2.9, can be obtained by computing $S_F^{(j)}$ from each sampled $Z^{(j)}$. Figure 2.3 was constructed using such generated predictive samples of S_F.

2.6 Recap and Readings

In this chapter we presented the main ingredients needed to accomplish Bayesian inference in a little more detail. These ingredients are conditional probability, Bayes' theorem, data generating distribution or likelihood, knowledge distributions of knowledge of unknowns both external (prior) and data-informed (posterior), and predictions. The books cited in Section 3.4 (Carlin and Louis [63], Gelman et al. [133], Christensen et al. [79], Robert [271], and Hoff [166]) also cover these topics.

We have postponed discussion of one topic considered early in many books. This topic is the so-called subjectivity of Bayesian methods as they require a prior distribution. Chapter 6 covers some ground in this area, and an accessible discussion can be found in a pair of articles by Berger and Goldstein [30, 146].

2.7   Exercises

EXERCISE 2.1.   An enzyme-linked immunosorbent assay (ELISA) test is performed to determine if the human immunodeficiency virus (HIV) is present in the blood of individuals. The test is not perfect. Suppose that it correctly indicates HIV 99% of the time, and the proportion of time it correctly indicates no HIV is 99.5%. Suppose that the prevalence of HIV among blood donors is known to be 1/10,000.

(a) What proportion of the blood that is donated will test positive for HIV using the ELISA test?
(b) What proportion of the blood that has tested negative on the ELISA test is actually infected with HIV? One minus this term, the proportion of blood that has tested negative on the ELISA and that is actually not infected, is termed the negative predictive value (NPV).
(c) What is the probability that a positive ELISA outcome is truly positive, that is, what proportion of individuals with positive test outcomes are actually infected with HIV? This probability is termed the positive predictive value (PPV).

EXERCISE 2.2.   Suppose that hospital surgeries are performed five days a week, with 15% of surgeries on Mondays, 25% on Tuesdays, 25% on Wednesdays, 25% on Thursdays, and 10% on Fridays. Suppose that Monday and Friday surgeries are successful 80% of the time, and that Tuesday–Thursday surgeries are successful 95% of the time.

(a) What proportion of surgeries are successful during a typical week?
(b) What proportion of non-successful surgeries occur on Monday? Tuesday? Wednesday? Thursday? Friday?

EXERCISE 2.3.   Suppose it is known that 7% of British children attend special schools that cater to privileged parents and that 75% of all hospital administrators are known to have attended such schools. Consider the implication that under-privileged but presumably intelligent and hard-working children might have been excluded from high-ranking professions such as hospital administration. We look at the relative probabilities of becoming a hospital administrator given that one did or did not attend an elite school.

Specifically, let E denote attending an elite school, with E^c the complement. Let H denote becoming a hospital administrator, with H^c the complement. Let $p = P(H)$ be the (unknown to us) proportion of hospital administrators among the populace of Great Britain. We are given that $P(E \mid H) = 0.75$ and $P(E) = 0.07$.

(a) Use the definition of conditional probability to find $P(H \mid E)$ and $P(H \mid E^c)$ as functions of p.

(b) Find an actual number for the (risk) ratio $P(H|E)/P(H|E^c)$.

(c) What can you say about the effect of availability of elite schooling on the prospects of becoming a hospital administrator in Great Britain?

(d) Let $q = P(E)$. What value of q corresponds to no effect of school type on the chances of becoming a hospital administrator later in life? No effect means that $P(H \mid E) = P(H \mid E^c) = P(H)$.

EXERCISE 2.4.   Reproduce Figure 2.3.

EXERCISE 2.5. *Model, prediction, and inference for conditionally geometric data.* Consider a sequence of independent Bernoulli trials with θ denoting the probability of success. The random variable Y = "number of failures before the first success" then has the geometric distribution:

$$p(y \mid \theta) = (1 - \theta)^y \theta, \quad y = 0, 1, \dots.$$

Let the data consist of $Y_1, \dots, Y_n$ conditionally independent and identically distributed as geometric with parameter θ. In the following, use a uniform prior on $(0, 1)$ for θ. The observed values are $y = (y_1, \dots, y_n)$.

(a) Derive the posterior pdf for θ. Identify the corresponding distribution precisely.

(b) For a future value $Z \sim p(z \mid \theta)$, independent of the observed data, derive the explicit form of the predictive density, $p(z \mid y)$.

(c) Suppose we are interested in the mean of the geometric distribution, $\mu = (1 - \theta)/\theta$. Using the usual transformation of variables technique from probability theory (see Appendix A), derive the posterior pdf for μ.

(d) *Extension to negative binomial data.* If in the definition of the geometric distribution above we change Y to "number of failures before the rth success" where r is a known number, we get the negative binomial distribution:

$$p(y \mid r, \theta) = \binom{r + y - 1}{y} \theta^r (1 - \theta)^y, \quad y = 0, 1, \dots.$$

Again with a uniform prior for θ, and using your results above, find the posterior and predictive densities given conditionally independent and identically distributed negative binomial data $y = (y_1, \dots, y_n)$.

EXERCISE 2.6.   A man with a prostate specific antigen (PSA) test value exceeding 4 will be suspected of having prostate cancer. Men over 50 are generally screened using the PSA test. Suppose it is known that the proportion of PSA values that will exceed 4 when such men do not have prostate cancer is 0.3; that for men who have stage I or II prostate cancer, the probability is 0.75; and that for men with higher than stage II prostate cancer, the probability is 0.85. Suppose that the proportion of men (over 50) who will ultimately be determined through various means to *not* actually have prostate cancer is 0.80, to have stages I or II is 0.15, and to be above stage II is 0.05.

(a) What proportion of men over 50 will be diagnosed based on their PSA values to have prostate cancer? Keep in mind that all this means is that their PSA is greater than 4; it does not mean that they necessarily have cancer.

(b) Under these made-up assumptions, suppose an individual has just been diagnosed as potentially having prostate cancer (PSA > 4). What are the chances that he actually has: stage I or II prostate cancer? above stage II cancer? prostate cancer? no prostate cancer?

(c) Now suppose he has just been diagnosed as potentially *not* having prostate cancer. What are the chances that he actually has: stage I or II prostate cancer? above stage II cancer? prostate cancer? no prostate cancer?

(d) Construct a table with rows corresponding to disease status and three columns of probabilities corresponding to (i) no PSA information, (ii) PSA > 4, and (iii) PSA ≤ 4. Comment on what you think of this PSA screening test.

EXERCISE 2.7. *Exercise 2.6, continued.* Generally, if the PSA outcome is positive, a follow-up test is performed that involves an invasive biopsy of the prostate. Biopsies are much more accurate in detecting cancer. While they also include information on the stage of cancer if present, for this exercise we consider only whether the biopsy is positive or negative for cancer. First suppose that such a biopsy is performed only on those that show PSA > 4, and that everyone with PSA > 4 undergoes a biopsy. Next suppose that biopsies for prostate cancer have the following properties: for those without cancer, it is cancer negative with probability 0.999; for those with disease stage I or II, it is cancer positive with probability 0.90; and for someone with disease stage higher than II, it detects cancer with 98% accuracy. Use this information and that in the question and answers for Exercise 2.6 to answer the following questions.

(a) As in Exercise 2.6(d), construct and fill a table with rows corresponding to disease status and three columns of probabilities corresponding to (i) no biopsy information for someone about to have this test, (ii) a positive biopsy for cancer, and (iii) biopsy negative for cancer. Comment on what you think of the value of a biopsy.

(b) Compute the probability that a randomly chosen man over 50 who is waiting for the result of his PSA test has a positive biopsy as a result of this two-step testing procedure.

(c) Compute the probability that a randomly chosen man over 50 who is waiting for the result of his PSA test has a negative biopsy as a result of this two-step testing procedure.

EXERCISE 2.8. Let X_1, X_2 be conditionally independent and distributed as exponential random variables with pdf $p(x \mid \theta) = \theta e^{-\theta x}$. Let $p(\theta) = e^{-\theta}$, namely $\theta \sim \exp(1)$. Let $x = (x_1, x_2)$ be the observed data.

(a) Write down and simplify the likelihood function $Lik(\theta) \propto p(x \mid \theta)$.

(b) Obtain the pdf for $p(\theta \mid x)$. There is a name for this distribution. Identify the precise distribution.

(c) Let $Z \mid \theta$ also be exponential, the same as the X_i, and conditionally independent of them. Obtain the precise form of the predictive density $p(z \mid x)$.

(d) Obtain the formula for the predictive probability $P(Z > c \mid x)$.

EXERCISE 2.9.   For the **VetBP** data discussed in Example 2.7, use R or some other program to determine the posterior median, mean, and a 95% probability interval for θ. Also obtain the posterior probability that θ is greater than 0.4 and 0.5.

Chapter 3

Fundamentals II: Models for Exchangeable Observations

In this chapter we discuss commonly used models for exchangeable observations. Measurements taken on individuals are regarded as exchangeable provided the individuals are sampled randomly from a particular population without regard to their individual characteristics beyond simply belonging to that population. This implies a symmetry about the role of individuals in the sampling. Technically, *exchangeable* means that the joint distribution of a collection, say $(Y_1, \ldots, Y_n)$, of random variables (RVs) is unaffected by any reordering of the observations. While exchangeable random variables are *not necessarily independent*, they are identically distributed. In other words, their marginal distributions are the same. If we start with $Y_i | \theta \overset{iid}{\sim} p(y \mid \theta)$ and then let $\theta \sim p(\theta)$, then the Y_i are exchangeable. In this instance, the Y_i are (unconditionally) dependent. Dependence in the context of exchangeable RVs allows us to learn from observing some outcomes in order to predict outcomes that are not yet observed. This kind of model is our common theme in this chapter for different choices of sampling distribution and prior.

A major purpose of this chapter is to establish familiarity with the mathematical manipulations in Bayesian analysis in relatively simple scenarios. Understanding these computations will be useful for building more complex and more realistic models in later chapters. We introduce Bernoulli, binomial, normal, Poisson and exponential models for data along with probability models that reflect pre-data knowledge about unknown quantities or parameters associated with these models. The presentation includes illustrations of standard Bayesian inferences that use these models in conjunction with mostly so-called conjugate priors.

Model specification consists of writing down a sampling distribution (likelihood) and specifying a suitable family of (prior) distributions to be used to represent knowledge about unobservable parameters in the sampling distribution. For the pre-data knowledge distributions in this chapter, we use what are called *conjugate families* in all but one instance. Conjugate families have the property that *both* knowledge distributions, data-excluded and data-informed, are in the same family. To derive the data-informed knowledge distribution (the posterior), we use expression (2.6) for Bayes' theorem in the proportionality form, and recognize that the product of prior and likelihood belongs to the same family as $p(\theta)$.

While conjugacy is rarely necessary in modern Bayesian statistics, it does allow for simple calculations that result in a known form for the posterior pdf, which results in a relative ease of illustration at this early stage of our development of Bayesian inference. Moreover, these simple calculations can also provide insight into the relative influence of the data compared with the prior on the posterior distribution.

The statistical model for the data is selected to be appropriate for the particular type of exchangeable data to be analyzed. The selected sampling distribution gives rise to a likelihood function, which gives rise to a possible form for the prior in the conjugate case. In later chapters, we often select families of pre-data distributions for the unknowns that are not conjugate.

The chapter concludes with a discussion of nonparametric models, which provide an alternative to the more constrained parametric models that are often used in data analysis. Required background material is in Appendix A.

3.1 Overview of Binomial, Normal, Poisson and Exponential Models

We consider four fundamental models for statistical data. The presentation at times will be somewhat technical as we focus on generic data of various types. However, scientific illustrations based on each type of data are given.

Bernoulli. The Bernoulli RV is named for the seventeenth-century mathematician Jacob Bernoulli. It occurs in the context of what is termed a Bernoulli trial, an experiment where there is a simple yes or no outcome. For example, we have performed a Bernoulli trial if we sample a blood donor at random from the population of Red Cross donors, test the donor's blood for HIV, and declare the outcome as yes or no. We also discussed Bernoulli trials in Example 2.7 in the previous chapter.

In general, if Y represents the outcome of a Bernoulli trial and the trial results in a "yes," we let $Y = 1$; if the answer is "no," we let $Y = 0$. Generic terminology designates $Y = 1$ as "success" and $Y = 0$ as "failure." With this specification, Y is a numerical outcome associated with the Bernoulli trial. Furthermore, let θ be the proportion of "successes" in the sampled population. We write $Y \mid \theta \sim Ber(\theta)$ where $P(Y = 1 \mid \theta) = \theta$ and $P(Y = 0 \mid \theta) = 1 - \theta$.

Binomial. From elementary probability, we know that the binomial distribution is just the sum of independent and identically distributed $Ber(\theta)$ random variables. Suppose there are n iid $Ber(\theta)$ random variables and S equals the sum of them. We then have $S \mid \theta \sim Bin(n, \theta)$. In other words, the binomial is the total number of yes answers for some characteristic out of a total of n independently sampled individuals from a single population.

As an illustration, suppose we place the names of all current Red Cross blood donors on a list and then randomly sample 100 names from that list. We then test each of the 100 sampled individuals for HIV and count the number of positive outcomes. If the actual population proportion of positive outcomes that we would observe if we tested everyone on the entire list were, say, 0.01, we would write $S \mid \theta \sim Bin(100, 0.01)$.

Given the fixed known value of n, the binomial is completely characterized by the unknown parameter θ, which will be the primary scientific unknown of interest for making statistical inferences in this setting. The wonderful thing about the binomial is that it is possible to think about the way the sampling was done and characterize the distribution of possible outcomes with the binomial distribution.

It is well known that

$$P(S = k \mid \theta) = \binom{n}{k} \theta^k (1 - \theta)^{n-k}, \quad k = 0, 1, \ldots, n,$$

and that $E(Y) = n\theta$ and $\text{Var}(Y) = n\theta(1 - \theta)$. We discuss Bernoulli and binomial outcomes in Section 3.2.1.

Normal. The normal or Gaussian distribution is ubiquitous in the world of data analysis. While it is possible *a priori* to reasonably assert that a random variable is binomial, it is not possible to know with any degree of certainty that a random variable is normal. It is possible, however, to check whether the assumption of normality is reasonable using various statistical techniques, such as by constructing a so-called quantile–quantile plot based on observed data. We make such considerations later in the book.

The normal distribution is a model for a continuous RV. In theory, a normal RV can take on any value in $\mathbb{R} \equiv (-\infty, \infty)$ to any degree of decimal accuracy. However, observed data can only be measured to a finite degree of accuracy. For example, if we measure the time to death from diagnosis with lung cancer, the time of observation would rarely be more accurate than to the minute, and data that biostatisticians analyze would generally only be accurate to the day of death. We would not generally model time-to-event data with a normal distribution, but one possibility is to take logs and to assume log times are approximately normal. When observed data can take on a sufficient number of possible values, somehow approximating a continuum over a large enough range of possibilities, they are usually modeled by a RV that is defined on the continuum, and this seems eminently reasonable in most instances. This assumption is made for all continuous RVs considered in this book.

When we write $Y \mid \mu, \sigma^2 \sim N(\mu, \sigma^2)$, we are asserting that the probability density function (pdf) of Y is bell-shaped, symmetric about μ, that 95% of the area under the curve is in the interval $(\mu - 1.96\sigma, \mu + 1.96\sigma)$, that its median and thus its mean are both μ, and that its standard deviation is σ. We know that the standardized version of Y, $Z \equiv (Y - \mu)/\sigma$, has a standard normal, $N(0, 1)$, distribution with pdf

$$f(z) = \frac{1}{\sqrt{2\pi}} e^{-z^2/2}, \quad z \in \mathbb{R}.$$

We discuss statistical inference for normal outcomes in Section 3.2.2.

Poisson. The Poisson distribution is named for the nineteenth-century mathematician and physicist Siméon Poisson. The Poisson random variable has the property that its mean, say λ, also equals its variance (λ). We use the notation $Y|\lambda \sim Po(\lambda)$. It is a count variable that Poisson originally used to characterize the distribution of the number of events occurring during a fixed time interval. The distribution has also found much use in other applications. Two examples are modeling the number of blood transfusions per month among cancer patients suffering chemotherapy-induced anemia and the number of tumors in the livers of mice exposed to a carcinogen. The Poisson distribution is similar to but different from the binomial.

The Poisson also arises as an approximation to the binomial when n is large and θ is small. Under these circumstances, if $Y \mid \theta \sim Bin(n, \theta)$, then we can show that $Y \mid \theta \overset{\cdot}{\sim} Po(n\theta)$, where $\overset{\cdot}{\sim}$ means *is approximately distributed as*. The Poisson approximation was historically important before the advent of fast computers.

Consider the following examples one might characterize via the Poisson distribution: (i) the number of lung cancer incidences (events) in New York City over the period of a year; (ii) the number of babies born in Los Angeles during a specified year; (iii) the number of unique incidences of individuals infected with the Zika virus (events) in the U.S. since January 2016. By "unique" we mean that if Zika was transmitted to a member of a family, we do not count additional incidences within the same family.

The assumptions for a variable Y to be $Po(\lambda)$ are as follows.

- Events occur independently of one another. Specifically, if it is known that a certain number of events occurred in a particular time window, this knowledge has no effect on the probability of any number of events occurring in a non-overlapping time window, conditional on λ.

- The probability of seeing a particular number of events in any given time window is the same for all time windows of the same length; this is called stationarity.

- The probability of exactly one event occurring in a small time window is proportional to λ times the length of the time window.

- The probability of two or more events occurring in a small time window is very small.

Examples (i)–(iii) above should at least approximately satisfy these assumptions. Observe that there is no fixed number of individuals that constitute a sample, as in the binomial case. In the cancer incidence case, there is no fixed number of individuals living in a city over the course of a year, since many people move into a city, many die, and many leave a city during any given year. The "babies being born" and the Zika examples clearly have no fixed ascertainable n.

Under the above assumptions, it can be shown that

$$P(Y = k \mid \lambda) = \frac{\lambda^k}{k!} e^{-\lambda}, \quad k = 0, 1, \ldots,$$

with $E(Y \mid \lambda) = \lambda$ and $\text{Var}(Y \mid \lambda) = \lambda$. In fact, under these assumptions, if we define $N(t)$ to be the number of events to occur by time t, it is true that $N(t) \sim Po(\lambda t)$. The collection of Poisson random variables $\{N(t) : t > 0\}$ is called a Poisson process with rate λ. We discuss inferences for Poisson outcomes in Section 3.2.3.

Exponential. If we let T be the waiting time for the first event in a Poisson process $\{N(t) : t > 0\}$, we must have $P(T > t \mid \lambda) = P(N(t) = 0 \mid \lambda) = e^{-\lambda t}$, since $\{T > t\} \Leftrightarrow \{N(t) = 0\}$. (The symbol $\Leftrightarrow$ means "if and only if.") This probability is called the *survival* (or *survivor*) *function* and is 1 minus the cumulative distribution function (cdf). The pdf for T is the derivative of the cdf and we obtain

$$p(t \mid \lambda) = \lambda e^{-\lambda t}, \quad t \geq 0.$$

We write $T \sim Exp(\lambda)$ and it is easy to show that $E(T) = 1/\lambda$ and $\text{Var}(T) = 1/\lambda^2$. It can also be shown that the waiting times between events in a Poisson process with rate parameter λ are independent and identically distributed as $Exp(\lambda)$. We discuss exponential models in Section 3.2.4.

We proceed to obtain posterior and predictive distributions and make inferences using these models.

3.2 Posterior and Predictive Inferences

3.2.1 Bernoulli and Binomial Models

In this section we first discuss statistical inferences for exchangeable Bernoulli RVs. We assume that n conditionally iid $Ber(\theta)$ RVs are observed. We also observe the sum of the Bernoullis. Since, conditional on the success probability θ, the sum of n iid $Ber(\theta)$ RVs is distributed as $Bin(n, \theta)$, and since the likelihood, $Lik(\theta)$, is identical whether only the sum is observed or if the individual Bernoullis are observed, Bayesian inferences based on the binomial and Bernoulli models will be identical if the same prior is used for θ.

Exchangeable Bernoulli Model. We already considered an illustration of this model in Example 2.7. Here, we present a general version of what was presented there.

With notation from the distribution table in Appendix B, we write the model as

$$Y_1, \ldots, Y_n \mid \theta \overset{\text{iid}}{\sim} Ber(\theta).$$

We need an analytical form for the distribution of the data given the parameter if we are to use Bayes' theorem. As discussed just above expression (2.6), the pdf for this *sampling distribution* of the data, when looked at as a function of the parameter for fixed observed data, is proportional to the likelihood function, $Lik(\theta)$. We have

$$Lik(\theta) = p(y_1, \ldots, y_n \mid \theta) = \prod_{i=1}^{n} \theta^{y_i}(1-\theta)^{1-y_i} = \theta^{\sum_{i=1}^{n} y_i}(1-\theta)^{n-\sum_{i=1}^{n} y_i}.$$

The next step is to specify an *external (or pre-data)* knowledge distribution (or prior) for θ, which must be obtained without looking at the data. We have argued throughout that such considerations must be made independently of the data to be analyzed. This means that the information could be obtained before the data are even collected, or simply obtained from sources that are separate from any information provided in the data.

The beta family of prior distributions is conjugate here. So let us assume that scientific knowledge about θ can be reasonably reflected by a $Be(a_0, b_0)$ distribution. Then by expression (2.6), and defining $s = \sum_{i=1}^{n} y_i$, we have

$$p(\theta \mid \boldsymbol{y}) \propto \theta^s (1-\theta)^{n-s} \theta^{a_0-1} (1-\theta)^{b_0-1} \propto \theta^{a_0+s-1} (1-\theta)^{b_0+n-s-1}$$

which is the kernel of a $Be(a_0 + s, b_0 + n - s)$ pdf. Then we say that

$$\theta \mid \boldsymbol{y} \sim Be(a_0 + s, b_0 + n - s).$$

The prior and the posterior are in the same family. This property has also been called "closed under sampling."

We note that the prior and posterior means are

$$E(\theta) = \frac{a}{a+b}, \quad \tilde{\theta} \equiv E(\theta \mid \boldsymbol{y}) = \frac{a_0 + s}{a_0 + b_0 + n} = w \frac{a_0}{a_0 + b_0} + (1-w) \frac{s}{n},$$

where $w = (a_0 + b_0)/(a_0 + b_0 + n)$. The posterior mean is a weighted average of the prior mean and the proportion of successes, s/n, in the sample. If $a_0 + b_0 = n$, each part gets equal weighting. Generally, we would expect $a_0 + b_0 < n$ so that more weight is given to the data than to the prior; $a_0 + b_0$ is often regarded as the "prior sample size" because of this weighting. Such estimators are called "shrinkage" estimators since they shrink away from the solely data-based estimate towards the prior guess.

The unique mode of a $Be(a_0, b_0)$ distribution is $(a_0 - 1)/(a_0 + b_0 - 2)$, provided $a_0 \geq 1$, $a_0 + b_0 > 2$. With $a_0 = b_0 = 1$, we have the uniform distribution, $U(0, 1)$; with $a_0 \leq 1$, $b_0 > 1$ the unique mode is 0; with $a_0 > 1$, $b_0 \leq 1$ the unique mode is 1. With $a_0 < 1$, $b_0 < 1$, there are two modes, at 0 and 1. The latter case implies that the scientist would have a belief that θ was more likely to be close to 0 or 1, and less likely to be in between. It would be unusual for real scientific information to follow this reasoning.

The posterior standard deviation is

$$\sqrt{\tilde{\theta}(1 - \tilde{\theta})/(a_0 + b_0 + n)}.$$

So the larger is $a_0 + b_0 + n$, the more concentrated the posterior for θ is about its mean. Since good approximations to the quantiles of the beta distribution are easily obtained in packages like R, it is simple to obtain a 95% probability interval (PI) for θ by obtaining the 0.025 and 0.975 quantiles of the specified beta distribution. The posterior median is also easily obtained in this way. For this kind of situation, the Monte Carlo-based computational methods are not needed.

Example 3.1. Here we continue with the **VetBP** illustration from Example 2.7. Recall that a $Be(1,1)$ (or $U(0,1)$) prior was used there. Since $n = 404$ and $a_0 + b_0 = 2$, estimates are primarily driven by the data. We obtain the posterior mean, $185/(185+221) = 0.457$, posterior mode, $184/(185+221-2) = 0.455$, and median,[1] 0.456, posterior standard deviation, 0.025, and 95% interval,[2] $(0.408, 0.504)$. We can also obtain $P(\theta < c \mid \boldsymbol{y})$, using R. For example, with $c = 0.5$, we find the probability that θ is less than 0.5 is about[3] 0.96.

As previously discussed, the median will actually be more appropriate as a point estimate if the corresponding posterior pdf is skewed since, in that instance, it may well represent the "middle" of the posterior distribution much better than the posterior mean, especially if highly skewed. Since mean, median, and mode are nearly identical in this illustration, it would make little difference which was used as a point estimate.

The interpretation for the probability interval is straightforward: conditional on the data, the probability is 0.95 that the unknown fraction of uncontrolled hypertension among hypertensive veterans in the target population is between 0.408 and 0.504. The interval is often called a 95% *credible interval*, but it is also called a 95% *posterior probability interval*, and often just a 95% *probability interval*. There are also 95% *prior probability intervals* that are simply based on the prior distribution. In this example, a 95% prior probability interval for θ is simply $(0.025, 0.975)$. We are using intervals that have 0.025 area to the left of the lower endpoint and to the right of the upper endpoint, under the prior or the posterior pdf, respectively. Other choices are possible; we discuss one possibility in the next paragraph. Point and interval estimates for the **VetBP** data are shown in Figure 3.1.

Another method of interval estimation involves calculation of the highest posterior density (HPD) interval. This is the interval with the correct area for which all points outside the interval have smaller density (or plausibility). If the posterior pdf is symmetric and unimodal, the interval obtained will be identical to the one described above. However, if the posterior were bimodal with modes at 0 and 1, for example with a $Be(0.5, 0.5)$ posterior, the 95% HPD would be $(0, 0.46) \cup (0.54, 1)$, where 0.46 is the 0.475 quantile and 0.54 is the 0.525 quantile. On the other hand, the interval corresponding to the 0.025 and 0.975 quantiles would be $(0.0015, 0.9985)$, which is radically different since all the ordinates outside the interval are more plausible than all the ordinates inside the interval. The HPD is obviously preferable in general and especially in this situation. However, it is doubtful that this particular posterior would arise, and if it did, we would use the HPD. Highly skewed posteriors also warrant HPD intervals. We generally use the equal-tail method unless the nature of the posterior demands otherwise.

Functions of Unknowns in the Model. As previously discussed, interest often lies in some function of the unknown used in the model. To illustrate, suppose we are interested in the *odds* of uncontrolled hypertension in addition to the fraction

---

[1] qbeta(0.5,185,221) in R.

[2] qbeta(c(0.025,0.975),185,221) in R.

[3] pbeta(0.5,185,221) in R.

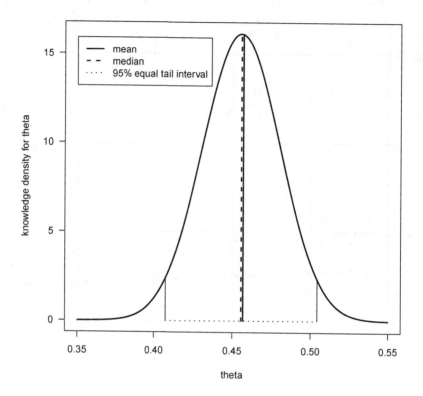

FIGURE 3.1: Posterior distribution with mean, median, and 95% equal-tail credible interval.

(or probability). With γ denoting odds, the relationship is

$$\gamma = \frac{\theta}{1 - \theta}.$$

The prior or posterior distribution of γ is induced from the specified distribution for θ. While an analytical derivation is possible using the calculus of probability (see Appendix A), inferences can be readily obtained by Monte Carlo sampling of a large number, say M, of values of θ from its distribution, $\{\theta^{(1)}, \theta^{(2)}, \ldots, \theta^{(M)}\}$, and calculating the corresponding values $\{\gamma^{(j)} = \theta^{(j)}/(1 - \theta^{(j)}) : j = 1, \ldots, M\}$. This effectively gives a large sample from the posterior distribution of γ that can be used to approximate the density of γ, as well as any summaries, such as mean, median, and PI for γ. Figure 3.2 displays the knowledge distributions for γ, both pre-data (obtained analytically) and post-data (obtained via sampling).

Moreover, since the function of θ above is monotone and increasing, the median of the posterior for γ is just the transformed median of θ, namely, $0.456/(1-0.456) = 0.84$, and the 95% posterior interval is $(0.69, 1.02)$. We are thus 95% certain that the odds of uncontrolled hypertension are between 0.69 and 1.02.

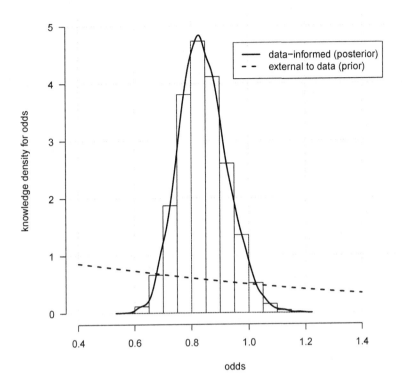

FIGURE 3.2: Prior and posterior distributions for γ, for the **VetBP** data, the posterior obtained via sampling.

Binomial Model. Let $Y \mid \theta \sim Bin(\theta)$ and assume that $Y = y$ is observed. We continue as above with a generic $Be(a_0, b_0)$ prior to model uncertainty about the binomial success probability θ. While it is convenient, it is by no means necessary to use a beta distribution as a model for the prior. The beta distribution is conjugate to the binomial distribution, the same as it was for exchangeable Bernoullis. The $Be(a_0, b_0)$ pdf is

$$p(\theta) = \frac{\Gamma(a_0 + b_0)}{\Gamma(a_0)\Gamma(b_0)} \theta^{a_0 - 1}(1 - \theta)^{b_0 - 1} I_{(0,1)}(\theta). \tag{3.1}$$

Here $\Gamma(\cdot)$ is the well-known *gamma* function; a_0 and b_0 are selected to reflect the researcher's beliefs and uncertainty.

Since

$$p(\boldsymbol{y} \mid \theta) = \binom{n}{y} \theta^y (1 - \theta)^{n-y} \propto \theta^y (1 - \theta)^{n-y} = Lik(\theta),$$

Bayes' theorem in proportionality form gives

$$p(\theta \mid y) \propto p(y \mid \theta)p(\theta)$$
$$\propto \theta^y(1-\theta)^{n-y}\theta^{a_0-1}(1-\theta)^{b_0-1}$$
$$\propto \theta^{a_0+y-1}(1-\theta)^{b_0+n-y-1},$$

which is the kernel of the $Be(a_0+y, b_0+n-y)$ distribution. Thus we have established that

$$\theta \mid y \sim Be(a_0+y, b_0+n-y),$$

which is identical to the result obtained when n exchangeable $Ber(\theta)$ RVs were observed; there y, the observed number of "successes," was denoted s.

*Prediction in the Binomial Model. We have just developed Bayesian estimation for the Bernoulli and binomial models, and we developed predictive inferences for a particular example in Chapter 2. We now extend the methodology to prediction of a generic binomial count. For example, if it is known that m blood units have been donated but have not yet been tested, we may be interested in using the data at hand to predict the number of those units that might test positive for HIV infection.

Let $Z \mid \theta \sim Bin(m, \theta)$ be a future binomial count of interest. Furthermore, suppose we have already observed data $Y = y$ that we take to be distributed as $Y \mid \theta \sim Bin(n, \theta)$ and that Y and Z are conditionally independent given θ. Assume the prior $\theta \sim Be(a_0, b_0)$. We showed above that the posterior was also beta distributed. Let us denote the updated parameters of the posterior beta distribution as (a_y, b_y), where $a_y = a_0 + y$ and $b_y = b_0 + n - y$. We can now obtain both pre-data and post-data prediction probabilities in one calculation:

$$\begin{aligned}
P(Z = r \mid y) &= \int_0^1 P(Z = r \mid y, \theta)p(\theta \mid y)d\theta \\
&= \int_0^1 \binom{m}{r}\theta^r(1-\theta)^{m-r}\frac{\Gamma(a_y+b_y)}{\Gamma(a_y)\Gamma(b_y)}\theta^{a_y-1}(1-\theta)^{b_y-1}d\theta \\
&= \binom{m}{r}\frac{\Gamma(a_y+b_y)}{\Gamma(a_y)\Gamma(b_y)}\int_0^1 \theta^{(a_y+r)-1}(1-\theta)^{b_y+m-r-1}\,d\theta \\
&= \binom{m}{r}\frac{\Gamma(a_y+b_y)}{\Gamma(a_y)\Gamma(b_y)}\frac{\Gamma(a_y+r)\Gamma(b_y+m-r)}{\Gamma(a_y+b_y+m)}.
\end{aligned}$$

If $m = 1$, the probability that the next observation will be $Z = 1$, given the current data, is $a_y/(a_y + b_y)$. This predicted probability follows from the factorial property of the *gamma* function: $\Gamma(a+1) = a\Gamma(a)$. The general r case simplifies by repeatedly using this property.

Example 3.2. Predicting HIV Infection. Let the proportion of infected blood units in the population be denoted as the prevalence of infection, or simply, the prevalence. Suppose that, before any blood units have been tested, we are tempted to assert that the prevalence is equally likely to be any number between 0 and 1.

As we have already seen, the $U(0,1)$ (or $Be(1,1)$) distribution would be a prime candidate in this instance. This prior reflects a belief that the prevalence is equally likely to be above or below 0.5. However, some reflection may lead us to think that such a prior would fail to represent scientific reality. If the population sampled involves units donated to the American Red Cross, it is difficult to imagine that the prevalence could even be 10%, let alone above 50%.

Let us assume that information is available that suggests that it is extremely unlikely that 10% or more blood donors could be HIV infected. A little calculus can be used to show that a $Be(1, 43.7)$ only admits a 1% chance for a value above 0.1. This prior has a mode of 0 and would be conservative if the likely prevalence is very much smaller than 0.1.

Suppose we examine 10,000 units of blood and test each for HIV. If 2 of the 10,000 units are infected, our posterior distribution for the proportion of infected units of blood will have a beta distribution with parameters $3 \ (= 1+2)$ and $10,041.7$ $(= 43.7+10,000-2)$. This posterior is quite skewed so we would choose the median of the posterior as a point estimate for the prevalence. The posterior median is 0.00027 and a 95% PI is $(0.000062, 0.00072)$. If asked to predict what proportion of future blood units we examine will be infected with HIV, our answer would be 0.027%, or about 27 in 100,000, and with 95% certainty, we would assert that the prevalence was between 6.2 and 72.0 per 100,000 units.

If we then plan to examine another 10,000 blood units, we find that the mean of the predictive distribution is 3, the median is 2, and a 95% prediction interval for the number of HIV infected units in the future sample is $[0, 9]$. This was performed using Monte Carlo methods, yet to be discussed.

These calculations were based on the assumption that the probability that each unit of blood is infected is essentially the same across all tested units, and that knowing the test outcome for any particular selection of units conveys no information about the chances that other units are infected, conditional on a given true value for the probability of infection. This all translates to the conditionally iid sampling assumption. These assumptions may be too strong. An example of how the binomial assumption could be wrong would be if our sample contained multiple units of blood from the same person, or if the sample was meant to include only men, and if units from one or more women were included by mistake.

3.2.2 Normally Distributed Exchangeable Observations

We now consider the $N(\mu, \sigma^2)$ distribution for exchangeable continuous observations. A new feature is the fact that there are two model parameters, the mean, μ, and the variance, σ^2. We will need to obtain the likelihood for this model, and we will need to specify one or more families of prior distributions for the model parameters. In this section it will be convenient, for technical reasons, to reparameterize the model. There are a variety of reasons in statistical modeling why reparameterization can be helpful and important. Therefore, in addition to making the presentation easier, we think it will be helpful to provide an in-depth example, so that subsequent experiences will seem more familiar.

For the development and presentation of the joint posterior, it will be much easier for us to use the parameter $\tau = 1/\sigma^2$, rather than σ^2; τ is the "precision" of the distribution. We thus proceed to discuss making inferences for (μ, τ). Once we have inferences for (μ, τ), it is a simple matter when using Monte Carlo methods to make inferences for (μ, σ^2), and for virtually any function, $\gamma = \gamma(\mu, \sigma^2)$. For example, we may be interested in the 90th percentile of the normal distribution, which is $\mu + 1.28\sigma = \mu + 1.28/\sqrt{\tau}$. Another parameter of interest might be the probability

$$P(Y < c \mid \mu, \sigma) = P\left(Z < \frac{c - \mu}{\sigma}\right) = \Phi\left(\frac{c - \mu}{\sigma}\right),$$

which can just as easily be written in terms of τ. It is equally easy to make inferences regardless of the model parameterization.

When it is time to place a normal *prior* distribution on, say, μ, which we will do, we find that it is considerably easier to leave the parameterization for that distribution alone. So our notation throughout this section will be $Y \sim N(\mu, 1/\tau)$ when modeling data. And when we model external knowledge about μ, we write $\mu \sim N(\mu_0, \sigma_0^2)$, where μ_0 is a prior guess for μ and σ_0 is the standard deviation of the prior for μ, which determines how precise the prior information is.

We now present some important technical details that will be needed for the rest of the section.

The Joint Likelihood and Posterior. With the data modeled as

$$Y_i | \mu, \tau \overset{\text{iid}}{\sim} N(\mu, 1/\tau), \quad i = 1, \ldots, n,$$

we have the likelihood function

$$Lik(\mu, \tau) \propto \prod_{i=1}^{n} \tau^{1/2} e^{-\frac{\tau}{2}(y_i - \mu)^2} = \tau^{n/2} e^{-\frac{\tau}{2} \sum_{i=1}^{n}(y_i - \mu)^2}.$$

One can easily show that

$$\sum_{i=1}^{n}(y_i - \mu)^2 = n(\mu - \bar{y})^2 + \sum_{i=1}^{n}(y_i - \bar{y})^2, \tag{3.2}$$

where $\bar{y} = \sum_{i=1}^{n} y_i / n$, the sample mean. Showing this result is left as an exercise. Using equation (3.2), we obtain

$$Lik(\mu, \tau) \propto \tau^{n/2} e^{-\frac{\tau}{2}\{n(\mu - \bar{y})^2 + \sum_{i=1}^{n}(y_i - \bar{y})^2\}}. \tag{3.3}$$

Specifying the joint prior for (μ, τ) as $p(\mu, \tau)$, the joint posterior is

$$p(\mu, \tau \mid \boldsymbol{y}) \propto Lik(\mu, \tau) p(\mu, \tau),$$

where $\boldsymbol{y}$ denotes the vector $(y_1, \ldots, y_n)'$. Two basic choices for prior families will be considered,

$$p(\mu, \tau) = p(\mu \mid \tau)p(\tau) \quad \text{and} \quad p(\mu, \tau) = p(\mu)p(\tau).$$

In the first instance, knowledge about μ is assumed to be dependent on the value of τ, while the second specification assumes independence.

Based on conjugacy considerations, we use gamma distributions for the marginal priors for τ in this section. We consider other types of priors later in the book. We also consider normal distributions for μ in both cases, where in the first case the prior for μ will depend on τ in a way that results in joint conjugacy, meaning that the joint posterior will be in the same form as the joint prior. In the second case, the conditional distribution $p(\mu \mid \tau, \boldsymbol{y})$ will be normal, and the conditional distribution $p(\tau \mid \mu, \boldsymbol{y})$ will be gamma, which results in what is termed "conditional conjugacy."

The advantage of the independence prior is that it is easier to think about the mean μ independently of the precision (or variance or standard deviation). The price paid for the assumption of independence is that there is no analytical solution for obtaining the precise joint posterior. The particular choice in the dependence case, on the other hand, results in a more difficult prior specification for μ.

In practice, we use the independence assumption, since there are computational methods that we discuss in Chapter 4 that make the analytical intractability disappear using Monte Carlo simulation. So why consider the analytically tractable but less practicable dependence prior if the independence prior is conceptually nicer and is computationally tractable? Part of the answer is that we present it for historical reasons. Before the advent of modern computational methods, the dependence prior was the only one that could be used. In addition, the dependence prior specification allows us to illustrate how the Bayesian method works when there is analytical tractability in a somewhat complex two-parameter problem.

Using the development above, we first present methods for the case with known precision or variance. While it would be extremely rare that the variance is known, the presentation further demonstrates how Bayesian methods work. We will see that the posterior mean is a weighted average of the sample mean, $\bar{y}$, and the prior guess, μ_0, and where the weights depend on the relative magnitudes of n and σ_0. If σ_0 is very small, it means that we basically believe, before seeing any data, that $\mu = \mu_0$, so the posterior mean should shrink to be very close to μ_0 for moderate n. On the other hand, if there is substantial prior uncertainty about μ, meaning σ_0 is large, and if n is moderate to large, the posterior mean should be relatively close to the sample mean.

Known Variance or Precision. Using expression (3.3), and with $\mu \sim N(\mu_0, 1/\tau_0)$, we have

$$p(\mu \mid \tau, \boldsymbol{y}) \propto e^{-\frac{n\tau}{2}(\mu-\bar{y})^2} e^{-\frac{\tau_0}{2}(\mu-\mu_0)^2} = e^{-\frac{1}{2}\{\tau_0(\mu-\mu_0)^2 + n\tau(\mu-\bar{y})^2\}}.$$

For conditional conjugacy to hold, this must be proportional to a normal density in μ, which is not at all obvious at this stage. A technique called "completing the square" results in the very useful formula

$$\tau_0(\mu-\mu_0)^2 + n\tau(\mu-\bar{y})^2 = (\tau_0 + n\tau)(\mu-\tilde{\mu})^2 + \frac{\tau_0 n\tau}{\tau_0 + n\tau}(\mu_0-\bar{y})^2, \qquad (3.4)$$

where

$$\tilde{\mu} = \frac{\tau_0}{\tau_0 + n\tau}\mu_0 + \frac{n\tau}{\tau_0 + n\tau}\bar{y}.$$

It follows immediately that

$$p(\mu \mid \tau, \boldsymbol{y}) \propto e^{-\frac{1}{2}\{(\tau_0+n\tau)(\mu-\hat\mu)^2 + \frac{\tau_0 n\tau}{\tau_0+n\tau}(\mu_0-\bar y)^2\}} \propto e^{-\frac{1}{2}\{(\tau_0+n\tau)(\mu-\tilde\mu)^2\}}, \qquad (3.5)$$

which implies that the conditional posterior is indeed normal, namely

$$\mu \mid \tau, \boldsymbol{y} \sim N\left(\frac{n\tau\,\bar y + \tau_0\,\mu_0}{n\tau + \tau_0}, \frac{1}{\tau_0 + n\tau}\right). \qquad (3.6)$$

As claimed above, conditional on knowing τ, the posterior mean $\tilde\mu$ is a weighted average of our pre-data guess for μ and the sample mean, $\bar y$. The weight on the latter is proportional to sample size, while the weight on the prior guess is proportional to $\tau_0 = 1/\sigma_0^2$.

This is another example of a shrinkage estimator; with larger sample sizes, the prior mean is downweighted in relation to the data, while with small σ_0, the estimator shrinks towards the prior guess. It is also interesting to note that the precision in the posterior is the sum of precisions, the precision for the prior and the precision for the sample mean of n observations, namely $n\tau$.

The posterior variance is $\mathrm{Var}(\mu \mid \sigma^2, \boldsymbol{y}) = \sigma_0^2\sigma^2/(n\sigma_0^2 + \sigma^2)$ with $\sigma_0^2 = 1/\tau_0$ and $\sigma^2 = 1/\tau$. Thus the posterior distribution of μ will be more concentrated about its posterior mean if n is large or σ is small compared to σ_0.

Both Mean and Variance (or Precision) Unknown. We consider two distinct priors when both μ and τ are unknown. The first is a joint prior in which μ and τ are dependent. The particular choice leads to a posterior in the same joint family (i.e., it is conjugate). The second prior uses independent μ and τ, which also has some useful properties of posterior *conditional* distributions of μ, τ being conjugate with simple parameter updates.

*Jointly Conjugate Dependence Prior.   Here, we assume a jointly conjugate prior for (μ, τ). Let

$$\mu \mid \tau \sim N\left(\mu_0, \frac{1}{k\tau}\right), \quad \tau \sim Ga(c, d).$$

We call this a normal-gamma distribution and denote it $NoGa(\mu_0, k, c, d)$. Recall that the pdf for a $Ga(c, d)$ RV is

$$p(\tau) = \frac{d^c}{\Gamma(c)}\tau^{c-1}e^{-\tau d}, \quad \tau > 0,$$

for $c, d > 0$. The mean of the $Ga(c, d)$ distribution using our parameterization is c/d, and its variance is c/d^2. The mode is $(c-1)/d$, provided $c \geq 1$ and is zero if $0 < c \leq 1$. If one has a prior guess for τ, such as $\tau = \tau_0$, one can set $c/d = \tau_0$ or $(c-1)/d = \tau_0$. Letting d be somewhat small gives a gamma distribution that is diffuse. We give a more nuanced discussion later.

A useful observation is that, since the gamma density is a density, we must have

$$\int \tau^{c-1}e^{-\tau d}d\tau = \frac{\Gamma(c)}{d^c}. \qquad (3.7)$$

This is the normalizing (or integration) constant for the gamma distribution as in the table in Appendix B. We will use such constants often.

The prior for μ depends on unknown τ, which was not the case in the previous discussion where there was no reference to τ_0 depending on τ. The specific reason for this choice of prior is that it leads to joint conjugacy, as we shall soon see.

Any joint distribution for a pair of RVs can be expressed as a marginal times a conditional. Here we have

$$p(\mu, \tau \mid \boldsymbol{y}) = p(\tau \mid \boldsymbol{y})p(\mu \mid \tau, \boldsymbol{y}).$$

We already know that $p(\mu \mid \tau, \boldsymbol{y})$ is the normal density given in expression (3.5), only with $k\tau$ replacing τ_0 in that formula, namely

$$\mu \mid \tau, \boldsymbol{y} \sim N\left(\tilde{\mu}, \frac{1}{(k+n)\tau}\right). \tag{3.8}$$

In this formula,

$$\tilde{\mu} = \frac{k\tau}{(k+n)\tau}\mu_0 + \frac{n\tau}{(k+n)\tau}\bar{y} = \frac{k}{k+n}\mu_0 + \frac{n}{k+n}\bar{y}.$$

We see that k and n play comparable roles in the analysis, for example if $k = n$, the prior guess and sample mean get equal weight. Observe that the conditional prior and posterior distributions for μ are in precisely the same form, normal with distinct means and with precisions $k\tau$ and $(k+n)\tau$, respectively.

Using expression (3.3) and defining $\sum_{i=1}^{n}(y_i - \bar{y})^2 = ns^2$, the joint posterior can be represented as

$$
\begin{aligned}
p(\mu, \tau \mid \boldsymbol{y}) &\propto \tau^{n/2}e^{-\frac{\tau}{2}\{n(\mu-\bar{y})^2+ns^2\}}\tau^{1/2}e^{-\frac{k\tau}{2}\{(\mu-\mu_0)^2\}}\tau^{c-1}e^{-\tau d} \\
&= \tau^{1/2}e^{-\frac{\tau}{2}\{(n+k)(\mu-\tilde{\mu})^2\}}\left[\tau^{c+n/2-1}e^{-\tau\{d+ns^2/2+\frac{nk}{n+k}(\mu_0-\bar{y})^2/2\}}\right] \\
&\propto p(\mu \mid \tau, \boldsymbol{y})p(\tau \mid \boldsymbol{y}),
\end{aligned}
$$

where the middle result follows from using the complete-the-square technique as in equation (3.4) with τ_0 replaced by $k\tau$, some simple algebra and a rearrangement of terms. The last expression follows since $\int p(\mu, \tau \mid \boldsymbol{y})d\mu = p(\tau \mid \boldsymbol{y})$, and since the expression just above is the product of the kernel for a $N(\tilde{\mu}, 1/[(k+n)\tau])$ density in μ times a function of only τ (in square brackets). Thus integrating with respect to μ results in a constant (not depending on τ or μ) times the term in brackets, which is the kernel of a gamma pdf; hence the joint posterior pdf is in conjugate normal-gamma form. Simplifying notation, we term it a $NoGa(\tilde{\mu}, k+n, c', d')$ distribution, with

$$c' = c + n/2, \quad d' = d + ns^2/2 + \frac{nk}{n+k}(\mu_0 - \bar{y})^2/2.$$

We are also interested in the marginal posterior for μ,

$$p(\mu \mid \boldsymbol{y}) = \int p(\mu, \tau \mid \boldsymbol{y})d\tau.$$

With our simplified notation, we have

$$p(\mu, \tau \mid \boldsymbol{y}) \propto \tau^{c'+1/2-1} e^{-\tau\{(n+k)(\mu-\tilde{\mu})^2/2+d'\}}$$

and thus

$$p(\mu \mid \boldsymbol{y}) \propto \int \tau^{c'+1/2-1} e^{-\tau\{(n+k)(\mu-\tilde{\mu})^2/2+d'\}} d\tau$$

$$\propto \frac{1}{\{(n+k)(\mu-\tilde{\mu})^2/2+d'\}^{c'+1/2}},$$

using the integration constant from equation (3.7), since the integrand is the kernel of a $Ga(c' + 1/2, \{(n + k)(\mu - \tilde{\mu})^2/2 + d'\})$ pdf. Multiplying the above expression and dividing by the constant $(d')^{c'+1/2}$ results in

$$p(\mu \mid \boldsymbol{y}) \propto \frac{1}{\{1 + c'(n+k)(\mu-\tilde{\mu})^2/(2c'd')\}^{(2c'+1)/2}},$$

which is the kernel of a $t(2c', \tilde{\mu}, \sqrt{d'/\{c'(n+k)\}})$ distribution. The parameters in the Student's distribution are $2c'$, called the degrees of freedom (df); $\tilde{\mu}$, the location; and $\sqrt{d'/\{c'(n+k)\}}$, the scale. For those unfamiliar with this distribution, it is a simple generalization of the usual t distribution. In fact,

$$\frac{\mu - \tilde{\mu}}{\sqrt{d'/[c'(n+k)]}} \mid \boldsymbol{y} \sim t_{2c'},$$

where $t_{2c'}$ is the usual t RV with $2c'$ df. In the table of distributions in Appendix B, this corresponds to $t(2c', 0, 1)$. The general form of the Student's t distribution is $t(\nu, \mu, \sigma)$ with pdf

$$p(s) \propto 1/\left\{1 + \frac{(s-\mu)^2}{\nu\sigma^2}\right\}^{(\nu+1)/2}, \quad s \in (-\infty, \infty).$$

The Student's distribution is similar to the normal distribution in that it is symmetric about its location parameter and its spread depends on its dispersion parameter. When df $= 1$, it is also called a Cauchy distribution. A peculiarity of the Cauchy distribution is that its mean and variance do not exist, which is why we use the terms "location" and "dispersion" rather than mean and variance. We get the standardized Student distribution by subtracting the location and dividing by the square root of the dispersion. Student's distribution approximates a normal distribution as the df parameter grows.

A posterior probability interval for μ is obtained as follows. The standardized Student distribution is symmetric about 0, allowing us to specify appropriate ends for the interval. For example, we might consider equal-tail percentiles, such as $-t_{0.025}$ and $t_{0.025}$, the 0.025 and 0.975 percentage points of the standard t distribution with $2c'$ df. Using these percentiles, we have a 95% posterior probability interval from the standardized distribution as

$$P\left(-t_{0.025} < \frac{\mu - \tilde{\mu}}{\sqrt{d'/[c'(n+k)]}} < t_{0.025} \mid \boldsymbol{y}\right) = 0.95.$$

We rewrite this interval using simple algebra as

$$P(\tilde{\mu} - t_{0.025}\sqrt{d'/[c'(n+k)]} < \mu < \tilde{\mu} + t_{0.025}\sqrt{d'/[c'(n+k)]} \mid \boldsymbol{y}) = 0.95$$

and have a 95% posterior probability interval for μ, namely,

$$\tilde{\mu} \pm t_{0.025}\sqrt{d'/c'(n+k)]}.$$

Remark. A considerably simplified prior distribution that has been used historically is described as follows. First, let c, d be very close to zero. Then we know $p(\tau) \propto \tau^{c-1}e^{-\tau d}$, but this is approximately equal to $1/\tau$. Moreover, if we let $\mu_0 = 0$ and k be approximately zero, we have $p(\mu \mid \tau) \propto e^{-k\tau(\mu)^2}$, which is approximately a constant in μ. Then under these conditions, we have $p(\mu, \tau) \propto 1/\tau$ approximately. There is a "small" issue with this approximation, which is that the approximate joint prior is not a pdf because $\int 1/\tau d\mu d\tau = \infty$. This is called an "improper" prior as a result, and thus using this approximation violates a key probability law.

Nonetheless, if we used this prior, following the same method just described, we would more easily get the following results:

$$\mu \mid \tau, \boldsymbol{y} \sim N\left(\bar{y}, \frac{1}{(k+n)\tau}\right), \quad \tau \mid \boldsymbol{y} \sim Ga\left(\frac{n-1}{2}, \sum_{i=1}^{n}(y_i - \bar{y})^2/2\right),$$

so the conditional posterior mean is simply the sample mean. The posterior mean of τ is

$$E(\tau \mid \boldsymbol{y}) = \frac{n-1}{\sum_{i=1}^{n}(y_i - \bar{y})^2} \equiv 1/(s')^2,$$

the reciprocal of the usual unbiased estimate of σ^2. In addition,

$$\mu \mid \boldsymbol{y} \sim t(n-1, \bar{y}, s'/\sqrt{n}),$$

so that a 95% PI for μ in this case is $\bar{y} \pm t_{0.025}s'/\sqrt{n}$, which is precisely the same interval that frequentists use in this setting. The only difference is that their interpretation of the interval is quite convoluted. The Bayesian interpretation is simply that we are 95% certain that μ is in the calculated interval based on observed data.

Moreover, since the posterior for $(n-1)(s')^2\tau \mid \boldsymbol{y} \sim Ga([n-1]/2, 1/2) = \chi^2_{n-1}$, we can derive a 95% posterior probability interval that is identical to the usual frequentist interval for σ^2.

Since this particular (improper) prior results in inferences that compare with frequentist inferences, it is often called a "reference" prior. Showing these results is left as exercises at the end of this chapter.

Independence Prior. We assume $p(\mu, \tau) = p(\mu)p(\tau)$. Since analytic tractability is not possible here, we proceed in a direction that leads to computational tractability. We make the same assumptions that we made when considering the known variance or precision case, namely, $\mu \sim N(\mu_0, 1/\tau_0)$. We also assume $\tau \sim Ga(c, d)$, as we did in the dependence case. We already know from expression (3.5) that the conditional posterior distribution is $\mu \mid \tau, \boldsymbol{y} \sim N(\tilde{\mu}, 1/(\tau_0 + n\tau))$, where $\tilde{\mu}$ is given in equation (3.6).

Try as we might, it would be impossible to obtain the marginal posterior for $\tau \mid \boldsymbol{y}$, under the assumption of prior independence that we have made. Thus the plan now is to obtain the conditional distribution of $\tau \mid \mu, \boldsymbol{y}$, which is quite easy, as we will soon see. As it turns out, if we can sample from the two conditional posterior distributions, we can obtain a sample from the joint posterior, $p(\mu, \tau \mid \boldsymbol{y})$, and consequently we can numerically approximate the joint posterior and various parameters of interest. Throughout the book, these will be called "full conditional distributions."

Using the joint likelihood, expression (3.3), times the prior for τ gives

$$
\begin{aligned}
p(\tau \mid \mu, \boldsymbol{y}) \;&\propto\; \tau^{n/2} e^{-\frac{\tau}{2}\{n(\mu-\bar{y})^2 + \sum_{i=1}^n (y_i - \bar{y})^2\}} \tau^{c-1} e^{-\tau d} \\
&=\; \tau^{c+n/2-1} e^{-\tau\{d + n(\mu-\bar{y})^2/2 + \sum_{i=1}^n (y_i-\bar{y})^2/2\}}
\end{aligned}
$$

which is the kernel of a gamma distribution. We thus have

$$
\tau \mid \mu, \boldsymbol{y} \sim Ga\left(c + n/2, d + n(\mu - \bar{y})^2/2 + \sum_{i=1}^n (y_i - \bar{y})^2/2\right). \qquad (3.9)
$$

As a preview of how this posterior distribution can be used for inference, consider the following algorithm. (i) Select initial values $(\mu^{(0)}, \tau^{(0)})$. (ii) Sample $\mu^{(1)} \mid \tau^{(0)}, \boldsymbol{y}$ from its normal distribution, followed by sampling $\tau^{(1)} \mid \mu^{(1)}, \boldsymbol{y}$ from its gamma distribution. (iii) Sample $\mu^{(2)} \mid \tau^{(1)}, \boldsymbol{y}$ from its normal distribution, followed by sampling $\tau^{(2)} \mid \mu^{(2)}, \boldsymbol{y}$ from its gamma distribution. Continue sampling from the two full conditional distributions using previous iterates for conditioning until you have a sample of size M, $\{(\mu^{(i)}, \tau^{(i)}) : i = 1, \ldots, M\}$. The later samples, after what is called a "burn-in," in this sequence will be random iterates from the joint posterior. This overall procedure is called Gibbs sampling, which we discuss thoroughly in Chapter 4. Gibbs sampling is a particular type of Markov chain Monte Carlo (MCMC) sampling that facilitates modern Bayesian methods, allowing one to carry out inference with many types of complex statistical models and inferential problems, including the present illustration.

*Prediction. We discuss both independence and dependence priors, with normal and gamma priors on μ and τ in the former case, and with normal-gamma priors in the latter case. We first consider the case under the independence prior with $\mu \mid \tau \sim N(\mu_0, 1/\tau_0)$. Simplifying notation, we denote the posterior distribution given in equation (3.6) as $N(\mu_1, 1/\tau_1)$. For further simplicity, we denote the predictive distributions with respect to the prior and the posterior as follows:

$$
\begin{aligned}
p(z \mid r, \tau) &= \int_{-\infty}^{\infty} p(z \mid \tau, \mu) p(\mu \mid r, \tau) \, d\mu \\
&= \int_{-\infty}^{\infty} \frac{\tau^{1/2}}{\sqrt{2\pi}} e^{-\frac{\tau}{2}(z-\mu)^2} \frac{\tau_r^{1/2}}{\sqrt{2\pi}} e^{-\frac{\tau_r}{2}(\mu - \mu_r)^2} \, d\mu,
\end{aligned}
$$

for $r = 0, 1$, respectively; namely, $p(\mu \mid r = 0, \tau) = p(\mu \mid \tau)$, $p(z \mid r = 0, \tau) = p(z \mid \tau)$, and $p(\mu \mid r = 1, \tau) = p(\mu \mid \tau, \boldsymbol{y})$, $p(z \mid r = 1, \tau) = p(z \mid \tau, \boldsymbol{y})$. We obtain

$$p(z \mid r, \tau) \propto \int_{-\infty}^{\infty} e^{-\frac{1}{2}\{\tau(z-\mu)^2 + \tau_r(\mu-\mu_r)^2\}} \, d\mu.$$

Recognizing the exponent as the sum of two quadratics in μ, we can apply the complete-the-square technique given in equation (3.4) but with the different components. We obtain

$$
\begin{aligned}
p(z \mid r, \tau) \ & \propto \ \int_{-\infty}^{\infty} e^{-\frac{1}{2}\{(\tau+\tau_r)(\mu-\tilde{\mu}(z))^2 + \frac{\tau\tau_r}{\tau+\tau_r}(z-\mu_r)^2\}} \, d\mu \\
& \propto \ e^{-\frac{1}{2}\{\frac{\tau\tau_r}{\tau+\tau_r}(z-\mu_r)^2\}} \int_{-\infty}^{\infty} e^{-\frac{1}{2}\{(\tau+\tau_r)(\mu-\tilde{\mu}(z))^2\}} \, d\mu \\
& \propto \ e^{-\frac{1}{2}\{\frac{\tau\tau_r}{\tau+\tau_r}(z-\mu_r)^2\}},
\end{aligned}
$$

where

$$\tilde{\mu}(z) = \frac{\tau}{\tau + \tau_r} z + \frac{\tau_r}{\tau + \tau_r} \mu_r,$$

which does not involve μ. The third line follows from the second, because the integrand in the second is just the kernel of a normal density for μ in which the mean and variance are free of μ, and the variance is free of z. The constant of integration for that density is $\sqrt{2\pi}/\sqrt{(\tau + \tau_r)}$, and dividing by it makes the integral equal to 1. Thus multiplying and dividing the integrand by the constant of integration results in just the constant of integration, which is free of z, and thus we have proportionality at line three. We recognize the final form in line three as the kernel of a normal density. We have thus established that

$$Z \mid r, \tau, \boldsymbol{y} \sim N(\mu_r, \sigma^2 + \sigma_r^2),$$

since the posterior precision is

$$\frac{\tau\tau_r}{\tau + \tau_r} = \frac{1}{1/\tau + 1/\tau_r}.$$

Thus the variance, given r, is $1/\tau + 1/\tau_r = \sigma^2 + \sigma_r^2$.

We now consider the case with unknown τ. We already know that this problem is analytically intractable in terms of identifying the joint posterior under the independence prior. This is also true in the $r = 0$ case. Our solution to analytical intractability is to sample from the full conditional distributions $p(\mu \mid r, \tau)$ and $p(\tau \mid r, \mu)$, resulting in the MCMC sample $\{(\mu^{(i)}, \tau^{(i)}) : i = 1, \ldots, M\}$, where we drop the subscript r to ease the notation. For the predictive distribution, we sample $Z^i \mid r, \mu^{(i)}, \tau^{(i)} \sim N(\mu^{(i)}, 1/\tau^{(i)})$ for $i = 1, \ldots, M$. This results in a sample, $\{Z^{BI+1}, Z^{BI+2}, \ldots, Z^M\}$ (BI is burn-in), from the marginal predictive distribution $p(z)$ when $r = 0$, and from the predictive distribution with pdf $p(z \mid \boldsymbol{y})$ when $r = 1$. This sample can be used to obtain a smoothed histogram as an approximation to the actual marginal predictive or predictive densities, respectively; the median of these iterates is a numerical approximation to the median of the appropriate predictive distribution, etc.

For the *conjugate* (dependence) prior for (μ, τ), we only consider the $r = 1$ (posterior) case. By expression (3.5) with $\tau_0 = k\tau$, we have $\mu \mid \tau, \boldsymbol{y} \sim N(\tilde{\mu}, 1/[(k + n)\tau])$. Then, since $Z - \mu \mid \tau, \mu, \boldsymbol{y} \sim N(0, 1/\tau)$, we know that $Z - \mu$ is independent of μ when τ is known, and thus

$$Z \mid \tau, \boldsymbol{y} \sim (Z - \mu) + \mu \mid \tau, \boldsymbol{y} \sim N\left(\tilde{\mu}, \frac{1}{\tau}\left(1 + \frac{1}{k + n}\right)\right).$$

Recall that $\tau \mid \boldsymbol{y} \sim Ga(c', d')$. Then we can calculate

$$
\begin{aligned}
p(z \mid \boldsymbol{y}) &= \int p(z \mid \tau, \boldsymbol{y}) p(\tau \mid \boldsymbol{y}) d\tau \\
&\propto \int \tau^{1/2} e^{-\frac{\tau}{2}(z - \tilde{\mu})^2/[1 + 1/(k+n)]} \tau^{c'-1} e^{-\tau d'} d\tau \\
&= \int \tau^{c'+1/2-1} e^{-\tau\{d' + (z-\tilde{\mu})^2/[2(1+1/(k+n))]\}} d\tau \\
&\propto 1/\{d' + (z - \tilde{\mu})^2/[2(1 + 1/(k + n))]\}^{(2c'+1)/2} \\
&\propto \frac{1}{\left\{1 + \frac{(z-\tilde{\mu})^2/2c'}{\{1+1/(k+n)\}d'/c'}\right\}^{(2c'+1)/2}},
\end{aligned}
$$

where we have used equation (3.7) to obtain the second to last term. The result is proportional to a Student's pdf, namely,

$$Z \mid \boldsymbol{y} \sim t\left(2c', \tilde{\mu}, \left\{1 + \frac{1}{k + n}\right\}\frac{d'}{c'}\right).$$

In the special case of the reference prior referred to above, we obtain $Z \mid \boldsymbol{y} \sim t(n - 1, \bar{y}, (s')^2(1 + 1/n))$. Here again, $(s')^2 = ns^2/(n - 1)$. In either case, we can obtain a 95% prediction interval for the future Z. With the reference prior, the interval is

$$\bar{y} \pm t_{0.025} s' \sqrt{1 + 1/n},$$

which is again the standard frequentist formula for a prediction interval in this setting. As we already indicated, Bayesian and frequentist interpretations of this interval are radically different. We simply say that we are 95% sure that the future value will reside in this fixed interval.

Remark. Observe that the conjugate case does not reduce to the reference prior case for any choice of parameters for the prior. If we let $k = c = d = 0$, we get $2c' = n, d' = ns^2$, which results in a $t(n, \bar{y}, s^2(1 + 1/n))$ predictive distribution.

Example 3.3. Data Analysis. In this example, we look again at the **VetBP** data set. We make inferences about average baseline systolic blood pressure of these veterans. We assume a $N(\mu, \sigma^2)$ sampling distribution for the baseline SBPs of these men. For illustration, we consider σ^2 to be known since the posterior distribution is available analytically. If the variance in the data is unknown, inference requires computational methods that were briefly discussed just after expression (3.9) and which we fully cover in the next chapter. We will show how to carry out inference for the unknown mean and variance case after presenting those methods.

We need a prior for our uncertainty about μ, and we need to specify a value for the *known* variance. There are surveys that provide information about the distribution of blood pressures among men in the U.S. The National Center for Health Statistics (NCHS) published a report with the distribution of blood pressures among U.S. adults during the beginning of the twenty-first century [355]. From this report, we gather that the mean SBP for men older than 18 years is around 124 mm Hg, based on a sample of 10,142 men.[4] Since the age distribution among our veterans may not be the same as that in the general U.S. population in 2000, we allow for greater uncertainty about the mean specification of 124 mm Hg.

The document reports a standard error of 0.3 mm Hg for the mean SBP. This standard error leads to a 95% confidence interval for the mean SBP among U.S. men older than 18 of $(123.4, 124.6)$ mm Hg. We choose to inflate the reported standard error by a factor of 25 to characterize greater uncertainty in mean SBP. This inflation of the standard error leads to a prior standard deviation equal to 7.5 mm Hg. Thus, we could choose a prior $N(124, 56.25)$ distribution for the mean SBP. Using the notation in expression (3.5), we have $\mu_0 = 124$ mm Hg, $\tau_0 = 1/56.25 = 0.0178$ in the prior specification for the mean SBP.

We specify the *known* variance of SBP in the population to be similar to the variance in the report from the NCHS. The latter also provides percentiles for blood pressures.[5] We obtain a robust *estimate* of σ based on the interquartile range (i.e., the difference between the 25th and 75th percentiles of the normal distribution). For a normal distribution, the interquartile range is $1.34\,\sigma$. The 25th and 75th percentiles of SBPs among U.S. males aged 18 years and older are 113 and 131 mm Hg, respectively. This leads to specifying known $\sigma = 13.43$ mm Hg, or $\sigma^2 = 180.44$.[6]

For this analysis, our model is given by

$$\text{Prior:} \quad \mu \sim N(124, 56.25),$$

$$\text{Sampling distribution:} \quad Y_i \mid \mu \overset{\text{iid}}{\sim} N(\mu, 180.44).$$

Using the formulas for a normal sampling distribution with known variance and normal prior for the mean given in equation (3.6), we can immediately write out

---

[4]The sample average is adjusted for the age distribution in the U.S. in the year 2000. Such adjustment makes it easier to make comparisons across time or place if one uses the same age distribution each time. In this way, any age-associated changes will not affect the comparison, even if one population is older than the other in the comparison.

[5]As with the means, these percentiles are age adjusted, but we assume that this makes little difference.

[6]This estimate is based on a much larger sample than the current sample. But we remind the reader that we are in effect pretending that we know σ for the purpose of illustration at this stage in the book.

the posterior distribution as

$$\mu \mid y \sim N\left(\frac{(404 \times 134.5/180.44) + (124/56.25)}{(404/180.44) + (1/56.25)}, \frac{1}{(404/180.44) + (1/56.25)}\right)$$

or

$$\mu \mid y \sim N(134.41, 0.44).$$

We see that the posterior mean is close to the SBP sample mean even though we started with a prior distribution centered at 124 mm Hg.

Another researcher may think that a sample of male veterans may tend to be older than the general population of adult men who are older than 18 years. In line with this thinking, the researcher may think that the average SBP for the veterans will likely be higher than the average in the NCHS report. This researcher may specify their prior distribution for the mean SBP as follows.

There are categories for SBP with ranges that allow for diagnosing hypertension. Health authorities suggest that "normal" SBP is 120 mm Hg or below, that so-called "pre-hypertension" is SBP in the range of 120 to 139 mm Hg, and hypertensive individuals have SBP of 140 mm Hg or higher. For our population of veterans, the new researcher might take 120 mm Hg as a lower bound of a likely mean SBP values among the **VetBP** sample and 140 mm Hg as an upper bound, to allow for an expected increase in SBP with age, giving $(120, 140)$ as a prior 95% credible interval for μ based on this information. Then a reasonable prior specification would have a mean of 130 mm Hg and standard deviation equal to $10/1.96 = 5.1$ mm Hg, resulting in a $N(130, 5.1^2)$ distribution.

Again, we will use the variance of the population SBPs (i.e., 180.44) that we calculated from the NCHS report as the variance in our **VetBP** data, treating it as known. For this researcher, the prior model in the notation of equation (3.5) is $\mu_0 = 130$ mm Hg and $\tau_0 = 1/26.01 = 0.0384$ in the prior for the mean SBP in our population, or $\mu \sim N(130, 26.01)$. We obtain the posterior distribution as

$$\mu \mid y \sim N\left(\frac{(404 \times 134.5/180.44) + (130/26.01)}{(404/180.44) + (1/26.01)}, \frac{1}{(404/180.44) + (1/26.01)}\right)$$

or

$$\mu \mid y \sim N(134.42, 0.44).$$

Again, the data dominate and the posterior mean is very close to the sample mean SBP.

What if we simply plug in the sample variance from the **VetBP** sample, treating it as *known*? This is not appropriate since it is an estimate based on the data we are analyzing.[7] However, we can see how changing the data variance changes the inference. In the data, the variance is 242.24 (mm Hg)^2, which is around 134% of the value we used in the previous calculation. In other words, our data show

---

[7] Using the **VetBP** data to specify σ amounts to using the current data in specifying the prior. Recall that prior information must be independent of the current data.

greater variability (less precision) than the survey's data in the report. Will this lower precision in the data lead to greater dominance of the prior in our inference?

Using calculations with the prior $\mu \sim N(130, 242.24)$, we obtain $\mu \mid y \sim N(134.39, 0.59)$. Despite the larger variance for the data in this calculation, posterior inferences hardly change. The posterior mean is still very close to the sample mean, and the posterior standard deviations change from 0.66 to 0.77, reflecting the greater variability we assumed to be in the data. This example illustrates an important lesson that, when there is a large sample size relative to the uncertainty in the prior distribution, the data will dominate the inference. In other words, the prior distribution has less influence on the inference as the sample size increases.

3.2.3 Poisson Distributed Exchangeable Count Observations

The Poisson distribution is often suitable as a model for count data, where each observation is a non-negative integer, especially when the counts are small and can equal zero with a non-zero probability. This type of count data arises frequently in biostatistical applications. Some examples are the number of doctor visits in a year paid to individuals on a patient panel, the number of ear infections during a six-month period among children between 2 and 4 years of age, and the number of lymph nodes examined during surgery for breast cancer.

The Poisson distribution has a single parameter, the rate at which "events" occur per unit interval. The unit interval could be time, if one is counting the number of events over a specified period of time; space, if one is counting the number of occurrences of some "event" over a length; area or volume, if within such units one is counting events. We say time to be specific, and let λ be the expected number of events per unit time. Assumptions for the Poisson were given in Section 3.1.

If we have a sample of n conditionally iid Poisson variates,

$$Lik(\lambda) \propto p(y_1, \ldots, y_n \mid \lambda) = \prod_{i=1}^{n} \frac{\lambda^{y_i}}{y_i!} e^{-\lambda} \propto \lambda^{\sum_{i=1}^{n} y_i} e^{-n\lambda}.$$

The form of likelihood suggests that the gamma family will be conjugate. With $Ga(a_0, b_0)$ as the prior, we get

$$\begin{aligned} p(\lambda \mid y) &\propto \lambda^{a_0-1} e^{-b_0\lambda} e^{-n\lambda} \lambda^{\sum_{i=1}^{n} y_i} \\ &\propto \lambda^{(a_0+\sum_{i=1}^{n} y_i)-1} e^{-\lambda(b_0+n)}, \end{aligned}$$

which is the kernel of a $Ga(a_1, b_1)$ distribution with $a_1 = a_0 + n\bar{y}$, $b_1 = b_0 + n$. (Note that $n\bar{y} = \sum_{i=1}^{n} y_i$.)

The posterior mean is

$$\frac{a_0 + \sum_{i=1}^{n} y_i}{b_0 + n} = \left(\frac{b_0}{b_0 + n}\right)\left(\frac{a_0}{b_0}\right) + \left(\frac{n}{b_0 + n}\right)\bar{y},$$

which is a weighted average of the prior mean and the sample mean (again a shrinkage estimator). The sample size and b_0 play comparable roles in the weighting. The posterior mode is $(a_1 - 1)/b_1$, and the posterior variance is a_1/b_1^2. The median and a 95% PI can be obtained using R with the command `qgamma(c(0.025, 0.5, 0.975), a1, b1)`.

Example 3.4. Women with tuberculosis receive multiple diagnostic chest X-rays to monitor their disease. Radiation exposure, however, is associated with a risk of developing cancer. A group of researchers set out to assess the risk of breast cancer among women who are exposed to radiation. We use a Poisson model for the number of incident breast cancers among a cohort of women with tuberculosis.

We note that incidence involves counts of the number of cases over time at risk, whereas prevalence simply involves counts of the number of cases among a group at a particular point in time. Thus, the unit of measurement for incident breast cancers in this example is a person-year of exposure to chest X-rays, rather than the number of cases per 1,000 women at a static point in time (which would be a measure of prevalence).

The total exposure for women in this study is the sum of individual exposures, measured as years for each woman. The researchers determined that this cohort's total exposure to diagnostic X-ray imaging, denoted E, was 28,010 person-years. Let Y be the number of incident breast cancers among these women with tuberculosis who received multiple X-rays of the chest. In this study, there were $y = 41$ cases of breast cancer. Let λ denote the rate of breast cancers per 10,000 person-years of exposure to diagnostic X-rays for tuberculosis. The observed breast cancer incidence rate for these women is $41/2.801 = 14.6$ cases per 10,000 person-years. The sampling distribution is $Y \mid \lambda \sim Po(\lambda E)$.

Based on information from the general population of women, the researchers assessed an *a priori* 95% probability that the rate would be between 5 and 17 cases per 10,000 person-years of exposure. If one treats these numbers as the 0.025 and 0.975 quantiles for prior distribution for λ, a $Ga(10, 1)$ distribution provides a reasonable approximation for characterizing this prior information about λ. In particular, `qgamma(c(0.025,0.975),10,1)` = (4.8, 17.1), which was obtained by trial and error using R.

With the prior distribution $\lambda \sim Ga(10, 1)$, the prior mean is 10 cases of breast cancer per 10,000 person-years of exposure and $P(4.8 \le \lambda \le 17.1) = 0.95$. With this prior and these data, the posterior distribution for the incidence rate of breast cancers among women with tuberculosis exposed to repeated diagnostic X-ray exams is $Ga(10 + 41, 1 + 2.801)$. The posterior mean is 14.7 cases per 10,000 person-years, the median is 13.4, and the posterior 95% credible interval is $(10.0, 17.3)$ cases per 10,000 person-years.

Of considerable interest is the comparison of this rate to the background rate of breast cancer in the general population. Suppose that there was a 95% *a priori* science-based belief that the background rate was in the interval (5, 11). Then we would have considerable evidence, reflected in the statement $P(\lambda > 11 \mid data) = 0.91$, that the rate among women exposed to this kind of radiation is higher than the background rate. In a later chapter, we consider the formal statistical comparison of rates of risk when we have data for both kinds.

*Prediction. The predictive density, $p(z \mid \boldsymbol{y})$, can be obtained as

$$
\begin{aligned}
p(z \mid \boldsymbol{y}) &= \int_0^\infty p(z \mid \lambda)\, p(\lambda \mid \boldsymbol{y})\, d\lambda = \int_0^\infty \frac{\lambda^z e^{-\lambda}}{z!} \frac{b_1^{a_1} \lambda^{a_1-1} e^{-b_1 \lambda}}{\Gamma(a_1)} d\lambda \\
&= \frac{b_1^{a_1}}{z!\,\Gamma(a_1)} \int_0^\infty \lambda^{a_1+z-1} e^{-(b_1+1)\lambda}\, d\lambda = \frac{b_1^{a_1}}{z!\,\Gamma(a_1)} \frac{\Gamma(z+a_1)}{(1+b_1)^{z+a_1}} \\
&= \frac{\Gamma(z+a_1)}{z!\,\Gamma(a_1)} \left(\frac{b_1}{1+b_1}\right)^{a_1} \left(1 - \frac{b_1}{1+b_1}\right)^z, \quad z = 0, 1, \ldots.
\end{aligned}
$$

This is the pdf with support on the non-negative integers, the same as a Poisson, and is known as the negative binomial distribution. It is easy to see that if we were interested in computing the *prior* predictive distribution $p(z)$ (i.e., the marginal distribution of z, also sometimes called the marginal likelihood), the calculation would be very similar. We would replace $p(\lambda \mid \boldsymbol{y})$ by $p(\lambda)$, leading again to a negative binomial distribution with a_1 and b_1 replaced by prior parameters a_0 and b_0, respectively.

3.2.4 Exchangeable Exponentially Distributed Time-to-Event Observations

Time-to-event data are commonplace in medical applications. Examples include time to death after bone marrow transplantation, time to recurrence after an initial treatment for breast cancer, and time to complete recovery after knee replacement surgery. Such data are also known as *survival-time data*, and statistical methodology in this context is called *survival analysis*. Historically, these methods first addressed time to death after treatment for some life-threatening conditions. While such studies abound, the techniques are more widely used to analyze the times to any event from a well-defined moment such as a surgical treatment.

A simple model for exchangeable time-to-event data is the exponential distribution. While this distribution is limited in flexibility for practical applications, it gives us a good starting point from which to build. This is a one-parameter distribution. Let $T \mid \lambda \sim Exp(\lambda)$, where $E(T \mid \lambda) = 1/\lambda$. This expectation has time units (e.g., hours, days, months). Suppose that we planned to observe a sequence of times until events for a series of patients. Denote the potential list of times to event as $T_1, T_2, \ldots$, with $T_j \mid \lambda \overset{iid}{\sim} Exp(\lambda)$ random variables. For example, these could be times until a patient is able to walk independently after undergoing hip replacement surgery, with T_1 the time until the first patient can walk independently, T_2 the time until the second patient can walk independently, etc.

Using the notation for the exponential distribution in the table of distributions in Appendix B, we write the likelihood as

$$
Lik(\lambda) \propto p(t_1, \ldots, t_n \mid \lambda) = \prod_{i=1}^n \lambda e^{-\lambda t_i} \propto \lambda^n e^{-\lambda \sum_{i=1}^n t_i}.
$$

This form clearly suggests that the gamma family will be conjugate. With $\lambda \sim$

$Ga(a_0, b_0)$, we have

$$p(\lambda \mid \boldsymbol{t}) \propto \lambda^{a_0-1} e^{-b_0 \lambda} \lambda^n e^{-\lambda \sum_{i=1}^n t_i}$$
$$\propto \lambda^{a_0+n-1} e^{-\lambda(b_0+\sum_{i=1}^n t_i)},$$

which is the kernel of a $Ga(a_1, b_1)$ distribution with $a_1 = a_0 + n$ and $b_1 = b_0 + n\bar{t}$, where $\bar{t}$ is the sample average of the follow-up times.

Inferential interest in time-to-event analysis will generally center on the median time and the survivor function, namely the probability of surviving (i.e., not experiencing the event) at least t years after diagnosis for various choices of t. The median survival time is obtained by solving

$$P(T > m \mid \lambda) = e^{-\lambda m} = 0.5 \quad \Leftrightarrow \quad m = \frac{\ln(2)}{\lambda}.$$

The survivor function is

$$S(t \mid \lambda) = e^{-\lambda t}.$$

While we could easily obtain formulas for $E(\lambda \mid \boldsymbol{t})$ and $E(e^{-\lambda t} \mid \boldsymbol{t})$, we can more easily find the median and a 95% PI for these quantities. First, we get the median and a 95% interval for λ using the command `qgamma(c(0.5, 0.025, 0.975),a1,b1)` in R. Then we simply transform these values, since all parameters of interest are monotone functions of λ.

For example, let $(\tilde{m}, l, u)$ be the posterior median and posterior lower and upper limits for λ. Let $\gamma = e^{-\lambda t}$ for a fixed value of t of interest. Then since

$$0.5 = P(\lambda > \tilde{m} \mid \boldsymbol{t}) = P(e^{-\lambda t} < e^{-\lambda \tilde{m}} \mid \boldsymbol{t}),$$

we must have the result that $e^{-\tilde{m}t}$ is the posterior median of γ. We similarly obtain the 95% interval for γ, (e^{-ut}, e^{-lt}), since the survivor function is monotone and decreasing in λ. Results are similarly obtained for the median and mean times to event.

The mean of the posterior for λ is $(a_0 + n)/(b_0 + n\bar{t})$. But we would make inferences for λ, the rate of events, using posterior quantiles as discussed above. The general topic of survival analysis is covered in Chapters 11 and 12.

Example 3.5. Leukemias are cancers that are associated with different types of blood cells. Many different types of blood cells are produced in the bone marrow, and one can classify them broadly into myeloid cells and lymphocytes. Lymphocytes are mature white cells that fight infections. Myeloid cells include white blood cells (other than lymphocytes), red blood cells, and cells that produce platelets (megakaryocytes). Whereas immature blood cells (called blasts) divide quickly to produce more mature cells that the body needs for normal functioning, leukemias are characterized by blasts continuing to divide rather than stopping to become normal healthy white blood cells. Acute myelogenous leukemia (AML) is a cancer that starts with immature myeloid cells and produces an overabundance of white blood cells. The disease progresses very quickly if left untreated, which is why it is called an "acute" leukemia.

Feigl and Zelen [107] provide data from a study of 33 patients who died of AML. The goal of the paper was to show how one might analyze the association between a baseline characteristic, such as white blood cell count (WBC) at the time of diagnosis, and time to death. In addition to WBC, the data also include a variable called POS, for positive. This is a variable that takes the value 1 or 0 and indicates the presence of so-called Auer rods or of leukemia cells having significant granulature (POS = 1). We will analyze the survival times of the 17 patients whose bone marrow at diagnosis had POS = 1. Analyses later in the book will account for the effect of WBC and POS on survival.

As we have seen, a gamma prior distribution is mathematically convenient for the rate parameter, λ, of the $Exp(\lambda)$ sampling distribution. We adopt a $Ga(a, b)$ prior.

Let T_i be the time (weeks) until death for the ith patient ($i = 1, \ldots, 17$). Since these patients have acute leukemias, a reasonable *a priori* estimate of the median time until death for similar patients, $\ln(2)/\lambda = 0.69/\lambda$, could be 6 months or 26 weeks. Since the survival times in these data are in weeks, the rate parameter λ is in units *deaths per week*. A reasonable prior estimate for λ is $\lambda_0 = 0.69/26 = 0.027$ deaths per week.

If we are 90% certain that the median time to death is somewhere between 3 months (approximately 13 weeks) and 18 months (around 78 weeks), we can find a $Ga(a, b)$ distribution that reasonably matches our prior uncertainty. We note that

$$0.9 = P(l < 0.69/\lambda < u) = P(0.69/u < \lambda < 0.69/l),$$

since the median time to death is a monotone and decreasing function of λ. Thus setting $l = 13, u = 78$, we obtain the prior 90% probability interval $(0.0089, 0.053)$ for λ.

Using a little trial and error in R looking for an a and b that result in gamma distribution quantiles that match these, we obtain the *a priori* median of 0.027 and a 90% PI of $(0.0089, 0.0521)$,[8] which gives numbers very close to the ones specified above. We thus take a $Ga(3.3, 110)$ prior for λ. Using this prior, and converting from rates of death per week back to median times to death, we get a prior median of 25.5 and a 90% PI for median time to death of $(11.3, 77.8)$,[9] which is quite close to our original specification on this scale.

The sum of the survival times among the 17 AG patients equals 1,062 weeks. Since we assume *a priori* that $\lambda \sim Ga(3.3, 110)$, we immediately determine that the posterior distribution for λ is $Ga(20.3, 1172)$. The posterior mean is $20.3/1172 = 0.0173$ deaths per week.

Using R again, we obtain the posterior median and a 95% interval for λ, namely, 0.0170 and $(0.0106, 0.0256)$.[10] So we have

$$0.95 = P(0.0106 < \lambda < 0.0256 \mid t) = P(26.9 < 0.69/\lambda < 65 \mid t).$$

---

[8] qgamma(c(0.05,0.5,0.95),3.3,110) = (0.0089, 0.0270, 0.0521)
[9] 0.69/qgamma(c(0.05,0.5,0.95),3.3,110) = (77.8, 25.5, 11.3)
[10] qgamma(c(0.025,0.5,0.975),20.3,1172) = (0.0106, 0.0170, 0.0256)

We are *a posteriori* 95% certain that the median time to death is between 26.9 and 65 weeks, or equivalently, between 0.52 and 1.25 years. The posterior median rate of deaths per week is 0.0170, so the posterior mean and median are virtually identical. While the median time to death can be obtained as $0.69/0.0170 = 40.6$,[11] it is not possible to obtain the posterior mean time to death using this output since the mean of $1/\lambda$ is not equal to 1 over the mean of λ. We could, however, easily approximate $E(1/\lambda \mid data)$ by a simple simulation from $Ga(20.3, 1172)$. For example, the R command `mean(1/rgamma(1000,20.3,1172))` resulted in $E(1/\lambda \mid data) \approx 61.4$. For the median time to death, $0.69/\lambda$, we get $E(0.69/\lambda \mid data) = 40.5$ and posterior 95% interval $(26.9, 65.0)$.[12]

In a similar fashion, we obtain inferences for the two-year survival rate, $e^{-104\lambda}$, using R functions `rgamma()`, `mean()`, and `quantile()` as $E(e^{-104\lambda} \mid data) = 0.17$ and $P(0.07 < e^{-104\lambda} < 0.33 \mid data) = 0.95$. So we are 95% certain that between 7% and 33% of individuals in this population will survive at least 2 years.

Since the natural purely data-based estimate of λ is $17/1062 = 0.016$, and our Bayesian estimate is 0.017, and since our prior estimate was 0.027, we see that even with just 17 patients, the data dominate the estimate over the prior distribution.

*Motivation for Exponential Distribution: Relationship to the Poisson.
Let $N(t)$ to be the number of "events" that have occurred by time $t > 0$ under the conditions described in Section 3.1 for the Poisson distribution to hold for count data.

Let T_i denote the time between the $(i-1)$th and ith events in this event generating process. For the sake of being concrete, suppose that the event of interest is a seizure in a patient with brain cancer and we are measuring the time between successive seizures. Then T_i is the time between the $(i-1)$th and ith seizures, and $N(t)$ is the number of seizures by time t. We have $N(t) = 0$ if $T_1 > t$, and $N(t) = 1$ if $T_1 \leq t$ and $T_1 + T_2 > t$. Generalizing, $N(t) = i$ if $\sum_{j=1}^{i} T_j \leq t$ and $\sum_{j=1}^{i+1} T_j > t$, for $i = 1, 2, \ldots$. Then

$$N(t) \mid \lambda \sim Po(\lambda t)$$

so that $E(N(t)) = \lambda t$, and if we let $t = 1$ unit of time, it follows that $E(N(1)) = \lambda$. The units for λ are "events per unit time," and the units for $1/\lambda$ are "time per event." Note that if the Poisson assumption holds, then

$$S(t \mid \lambda) = P(T_1 > t \mid \lambda) = P(N(t) = 0 \mid \lambda) = e^{-\lambda t},$$

since the only way that a wait time for an event can be longer than t is if no events occur before time t. The pdf of T_1 is the derivative of this expression for the cdf and is

$$p(t \mid \lambda) = \lambda e^{-\lambda t} I_{(0,\infty)}(t).$$

The collection $\{N(t) : t > 0\}$ is called a Poisson process with rate λ, and the result implied here is that the waiting times, T_i, between events in a Poisson

---

[11] There is rounding error here since we rounded all quantiles to four decimal places
[12] `0.69/qgamma(c(0.025,0.5,0.975),20.3,1172)` = (65.0, 40.5, 26.9)

process are iid $Exp(\lambda)$ conditional on λ. The reverse implication is also true: in an infinite sequence of waiting times with $T_i \overset{iid}{\sim} Exp(\lambda)$, if $N(t)$ is the count of event occurrences up to time t, $\{N(t) : t > 0\}$ is a Poisson process with rate λ (Ross, 2014 [275]).

*Prediction. A future observation, Z, can be predicted using $p(z \mid t)$, where

$$
\begin{aligned}
p(z \mid \boldsymbol{t}) &= \int_0^\infty p(z \mid \lambda)\, p(\lambda \mid \boldsymbol{t})\, d\lambda = \int_0^\infty \lambda e^{-\lambda z}\, \frac{b_1^{a_1}}{\Gamma(a_1)}\, \lambda^{a_1-1} e^{-b_1 \lambda}\, d\lambda \\
&= \frac{b_1^{a_1}}{\Gamma(a_1)} \int_0^\infty \lambda^{1+a_1-1} e^{-(z+b_1)\lambda}\, d\lambda = \frac{b_1^{a_1}}{\Gamma(a_1)} \frac{\Gamma(1+a_1)}{(z+b_1)^{1+a_1}} \\
&= \frac{a_1}{b_1} \left(1 + \frac{z}{b_1}\right)^{-(a_1+1)}, \quad z > 0,
\end{aligned}
$$

which is the pdf of a Pareto distribution of the second kind.

Perhaps of greater interest is the predictive survival distribution

$$
p(Z > z \mid \boldsymbol{t}) = \int_0^\infty p(Z > z \mid \lambda) p(\lambda \mid \boldsymbol{t}) d\lambda = \int_0^\infty e^{-\lambda z} p(\lambda \mid \boldsymbol{t}) d\lambda
$$

where we assume, as usual, conditional independence of future data and past data given λ. Then

$$
\begin{aligned}
p(Z > z \mid \boldsymbol{t}) &= \frac{b_1^{a_r 1}}{\Gamma(a_1)} \int_0^\infty \lambda^{a_1-1} e^{-\lambda(z+b_1)} d\lambda \\
&= \frac{b_1^{a_1}}{\Gamma(a_1)} \frac{\Gamma(a_1)}{(b_1+z)^{a_1}} \\
&= \left(1 + \frac{z}{b_1}\right)^{-a_1}, \quad z > 0.
\end{aligned}
$$

We note again that the prior predictive calculation would be very similar, replacing $p(z \mid t)$ and $p(\lambda \mid t)$ by $p(z)$ and $p(\lambda)$, respectively. The result is again a Pareto of the second kind with (a_1, b_1) replaced by prior parameters (a_0, b_0).

3.3 *More Flexible Models

All of the models considered in the previous section are termed *parametric*, and except for the Bernoulli, they have some restrictions. The normal distribution, for example, is unimodal and symmetric, and the exponential pdf has a mode of 0 and is monotone and decreasing; both models are very restrictive for many types of data arising in practice. The Poisson model is restricted in the sense that the mean and the variance are the same. In this section we briefly consider a broad class of distributions for data with few restrictions. In other words, we discuss a flexible class of models that is often termed *nonparametric*. But "nonparametric" is actually a historical misnomer, since more flexible models are actually "richly parametric," meaning that they have many more parameters than traditional parametric models.

3.3.1   Mixture Distributions

To gain more flexibility, mixing distributions to generate other distributions is a fairly straightforward and highly useful idea. Consider two densities, $f_1(\cdot)$ and $f_2(\cdot)$, with a common domain where the densities are strictly greater than zero. Then $pf_1(\cdot) + (1-p)f_2(\cdot)$ is also a density on this domain for $0 \leq p \leq 1$. While mixtures can be made from any two densities on a common domain, it is useful to choose the components of the mixture from a parametric family. The normal family is particularly fruitful in this regard. Figure 3.3 shows some mixture densities made with two or three components. The thickest line represents the mixture density and all other lines the components. It is clear that much flexibility in the shape of the density is gained by mixing just a few normals. In general, we can make a finite

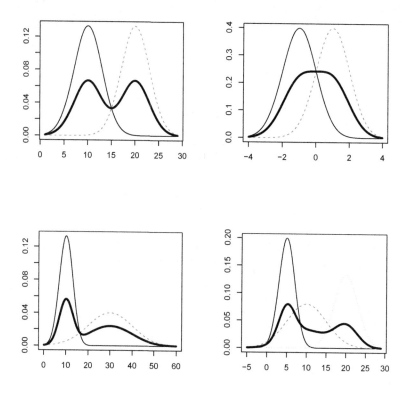

FIGURE 3.3: Some mixtures of normal densities.

mixture of m parametric pdfs and write

$$p(y \mid p_1, \ldots, p_m, \theta_1, \ldots, \theta_m) = \sum_{i=1}^{m} p_i \, p(y \mid \theta_i).$$

We would need to place prior distributions on the θ_i and the p_i. Since the p_i must sum to 1, a natural choice would be an m-dimensional Dirichlet distribution $D_m(\alpha_1, \ldots, \alpha_m)$ (see Appendix B); in the $m = 2$ case, the Dirichlet is simply a beta distribution, $Be(\alpha_1, \alpha_2)$.

A possible choice for the prior on the θ_i might be $\theta_i \stackrel{iid}{\sim} G$ for a fixed known distribution G that is defined on Θ. There are many possible choices. The idea here is to convey the sense of flexibility that is possible when making a mixture of parametric distributions.

If we pick a common $\alpha > 0$, and select the $D_m(\alpha/m, \alpha/m, \ldots, \alpha/m)$ distribution for the vector of weights, and if we consider an indefinitely large m, we obtain an amazing result: the induced prior distribution on the unknown G is approximately distributed as a Dirichlet process [108]. The next subsection describes some details of such a fruitful way of specifying mixtures to gain great flexibility.

3.3.2 Dirichlet Process Mixtures

As before for parametric models, consider a family of distributions, $p_\theta(\cdot)$, indexed by a parameter θ. As an example, we can think of the normal family $N(\mu, \sigma^2)$ indexed by the two-dimensional parameter $\theta = (\mu, \sigma^2)$. We now model successive observations as

$$y_i | \theta_i \stackrel{iid}{\sim} p_{\theta_i}(y_i), \quad i = 1, 2, \ldots,$$
$$\theta_i | G \stackrel{iid}{\sim} G(\cdot), \quad i = 1, 2, \ldots,$$

where G is unknown and needs a prior. This specification of G, or its prior, will determine how flexible the mixture density will be. One particular choice for G has proved to be very useful in practice. It is called the *Dirichlet process* (DP) [108]. It generates θs from a *random distribution* G on Θ (the space of possible values of θs).

We now give a heuristic and constructive description of the DP. Begin with a single fixed distribution G_0 on Θ and a scalar variability or concentration parameter $\alpha > 0$. G_0 is called the "base" distribution. We need two more ingredients to proceed. Let

$$\theta_1, \theta_2, \ldots \mid G_0 \stackrel{iid}{\sim} G_0 \quad \text{and} \quad V_1, V_2, \ldots \mid \alpha \stackrel{iid}{\sim} Be(1, \alpha).$$

Both are sequences of iid random variables, and these two sequences are independent of each other. The first sequence is a sample of θs from the base distribution, and the second is a sequence of random variates that will be used to construct the weights, $p_1, p_2, \ldots$. Consider any event A in Θ. The DP generates a random distribution G, and we start by thinking about the random probability of the event A, $G(A)$. We can describe the distribution of $G(A)$ by writing

$$G(A) \stackrel{d}{=} \sum_{k=1}^{\infty} p_k \, \delta_{\theta_k}(A),$$

where $\stackrel{d}{=}$ means "equal in distribution," and $\delta_\theta(A)$ is an indicator function that equals 1 if $\theta \in A$ and 0 otherwise. The weights in this expression are given by

$$p_1 = V_1, p_2 = V_2(1 - V_1), \ldots, p_k = (1 - V_1)(1 - V_2) \cdots (1 - V_{k-1})V_k, \ldots.$$

Since the V_k and θ_k are independent of each other, the p_k are independent of the θ_k, leading to

$$E(p_k \delta_{\theta_k}(A)) = E(p_k)E(\delta_{\theta_k}(A)) = E(p_k)E(I_A(\theta_k)) = E(p_k)G_0(A)$$

for all k. We argue below that $\sum_k p_k = 1$, so that

$$E(G(A)) = G_0(A)E\left\{\sum_{k=1}^{\infty} p_k\right\} = G_0(A)$$

since the expected value of a sum is the sum of expected values when these expectations are finite.

While it is not easy to show, it is true that

$$G(A) \sim Be(\alpha G_0(A), \alpha G_0(A^c)),$$

which obeys $E(G(A)) = G_0(A)$. In addition, $\text{Var}(G(A)) = G_0(A)(1 - G_0(A))/(\alpha + 1)$. We say that the random G is "centered" on the fixed distribution G_0 and that $G \sim \text{DP}(\alpha, G_0)$. Observe that the magnitude of α determines how concentrated the random G is about G_0. If α is very large, then G will be very close to G_0.

The expression above is called the Sethuraman "stick-breaking" representation of the DP [291]. It is a randomly weighted average of random point masses. The random weights (p_i) are obtained by randomly breaking a stick (of original length 1) and its successive remnants after keeping one piece of each successive break. Specifically, V_1 is the first break of the $(0, 1)$ stick, and $1 - V_1$ is length of the first remnant. We keep the V_1 piece, call it p_1, and break the remnant of length $1 - V_1$ in two, according to the proportion V_2. We keep the new piece of length $V_2(1 - V_1)$, call it p_2, and break the remaining piece, which has length $(1 - V_2)(1 - V_1)$. We continue in this fashion, keeping one piece and breaking the remaining piece, so that at the ith break we have pieces of length $\{V_1, V_2(1 - V_1), V_3(1 - V_2)(1 - V_1), \ldots, V_i \prod_{j=1}^{i-1}(1 - V_j)\}$. The elements of this sequence are $\{p_1, p_2, \ldots, p_i\}$. After the ith break, the remnant has length $\prod_{j=1}^{i}(1 - V_j)$. It is not surprising that by breaking off enough sticks, the p_j will sum to 1.

We thus have a model for datum Y that has random pdf

$$p(y \mid \alpha, G) = \sum_{i=1}^{\infty} p_i p(y \mid \theta_i), \tag{3.10}$$

which is an infinite mixture of randomly weighted parametric densities that have parameters that are randomly selected from a random G centered on G_0. This model for the observable Y is called a *Dirichlet process mixture* (DPM) model.

In general, mixtures of densities have great flexibility. Finite mixtures are often used to achieve that flexibility, but it is necessary to select the number of terms in the mixture. It turns out that in practice we will have to truncate the above sum to be finite, but that this particular choice of mixture model allows the data to decide how many terms in the mixture will matter. Alternatively, we can use the approximation by Ishwaran and Zarepour [174] that was mentioned above.

The full model for a sample of n exchangeable Y_i is

$$Y_i \mid \theta_i \overset{\text{ind}}{\sim} p(\cdot \mid \theta_i), \quad \theta_i \mid G \overset{\text{iid}}{\sim} G, \quad G \sim \mathrm{DP}(\alpha, G_0).$$

Inference and prediction for such models can be carried out by computational methods, mainly relying on sampling any unknowns of interest conditioned on the data. There are many additional uses of the DP and the DPM; this one has been presented to give the basic ideas involved.

3.3.3 Computation via DPpackage

Computation for many nonparametric models is now available from several evolving resources distributed by academic researchers. One such resource is the R package named DPpackage [176, 175] originated and maintained by Alejandro Jara with contributions by several other authors. For time-to-event data, the package named DPWeibull [294] is useful.

Example 3.6. Let us return to the leukemia data in Example 3.5. We modeled the data with an exponential distribution there. Using the 17 observations available, we constructed a 95% posterior probability interval for the median from 26.9 weeks to 65 weeks. The posterior mean survival probabilities and pointwise 95% intervals for these are shown in Figure 3.4a. Using the flexible models of this section, we obtain the corresponding plot shown in Figure 3.4b. We can see that the shape of the curves in (a) is dictated by the exponential model, whereas the shape in (b) is more responsive to the local variation in the data points. Notice that there are appreciable differences early on the time axis. Also, a 95% posterior probability interval for the median now is 38.8 weeks to 80.8 weeks. The exponential model is too restrictive and unsuitable for data of this type. We postpone until a later chapter the details of how such computations can be carried out.

3.4 Recap and Readings

This chapter and the previous chapter have introduced the essential concepts and mathematical tools needed for Bayesian analysis in biostatistics. Probability models

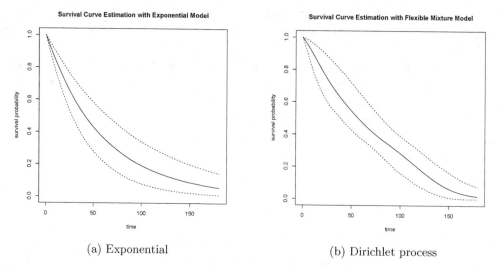

(a) Exponential   (b) Dirichlet process

FIGURE 3.4: Survival function estimation with leukemia data, based (a) on the exponential distribution, (b) on the Dirichlet process.

for data, knowledge distributions for unknowns, conditional probability, and Bayes' theorem are central to Bayesian thinking. Bayesian theory and methods in general are introduced and discussed in many other excellent textbooks, including those by Carlin and Louis [63], Gelman et al. [133], Christensen et al. [79], Robert [271], and Hoff [166]. Most of these books also address, to varying degrees, two topics that we do not cover here. These are: why we might choose Bayesian analysis over more traditional (or frequentist) methods, and a comparison of Bayesian and other approaches. Robert's book most directly addresses the first and emphasizes a decision-theoretic approach. More advanced readings in this regard would include books and monographs by Berger and Wolpert [33], Bernardo and Smith [35], Berger [29], Savage [279], Kadane [196], and a volume in honor of James Berger [70]. Most of these require a good degree of mathematical preparation.

3.5 Exercises

EXERCISE 3.1. *Conditionally iid Poisson data.* In the **LE** data for Dr. Yen's study, the variable `exam` contains the number of lymph nodes examined during breast cancer surgery for 1,307 patients. For illustration, suppose these observations arise from a conditionally iid Poisson distribution. Suppose that the mean of this variable is 7.5 for these patients. Let $\mu \sim Ga(2.58, 0.32)$ be the prior for the unknown Poisson mean μ of the population from which the 1,307 patients can be considered a random sample.

(a) Plot the posterior and prior pdf for μ on the same plot, and obtain the posterior mean, median, and a 95% probability interval for μ.

(b) Plot the predictive density for the number of nodes examined in a future randomly chosen breast cancer patient from this population, and then obtain a Monte Carlo sample from the predictive distribution by first sampling from the posterior for μ and then sampling from the conditional distribution for $Z \mid \mu$. (You might use R or some statistical package.) Use this sample to obtain a numerical approximation to the predictive mean, median, and 95% prediction interval for a future value, Z.

EXERCISE 3.2. *Conditionally iid normal data.* In the **VetBP** data set, consider the 404 baseline systolic blood pressure (variable SBP_00) observations to arise from the normal model. The data show a mean of 134.5 and a variance of 242.2.

(a) For illustration only, consider that the population variance is known to be 242.2. Use a normal prior for the population mean, $\mu \sim N(130, 100)$, and with $\bar{y} = 134.5$, plot the posterior and prior distributions of μ on a common set of axes, and obtain the posterior mean and median, and a 95% posterior probability interval for μ.

(b) Plot the predictive density for the systolic blood pressure of a future randomly chosen veteran from this population, and obtain a random sample from the predictive distribution for a future Z to obtain a numerical approximation to the predictive mean, median, and 95% prediction interval.

EXERCISE 3.3. *Conditionally iid normal data.* In the **VetBP** data set, consider again the 404 baseline systolic blood pressure (variable SBP_00) observations to arise from the normal model. Assume that the population mean is known to be 134.5. Assume the prior $\tau \sim Ga(4, 1000)$, and that $\sum_{i=1}^{404}(y_i - \mu)^2 = 403 \times 242.2$ is observed.

(a) Plot the posterior and prior pdfs for τ on a common set of axes, and obtain the posterior mean, mode, and a 95% probability interval for τ.

(b) Plot the posterior and prior distributions of σ on a common set of axes. You will need to transform to $\sigma = 1/\sqrt{(\tau)}$ to obtain the precise pdfs for σ.

(c) Plot the predictive distribution for the systolic blood pressure of a future randomly chosen veteran from this population by first sampling from the posterior for τ and then sampling from the sampling distribution for $Z \mid \tau$, to obtain a sample from the predictive distribution. Use that sample to obtain a numerical approximation to the predictive mean, median, and 95% prediction interval.

*EXERCISE 3.4. Consider again the **VetBP** data set and the information from it, namely, the sample mean is 134.5 mm Hg and the sample variance is 242.2, for a sample of 404 vets. In the following, use the $NoGa(130, 1/3, 4, 1000)$ prior on (μ, τ).

(a) Plot the marginal posterior pdf for μ.

(b) Compute the posterior probability that μ is between 132.5 and 135.5.

(c) Plot the posterior pdf for σ. Use the usual transformation technique for $\sigma = 1/\sqrt{\tau}$.

(d) Compute the posterior probability that σ is between 14.5 and 16.5.
(e) Simulate a Monte Carlo sample from the joint posterior for (μ, τ). Using that sample, obtain the approximate posterior probability that μ is between 132.5 and 135.5 and that σ is between 14.5 and 16.5. Comment on how the answer here relates to parts (b) and (d).

EXERCISE 3.5. Show that $\sum_{i=1}^{n}(y_i - \mu)^2 = n(\bar{y} - \mu^2) + \sum_{i=1}^{n}(y_i - \bar{y})^2$.

EXERCISE 3.6. Let Y_1, Y_2, Y_3 be iid $N(0, 1/\tau)$, and assume the prior specification $\tau \sim Ga(2, 2)$.

(a) Obtain and identify the precise posterior distribution for τ.
(b) Suppose the sum of the squares of the observed y_i is 10. Plot the prior and posterior pdfs on the same graph. Comment.
(c) Now plot the prior and posterior pdf for $\sigma = 1/\sqrt{\tau}$ on the same graph. Comment.

EXERCISE 3.7. Let $X \sim Ga(a, b)$.

(a) Show that the transformed random variable $cX \sim Ga(a, b/c)$ for $a, b, c > 0$.
(b) Argue that if a' is a positive integer then a $Ga(a'/2, 1/2)$ random variable is the same as a $\chi^2_{a'}$ random variable.
(c) Assume that $\theta \sim Ga(10, 20)$. Use the facts in parts (a) and (b) to derive an exact formula for a 95% probability interval for θ that uses the appropriate quantiles of the appropriate χ^2 distribution.
(d) Obtain an exact 95% interval for θ and for $\sqrt{\theta}$ (e.g., with R).

*EXERCISE 3.8. Let $Y_1, Y_2, \ldots, Y_n$ be iid $N(\mu, 1/\tau)$, and let $p(\mu, \tau) \propto 1/\tau$, which is of course an improper diffuse prior.

(a) Derive the conditional posterior for $\mu \mid \tau$.
(b) Obtain the marginal posterior for μ and identify it precisely.
(c) Using part (b), obtain a 95% probability interval formula using appropriate notation.
(d) Now obtain the marginal posterior for τ, identify its distribution, and, using results in Exercise 3.6, obtain a 95% probability interval formula for τ using the appropriate χ^2 distribution.
(e) Using part (d), obtain a probability interval formula for $\sigma = 1/\sqrt{\tau}$.

EXERCISE 3.9. Let $\theta \sim Ga(a, b)$ and $Y \mid \theta \sim Po(\theta)$. Also let $Z \mid \theta \sim Po(\theta)$, independently of Y, conditional on knowing θ.

(a) Derive the posterior pdf for $\theta \mid y$ and identify it.
(b) Obtain a simple formula for the marginal predictive probability, $P(Z = k) = \int \theta^k e^{-\theta}/k! p(\theta) d\theta$ for $k \geq 0$.
(c) Obtain the predictive probability $P(Z = k \mid y)$. Write this in a neat simple formula that can be interpreted.

EXERCISE 3.10. Let $\theta \sim Be(a,b)$ and $Y \mid \theta \sim Ber(\theta)$. Also let $Z \mid \theta \sim Ber(\theta)$, independently of Y, conditional on knowing θ.

(a) Derive the posterior pdf for $\theta \mid y$ and identify it.
(b) Obtain a simple formula for the marginal predictive probability, $P(Z = k) = \int \theta^k (1 - \theta)^{1-k} p(\theta) d\theta$ for $k = 0, 1$.
(c) Obtain the predictive probability $P(Z = k \mid y)$. Write this in a neat simple formula that can be interpreted.

EXERCISE 3.11. Let $\theta \sim Be(1,b)$ for $b > 0$. Find b such that $P(\theta \leq 0.1) = c$ for $c = 0.1, 0.2, 0.5$. Using R or some other program, find $P(X \leq c)$ for the three values of b obtained, where $X \sim Be(1,b)$.

EXERCISE 3.12.

(a) Find a $Be(a,b)$ prior that has a mean of 0.5 and a 95th percentile of 0.8. So $a/(a+b) = 0.5$ and 0.8 is 95th percentile of the $Be(a,b)$ distribution. Use trial and error.
(b) Repeat (a) but set the mode equal to 0.5. How different are the priors?
(c) Now repeat (a) but set the median equal to 0.5. How different are the priors?

EXERCISE 3.13.

(a) Find a $Ga(a,b)$ prior that has a mean of 10 and a 95th percentile of 20. So $a/b = 10$ and, in R, `qgamma(0.95,a,b)` $= 20$. Use trial and error.
(b) Repeat (a) but set the mode equal to 10. How different are the priors?
(c) Now repeat (a) but set the median equal to 10. How different are the priors?

Chapter 4

Computational Methods for Bayesian Analysis

Bayesian inference statements stem from the data-informed knowledge distribution (or posterior distribution) of the unknown quantities in the model. As introduced in Chapters 2 and 3, computing this distribution involves integration, often in a multi-dimensional space. This chapter addresses how this can be accomplished, especially in the vast majority of models where closed-form integrals are not available. Sections 4.1.1–4.3 introduce analytical, asymptotic (large-sample) and Monte Carlo sampling methods, respectively. Section 4.4 discusses the ground-breaking Gibbs sampling method and its generalization, Markov chain Monte Carlo (MCMC). Section 4.4.5 deals with the issue of whether or not the Markov chain generated samples can be considered as "random" samples from the target (posterior) distribution. Section 4.5 concludes the chapter with a recap and recommendations for further reading. Appendix C provides a brief introduction to software that makes it possible to carry out Bayesian inference in practice.

Bayesian inference statements all flow from the posterior distribution in various forms. Posterior expectations, medians and other percentiles and standard deviations of unknowns are often of interest. We now address the three main approaches to calculating such quantities.

Whenever possible, it is useful to obtain the data-informed distribution in a closed-form expression as this generally simplifies computation. For likelihoods arising from some models, one can design a prior that leads to a posterior of the same form. Such priors are termed *conjugate*, as discussed in Chapter 3. There we encountered several such cases involving normal data, binary and Poisson count data, and exponentially distributed time-to-event data. In all of the conjugate cases considered in Chapter 3, we were able to obtain closed-form analytical methods for making statistical inferences. Recall that in non-conjugate cases, we indicated that Monte Carlo methods would be needed. Here we consider two additional models where purely analytical methods are not possible.

4.1   Additional Sampling Distributions

4.1.1   Gamma Distributed Data

The gamma distribution (see the table of common distributions in Appendix B) is a generalization of the exponential as well as the chi-square distribution. It has a shape parameter α and a rate parameter λ, and is denoted by $Ga(\alpha, \lambda)$. With conditionally iid observations $(Y_1, \ldots, Y_n)$,

$$p(y_1, \ldots, y_n \mid \alpha, \lambda) \propto \prod_{i=1}^{n} \frac{\lambda^\alpha}{\Gamma(\alpha)} y_i^{\alpha-1} e^{-\lambda y_i} \propto \frac{\lambda^{n\alpha}}{\Gamma(\alpha)^n} \left\{ \prod_{i=1}^{n} y_i \right\}^{\alpha-1} e^{-\lambda \sum_{i=1}^{n} y_i}.$$

Note that, with α fixed, the last expression can be recognized as the kernel of the gamma distribution. Also note that with λ fixed, there is no recognizable kernel in α. We claim that there is no obvious conjugate prior for (α, λ), and therefore, there is no nice analytical formulation for the joint posterior. Consequently, we first specify an independence joint prior, and then consider obtaining full conditional distributions as we did in Section 3.2.2 for the normal distribution.

We thus specify $p(\alpha, \lambda) = p(\alpha)p(\lambda)$ and we take $\lambda \sim Ga(a, b)$. Then

$$
\begin{aligned}
p(\lambda \mid \alpha, \boldsymbol{y}) &\propto \left\{ \lambda^{a-1} e^{-b\lambda} \right\} \left\{ \lambda^{n\alpha} e^{-\lambda \sum_{i=1}^{n} y_i} \right\} \\
&\propto \lambda^{a+n\alpha-1} e^{-\lambda(b + \sum_{i=1}^{n} y_i)},
\end{aligned}
$$

which is the kernel of a $Ga(a + n\alpha, b + n\bar{y})$ distribution. We say that the gamma prior here is *conditionally conjugate*. The full conditional for α is

$$p(\alpha \mid \lambda, \boldsymbol{y}) \propto \frac{\lambda^{n\alpha}}{\Gamma(\alpha)^n} \left\{ \prod_{i=1}^{n} y_i \right\}^{\alpha-1} p(\alpha),$$

which is not recognizable for any known choice of $p(\alpha)$, so we do not even have conditional conjugacy in this instance. We address how to handle situations like this later in this chapter. As discussed for the normal distribution with an independence prior in Chapter 3, we will sample iteratively from these two full conditional distributions to obtain a Monte Carlo sample from the joint posterior.

4.1.2   Weibull Distributed Data

The Weibull distribution (see the table of common distributions in Appendix B) is another generalization of the exponential, often used in describing time-to-event data (see Section 3.2.4). It also has a shape parameter α and a rate parameter λ, and is denoted by $Weib(\alpha, \lambda)$. With conditionally iid observations,

$$p(y_1, \ldots, y_n \mid \alpha, \lambda) \propto \prod_{i=1}^{n} \alpha \lambda y_i^{\alpha-1} e^{-\lambda y_i^\alpha} \propto \alpha^n \lambda^n \left\{ \prod_{i=1}^{n} y_i \right\}^{\alpha-1} e^{-\lambda \sum_{i=1}^{n} y_i^\alpha}.$$

Once again with α known, multiplicative terms in α can be omitted in this sampling distribution when viewed as a likelihood function in λ. The last expression can be recognized as the kernel of a gamma distribution for λ. Thus, as in the gamma distribution case, we assume $p(\alpha, \lambda) = p(\alpha)p(\lambda)$ and we take $\lambda \sim Ga(a, b)$. We obtain

$$
\begin{aligned}
p(\lambda \mid \alpha, \boldsymbol{y}) &\propto \left\{\lambda^{a-1} e^{-b\lambda}\right\} \left\{\lambda^n e^{-\lambda \sum_{i=1}^n y_i^\alpha}\right\} \\
&\propto \lambda^{a+n-1} e^{-\lambda(b+\sum_{i=1}^n y_i^\alpha)},
\end{aligned}
$$

which is the kernel of a $Ga(a + n, b + \sum_{i=1}^n y_i^\alpha)$ distribution. So we again have conditional conjugacy. The full conditional for α is

$$
p(\alpha \mid \lambda, \boldsymbol{y}) \propto \alpha^n \left\{\prod_{i=1}^n y_i\right\}^{\alpha-1} e^{-\lambda(\sum_{i=1}^n y_i^\alpha)} p(\alpha),
$$

which again is not recognizable for any known choice of prior on α.

4.2 Asymptotics: Normal and Laplace Approximations

Historically, large-sample approximations have played an important role in statistics. Before the advent of Monte Carlo (MC) methods, and more particularly, Markov chain Monte Carlo methods (MCMC), large-sample approximations were crucial in Bayesian statistics. We present these approximations in order to give a historical perspective, and also because aspects of these approximations have continued to play an important role in some implementations of Bayesian methods—in particular, they are used in the implementation of certain MCMC procedures.

Assume that $\boldsymbol{Y} = (Y_1, Y_2, \ldots, Y_n)$ are conditionally iid with probability density $p(\cdot \mid \theta)$, where $\theta = (\theta_1, \theta_2, \ldots, \theta_p)' \in \mathbb{R}^p$. Then the joint pdf for $\boldsymbol{Y}$ is $p(\boldsymbol{y} \mid \theta) = \prod_{i=1}^n p(y_i \mid \theta)$. Assume a knowledge-based pdf for θ, $p(\theta)$. Then, as always, the posterior pdf is $p(\theta \mid \boldsymbol{y}) \propto p(\boldsymbol{y} \mid \theta)p(\theta) \propto Lik(\theta)p(\theta)$.

Normal Approximation to the Joint Posterior. In the case $p = 1$, if $p(\theta \mid \boldsymbol{y})$ is unimodal and symmetric, we might think that it could be approximated by a normal distribution with mean equal to the posterior mean, and variance equal to the posterior variance. If the sample size is large, we can consider the following approximation in the arbitrary p case.

Let $\ell(\theta) = \ln(p(\theta \mid \boldsymbol{y}))$, and let $\dot{\ell}(\theta)$ be the vector of p partial first derivatives and $\ddot{\ell}(\theta)$ be the matrix of second partials of $\ell(\theta)$, namely

$$
\dot{\ell}(\theta) = \left\{\frac{\partial}{\partial \theta_i} \ell(\theta)\right\}, \quad \ddot{\ell}(\theta) = \left\{\frac{\partial^2}{\partial \theta_i \partial \theta_j} \ell(\theta)\right\}.
$$

We are, of course, assuming all of these derivatives exist. Further, suppose the posterior mode, $\hat{\theta}$, exists and that it is not on the boundary of the parameter space. It follows that $\dot{\ell}(\hat{\theta}) = 0$, the zero vector. Then under some regularity conditions,[1] we can take a second-order Taylor series approximation of $\ell(\theta)$ as

$$\ell(\theta) \doteq \ell(\hat{\theta}) + \dot{\ell}(\hat{\theta})(\theta - \hat{\theta}) + \frac{1}{2}(\theta - \hat{\theta})'\ddot{\ell}(\hat{\theta})(\theta - \hat{\theta}).$$

Then, using the facts that $\dot{\ell}(\hat{\theta}) = 0$ and that $\ell(\hat{\theta})$ is free of the parameter vector θ, we obtain

$$p(\theta \mid \boldsymbol{y}) \,\dot{\propto}\, e^{-\frac{1}{2}(\theta-\hat{\theta})'(-\ddot{\ell}(\hat{\theta}))(\theta-\hat{\theta})}.$$

Thus the joint posterior is distributed as approximately multivariate normal in large samples, namely

$$\theta \mid y \,\dot{\sim}\, N_p\left(\hat{\theta}, (-\ddot{\ell}(\hat{\theta}))^{-1}\right),$$

with mean vector equal to the posterior mode and large-sample[2] covariance matrix $(-\ddot{\ell}(\hat{\theta}))^{-1}$.

The negative of second derivative matrix evaluated at the mode provides a measure of the curvature of the joint posterior around $\hat{\theta}$. For example, with $p = 1$, if it is "large," the posterior pdf will be highly concentrated about $\hat{\theta}$, while if it is small, the posterior will be diffuse while still centered on the mode.

Most statistical software packages have routines that will find the posterior mode vector and covariance matrix. Approximations can sometimes be improved by transforming the parameters. For example, a posterior distribution for a log odds ratio is more likely to be approximately normal than the posterior of the odds ratio itself. The log odds of a binomial proportion is more likely to have a normal posterior than the binomial proportion itself. The log mean volume of a tumor in an animal study of anticancer drugs is more likely to have a normal posterior than the mean volume itself, etc. Normal approximations will not be useful if there is skewness or multimodality in the posterior distribution.

*Laplace Approximation to a Posterior Expectation. Another large-sample approximation is based on the Laplace transform [328, 329]. Suppose we wish to approximate the posterior expected value of a positive function, $g(\theta) > 0$, namely

$$E\left[g(\theta) \mid \boldsymbol{y}\right] = \frac{\int g(\theta)Lik(\theta)p(\theta)d\theta}{\int Lik(\theta)p(\theta)d\theta}.$$

---

[1]Similar to those needed for the large-sample normal approximation of maximum likelihood estimators. See, for example, [65].

[2]This is analogous to the inverse of the Fisher observed information (FOI) matrix, which serves as the large-sample covariance matrix estimate for the maximum likelihood estimate (MLE) for θ. In fact, if we set $p(\theta)$ to be constant in θ, the posterior mode is the MLE and the large-sample covariance matrix is exactly equal to the inverse of the FOI. Thus large-sample posterior inferences will be exactly the same as large-sample MLE inferences.

The Laplace method involves rewriting this as

$$E\left[g(\theta) \mid \boldsymbol{y}\right] = \frac{\int \exp\{\ln(g(\theta)) + \ln(Lik(\theta)) + \ln(p(\theta))\}d\theta}{\int \exp\{\ln(Lik(\theta)) + \ln(p(\theta))\}d\theta}$$

$$\equiv \frac{\int \exp\{L^*(\theta)\}d\theta}{\int \exp\{L(\theta)\}d\theta}.$$

Suppose $L^*(\theta)$ and $L(\theta)$ have unique maxima, θ^* and $\hat{\theta}$, respectively. Then expand each in a second-order Taylor series expansion. We obtain

$$E\left[g(\theta) \mid \boldsymbol{y}\right] \doteq \frac{\int \exp\{L^*(\theta^*) + 0.5(\theta - \theta^*)'\ddot{L}^*(\theta^*)(\theta - \theta^*)\}d\theta}{\int \exp\{L(\hat{\theta}) + 0.5(\theta - \hat{\theta})'\ddot{L}(\hat{\theta})(\theta - \hat{\theta})\}d\theta}$$

$$= \exp\{L^*(\theta^*) - L(\hat{\theta})\}\frac{\int \exp\{-0.5(\theta - \theta^*)'(-\ddot{L}^*(\theta^*))(\theta - \theta^*)\}d\theta}{\int \exp\{-0.5(\theta - \hat{\theta})'(-\ddot{L}(\hat{\theta}))(\theta - \hat{\theta})\}d\theta}$$

$$= \exp\{L^*(\theta^*) - L(\hat{\theta})\}|\ddot{L}(\hat{\theta})|^{1/2}|\ddot{L}^*(\theta^*)|^{-1/2}.$$

The last equality follows by recognizing the integrands as kernels of multivariate normal distributions (Appendix B). The advantage of this method of approximation is that it tends to the actual posterior expectation very quickly (on the order of $1/n^2$).

4.3 Approximating Posterior Inferences using Monte Carlo Sampling

As indicated in Chapter 3, numerical approximations to posterior distributions and their characteristics may be necessary in order to obtain statistical inferences due to lack of analytical tractability. In some situations, when data sample sizes are sufficiently large, large-sample approximations like those discussed above may be useful and even desirable. However, it will usually be preferable to obtain a Monte Carlo sample from the posterior. This is certainly the case when n is small or when it is not known whether it is large enough to justify a large-sample approximation, when the dimension of the parameter vector is large and we are interested in making inferences for complicated functions of θ, and when there is a lack of analytical tractability. We will see many such examples throughout the book. As indicated in Chapter 3, an appropriate Monte Carlo sample can be used to approximate the posterior density for any $g(\theta)$ and its characteristics, such as posterior quantiles, means and standard deviations.

We proceed to discuss some useful methods of simulating samples from various distributions.

4.3.1   Random Number Generation

Simulating samples from a distribution requires random number generation. Most statistical packages provide one or more random number generators, along with several functions to simulate from common families of distributions.

Computer generated random numbers are more properly called "pseudorandom numbers." The algorithm that outputs a sequence of these is deterministic, following some fixed rules to compute the next number given the current one; yet the sequence behaves in the same way as a truly random sequence. The mathematics of these algorithms has been well developed over the past decades, along with statistical techniques to test whether an algorithm generates sequences that mimic random numbers. While most generators produce random integers, these are easily rescaled to the interval $(0, 1)$, resulting in pseudo-samples from the uniform distribution on this interval. In R, for example, the simple expression `runif(n)` produces a sequence of n such $U(0, 1)$ random numbers. Starting with such uniforms, one can generate samples from a rich variety of distributions via transformations and other methods.

For example, if $U \sim U(0, 1)$, then $W = -\ln(U) \sim Exp(1)$. Moreover, $V = W/\lambda \sim Ga(1, \lambda)$. Then we can obtain an $S \sim Ga(k, \lambda)$ variate by first simulating $(U_1, \ldots, U_k)$ as iid $U(0, 1)$, then calculating $V_i = -\ln(U_i)$ and finally calculating $S = \sum_{i=1}^{k} V_i$. We obtain a pair of independent standard normals using the Box–Muller transformation, $(Z_1, Z_2) = (\sqrt{-2\ln(U_1)}\cos(2\pi U_2), \sqrt{-2\ln(U_1)}\sin(2\pi U_2))$, where the U_i are independent $U(0, 1)$. A normal $N(\mu, \sigma^2)$ variate is obtained as $X = \mu + \sigma Z$ from a standard normal Z. We can simulate a $Ber(\theta)$ variate as $Y = I_{(0,\theta)}(U)$, and a $Bin(n, \theta)$ is simulated as the sum of n iid $Ber(\theta)$s. There are many more distributions that can be simulated along these lines. All of the standard types of well-known distributions can be simulated in most statistical programs. For example, in R the command `X = norm(100, 10, 5)` will simulate 100 $N(10, 25)$ random variates.

In the next subsections, we discuss additional methods of simulation, including distributions that are not necessarily known, meaning that they do not have a name, or their normalizing constant is not known or there is no known simple way to simulate from them directly via transformations.

4.3.2   Inverse cdf Method

This method is based on the probability integral transform $U = F(X)$, so called because the cdf, $F(x) = \int_{-\infty}^{x} p(s)ds$, is the integral of the density that yields the cumulative probability up to and including x. For a continuous cdf F, a random variable X having this cdf, when transformed to $U = F(X)$, will result in U having a $U(0, 1)$ distribution. When F has an inverse, this is easy to see:

$$P(U \leq u) = P(F(X) \leq u) = P\left(X \leq F^{-1}(u)\right)$$
$$= F\left(F^{-1}(u)\right) = u, \quad 0 < u < 1.$$

Reversing this process generates X having cdf F via $X = F^{-1}(U)$. This method works well when we have a simple analytic form for F^{-1}. For example, $X \sim Exp(\lambda)$

has cdf $1 - e^{-\lambda x}$. Setting this to u and solving for x yields $x = -\ln\{(1-u)\}/\lambda$. In R, we can generate n $Exp(\lambda)$ variates as `-log(runif(n))/lambda`, since $U \sim U(0,1)$ if and only if $1 - U \sim U(0,1)$. R also provides the function `rexp()` directly for this purpose.

4.3.3 Importance Sampling

The situation considered here involves the need to sample from a distribution, say $p(\cdot)$, that is intractable, but where it is possible to find a "mimicking" distribution that can be sampled directly, say $g(\cdot)$, as in those cases discussed above.

Our discussion begins with an approach to computing the expectation of a function of a RV, X, say $h(X)$, where $X \sim p(\cdot)$. We assume that, in some sense, $g(\cdot)$ behaves in a similar way to $p(\cdot)$, and that we know how to sample from $g(\cdot)$. Then we note that

$$E_p\{h(X)\} = \int h(x)p(x)dx = \int h(x)\left\{\frac{p(x)}{g(x)}\right\}g(x)dx = E_g\{h(X)w(X)\},$$

where $w = f/g$ can be seen as a weight function, and the expectations are subscripted according to the distribution with respect to which the expectation is taken. Thus, if we sample $(X^{(1)}, \ldots, X^{(M)})$ with $X^{(t)} \overset{iid}{\sim} g(\cdot)$, we obtain

$$E_p\{h(X)\} \doteq \sum_{t=1}^{M} h(x^{(t)})w(X^{(t)})/M$$

for large M by the strong law of large numbers. The method works well when the weight function is stable in the sense that it does not grow wildly in the tails of p, which can occur if the tail ordinates of g are relatively much smaller than those for p. Thus the tails for g should be somewhat "fat" compared to those for p for this to work well.

The use of this technique in Bayesian statistics must be modified slightly. Let $p(\theta \mid \boldsymbol{y})$ be the posterior pdf for a parameter (vector) θ. We are interested in the posterior expectation

$$\int h(\theta)p(\theta \mid \boldsymbol{y})d\theta,$$

but the integral is intractable due to the fact that we may only know the posterior up to the constant of integration, that is, all we know is that $p(\theta \mid y) \propto Lik(\theta)p(\theta)$. Thus rewrite

$$
\begin{aligned}
\int h(\theta)p(\theta \mid y)d\theta &= \frac{\int h(\theta)Lik(\theta)p(\theta)d\theta}{\int Lik(\theta)p(\theta)d\theta} \\
&= \frac{\int h(\theta)\frac{Lik(\theta)p(\theta)}{g(\theta)}g(\theta)d\theta}{\int \frac{Lik(\theta)p(\theta)}{g(\theta)}g(\theta)d\theta} \\
&\equiv \frac{\int h(\theta)w(\theta)g(\theta)d\theta}{\int w(\theta)g(\theta)d\theta},
\end{aligned}
$$

Suppose we now have an iid sample $\{\theta^{(1)}, \ldots, \theta^{(M)}\}$ from $g(\cdot)$. Then a numerical approximation to the posterior expectation is

$$E(h(\theta) \mid \boldsymbol{y}) \;\doteq\; \frac{\sum_{t=1}^{M} h(\theta^{(t)}) w(\theta^{(t)})}{\sum_{t=1}^{M} w(\theta^{(t)})}$$

$$= \sum_{t=1}^{M} h(\theta^{(t)}) \tilde{w}(\theta^{(t)}),$$

where $\tilde{w}(\theta^{(t)}) = w(\theta^{(t)}) / \sum_{j=1}^{M} w(\theta^{(j)})$. This is again justified by the strong law of large numbers. Observe that $w(\theta)$ need only be specified up to a constant, since any constant will cancel in the calculation of $\tilde{w}(\theta)$.

Now we return to the main problem of interest, namely, obtaining a sample from the posterior, $p(\theta \mid \boldsymbol{y})$. Observe that the collection $\{(\theta^{(t)}, \tilde{w}(\theta^{(t)})) : t = 1, \ldots, M\}$ defines a discrete distribution with the sampled $\theta^{(t)}$ as discrete points with probabilities $w(\theta^{(t)})$. It is not difficult to show that this discrete distribution tends to the continuous distribution with pdf $p(\theta \mid \boldsymbol{y})$, and so it is a discrete approximation to the posterior.

The method can be taken a step further to convert samples from one density into those from another by resampling from this discrete approximation. To illustrate, suppose the posterior for scalar θ is $Ga(1.5, 0.5)$. The mean and variance of this distribution are 3 and 6, respectively. We select $g(\theta) = 0.25 e^{-0.25\theta} I(\theta > 0)$, which is an $Exp(0.25)$ pdf. We obtain samples from this exponential distribution by obtaining $\theta^{(t)} = -\ln(U^{(t)})/0.25$ for $U^{(t)} \sim U(0, 1)$, $t = 1, \ldots, M$. Then with

$$w(\theta) = \frac{\theta^{1.5-1} e^{-0.5\theta}}{e^{-0.25\theta}} = \theta^{0.5} e^{-0.25\theta},$$

we obtain the $\tilde{w}(\theta^{(t)})$. Then sample M^* values (with replacement) from the discrete approximation to the $Ga(1.5, 0.5)$ distribution to obtain $\{\tilde{\theta}^{(t)} : t = 1, \ldots, M^*\}$, where we now have $\tilde{\theta}^{(t)} \dot{\sim} Ga(1.5, 0.5)$. This method of generating samples is known as the SIR (sampling-importance resampling) algorithm.

The following short R code generates samples for this illustration and verifies that the histogram matches the true density.

```
theta <- -log(runif(10000))/0.25
weights <- theta^(0.5)*exp(-0.25*theta)
ttheta <- sample(theta,10000,replace=TRUE,prob=weights)

xx <- seq(min(ttheta),max(ttheta),length.out=200)
yy <- dgamma(xx,1.5,0.5)
breaks <- quantile(ttheta,probs=seq(0,1,0.02))
hist(ttheta,breaks=breaks,probability=TRUE)
lines(xx,yy,lty=1)
```

While this illustrates the SIR algorithm, we note that gamma random variates can be generated by other more efficient methods. For example, R provides the function `rgamma()` for this purpose.

4.3.4 Rejection Sampling

This method also substitutes an easily sampled density function to achieve sampling from a more difficult density under some conditions, this time by rejecting samples with the "correct" frequencies dictated by a ratio. To understand this method, first imagine that you are able to throw darts at a cut-out of the *target density* in such a way that you will always hit the picture and that you are equally likely to hit regions with equal areas, namely, according to a uniform distribution on the target itself. Then taking the horizontal coordinate of the dart's position results in a randomly sampled value from the target density.

Correspondingly, generating a random value, $\theta \sim p(\theta)$, followed by drawing a value, $U = u$, from the uniform distribution on $(0, p(\theta))$, results in the coordinate location (θ, u), that is equivalent to throwing a dart uniformly at the cut-out of the density. This is true since the joint pdf is just

$$p(\theta, u) = p(\theta)p(u \mid \theta) = p(\theta)\frac{1}{p(\theta)}I(u \leq p(\theta)) = 1$$

over the graph of $(\theta, p(\theta))$, which has total area 1. Of course if we could sample from $p(\cdot)$, we would not need to take this extra step of simulating the uniform variate. But the idea of sampling from the cut-out graph leads us to the following parallel argument that allows us to obtain samples from $p(\cdot)$.

The target density of interest for us is again the posterior $p(\theta \mid \boldsymbol{y})$, where, for easy visualization, we think of θ as a scalar. We often do not know the constant of integration (i.e., we know a kernel $f(\theta)$ that is proportional to $p(\theta|y)$). Let $\int_{-\infty}^{\infty} f(\theta)d\theta = c_f$, with this normalizing constant c_f typically unknown. We continue the dart throwing scenario, only now we consider the cut-out of the plot of $f(\theta)$, which does not integrate to 1. With the help of Figure 4.1 we can describe the actual algorithm as follows.

Our goal is to sample $\theta \sim p(\theta) = f(\theta)/c_f$. Suppose we can find another kernel, $g(\theta)$, such that $f(\theta) \leq g(\theta)$ for all θ and we can sample easily from $g(\theta)/c_g$, where $c_g = \int_{-\infty}^{\infty} g(\theta)d\theta$ is the normalizing constant for g, possibly also not known. Then the following algorithm generates the desired samples from the distribution with pdf $p(\theta)$:

- Step 1: Generate θ from $g(\cdot)$.

- Step 2: Generate $U \sim U(0, 1)$.

- Step 3: If $U \leq \frac{f(\theta)}{g(\theta)}$ then accept θ; else reject θ and go to Step 1.

Step 3 follows from observing that $(\theta, g(\theta))$ is a dart thrown at the function $g(\cdot)$ uniformly, and when its vertical coordinate is greater than $f(\theta)$, we discard darts landing in the sliver between $g(\cdot)$ and $f(\cdot)$. This leaves darts thrown uniformly under $f(\cdot)$. It will be seen below that, despite the fact that $f(\cdot)$ is only the kernel and not the actual pdf, the accepted value of θ is still coming from the distribution with pdf $p(\theta)$.

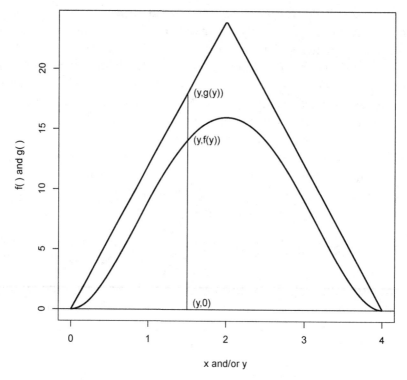

FIGURE 4.1: Illustration showing how the rejection sampling algorithm emulates a dart thrown randomly and uniformly in the area under $f(\cdot)$ by throwing such a dart under $g(\cdot)$ and keeping it if it is under $f(\cdot)$.

It is clear from Figure 4.1 that the rejected proportion of samples from $g(\cdot)$ equals the ratio of the area between the functions $g(\cdot)$ and $f(\cdot)$ (i.e., $c_g - c_f$) to that under $g(\cdot)$ (i.e., c_g). To make this area smaller, and thus to make the sample acceptance probability c_f/c_g larger, let $S = \sup_\theta \{f(\theta)/g(\theta)\} \le 1$ and set $g^*(\theta) = Sg(\theta)$. The acceptance probability is now $c_f/c_{g^*} = c_f/(Sc_g) = (c_f/c_g)/S$. This choice of g^* simply means the envelope defined by g^* is closer to f than that defined by g, and improves the sample acceptance probability by a factor of $1/S$ which is clearly greater than or equal to 1.

The proof that the accepted value is from the correct distribution follows as

$$
\begin{aligned}
P(\theta \le c \mid \text{Accept}) &= P\left(\theta \le c, U \le \frac{f(\theta)}{g(\theta)}\right) \Big/ P\left(U \le \frac{f(\theta)}{g(\theta)}\right) \\
&= \frac{\int_{-\infty}^{c} P\left(U \le \frac{f(\theta)}{g(\theta)} \mid \theta\right)(g(\theta)/c_g)d\theta}{\int_{-\infty}^{\infty} P\left(U \le \frac{f(\theta)}{g(\theta)} \mid \theta\right)(g(\theta)/c_g)d\theta} \\
&= \frac{\int_{-\infty}^{c} \frac{f(\theta)}{g(\theta)}g(\theta)d\theta}{\int_{-\infty}^{\infty} \frac{f(\theta)}{g(\theta)}g(\theta)d\theta} \qquad \{f(\theta) \text{ must be } \le g(\theta)\}
\end{aligned}
$$

$$= \frac{\int_{-\infty}^{c} f(\theta)d\theta}{\int_{-\infty}^{\infty} f(\theta)d\theta}$$

$$= \int_{-\infty}^{c} p(\theta)d\theta,$$

which is the cdf corresponding to pdf $p(\theta)$. We used the law of total probability and the property that $P(U \leq v) = v$.

Example 4.1. Truncated Normal. To generate θ from the truncated normal distribution, say $N(0,1)I_{(c,\infty)}(\theta)$ for $c \geq 1$, let

$$f(\theta) = e^{-\frac{1}{2}\theta^2} I_{(c,\infty)}(\theta).$$

Take $g(\cdot)$ to be proportional to a truncated Weibull density with shape parameter $a = 2$ and rate parameter $b = \frac{1}{2}$ (Appendix B). We have

$$g(\theta) = \theta^{a-1}e^{-b\theta^a}, \quad \theta > c.$$

Then

$$\frac{f(\theta)}{g(\theta)} = \frac{e^{-\frac{1}{2}\theta^2}}{\theta^{a-1}e^{-b\theta^a}} = \frac{1}{\theta}, \quad \theta > c.$$

Clearly this ratio is no greater than 1 since $c \geq 1$. Now $c_f = \int_c^{\infty} e^{-\frac{1}{2}\theta^2} d\theta = \sqrt{2\pi}(1 - \Phi(c))$, where Φ denotes the standard normal cdf. We also have $c_g = \int_c^{\infty} \theta e^{-\frac{1}{2}\theta^2} d\theta = \int_{c^2}^{\infty} \frac{1}{2}e^{-t}dt = e^{-\frac{1}{2}t^2}$, and $S = 1/c$ so that the sample acceptance probability (SAP) is

$$P(\text{Accept Sample}) = (c_f/c_g)/S = \sqrt{2\pi}(1 - \Phi(c))ce^{\frac{1}{2}c^2}$$

if we generate the truncated Weibull and accept it if $U \leq \frac{c}{\theta}$. Numerically, we get the following:

c	1	2	3	4	5	10	50
SAP	0.6557	0.8427	0.9138	0.9466	0.9640	0.9903	0.9996

Truncated Weibull samples can be obtained easily by the inverse cdf method. This and similar examples appear in [214].

4.3.5 Adaptive Rejection Sampling for Log-Concave Densities

Rejection sampling works well with the large class of densities in which the logarithm of the density (or kernel of the density) is a concave function. Such densities are unimodal and the second derivative of the log-density is non-positive. For such densities, we work with the kernel since the constant of integration is usually not known. A good envelope can be constructed by first finding two tangent lines to the log kernel, one on each side of the mode. Then transform the kernel and the tangent lines by exponentiating. The method is adaptive in the sense that the rejected samples can be used to construct additional tangent lines, thus creating a more efficient envelope. As just discussed, the target distribution is p with kernel f, and the envelope described here is g which can be sampled from.

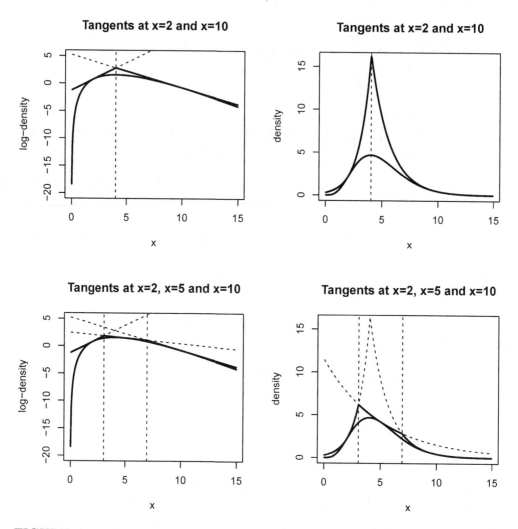

FIGURE 4.2: The top row shows the target and envelope with two initial points. The second row shows how the addition of a rejected point improves the envelope.

To illustrate, consider the target kernel $f(x) = x^4 e^{-x}$. It is easy to verify that this is a log-concave function. Working initially with tangents at two points, $x = 2$ and $x = 10$, an envelope is constructed for the log of the kernel. This is shown in the top left plot of Figure 4.2, and the corresponding envelope for the kernel itself is shown to its right. If we now pretend that sampling from the envelope generated the value 5, and this value was rejected, we can add this point to the initial two to improve the SAP. This is shown by the plots in the second row of the figure.

Log-concave kernels arise as so-called full conditional distributions for joint posteriors for many statistical models. Bayesian software packages use versions of this method widely. The tangent-based method described above requires evaluation of the derivative of the log-kernel. A derivative-free version constructs an envelope for the log-kernel using cords in place of tangents. In R the `arms` function in the package HI implements this version. We use it in Example 4.3 below. Observe that the constructed envelope gives a non-negative function that could be integrated to find the area underneath it. A "good" envelope constructed in this way would closely track, from above, the kernel of the pdf that we are attempting to sample.

4.4 Markov Chain Monte Carlo Sampling

Thus far in this chapter, we have considered how to obtain independent random samples from a distribution where the target is univariate. In most statistical models, we have more than one parameter. This means the posterior distribution is multivariate. In the case of exchangeable normal observations, we have encountered a bivariate parameter $\theta = (\mu, \tau)$. In Section 3.2.2, with both parameters unknown, we used a $N(\mu_0, \sigma_0^2)$ prior for μ, independent of a $Ga(c, d)$ prior for τ. This resulted in conditional conjugacy, that is, the full conditional for μ was normal and the full conditional for τ was gamma. The fully conjugate normal-gamma prior was also discussed in a section marked with an asterisk (*). We briefly introduced the concept of Gibbs sampling there, which involves sampling successively from these full conditional distributions to obtain, ultimately, a sample from the joint posterior.

Two other examples of unfamiliar bivariate posteriors are inherent in Sections 4.1.1 and 4.1.2 where we considered two-parameter distributions for which there is no nice form for the joint posterior, and where one full conditional is nice and the other is not. Nonetheless, Gibbs sampling is a method that will allow us to obtain samples from such analytically intractable posteriors.

To understand Gibbs sampling and other methods to be discussed in this chapter, we begin with some notation and concepts. We gave some introduction to this topic in the previous two chapters, but we give a more formal and more general treatment here. Suppose we need samples from a joint posterior distribution for a parameter vector θ with components $\theta_1, \ldots, \theta_k$. We had $k = 2$ in the three examples above. Under mild conditions, Gibbs sampling generates a sequence of iterates, $\theta^{(1)}, \theta^{(2)}, \ldots$, where eventually iterates are from the joint posterior.

Unlike the methods of Section 4.3, the sequence does not result in iid samples from the posterior distribution. In fact, the first iterate will not be from the posterior; and successive iterates in the sequence are not independent since the method of sampling uses the value of a current iterate, say $\theta^{(t)}$, to generate the next iterate, $\theta^{(t+1)}$, for every t. Such a stochastic sequence is termed a Markov chain. Gibbs sampling uses the realization of a particular type of Markov chain to achieve its goal.

A Markov chain is defined on a state space, in our case the parameter space Θ for θ. In the normal data example, this is a half-plane defined by $\mu \in (-\infty, \infty)$, $\tau \in (0, \infty)$. For the gamma and Weibull data examples, the state space is the first quadrant of the coordinate plane, as the parameter components are both positive in each case. To construct a Markov chain, we must specify what is termed in the stochastic process literature as a *transition kernel*. It is just a conditional density that governs how to sample the next iterate given the current iterate, which we represent as $r(\theta^{(t+1)} \mid \theta^{(t)})$. Our goal is to sample from the posterior distribution for θ, which we simply write here as $p(\theta)$. The joint posterior is used to obtain the transition kernel in a variety of different ways in general, but for Gibbs sampling it is obtained in a very particular way involving the full conditional distributions of the joint posterior. We formally define this in Section 4.4.1.

Markov Chain Concepts. The theory of Markov chains contains results about the distribution of $\theta^{(t)}$ as t grows indefinitely. In brief, under some conditions, the distribution of $\theta^{(t)}$ converges to the joint posterior as t grows, regardless of where the chain was initiated. The main condition is that the transition kernel satisfies

$$p(\theta) = \int_\Theta r(\theta \mid \theta^*) p(\theta^*) d\theta^*. \tag{4.1}$$

When $r(\cdot \mid \cdot)$ satisfies this condition, it is called a *stationary transition kernel*. This is a necessary condition for the iterates to ultimately be sampled from the joint posterior. Transition distributions satisfying (4.1) are called "stationary transition kernels of the chain," and the target distribution, p, is called the "stationary distribution of the chain." There can be more than one such r that satisfies this condition, which means that there can be different chains, generated by different rs, that lead to samples from the same target $p(\cdot)$.

If we generate the first iterate in the sequence by sampling, say $\theta^0 \sim p(\theta)$, then it is easy to show using the law of total probability that $\theta^{(1)} \sim p(\theta)$, and then by induction that $\theta^{(t)} \sim p(\theta)$. This is precisely what it means for p to be the stationary distribution.

There is a rather large practical issue associated with this fact, namely, that we are looking for a method of sampling from p when we do not already know how to do it. Thus, since we cannot sample the initial iterate from the target distribution, the result is practically useless, though it does give us some hope that if we start with some initial we might eventually obtain a sample from p and that subsequent samples will be from p.

In practice, we select some reasonable initial iterate, $\theta^{(0)}$, possibly by sampling from the prior distribution or possibly by just selecting values that seem reasonable in view of any scientific interpretations or knowledge about θ. Then indeed, under mild conditions on the kernel and stationary distribution, there is Markov chain theory that asserts that we will eventually sample from the target posterior distribution. In other words, for a sufficiently large number, BI, if $t \geq BI$ then $\theta^{(t)} \overset{.}{\sim} p(\theta)$; BI is termed the "burn-in." Moreover, it also asserts that for any integrable function $g(\cdot)$,

$$\sum_{t=1}^{M} g(\theta^{(t)})/M \to \int_{\Theta} g(\theta)p(\theta)d\theta$$

as $M \to \infty$, meaning that the Markov chain Monte Carlo average above will become arbitrarily close to the posterior mean of $g(\theta)$ (almost surely) as M grows. This is called an "ergodic" theorem. It is analogous to the strong law of large numbers, which is identical to this one if the iterates are obtained as an iid sequence.

The major implication of this result is that MCMC iterates can be treated almost the same as MC iterates that might be obtained by other means. There are two issues here that are different. We will need to study what is called the convergence aspect of the chain, which amounts to selecting a suitable value for BI. The second issue is that the total number of MCMC samples after the burn-in, $M - BI$, may need to be larger than for other methods, due to the correlation between iterates that is implied by the Markov property of the chain.

Markov chain theory applies to a number of situations that we now discuss. The Gibbs sampler employs precisely one such chain, and another type is introduced subsequently.

4.4.1   Gibbs Sampler

With this background, we describe the Gibbs sampler for vector $\{\theta_1, \ldots, \theta_k\}$:

- Select an initial value $\theta^{(0)}$.

- Denote the target distribution by $p(\theta)$ and the full conditional distributions as $p(\theta_i \mid \theta_{-i})$, where θ_{-i} is shorthand for $\theta_1, \ldots, \theta_{i-1}, \theta_{i+1}, \ldots, \theta_k$.

- Simulate $\theta_1^{(1)} \sim p(\theta_1 \mid \theta_{-1}^{(0)})$.

- Simulate $\theta_2^{(1)} \sim p(\theta_2 \mid \theta_1^{(1)}, \theta_3^{(0)}, \ldots, \theta_k^{(0)})$.

- Continue simulating from the conditional distributions $p(\theta_i|\theta_{-i})$, always using the most recently generated component iterates in the conditioning set. With the generation of the kth component, the vector $\theta^{(1)}$ is complete.

- Using this procedure, generate a sequence $\theta^{(1)}, \theta^{(2)}, \theta^{(3)}, \ldots, \theta^{(M)}$ for some sufficiently large M.

- The stationary distribution of this Markov chain on Θ is the target distribution $p(\theta)$, that is, the transition kernel implied by this procedure satisfies (4.1).

Consider the $k = 2$ case. We have

$$r(\theta^{(t+1)} \mid \theta^{(t)}) = p(\theta_2^{(t+1)} \mid \theta_1^{(t)})p(\theta_1^{(t+1)} \mid \theta_2^{(t+1)}).$$

It is not difficult to show that this satisfies equation (4.1). We illustrate the sampler with some examples.

Example 4.2. Normal Data. Consider the joint likelihood of Section 3.2.2, with independent priors on μ and τ. The full conditional distributions for this case were derived before, and given in expressions (3.5) and (3.9), respectively. We set $\mu \sim N(0, 100)$ and $\tau \sim Ga(1, 1)$. Gibbs sampling can be easily coded in R as a function and used to obtain samples from the joint posterior (after the burn-in) as follows:

```
gibbsnormal <- function(
  y=rnorm(100),           # default data
  mu0=0,                  # prior mean for mu
  tau0=0.01,              # prior precision for mu
  a0=1.0,               # shape parameter in prior for tau
  b0=1.0,               # rate parameter in prior for tau
  burnin=100,             # initial iterations to discard
  thin=1,                 # thinning factor; no thinning by default
  M=1000,                 # number of samples returned
  muinit=NULL,            # initial value for mu
  tauinit=NULL            # initial value for tau
  )
{
  if(length(muinit)==0) muinit <- mu0
  if(length(tauinit)==0) tauinit <- a0/b0
  mus <- rep(0,M);  taus <- rep(1,M)
  mu <- muinit;  tau <- tauinit
  n <- length(y);  nybar <- sum(y)
  tm <- tau0*mu0;  a1 <- a0+n/2
  for(g in (1-burnin):(M*thin)){ # begin Gibbs loop
    precision <- n*tau+tau0
    mu <- rnorm(1)/sqrt(precision) + (nybar*tau+tm)/precision
    b1 <- b0+sum((y-mu)^2)/2
    tau <- rgamma(1,shape=a1,rate=b1)
    if(g>0 & (g%%thin)==0){       # save posterior sample
      mus[g] <- mu;  taus[g] <- tau
    }
  }                               # end Gibbs loop
  return(list(mu=mus,tau=taus))
}

samples <- gibbsnormal()
summary(samples$mu)
summary(samples$tau)
summary(1/sqrt(samples$tau))     # summary of posterior sd
```

Example 4.3. Gamma Data. Returning to the likelihood of Section 4.1.1, with $\lambda \sim Ga(a, b)$ as before, and an independent prior on α, $p(\alpha)$, we can write down the joint posterior for λ, α as

$$p(\lambda, \alpha \mid \boldsymbol{y}) \propto \frac{\lambda^{n\alpha}}{\{\Gamma(\alpha)\}^n} \left\{ \prod_{i=1}^{n} y_i \right\}^{\alpha-1} e^{-\lambda \sum_{i=1}^{n} y_i} \lambda^{a-1} e^{-b\lambda} p(\alpha),$$

where, for the moment, the prior for α is unspecified. From this, we recognize the kernel of the full conditional for λ, and thus

$$\lambda \mid \alpha, \boldsymbol{y} \sim Ga(a + n\alpha, b + n\bar{y}).$$

Since there is no obvious choice for a prior on α, we will pick a clever one that allows us to sample from it, even though it is not conditionally conjugate. We later discuss how one would be able to make the prior diffuse in a way that maintains the balance between prior and data-based information. When scientific input is available, we might elicit information for the mean, α/λ, or mode, $(\alpha - 1)/\lambda$, and a quantile of the $Ga(\alpha, \lambda)$ distribution. Since this is a chapter on computation, however, we postpone that discussion.

The clever prior that leads to full conditionals that we know how to sample involves the specification of a joint distribution on α, and an "auxiliary" parameter, say ϕ, which will be specified as $p(\alpha, \phi) = p(\alpha \mid \phi)p(\phi)$. This induces a prior on α, $p(\alpha) = \int p(\alpha, \phi)d\phi$. For our particular choice, it will turn out that the full conditional for $\phi \mid \alpha, \lambda, \boldsymbol{y}$ is easy to sample and that the full conditional for $\alpha \mid \phi, \lambda, \boldsymbol{y}$ is log-concave and can thus be sampled using adaptive rejection sampling (ARS). We are thus able to obtain a sample from the joint posterior, $p(\alpha, \lambda, \phi \mid \boldsymbol{y})$, but where the samples for ϕ are superfluous to the Bayesian analysis and are thus discarded. The samples for (α, λ) are indeed from the marginal target distribution, $p(\alpha, \lambda \mid \boldsymbol{y})$, using this technique of auxiliary parameters. It turns out that this is useful in other contexts as well, as we shall see when the opportunity arises.

The particular choice of hierarchically specified prior that works here is

$$p(\alpha \mid \phi)p(\phi) \propto \left\{ \frac{1}{\phi} I_{(0,\phi)}(\alpha) \right\} \frac{I_{(c,\infty)}(\phi)}{\phi^{(d+1)}}, \quad c > 0, \, d > 0 \ .$$

Conditioned on ϕ, α is uniformly distributed on $(0, \phi)$ and the marginal of ϕ has what is known as a Pareto distribution of the first kind on the interval (c, ∞). Multiplying the likelihood by this prior, we have

$$p(\alpha, \phi \mid \lambda, \boldsymbol{y}) \propto \frac{\lambda^{n\alpha}}{\{\Gamma(\alpha)\}^n} \left\{ \prod_{i=1}^{n} y_i \right\}^{\alpha-1} \phi^{-(d+2)} I_{(0,\phi)}(\alpha) I_{(c,\infty)}(\phi).$$

Observing that the product of the two indicator functions can be written as $I_{(\max\{c,\alpha\},\infty)}(\phi)$, we can obtain the separate Gibbs conditionals

$$p(\phi \mid \alpha, \lambda, \boldsymbol{y}) \propto \phi^{-(d+2)} I_{(\max\{c,\alpha\},\infty)}(\phi),$$

$$p(\alpha \mid \phi, \lambda, \boldsymbol{y}) \propto \frac{\lambda^{n\alpha}}{\{\Gamma(\alpha)\}^n} \left\{ \prod_{i=1}^{n} y_i \right\}^{\alpha-1} I_{(0,\phi)}(\alpha) \ .$$

The first of these is a Pareto distribution, $Par(\max\{c, \alpha\}, d + 1)$. It has a simple inverse cdf, so ϕ can be generated using it. The second, although not in a simple form, is log-concave and can be sampled using ARS. The R code in the file named `GibbsGamma.R` under Chapter 2 on the book's website shows how this Gibbs sampler can be implemented.

Example 4.4. Weibull Data. For the likelihood here, we return to that in Section 4.1.2, with the prior for λ as before and an independent hierarchical uniform-Pareto prior on (α, ϕ) as in Example 4.3. This yields

$$p(\lambda, \alpha \mid \boldsymbol{y}) \propto (\lambda\alpha)^n \left\{ \prod_{i=1}^{n} y_i \right\}^{\alpha-1} e^{-\lambda \sum_{i=1}^{n} y_i^\alpha} \lambda^{a-1} e^{-b\lambda} p(\alpha) \ .$$

Again, for the Gibbs conditional for λ, we reuse our previous derivation in Section 4.1.2 with α considered known: $\lambda \mid \alpha, \boldsymbol{y} \sim Ga(a + n, b + \sum_{i=1}^{n} y_i^{\alpha})$. Derivation of the other Gibbs conditional follows in the same manner as in Example 4.3, namely

$$p(\alpha, \phi \mid \lambda, \boldsymbol{y}) \propto \alpha^n \left\{ \prod_{i=1}^{n} y_i \right\}^{\alpha-1} e^{-\lambda \sum_{i=1}^{n} y_i^{\alpha}} \phi^{-(d+2)} I_{(0,\phi)}(\alpha) I_{(c,\infty)}(\phi),$$

from which we get the separate Gibbs conditionals

$$p(\phi \mid \alpha, \lambda, \boldsymbol{y}) \propto \phi^{-(d+2)} I_{(\max\{c,\alpha\},\infty)}(\phi),$$

$$p(\alpha \mid \phi, \lambda, \boldsymbol{y}) \propto \alpha^n \left\{ \prod_{i=1}^{n} y_i \right\}^{\alpha-1} e^{-\lambda \sum_{i=1}^{n} y_i^{\alpha}} I_{(0,\phi)}(\alpha).$$

Again, the first of these is a Pareto distribution, $Par(\max\{c,\alpha\}, d+1)$. Samples of ϕ can be generated using the inverse cdf method. The second can be shown to be log-concave. The R code is similar to that in the previous example. It is in a file named GibbsWeibull.R in the same folder as the file GibbsGamma.R.

4.4.2 Metropolis–Hastings Algorithm

The Gibbs sampler in the previous section iterates through the components (or blocks of components) of a multidimensional vector to generate the successive realizations of a Markov chain. In contrast, the Metropolis–Hastings algorithm generates the next multivariate iterate in the chain directly as a whole, without needing the conditionals of the target density as in the Gibbs sampler. On the other hand, it requires another distribution called the proposal (or candidate-generating) distribution as we describe below. The chain is then constructed in such a way that its stationary distribution equals the target density. The algorithm was first developed in the physics literature as the Metropolis algorithm [242], and later generalized by Hastings [160] in the statistics literature. The Gibbs sampler turns out to be a special case of this algorithm. We present Hastings' generalization first, pointing out the simpler Metropolis case immediately after.

As before, consider a space Θ with target distribution $p(\theta)$ from which we wish to draw random samples. Suppose $q(\theta; \theta^*)$ is a family of probability densities on Θ indexed by θ^*, that is, $q(\cdot\, ; \theta^*)$ is a probability density on Θ for each θ^*. This is called the "proposal density," as it is used to generate a candidate value for the next iteration of the chain when it is currently in state θ^*. This candidate value is accepted as the next one in the chain with a specified probability. The transition kernel for this chain can be shown to satisfy the stationarity condition (4.1), which means that, eventually, samples obtained in this way will be from the target distribution, $p(\theta)$. We state the algorithm.

- With iteration index t and the chain in state $\theta^{(t)}$, generate θ from the proposal distribution $q(\cdot\, ; \theta^{(t)})$.

- Set $\theta^{(t+1)} = \theta$ with acceptance probability

$$\alpha(\theta, \theta^{(t)}) = \min\left\{1, \frac{p(\theta)q(\theta^{(t)};\theta)}{p(\theta^{(t)})q(\theta;\theta^{(t)})}\right\}. \tag{4.2}$$

Otherwise set $\theta^{(t+1)} = \theta^{(t)}$.

- Advance the iteration index to $t+1$ and go to first bullet.

The Metropolis algorithm requires $q(\cdot;\cdot)$ to be symmetric, that is, $q(\theta;\theta^{(t)}) = q(\theta^{(t)};\theta)$. This leads to the simplification

$$\alpha(\theta, \theta^{(t)}) = \min\left\{1, p(\theta)/p(\theta^{(t)})\right\}. \tag{4.3}$$

In either case, notice that the chain either stays in place or moves to a new value. If the ratio in the definition of acceptance probability is greater than or equal to 1, the chain moves to the generated candidate. If the ratio is less than one, we generate a $U(0,1)$ variate and accept the candidate if the random variate is less than the ratio. Also, because the ratio contains a ratio of $p(\cdot)$ at two values of θ in both numerator and denominator, it is only necessary to know this density up to a multiplicative constant (i.e., $p(\cdot)$ can be replaced by a kernel).

The Markov chain resulting from this algorithm has $p(\theta)$ as its stationary distribution under conditions that are typically satisfied if we pick $q(\cdot;\theta^*)$ to be positive everywhere that $p(\cdot)$ is positive, for each θ^*. In most applications this is easy to accomplish. One special class of $q(\cdot;\cdot)$ leads to what is termed an "independence chain." Here $q(\theta;\theta^*) \equiv q_0(\theta)$ so that the proposal density does not depend on the current state.

Another popular class uses $q(\theta;\theta^*) \equiv q_0(\theta - \theta^*)$, where now the candidate value will depend on θ^* in that the new value will be the current iterate plus or minus an increment where the increment has density $q_0(\cdot)$. This is called the "random walk chain," since it "steps" forward or backward from the current iterate at each iteration. The candidate generating distribution of the increment is often taken to be multivariate-normal or Student with location θ^*. Since these distributions are symmetric about their location vectors, we must have $q(\theta;\theta^*) = q(\theta^*;\theta)$, or equivalently $q_0(\theta) = q_0(-\theta)$. In this case the acceptance probability takes the simpler form $\alpha(\theta, \theta^{(t)}) = \min\{1, p(\theta)/p(\theta^{(t)})\}$ due to cancellation of the generating densities in numerator and denominator of the acceptance probability formula. In this instance it is easy to see that the new value is accepted with probability 1 if the candidate value is more plausible than the previous iterate, under the target posterior distribution. The greater the plausibility of the candidate relative to the previous iterate, the higher the probability of acceptance.

In practice, it is recommended that the acceptance rate for the chain should be between 0.2 and 0.5. To control this rate, it is convenient to put a tuning parameter σ_0, typically a scale, in $q_0(\theta \mid \sigma_0)$. We illustrate with a univariate and a bivariate example.

Example 4.5. Suppose we want to simulate from the $Ga(0.5, 1)$ distribution, whose density is proportional to $x^{-1/2}e^{-x}$. Let $Y = \ln(X)$ so that $p(y) \propto \exp\{y/2 - e^y\}$. We simulate Y using the random walk chain and $N(0, \sigma_0^2)$ as the density for the increment. Note that the log-gamma and the normal distributions both have the entire real line as support. The acceptance probability is a simple ratio of the density for Y at the proposed value and the density for Y at the current state. Once a value for $Y = y$ is accepted, we obtain a value for $X = x = e^y$.

In the following R code we implement the Metropolis–Hastings algorithm. Notice that the implementation uses the log of the acceptance probability, $\ln(\alpha(\cdot, \cdot))$. This is often computationally convenient.

```
MHgamma <- function(
  burnin=100,
  thin=1,
  M=1000,
  sigma=5        # tuning parameter; after trial and error
  )
{
  samples <- rep(0,M)
  reject <- 0
  current <- rnorm(1)
  for(g in (1-burnin):(M*thin)){
    candidate <- current+sigma*rnorm(1)
    if(log(runif(1))<((0.5*candidate-exp(candidate))
                     -(0.5*current-exp(current))))
      current <- candidate
    else reject <- reject+1
    if(g>0 & (g%%thin)==0) samples[g/thin] <- exp(current)
    }
  acceptprob <- 1-reject/(burnin+thin*M)
  return(list(acceptprob=acceptprob,samples=samples))
}

out <- MHgamma(sigma=5,M=1000,thin=2)
out$acceptprob
summary(out$samples)
```

The value $\sigma_0 = 5$ was arrived at by trial and error to tune the acceptance ratio to be in the desirable range. The additional code

```
x <- out$samples
par(mfrow=c(1,2))
xx <- seq(min(x),max(x),length.out=200)
yy <- dgamma(xx,0.5,1)
breaks <- quantile(x,probs=seq(0,1,0.05))
hist(x,breaks=breaks,probability=TRUE)
lines(xx,yy,lty=1)
b <- quantile(x,probs=0.75)
x <- x[x<b]
xx <- seq(min(x),b,length.out=200)
yy <- dgamma(xx,0.5,1)/pgamma(b,0.5,1)
breaks <- quantile(x,probs=seq(0,1,0.05))
hist(x,breaks=breaks,probability=TRUE)
lines(xx,yy,lty=1)
```

produces Figure 4.3 to verify that the samples come from the target density. The trimmed sample plot takes a closer look at the density agreement up to the 75th percentile in the sample.

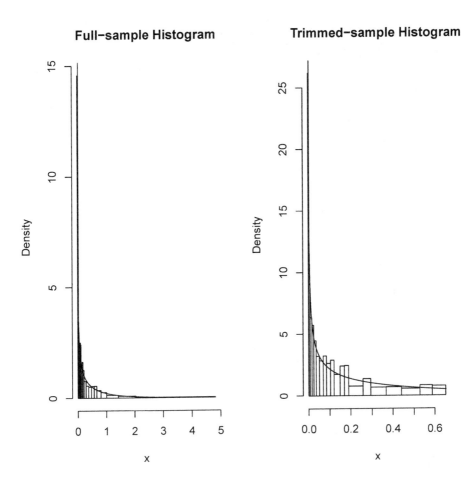

FIGURE 4.3: Histogram and gamma target density for samples using the Metropolis–Hastings algorithm.

Example 4.6. In Example 4.2 we discussed sampling (μ, τ) pairs from the joint posterior with an independence prior for parameters of the normal model using the Gibbs sampler. Here we use the Metropolis–Hastings algorithm on the bivariate pair $(\mu, \eta = \log(\tau))$ and recover $\tau = e^{\eta}$ by back transformation. We obtain

$$\ln(p(\mu, \eta \mid \boldsymbol{y})) = \text{const} + \left(a + \frac{n}{2}\right)\eta - \left\{b + \frac{1}{2}\sum_{i=1}^{n}(y_i - \mu)^2\right\}e^{\eta} - \frac{\tau_0}{2}(\mu - \mu_0)^2.$$

The R code below uses the random walk chain with independent normals for increments in (μ, η):

```
MHmutau <- function(
  y=rnorm(100),         # default data
  mu0=0,                # prior mean for mu
  tau0=0.01,            # prior precision for mu
  a0=1.0,            # shape parameter in prior for tau
  b0=1.0,            # rate parameter in prior for tau
```

```
  burnin=100,           # initial iterations to discard
  thin=1,               # thinning factor; no thinning by default
  M=1000,               # number of samples returned
  sigma1=0.2,           # tuning parameters; after trial and error
  sigma2=0.2
  )
{
  mus <- rep(0,M)
  taus <- rep(0,M)
  reject <- 0
  currmu <- rnorm(1)
  curreta <- rnorm(1)
  a <- a0+length(y)/2
  b <- tau0/2
  for(g in (1-burnin):(M*thin)){
    candmu <- currmu+sigma1*rnorm(1)
    candeta <- curreta+sigma2*rnorm(1)
    if(log(runif(1))<
        ((a*candeta-exp(candeta)*(b0+sum((y-candmu)^2)/2)
          -b*(candmu-mu0)^2)
        -(a*curreta-exp(curreta)*(b0+sum((y-currmu)^2)/2)
          -b*(currmu-mu0)^2)))
      {currmu <- candmu
        curreta <- candeta}
    else reject <- reject+1
    if(g>0 & (g%%thin)==0) {mus[g/thin] <- currmu
                            taus[g/thin] <- exp(curreta)
    }
  }
  acceptprob <- 1-reject/(burnin+thin*M)
  return(list(y=y,acceptprob=acceptprob,mu=mus,tau=taus))
}

out <- MHmutau(M=2000,thin=2,sigma1=0.2,sigma2=0.2)
out$acceptprob
summary(out$y)
summary(out$mu)
summary(out$tau)
```

4.4.3 Slice Sampling

Slice sampling uses a Markov chain to sample from a *univariate* distribution with density $p(\theta)$. Since we generally will not know the constant of integration, we work with the kernel of the posterior, $q(\theta)$. Imagine the two-dimensional graph of $q(\theta)$. Slice sampling takes a random walk through the area under the graph of $q(\theta)$, alternating steps along the two axes. To sample a slice, proceed as follows:

- Choose an arbitrary $\theta^{(0)}$ in the support of $p(\theta)$ to initialize the chain. The random walk starts at $(\theta^{(0)}, 0)$.

- Given $\theta^{(0)}$, *step up* by simulating $u^{(0)} \sim U(0, q(\theta^{(0)}))$ and move to $(\theta^{(0)}, u^{(0)})$. Then continue as follows.

- (i) With a *unimodal* $q(\theta)$, and starting with $(\theta^{(t)}, u^{(t)})$, step along the θ-axis by finding the two points $\theta_{t1} < \theta_{t2}$ that satisfy $u^{(t)} = q(\theta_{t1}) = q(\theta_{t2})$ and then simulate $\theta^{(t+1)} \sim U(\theta_{t1}, \theta_{t2})$. Move to $(\theta^{(t+1)}, u^{(t)})$. (ii) For *non-unimodal* densities, find $\{\theta : q(\theta) \geq u^{(t)}\}$ and sample from a uniform distribution on that set. The main difficulty in slice sampling is finding this set when $q(\theta)$ is not unimodal.

- Simulate $u^{(t+1)} \sim U(0, q(\theta^{(t+1)}))$ and move to $(\theta^{(t+1)}, u^{(t+1)})$.

The random walk used for slice sampling is a special case of Gibbs sampling, since we alternate between sampling $U \mid \theta = \theta^* \sim U(0, q(\theta^*))$ and $\theta \mid U = u \sim$ uniform on the set $(\theta' : q(\theta') \geq u)$.

4.4.4 Hamiltonian Markov Chain Monte Carlo Sampling

This section discusses a very important and useful special case of the Metropolis et al. [242] algorithm for simulating blocks of random variables. This approach does not require the modification of Hastings [160], so it is in fact simpler. It uses Hamiltonian dynamics from physics to generate new candidate iterates that will either be accepted or rejected according to the Metropolis acceptance probability in equation (4.3). In Section 4.4.2, a "candidate generating distribution" was used to simulate a new candidate. We next explain how first, in theory, candidates can be conceptualized deterministically using Hamiltonian dynamics, and then implemented in practice by an approximation.

4.4.4.1 Overview

First, the Hamiltonian MCMC method expands the parameter space of the parameters in the model, much like the method of auxiliary variables first introduced in Example 4.5. This leads to more efficient exploration of both parameter spaces. It is especially helpful in high-dimensional spaces, which are notoriously difficult to handle with methods presented up to now. These auxiliary variates are discarded after each full iteration of the procedure, since their only purpose is in facilitating the computational aspects of Bayesian inferences. In this expanded space, Hamiltonian dynamics is used to "generate" a deterministic candidate for the next iteration.

Next, upon realizing the impracticality of actually implementing this generation, we discuss an approximation that combines deterministic theory and random simulation of candidates. It has been argued that this method, if properly optimized, can be much more efficient than the usual random-walk Metropolis–Hastings method of generating MCMC samples from the target distribution.

The main reason for the development of this method is that it has the potential to be much faster and more efficient in exploring the support of posterior and/or predictive distributions. The method was first introduced by Duane et al. [99], who called it "hybrid Monte Carlo." More recently, Neal [248] provided a substantial review of this method with many illustrations and advice for implementation. Betancourt [42] has also given a lengthy introduction to the topic and has presented numerous graphical representations of the geometry involved in connecting the physics to the statistical problem of obtaining high-quality proposals with high acceptance probability in the Metropolis procedure. Both authors give arguments for why the target distribution is indeed the stationary distribution of the chain and address technical details for the implementation of the procedure. Other references of interest are Shahbaba et al. [292], Hoffman and Gelman [167], and Nishimura and Dunson [250]. Here, we give a brief summary of the procedure and refer readers to these works for a much broader and more detailed perspective on the topic.

The method proposes states that are distant from the current state, but which still have a high probability of acceptance. These proposals are found by using Hamiltonian dynamics, much used in physics and astronomy. Since we do not expect most readers to be familiar with the physics, we instead describe the method as a very clever way of making proposals for acceptance or rejection in the Metropolis algorithm. While the procedure is more general, we focus directly on obtaining Hamiltonian proposals that will be used in the Metropolis algorithm.

4.4.4.2 Expanding the Parameter Space

Suppose we have a statistical model with parameter $\theta \in \Omega$, with prior $p(\theta)$ and data generating distribution $p(y \mid \theta)$, resulting in the posterior $p(\theta \mid y)$. There may be covariates and the data components may be conditionally independent or not. The model may be nonlinear in the parameters. The goal is to obtain posterior samples of θ. Let the dimension of θ be r, which is allowed to be large.

Next define the *auxiliary* random variables $\delta \sim N_r(0, D)$ with $D = \text{diag}\{d_i : i = 1, \ldots, r\}$, and we assume that δ is independent of (θ, y), which implies that δ is independent of θ given y. Thus we can define the joint pdf

$$p(\theta, \delta \mid y) = p(\theta \mid y)p(\delta). \tag{4.4}$$

By auxiliary, we mean that these variates, δ, have nothing to do with the model for the data or the prior information about it. They are constructed as a clever device that will facilitate good proposals that can be used to obtain iterates from the target distribution, $p(\theta \mid y)$. The way this is done is to regard the joint distribution in equation (4.4) as the target distribution. Once we have samples from it, we simply disregard the iterates for r-dimensional δ, and use the iterates for θ to make inferences. In fact, the iterates for δ are removed after each full iteration of the algorithm; there is no need to waste space storing them.

4.4.4.3 Basics of Hamiltonian Dynamics

For this setup, the Hamiltonian function is defined as $p(\theta, \delta \mid y) \propto \exp\{-H(\theta, \delta)\}$, where

$$\begin{aligned} H(\theta, \delta) &= -\log(p(\theta, \delta \mid y)) \\ &= -\log(p(\theta \mid y)) - \log(p(\delta)) \\ &\equiv U(\theta) + K(\delta). \end{aligned} \tag{4.5}$$

In physics, the function $U(\theta)$ is called the potential energy that corresponds to the "position," θ, and the function $K(\delta)$ is called the kinetic energy, which is determined by the "momenta," δ. Momentum would have physical meaning in a real physical problem, but here it is used as a device, so we do not discuss its meaning. The Hamiltonian function H is termed the total energy.

These terms are very much related to the mechanics of physical systems that involve objects or particles moving in space, water or on surfaces. Different choices for U and K correspond to different physical systems. Here, we are focused on sampling from the support of the distribution $p(\theta \mid y)$.

The range of the mapping $\theta \to U(\theta)$ defines a space. For a log-concave posterior with $\dim(\theta) = 2$, $U(\theta)$ looks like a bowl, perhaps somewhat irregular in shape but still having a smooth surface, due to its convexity, sitting on top of a table or floor that corresponds to the support of the posterior. The bottom of the bowl corresponds to values in the support that have highest posterior density. There are contours of the bowl that correspond to level sets in the support, namely, $\{\theta \in \mathbb{R}^2 : p(\theta \mid y) = c\} = \{\theta \in \mathbb{R}^2 : U(\theta) = -\log(c)\}$. Our goal is to "explore" the entire space by iterating through values for θ that will be accepted by the Metropolis procedure.

Here is where the magic comes in. In order to explore this space, an expanded space, called *phase space*, is considered. The expanded space is the support of the mapping $(\theta, \delta) \to H(\theta, \delta)$. This is a mapping from $\mathbb{R}^{2r}$, the $2r$-fold Cartesian product of the real line, $\mathbb{R}$. Note that the parameter space Ω is a subset of this space. The mapping that actually defines how we would obtain candidate iterates is determined by a set of differential equations, called Hamilton's equations.

The mechanics of physical systems involves the evolution of particles or masses in space, here (θ, δ), and time, t. So far there has been no mention of time; this would be obvious to physicists in the context of a real physical mechanistic system. Here, time is fictitious. But we insert it into the problem in order to use the Hamiltonian physics. The Hamilton equations are

$$
\begin{aligned}
\frac{d\theta(t)}{dt} &= \frac{\partial H(\theta(t), \delta(t))}{\partial \delta} = \frac{\partial K(\delta(t))}{\partial \delta} = D^{-1}\delta(t), \\
\frac{d\delta(t)}{dt} &= -\frac{\partial H(\theta(t), \delta(t))}{\partial \theta} = -\frac{\partial U(\theta(t))}{\partial \theta} = \dot{\ell}(\theta(t)),
\end{aligned}
\tag{4.6}
$$

where $\dot{\ell}(\theta) = \partial \log(p(\theta \mid y))/\partial \theta$. Note that we have taken the Hamiltonian that did not depend on t and forced it to depend on t. Derivatives are with respect to the fictitious t, which implies that the solution to these equations is a deterministic process in t.

The solution of Hamilton's equations of motion will yield a trajectory in terms of positions, $\theta(t)$, and momenta, $\delta(t)$, as functions of time, say $T_t\{(\theta(t), \delta(t))\} : t > 0$, which is only implicitly defined. There are three major properties of the system that correspond to these equations:

- $H(\theta(t), \delta(t)) = H(\theta(t+s), \delta(t+s))$ for all $t, s \geq 0$. This follows since $\frac{dH}{dt} = 0$, which holds by using the chain rule and equations (4.6). This is termed conservation of energy, since the total energy is conserved by the Hamiltonian along its path. This then implies that the joint pdf, $p(\theta, \delta \mid y)$, is constant along this path as well. In other words, the level sets of the target density are the same as the level sets of the Hamiltonian.

- Consider a region, E, of the phase space that is the support of $p(\theta, \delta \mid y)$. Then consider the transformation of that region to the set, say E', by the mapping $T_s : (\theta(t), \delta(t)) \to (\theta(t+s), \delta(t+s))$, which was determined by Hamilton's equations. Then the volume of E is the same as the volume of E'. This is termed conservation of volume in Hamiltonian dynamics.

- The mapping $T_s : (\theta(t), \delta(t)) \to (\theta(t+s), \delta(t+s))$ is one-to-one. This implies that Hamiltonian dynamics are reversible. What does reversibility mean? Since the transformation T_s is one-to-one, it has an inverse, which is termed T_{-s}. Reversibility in this context means that this process can be run in reverse time and that it will maintain the same properties as the original.

We are now in a position to generate candidates that can be tested for acceptance using the Metropolis sampler. We observe from the first bullet, however, that no matter what increment of time, s, is selected, $p(\theta(t), \delta(t) \mid y) = p(\theta(t+s), \delta(t+s) \mid y)$, and so the Metropolis acceptance probability will always be 1. This sounds like a really nice feature provided that, as argued in Neal [248] and in Betancourt [42], the value would behave as if it were a random iterate from the target distribution. But this is only a single iterate. We could continue obtaining values for $s = 1, 2, \ldots$, up to some finite number, but we would only be sampling values from the level set corresponding to whatever initial values we used for (θ, δ).

In order to sufficiently explore the phase space, we would need to construct an appropriate mechanism for moving from one level set to another. Moreover, we have assumed that we could solve Hamilton's equations analytically, which would rarely be the case. So it is time to discuss the approximation that we mentioned above.

4.4.4.4 Approximation to Generate Candidate

While Neal [248] gives a simple example in which an analytical solution to equations (4.6) is easily obtained, such analytic solutions are not possible in general. So why have we spent this much effort to end up at an apparent dead end? A lesson for everyone is that exact solutions are often not possible, but good, useful approximate solutions often are. This is indeed the case here. For the approximation to work well, it must satisfy the properties discussed above, and the approximation can obviously be better understood by knowing what it is approximating.

We now switch to more familiar notation for MC iterates. The goal is to obtain $\{(\theta^{(t)}, \delta^{(t)}) : t = 0, 1, \ldots, M\}$, starting with an initial value and obtaining M iterates from a Metropolis Markov chain with target distribution $p(\theta, \delta \mid y)$. We regard the current iterate as $(\theta^{(t)}, \delta^{(t)})$, and the goal is to describe how we obtain the next iterate, $(\theta^{(t+1)}, \delta^{(t+1)})$, using an approximate Hamiltonian technique.

The approximation has two phases for obtaining a new iterate given the current iterate. The first phase randomly selects a new vector for δ, say $\delta^* \sim N_r(0, D)$, and replaces the current iterate with $(\theta^{(t)}, \delta^*)$. The reason for doing this is that, as discussed earlier, the exact Hamiltonian dynamics resulted in the next iterate being restricted to the same level set as the current iterate. By randomly selecting δ^* and replacing $\delta^{(t)}$ with it, this problem is avoided. The question arises as to whether modifying the current iterate in this way will affect the stationarity of iterates, that is, can they still be regarded as having come from the target distribution?

Since δ is independent of θ given y at every iteration, sampling $\delta^* \sim N_r(0, D)$ can be regarded as sampling from the conditional distribution of $\delta \mid \theta, y$. Then since $p(\theta, \delta \mid y) = p(\theta \mid y)p(\delta \mid \theta, y)$ is the target distribution at every iteration of the Metropolis sampler, and since the current value $\theta^{(t)}$ can be regarded as having come from the marginal for $\theta \mid y$, the new pair $(\theta^{(t)}, \delta^*)$ can also be regarded as coming from the stationary distribution (of course, after some burn-in). We now relabel $(\theta^{(t)}, \delta^*) = (\theta^{(t)}, \delta^{(t)})$ for the sake of notation, recognizing that what used to be $\delta^{(t)}$ was replaced by the new vector δ^* that has now been relabeled as $\delta^{(t)}$.

The second phase involves approximating Hamilton's equations by considering discrete time and by incrementally using some small step size ϵ, repeatedly L times, in order to obtain a candidate for $(\theta^{(t+1)}, \delta^{(t+1)})$. For dealing with Hamiltonian mechanics, we revert temporarily to the notation $(\theta(t), \delta(t))$, which for fixed t equals $(\theta^{(t)}, \delta^{(t)})$, and where we consider time that is local to that value and can be considered in steps of size ϵ. The method is termed *leapfrog*. It consists of iterating the steps

$$
\begin{aligned}
\delta(t + \epsilon/2) &= \delta(t) - (\epsilon/2)\frac{dU}{d\theta}(\theta(t)), \\
\theta(t + \epsilon) &= \theta(t) + \epsilon\frac{dK}{d\delta}(\delta(t + \epsilon/2)), \\
\delta(t + \epsilon) &= \delta(t + \epsilon/2) - (\epsilon/2)\frac{dU}{d\theta}(\theta(t + \epsilon))
\end{aligned}
\tag{4.7}
$$

L times in order to obtain one candidate in the overall Metropolis scheme. Here $dU/d\theta$ and $dK/d\delta$ are both r-dimensional vectors of partial derivatives, and we have selected $K(\delta) = 0.5\sum_{i=1}^{r} \delta_i^2/d_i$. The main reason for taking multiple steps is to *leap* to a further point in the space, resulting in less autocorrelation and ultimately exploring the space more broadly.

At the end of phase two, we ultimately obtain a single final iterate of the leapfrog procedure at local time $L\epsilon$. This iterate is taken as the new proposal for $(\theta(t + 1), \delta(t + 1))$. We label this final local iterate as (θ^*, δ^*), and either accept or reject it, with the acceptance probability

$$
\min[1, p(\theta^*, \delta^* \mid y)/p(\theta(t), \delta(t)) \mid y)].
$$

Neal [248] gives R code for implementing the leapfrog and gives illustrations of the implementation. A nice illustration is also given in Shahbaba et al. [292] in the introductory part of their paper, before they move on to discuss a potential improvement in the Hamiltonian procedure by splitting the Hamiltonian. For practical Bayesian computations, the software **Stan**, discussed and illustrated in Appendix C, makes extensive use of Hamiltonian Monte Carlo.

Remark. The initial approximation that was used to approximate the exact Hamiltonian equations (4.6) was to simply approximate each equation with a first-order Taylor series approximation to $\theta(t + \epsilon)$ and to $\delta(t + \epsilon)$, expanding each as a function of (small) ϵ for fixed t. The Hamiltonian derivatives in equation (4.6) were used to obtain the first-order derivatives in the expansions. But the approximation was poor. The leapfrog equations replaced this first attempt, and iterates obtained from using them have been found to satisfy all of the properties that were discussed for the exact approach. These features are ultimately responsible, according to Neal [248] and Betancourt [42], for approximate Hamiltonian iterates to move rapidly through the phase space, with appropriate choice of (ϵ, L).

Remark. It was mentioned that the step where δ was simulated from the $N_r(0, D)$ distribution was crucial for moving from one level set to another at each full iteration. It should also be mentioned that conservation of energy dictates that if $K(\delta)$ is larger in a new iteration, then $U(\theta)$ must be smaller so that the sum remains the same. The sum of the kinetic and potential energies is conserved.

4.4.5   Convergence Diagnostics

Most methods for assessing convergence rely on informal evaluations of individual parameters or functions of parameters. With a small number of parameters of interest, monitoring each individually is not too burdensome. On the other hand, if there are many parameters and one does not monitor all of them, one may be fooled into thinking that the process has converged based on the apparent convergence of the subset under examination.

Many convergence diagnostics are available in the R packages coda and boa. Several of the routines that are part of coda are built into OpenBUGS. Aside from providing built-in tools for assessing convergence, both of these packages also include functions to simplify the process of loading saved iterates from an MCMC program into R. The purpose of moving MCMC iterates into an analysis environment like R is to be able to manipulate the output when creating summary Bayesian inferences and/or to create pretty pictures of numerical approximations to posterior and predictive distributions.

Trace and History Plots. After we carry out an iterative method to generate samples from the posterior distribution, we will be interested in showing that the method did, in fact, converge. If the algorithm has not converged, then the generated values may not be random samples from the posterior distribution.

We first give an illustration of what a (non-Markov chain) iid Monte Carlo sample from a known bivariate distribution looks like as the sample size increases. Figure 4.4 illustrates an example in which we generated random samples from a bivariate normal distribution. Since we know how to sample bivariate normals exactly, all pairs are exact and there is no need for a burn-in. In the figure, there are separate graphs showing what happens after 5, 10, 25, and 100 iterations. Each graph shows sequential iterates for four sequences of bivariate normals, which is analogous to what we will do when we have actual MCMC iterates. This example illustrates how iterates should look in a *vanilla* setting where we can sample directly from the target distribution.

When thousands of iterates are generated from the posterior distribution, a plot such as Figure 4.4 will show a thick cluster of points piling up in the center but it will not be too helpful in terms of evaluating a trend towards convergence. There

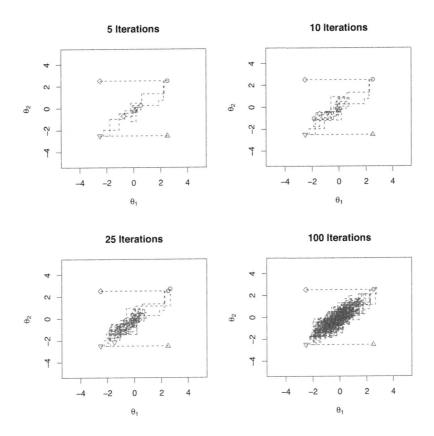

FIGURE 4.4: Paths taken by four different sequences, with different symbols indicating the initial points. Each path represents MCMC samples from the same joint posterior distribution.

are several ways we can monitor convergence. The easiest way involves plotting the history of the generated iterates for each parameter or variable, starting with the first saved value. We produce these trace or history plots by graphing the iterates as a time series, with iteration number on the X-axis and the iterate itself on the Y-axis, to show the history of the consecutively generated random samples. The trajectories should eventually look like *white noise* without a discernible trend or *hiccup*.

Starting chains at different initial values is a way to show that we have reached convergence. That is, we should run two or more parallel chains, each starting from a different initial value. If the algorithm converges, then regardless of the initial values, all of the chains will generate random samples from the same target distribution. If plotted on the same graph, the individual trace or history plots should merge together at some point and then stay together. If the chains remain separate after several thousand iterations, then there is potential for a convergence problem.

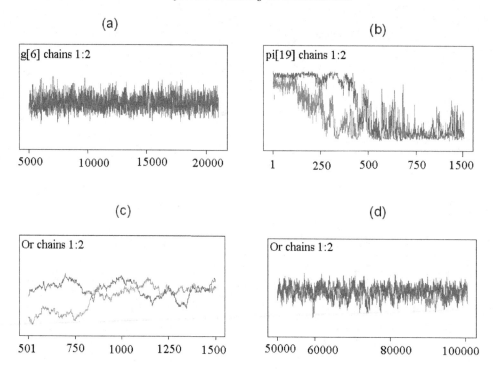

FIGURE 4.5: Four history plots each with two chains that start at different values. Plot (a) shows chains merging sometime before 5000 iterations. Plot (b) shows chains that separate and then start to merge. Plot (c) shows chains that are wildly distinct and which show high autocorrelation (see next section). Plot (d) shows chains that appear to be merging after 50,000 iterations, but where it is not quite clear if they have really merged yet.

Figure 4.5 shows four plots of histories where plots (a) and (d) are reasonably well behaved and plots (b) and (c) are not. The chains in (a) are well behaved and appear to have converged before 5,000 iterations. Plot (b) shows possible merging of chains at around 500 iterations, but we would want to see more iterations to be comfortable. The chains in (c) are wild up to 1,500 iterations and display strong autocorrelation, which is discussed next. The chains in (d) are continuations of the chains in (c) and they appear to have merged reasonably well by 50,000 iterations, but there may still be some doubt about convergence.

Quantile Plots. An additional type of plot involves plotting running estimates of the mean and the 0.025 and 0.975 quantiles of the iterates for each variable that is monitored. These are numerical approximations to the posterior mean and the values that would ultimately give 95% posterior probability intervals. The running estimates are based on iterates up to fixed numbers of iterations, as this number grows. Approximating these quantiles based on a small number of iterates is inevitably unstable, while the more iterates there are, the more stable the quantile

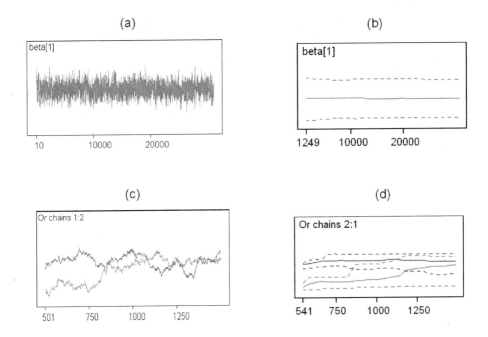

FIGURE 4.6: Two history plots of two chains that start at different values and their corresponding quantile plots. Plot (a) shows a well-behaved history plot after 10 iterations, while plot (b) shows the corresponding well-behaved quantile plot. Plot (c) shows a badly behaved history plot, while plot (d) shows the corresponding badly behaved quantile plot.

approximations should be. If there is a lack of convergence, the running quantiles should be unstable until convergence has occurred.

Figure 4.6 shows history plots for two chains and their corresponding running quantile plots. Plot (a) shows a very well-behaved chain and plot (b) shows the corresponding very well-behaved quantile plots. Plot (c) shows badly behaved histories and plot (d) shows the corresponding badly behaved quantiles.

Autocorrelation Plot. Many MCMC methods generate samples from the posterior distribution (after a burn-in period), but these samples are often autocorrelated. For example, the Metropolis–Hastings method allows the iterate (i.e., sample) at the next iteration of the sampler to remain at the same value as the current iterate. A graphical illustration of the autocorrelation as a function of the *lag* between iterates is often helpful. The sample autocorrelation for lag k in a sequence of M saved samples of θ is

$$\rho_k = \frac{\sum_{j=1}^{M-k} \left[(\theta^{(j+k)} - \bar{\theta})(\theta^{(j)} - \bar{\theta}) \right]}{\sum_{j=1}^{M} (\theta^{(j)} - \bar{\theta})^2}.$$

So with $k = 1$, ρ_1 is the Pearson correlation between running adjacent pairs of iterates. We expect the autocorrelation to decrease as the lag increases. In other words, if the chain is *mixing* well, then there should be less correlation—hopefully much less—between values 20 iterations apart than between values only one iteration apart.

Figure 4.7 shows two chains and their corresponding autocorrelations. Plot (a) shows a well-behaved chain with modest autocorrelation, shown in plot (b), which has virtually disappeared by lag 10. Plot (c) shows a reasonably well-behaved chain but with exceptionally high autocorrelation, shown in plot (d).

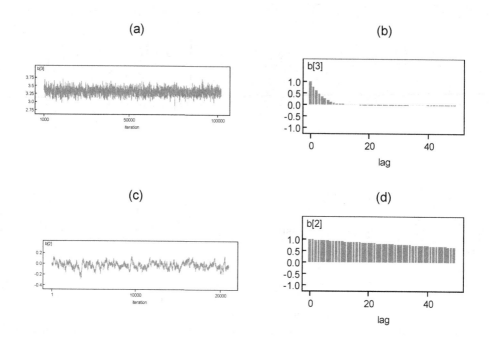

FIGURE 4.7: Plot (a) shows a history plot for a well-behaved chain, and plot (b) shows the corresponding autocorrelation plot. Plots (c) and (d) give the same plots for a chain with high autocorrelation.

A problem caused by autocorrelation in the sample is that the *effective* sample size (i.e., the *effective* number of independent samples from the posterior) is generally smaller, and sometimes much smaller, than the number of samples that are kept ($M' = M - \text{burn-in}$).

We illustrate by considering a hypothetical situation. Suppose our target distribution is the posterior for a parameter θ. Then assume that samples based on a particular MCMC approach are first-order autocorrelated. This means that the true correlation between samples k units apart is ρ^k, for $k = 1, 2, \ldots$. So the true first-order autocorrelation is just $\rho \geq 0$. Then, using time series theory, one can show that the standard error of the MC sample mean[3] of M' kept iterates for θ is

$$\sqrt{\frac{\sigma_\theta^2}{M'}\frac{1+\rho}{1-\rho}},$$

where σ_θ is the posterior standard deviation of θ. The smaller this is, the better is the numerical approximation. Note that with $\rho = 0$, the standard error follows the usual formula, $\sigma_\theta/\sqrt{M'}$.

Consider a sample mean approximation to the posterior mean based on an uncorrelated sample of size M^*. It will have standard error $\sigma_\theta/\sqrt{M^*}$. Then equate this to the above correlated sample's standard error and solve for the sample size M' that will give the same standard error as the uncorrelated sample. The solution is $M' = [(1+\rho)/(1-\rho)]M^*$. Since the multiple of M^* is greater than or equal to 1, this shows how much larger the correlated MCMC sample must be in order to achieve the same standard error as one would achieve with a sample of M^* uncorrelated samples. For example, if $\rho = 0.5$, one would need three times as large a sample. If $\rho = 0.75$, the required number increases to sevenfold.

One approach to reducing autocorrelation is to re-parameterize the model and thereby reduce the correlation among the parameters. An example of this approach is centering the covariates (Figure 4.8b) in a regression model, which will also improve mixing from Figure 4.8a.

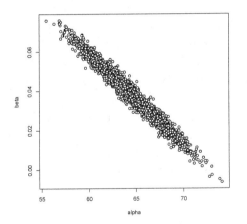

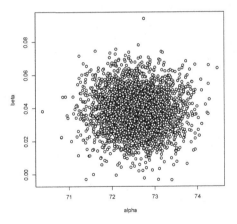

(a) Uncentered covariate in linear regression   (b) Centered covariate in linear regression

FIGURE 4.8: Centering covariates, plot (b), reduces correlation between slope and intercept and improves mixing, compared to the model without centering the covariate, plot (a).

Another way to reduce autocorrelation is by thinning. This means keeping the value generated by every rth iteration after convergence is reached. In general, then,

---

[3]Numerical approximation to the posterior mean is $\bar{\theta} = \sum_{i=1}^{M'} \theta^{(i)}/M'$.

if $z^{(l)}$ $(l = BI + 1, \ldots, M)$ is a sequence of $M' = M - BI$ values generated by an MCMC method (e.g., Metropolis–Hastings) after discarding the first BI iterations as burn-in, and if one wishes to thin by $r = 10$, then one would retain iterates $z^{(BI+1)}, z^{(BI+11)}, z^{(BI+21)}, \ldots$. One can determine a useful value of r by examining plots of the autocorrelation in the MCMC sample for different choices.

We caution the reader that thinning amounts to reducing the information in the MCMC sample, so that MC standard errors for posterior mean approximations may increase. Moreover, reducing autocorrelation does nothing to help convergence. There is an advantage, however, if iterates are to be used to subsequently make plots of posterior or predictive distributions. Huge MCMC sample sizes can make this task unpleasant, so thinning can be useful for this purpose.

Are We There Yet? Beyond plots, there are some recommended and useful statistics we can compute to judge if we have reasonably arrived at convergence. Two such are by Geweke [142] and Brooks, Gelman, and Rubin [138, 56]. There is also a method developed by Raftery and Lewis [266] that estimates how many additional samples may be needed to achieve convergence.

Geweke. If the Markov chain leading to random samples from the posterior distribution has converged, then random subsets of the realized iterates should behave like random samples from the posterior and, thus, be similar to one another. Geweke [142] proposed carrying out a modified two-sample test to compare means between subsets.

For example, one can take the first 20% of the sample iterates for θ (after a trial burn-in) and the last 50% of the sample and test for equality of the means. If each batch is a random sample from the same distribution, the resulting test statistic should not show a "significant" difference in the frequentist sense. Geweke's procedure is like the normal Z test to compare two means (provided the two sample sizes are large), except that the standard error of the difference accounts for autocorrelation in the subsets. Asymptotically, the standardized difference follows a standard normal distribution, allowing one to assess indirectly whether the sampled values follow the same distribution. Rejection of the null hypothesis that the means are the same will imply that the chain may not have converged, that is, a larger burn-in is needed. Of course if the sample sizes are *too* large, then the rejection may involve only a slight difference in the two means that would be of little or no practical import.

Brooks–Gelman–Rubin. Alternatively, as mentioned earlier, an intuitive approach to assessing convergence is to start several independent and parallel chains at different widely dispersed initial values and to see if the iterates from the separate chains manage to be distributed around the same central value and have the same amount of variability after sufficiently many iterations. The Brooks–Gelman–Rubin (BGR) method [138, 56] formalizes this notion by comparing the between-chain variation to within-chain variation.

Consider a parameter of interest, say θ, which may be a function of one or several model parameters. Suppose that J independent MCMC sequences have been sampled, each starting at a different value. Also, suppose that M' iterates remain for each chain. Let $\theta_j^{(i)}$ be iterate i from chain j, $i = 1, \ldots, M'$; $j = 1, \ldots, J$. Also let

$$\bar{\theta}_j = \sum_{i=1}^{M'} \theta_j^{(i)}/M', \quad \bar{\theta}. = \sum_{j=1}^{J} \bar{\theta}_j/J,$$

which are each numerical approximations to the posterior mean of θ, the first based on only chain j and the second based on all J chains. If all iterates are from the target distribution, both are appropriate approximations to the posterior mean, but the overall mean would be preferred since it is based on a larger MC sample size, $J \times M'$.

Throughout, we suppose that a particular *test* burn-in value has been specified and the corresponding iterates discarded for all J chains. We discuss two different approaches to the BGR method.

The simplest approach proceeds as follows. For each parameter, obtain a plot of the running ratio (as a function of M') of the width of an 80% credible interval based on pooling the chains to the average of J 80% interval widths for the J chains. Thus the numerator interval approximation is based on all of the $\{\theta_j^{(i)} : i = 1, \ldots, M'; j = 1, \ldots, J\}$ values considered as a single sample of size $J \times M'$, and the denominator interval is based on the average of the J intervals, with interval j based on $\{\theta_j^{(i)} : i = 1, \ldots, M'\}$, across $j = 1, \ldots, J$. If the chains have converged before the selected burn-in, this ratio should be close to 1, since all of the 80% intervals are valid approximations to the actual posterior 80% interval for θ. Using different test burn-in values, one finds the value where this ratio is subsequently close enough to 1. WinBUGS and OpenBUGS, in particular, provide this type of diagnostic plot.

The second approach recognizes that the structure here is like that of a balanced one-way analysis of variance (ANOVA) with J *factors* and M' observations per factor. The between-chain variation estimator is defined as

$$\text{MSB} = \frac{M'}{J-1} \sum_{j=1}^{J} \left(\bar{\theta}_{.j} - \bar{\theta}.. \right)^2 \equiv \frac{\text{SSB}}{J-1},$$

where SSB is the sum of squares *between* chains, and MSB is the between-chain mean square, by direct analogy with ANOVA. If the all samples are from the actual posterior distribution, namely if the test burn-in is large enough, then MSB is an unbiased estimate of σ_θ^2, the posterior variance of θ.

Within-chain variation is defined as

$$W = \frac{1}{J} \sum_{j=1}^{J} s_j^2, \quad s_j^2 = \frac{1}{M'-1} \sum_{i=1}^{M'} \left(\theta_j^{(i)} - \bar{\theta}_j \right)^2,$$

where s_j^2 is the usual (frequentist unbiased) estimate of the variance of the iterates from chain j. If all chains are being sampled from the posterior for θ, then W is a pooled (unbiased) estimate of the common posterior variance of θ, σ_θ^2. In fact, W is the usual pooled estimate of the common variance in an ANOVA setting, referred to as the within-chain mean square (MSW) variability. If the iterates were from normal distributions with common variance, the ratio $F \equiv \text{MSB}/\text{MSW}$ is the usual Fisher F statistic for testing that all J means are the same.

Remark. It is not difficult to show that the expected value of MSB under general assumptions is $\sum_{j=1}^{J} e'_J \Sigma_j e_J/[JM'] + M' \sum_{j=1}^{J} (\mu_j - \bar{\mu})^2$, where e_J is a column vector of J ones, Σ_j is the $M' \times M'$ variance covariance matrix of M' iterates from chain j, μ_j is the expectation of $\bar{\theta}_j$, and $\bar{\mu} = \sum_{j=1}^{J} \mu_j/J$. Let $I_{M'}$ be the M'-dimensional identity matrix. Then if $\Sigma_j = I_{M'}\sigma_j^2$ for all j, namely if the iterates for each chain were independent with distinct variances, and defining $\bar{\sigma}^2 = \sum_j \sigma_j^2/J$, we find that the simplified expected value of MSB is $\bar{\sigma}^2 + M' \sum_{j=1}^{J} (\mu_j - \bar{\mu})^2$. Finally, if the σ_j^2 are equal to σ_θ^2 and the μ_j are all equal, which they will be after convergence, we see that the expected value of MSB is indeed σ_θ^2. The case with dependent iterates (e.g., $\Sigma_j \neq I_{M'}\sigma_j^2$) is more difficult to show.

Another numerical approximation to σ_θ^2 is given by BGR as the weighted average

$$\hat{\sigma}_\theta^2 = \left(1 - \frac{1}{M'}\right) W + \frac{1}{M'}\text{MSB}.$$

If the chain has already converged and the burn-in discarded, this is an unbiased estimate of σ_θ^2. Both W and MSB will converge to σ_θ^2 as M' grows. However, before convergence, it is generally expected that the weighted average will be large and thus exceed σ_θ^2. This will certainly be the case in the beginning of the chain due to overdispersed initial values and since it is generally expected that the MCMC means for different chains will be somewhat different for the early part of the chains.

A slight modification of the BGR criterion for convergence is based on the ratio

$$\hat{R} = \frac{\hat{\sigma}_\theta^2}{W} = 1 - \frac{1}{M'} + \frac{F}{M'},$$

where $F = \text{MSB}/\text{MSW} = \text{MSB}/W$. Thus a large value for the Fisher F statistic is an indication of lack of convergence. BGR anticipate this ratio to be greater than 1 before convergence, but under the appropriate assumptions for the Markov chain to converge, it will approximate 1 as M' grows. The user would increase the test burn-in until the value of $\hat{R}$ is sufficiently close to 1 (say, no greater than 1.2) for all iterates after a selected value.

How many iterations until convergence? Raftery–Lewis method. An approach proposed by Raftery and Lewis [266] provides an estimate of the number of additional iterations one needs before one can be confident that convergence has been achieved. The method requires that one choose a tail quantile q (e.g., 2.5%, 5%, 97.5%), a level of accuracy ε, and a power for reaching this degree of accuracy for the quantile of interest. One then forms a sequence of 0s and 1s by comparing the saved samples, $\theta^{(j)}$, to the quantile q. That is, the jth element of the sequence is 1 if $\theta^{(j)} \leq q$ and 0 otherwise.

The method then involves thinning the sample, say by keeping every rth sampled value, where r is selected to be large enough that autocorrelation for the θ chain is approximately of order 1, meaning that the transition probability involving the next iterate given all previous iterates only depends on the current one. Consequently, the sequence of 0s and 1s is an approximate two-state Markov chain. Using the thinned series of 0/1 iterates, transition probabilities can be estimated. For example, the estimated (approximate) conditional probability of transitioning from state 0 (corresponding to $\theta^{(j)} > q$) to state 1 (corresponding to $\theta^{(j)} \leq q$) is just the number of times the thinned chain has a 0 followed by a 1 divided by the number of thinned iterates that equal 0.

The Raftery–Lewis method uses these estimated transition probabilities to (i) suggest the number of additional burn-in iterations required before one can be confident about convergence to stationarity, (ii) to assess the fraction of intermediate saves to discard (i.e., thinning), and (iii) to determine a value for the length of the chain (i.e., the number of saved samples) that one will need to achieve the desired degree of accuracy. The computation is based on estimating the quantile to a prespecified level of precision.

One may wish to evaluate several quantiles of the quantity of interest and then choose the largest number of iterations recommended by the procedure. Clearly, if one is interested in making inferences for several model characteristics, then one will need to evaluate this statistic for each. The number of such evaluations can become large.

To summarize, overall in practice, it is important to check sufficient burn-in and avoid long persisting autocorrelations. Then, with sufficient burn-in and moderate to low autocorrelations (after thinning if needed), one should routinely compute the Monte Carlo error for all quantities of interest while taking into account the residual correlations.

4.5   Recap and Readings

In this chapter we focused on how to accomplish calculation of quantities needed for inference. Although we began with some analytic methods, the main workhorse of Bayesian inferential computations is simulation of samples from the posterior distribution. Not only are such methods widely applicable, they are often more useful than analytic forms as they allow easy inference for functions of original parameters. The transition to sampling-based inference began in earnest with the advent of the Gibbs sampler, as described in the seminal paper by Gelfand and Smith [132]. Although the Metropolis and Metropolis–Hastings algorithms existed long before, the role of Markov chains in Monte Carlo simulations was clarified by Tierney [327], leading to much development and usage in Bayesian inference. Two accessible and well-written articles explain the Gibbs sampler and the Metropolis–Hastings algorithm. The first is by Casella and George [66], and the second is by Chib and Greenberg [73].

As we have seen, all these methods depend on simulating random variates with various specified distributions. A classic and excellent book discussing such simulation is by Devroye [95]. The adaptive rejection sampler for log-concave densities is described by Gilks and Wild [143, 354]. Development of BUGS and WinBUGS followed soon after. This enabled Bayesian data analysis for a wide range of statistical models. The evolution and direction of the BUGS project is described by Lunn et al. [232, 233], all of whose co-authors played key roles in its origination and growth.

4.6   Exercises

EXERCISE 4.1.   Let $Y \mid \theta \sim Bin(n, \theta)$. Let $p(\theta) \propto \theta^{a-1}(1 - \theta)^{b-1}$, with $a, b > 0$.

(a) Using the method discussed in Section 4.2, obtain an explicit formula for the normal approximation to the posterior for θ and identify the corresponding distribution.

(b) Now with $a = b = 1$, let observed $y/n = 0.5$. Then, for $n = 10, 20, 50$, plot the true posterior and the approximate posterior together on three separate plots. Comment on the quality of the approximation as n increases.

(c) Again with $a = b = 1$, let observed $y/n = 0.10$. Find the smallest n such that the normal approximation has 99.5% actual posterior probability that $\theta > 0$. Then compare that approximate posterior to the true one on the same graph.

EXERCISE 4.2.   Let $Y_1, \ldots, Y_n \mid \theta \sim Po(\lambda)$, independently. Let $p(\lambda) \propto \lambda^{a-1} e^{-b\lambda}$, $a, b > 0$. And let $S = \sum_i Y_i$, the sum of the Poisson random variables.

(a) Recall that $S \mid \lambda \sim Po(n\lambda)$. Show that the likelihood based on the sample of n observations, $y_1, \ldots, y_n$, is the same as the likelihood based on the observed $S = s$ provided $s = \sum_i y_i$. We say that the sum, S, is sufficient for making inferences about θ so that it is unnecessary to know the actual values of the y_i. Technically, when the likelihood factorizes in this way, the statistic S is termed Fisher sufficient, in honor of Sir Ronald Fisher.

(b) Using the method discussed in Section 4.2, obtain an explicit formula for the normal approximation to the posterior for λ and identify the corresponding distribution.

(c) With $a = b = 1$, let $s/n = 1$. Then, for observed $n = 10, 20, 50$, plot the true posterior and the approximate posterior together on three separate plots. Comment on the quality of the approximation as n increases.

(d) Again with $a = b = 1$, let observed $y/n = 0.10$. Find the smallest n such that the normal approximation has 99.5% actual posterior probability that $\lambda > 0$. Then compare that approximate posterior to the true one on the same graph.

*EXERCISE 4.3.   For the data and model described in Exercise 4.1, obtain the Laplace approximation to the posterior mean for θ. Compare the approximation to the known posterior mean for this situation.

*EXERCISE 4.4.   For the data and model described in Exercise 4.2, obtain the Laplace approximation to the posterior mean for λ. Compare the approximation to the known posterior mean for this situation.

EXERCISE 4.5   Suppose you have a black-box simulator that can give you independent $Exp(1) = Ga(1,1)$ random values. Recall that if $X \sim Ga(a,b)$, then $cX \sim Ga(a,b/c)$ for $a,b,c > 0$. Then explain how you would use those values to obtain the following RVs.

(a) $Ga(10,1)$ and $Ga(10,1/2)$.
(b) χ^2_{10}, a chi-square with 10 degrees of freedom.
(c) The Fisher $F_{(r,k)}$, an F distribution with numerator and denominator degrees of freedom r and k, respectively, for positive integers r and k.
(d) A Student's t distribution with k degrees of freedom.

EXERCISE 4.6   Let $Y \mid \alpha, \lambda \sim Weib(\alpha, \lambda)$. Recall that the cdf for Y is $F(y) = 1 - e^{-\lambda y^\alpha}$. Using the inverse cdf method for simulating variates, explain how to simulate from this distribution.

EXERCISE 4.7.   Generate samples from $Ga(0.6, 0.5)$ by using the SIR algorithm with $Ga(0.5, 0.5)$ as the initial sampling distribution. Note that $Ga(0.5, 0.5)$ is $\chi^2(1)$, which you can generate by squaring standard normal samples. Make plots as in Figure 4.3 to verify your sampling.

EXERCISE 4.8   Code the truncated normal algorithm of Example 4.1. Generate samples with $c = 2$ and $c = 10$. Empirically verify the corresponding sample acceptance probabilities given in the table of Example 4.1. Plot a sample histogram and the target density for the $c = 2$ case.

EXERCISE 4.9.   Consider the rejection sampling algorithm to generate samples from $Be(1.5, 1.5)$, which has density proportional to $f(x) = x^{0.5}(1 - x)^{0.5}I_{(0,1)}(x)$, using $g(x) = I_{(0,1)}(x)$, that is, a uniform.

(a) Specify the steps of the algorithm.
(b) Derive the sample acceptance probability.
(c) Code the algorithm. (i) Generate samples and empirically verify your answer to (b). (ii) Plot a histogram of samples and superimpose the target density on it.

EXERCISE 4.10.   Show log-concavity of $p(\alpha \mid \lambda, data)$ in the Weibull model of Section 4.1.2 where $p(\alpha)$ is taken to be log-concave.

EXERCISE 4.11.   With the exchangeable normal model for observations and independent priors $\mu \sim N(\mu_0, \tau_0)$, $\tau \sim Ga(a, b)$, show that the log of the joint posterior density is as given in Example 4.6. Recall that the $N(\mu_0, \tau_0)$ distribution has variance $1/\tau_0$.

EXERCISE 4.12.   Assume equation (4.1) holds.

(a) Prove that if an initial sample is taken from the target distribution and then a new sample is taken from the transition kernel, then the new observation will be from the target distribution. More specifically, prove that if $\theta^0 \sim p(\cdot)$, and if $\theta^1 \mid \theta^0 \sim r(\cdot \mid \theta^0)$ (e.g., according to the transition kernel with given θ^0), then the marginal pdf for θ^1 is just $\theta^1 \sim p(\cdot)$.

(b) Using induction, prove that under this sampling scheme, $\theta^t \sim p(\cdot)$ for $t = 0, 1, \ldots$.

EXERCISE 4.13.   The general algorithm for the Gibbs sampler is given in Section 4.4.1. In the two-parameter case, the transition kernel for moving from $\theta^{(t)}$ to $\theta^{(t+1)}$ is given by

$$r(\theta^{(t+1)} \mid \theta^{(t)}) = p(\theta_2^{(t+1)} \mid \theta_1^{(t)})p(\theta_1^{(t+1)} \mid \theta_2^{(t+1)}),$$

where the second coordinate was sampled first, given the current value of the first coordinate, followed by sampling the first coordinate, given the newly sampled value of the second coordinate. Prove that this choice of kernel satisfies equation (4.1), where $p(\cdot, \cdot)$ is the joint pdf of the target distribution that was used to obtain the full conditionals $p(\theta_2 \mid \theta_1)$ and $p(\theta_1 \mid \theta_2)$ that were used in the definition of $r(\cdot \mid \cdot)$ above. Of course we could have reversed the sampling order and the same result would obtain.

EXERCISE 4.14. *Weibull data.*   Suppose a random sample of 10 bone marrow transplants done in 2005 showed the following survival times (available in datafor-Weibull.csv on the book's website):

$$7.64, \ 7.21, \ 1.05, \ 0.73, \ 6.76, \ 0.85, \ 1.20, \ 3.29, \ 3.29, \ 6.29.$$

Modeling these as exchangeable Weibull observations, and using priors as in Example 4.4, use OpenBUGS, JAGS or Stan to obtain posterior inferences that can be used to address the questions below. Take $\alpha_0 = 0.1, \lambda_0 = 0.05$; this yields a prior mean of 2 and a standard deviation of $\sqrt{40}$ for λ. Further, take $a = 1.62$ and $b = 3.32$; this corresponds to a prior median of 2 and a 95th percentile of 10 for ϕ.

(a) Perform convergence diagnostics for posterior samples of α and λ.

(b) Plot posterior densities for α and λ.

(c) Plot the posterior density for median survival in the population from which this sample was taken. Compute a 95% probability interval for the median.

(d) Plot the posterior density for the probability of surviving 5 years. Also give a 95% probability interval for this probability.

(e) It turns out that these data are not real data from patients! These numbers were generated from a Weibull with $\alpha = 1.7$ and $\lambda = 0.2$. Plot this true density and a density that you would estimate from the data on the same graph. Justify your estimate of the density. You may use R for this part, with samples saved from OpenBUGS, JAGS or Stan.

(f) How would you obtain an estimate of the density that included pointwise 95% probability intervals over a grid of ordinates for it?

(g) Show that the prior for ϕ above has median 2 and 95th percentile 10.

EXERCISE 4.15. *Gamma data.* Data for this exercise are in dataforGamma.csv on the book's website. Model these 300 observations as arising from a gamma density. Use the same priors as in the previous problem, as these represent very little prior information in this setting also. Answer the following questions (e.g., with OpenBUGS, JAGS, or Stan).

(a) Perform convergence diagnostics for posterior samples of α and λ.
(b) Plot posterior densities for α and λ.
(c) Plot the posterior density for median survival in the population from which this sample was taken. Compute a 95% probability interval for the median.
(d) Plot the posterior density for the probability of surviving 5 years. Also give a 95% probability interval for this probability.
(e) The data here were generated from a gamma with $\alpha = 1.5$ and $\lambda = 0.3$. Plot this true density and the density you would estimate from the data on the same graph. Justify your estimate of the density.
(f) Construct an estimate of the survival function (probability) at each point on the grid (0, 1 ,2, 5, 8, 10, 12, 15) and corresponding pointwise 95% probability intervals.

EXERCISE 4.16. Let $Y \mid \theta \sim Exp(\theta)$.

(a) Give an explicit algorithm for sampling from this distribution using the slice sampler.
(b) Sample 5,000 iterates with $\theta = 1$ using this algorithm. Then plot the history of the iterates. Does it look like there is convergence? If not, try deleting some initial iterates until the history looks like it might have converged. Take a larger MC sample size if needed to be superficially confident that the series has converged.
(c) For your final selection of iterates, give a histogram and a plot of the exact pdf on the same plot. How well did you do?

EXERCISE 4.17. Let $p(\theta \mid u)$ and $p(u \mid \theta)$ be the full conditional distributions for the slice sampler. These distributions can be inferred from the sampling algorithm that is given in Section 4.4.3. Specify these distributions. They are both obviously uniform distributions, but care is needed in writing them down precisely. Since the slice sampler is implemented as a particular Gibbs sampler, Exercise 4.13 establishes that the corresponding transition kernel satisfies equation (4.1), and consequently, that sampling using the slice sampler results in samples from the target distribution, eventually, after some burn-in.

EXERCISE 4.18. Suppose that X and Y are random variables for which $\{(x, y) : p(x \mid y) > 0\} = \{(x, y) : p(y \mid x) > 0$, and where these conditional distributions have been obtained by some means, not necessarily from a known joint pdf—for example, as illustrated in Exercise 4.17 with the slice sampler. We say that these conditional distributions are compatible if the ratio

$$p(y \mid x)/p(x \mid y) \propto g(y)h(x), \quad \int g(y)dy < \infty,$$

holds for some functions $g(\cdot)$ and $h(\cdot)$. It has been shown by Arnold and Press [12] that *there exists a joint, possibly generalized, probability density function for the pair (X, Y) if and only if the conditional distributions are compatible.* Thus in this instance, there is a joint pdf, say $p(x, y)$, that can be used to obtain the same conditional distributions above. On the other hand, if the conditional densities are not compatible, then there is an obvious problem. Suppose, for example, that we were to iteratively sample incompatible full conditionals using Gibbs sampling.

(a) Explain precisely what is problematic in probabilistic terms. Then discuss what might be problematic with the samples.

(b) Let $Y \mid X = x \sim Exp(x)$ and $X \mid Y = y \sim Exp(y)$. Show that these two distributions are incompatible.

(c) Iteratively sample the full conditionals in (b) and monitor the histories for X and Y. Are they well behaved? What can be said about any possible target distribution?

EXERCISE 4.19.   (a) Using Exercises 4.17 and 4.18, argue that the full conditionals in Exercise 4.17 are compatible and thus that there exists a joint density, $p(\theta, u)$, that gives rise to those full conditionals for the generic slice sampler. This means that $p(\theta \mid u) = p(\theta, u)/p(u)$ and $p(u \mid \theta) = p(\theta, u)/p(\theta)$, where we have $p(\theta) = \int p(\theta, u) du$ and $p(u) = \int p(\theta, u) d\theta$. *Note that no such joint pdf has been given.* It immediately follows that $p(\theta \mid u)/p(u \mid \theta) = p(\theta)/p(u) \propto p(\theta)$. Thus, there has been cancellation of parts that involve both θ and μ in order for the ratio to be a simple function of θ alone divided by a simple function of u alone.

(b) Taking the ratio of full conditional densities for the slice sampler, obtain the kernel of the marginal pdf for θ and identify it. For this problem, the parts in numerator and denominator that involve both parameters mixed up together are indicator functions. The goal is to show that these indicator functions are identical and thus cancel out in the sense that either both are 1 or both are 0. Just ignore the 0/0 issue.

EXERCISE 4.20.   Modify the code in Example 4.2 to obtain inferences μ, σ, for the coefficient of variation, σ/μ, and for $\Phi[(2 - \mu)/\sigma]$, the proportion of samples from the population that would be less than 2.

(a) Obtain posterior medians and 95% probability intervals for all parameters. Compare inferences with the truth since the actual sampling distribution is given in the code.

(b) Repeat (a) after changing the prior on τ to $Ga(20, 10)$. Comment on any changes in inferences.

(c) Let $\tau \sim Ga(20, 10)$. Plot the induced prior on σ. Would this be a reasonable prior for σ if it was believed that the standard deviation of the data might be in a neighborhood of 1?

EXERCISE 4.21   Modify and run the code in Example 4.3 to make inferences about the population mean and standard deviation, $\mu = \alpha/\lambda$ and $\sigma = \sqrt{\alpha}/\lambda$, respectively.

Give posterior medians and 95% probability intervals. Compare inferences with the truth since the actual sampling distribution is given in the code.

EXERCISE 4.22   Modify the code in Example 4.4 to make inferences about the population median, $m = (\log(2)/\lambda)^{1/\alpha}$, and the survival probability $S = P(Y > 2 \mid \alpha, \lambda) = e^{-\lambda 2^\alpha}$. Give posterior medians and 95% probability intervals. Compare inferences with the truth, since the actual sampling distribution is given in the code.

EXERCISE 4.23   Run the code in Example 4.5. Try different values of σ_0 and compare acceptance probabilities to the choice $\sigma_0 = 5$.

EXERCISE 4.24   Run the code in Example 4.6. Obtain the proportion of accepted samples and estimate the autocorrelation in the chains for μ and σ up to order 10. Give an autocorrelation plot. Plot histories for μ and σ and comment.

EXERCISE 4.25   Write BUGS, JAGS or Stan code to analyze the data generated in Example 4.2 and considered in Exercise 4.20. Write the code to provide basic inferences for μ, σ, σ/μ and $\Phi[(2 - \mu)/\sigma]$. Run two chains to obtain history plots, quantile plots, BGR plots and autocorrelation plots.

(a) Give inferences.
(b) Comment on the plots.
(c) If you did Exercise 4.20, compare results with those obtained there.

EXERCISE 4.26   Write BUGS, JAGS or Stan code to analyze the data generated in Example 4.3 and considered in Exercise 4.21. Write the code to provide basic inferences for $\mu = \alpha/\lambda$ and $\sigma = \sqrt{\alpha}/\lambda$. Run two chains to obtain history plots, quantile plots, BGR plots and autocorrelation plots.

(a) Give inferences.
(b) Comment on the plots.
(c) If you did Exercise 4.21, compare results with those obtained there.

EXERCISE 4.27   Write BUGS, JAGS or Stan code to analyze the data generated in Example 4.4 and considered in Exercise 4.22. Write the code to provide basic inferences for the median, m, and the survival probability, S, both defined in Exercise 4.22. Run two chains to obtain history plots, quantile plots, BGR plots and autocorrelation plots.

(a) Give inferences.
(b) Comment on the plots.
(c) If you did Exercise 4.22, compare results with those obtained there.

∗EXERCISE 4.28 *Derivation of E(MSB) in Section 4.4.5.*   Let $X \sim \tilde{D}_p(\mu, \Sigma)$, that is, a p-variate from some possibly unknown distribution $\tilde{D}$ with mean vector μ and covariance matrix Σ. Let A be a $p \times p$ fixed matrix. Then consider taking the expectation of the quadratic form, $Q = X'AX$. Since Q is a scalar, it is a 1×1 matrix.

Recall that the trace of a matrix is just the sum of its diagonal elements. Moreover, it is easy to show that the trace of the product of two compatible matrices, say A and B, is $tr(AB) = tr(BA)$. "Compatible" simply means that it is possible to both multiply A times B and vice versa. Thus we have $Q = tr(Q) = tr(AXX')$, and

$$E(Q) = tr(AE(XX')) = tr(A(\text{Cov}(X) + \mu\mu')) = tr(A\Sigma) + \mu'A\mu.$$

This is a standard formula from mathematical statistics.

Now referring to the section that discusses the Brooks–Gelman–Rubin statistic, let $\tilde{\theta}_j = (\theta_j^{(1)}, \theta_j^{(2)}), \ldots, \theta_j^{(M')})'$ be the collection of iterates from chain j. Then let $\tilde{\theta} = (\tilde{\theta}_1', \ldots, \tilde{\theta}_J')'$ be the vector that contains all iterates from all J chains. Let $\tilde{\mu}_j = E(\tilde{\theta}_j)$ and $\text{Cov}(\tilde{\theta}_j) = \Sigma_j$. We note that $\tilde{\mu}_j = \mu_j e_{M'}$, where $e_{M'}$ is a vector of 1s of dimension M'. We observe that the $\tilde{\theta}_j$ will be independent, but that the variates within each chain will generally not be independent. So the covariance matrix Σ must be block diagonal with the jth block being Σ_j.

Now let C be a block diagonal matrix with jth block equal to $e_{M'}e_{M'}'/J$, and D the matrix $e_{(M'J)}e_{(M'J)}'/(M'J)$, where the vector e_k is a vector of 1s of dimension k. Define the matrix $A = C - D$.

(a) Show that

$$Q \equiv \tilde{\theta}'A\tilde{\theta} = M' \sum_{j=1}^{J} (\bar{\theta}_{\cdot j} - \bar{\theta}_{\cdot\cdot})^2.$$

(b) Let $\tilde{\mu} = (\tilde{\mu}_1', \ldots, \tilde{\mu}_J')'$. Show that $\tilde{\mu}'A\tilde{\mu} = M' \sum_j (\mu_j - \bar{\mu})^2$.

(c) Using the above results, show that

$$E(Q) = (J-1) \sum_j e_{M'}\Sigma_j e_{M'}/(JM') + M' \sum_j (\mu_j - \bar{\mu})^2.$$

Finally, we have $E(\text{MSB}) = E(Q)/(J-1)$.

Chapter 5

Comparing Populations

In this chapter we revisit the binomial, normal, and Poisson distributions, which we use as models for two-sample data. The goal, as the chapter title suggests, is to compare populations, a much more interesting topic than merely estimating a single parameter from a single population. Population comparisons are usually accomplished by contrasting scientifically relevant parameters. For example, we might be interested in comparing the proportion of HIV infections in two large cities, or in comparing rates of infection with malaria in different regions in Africa. A general theme here and throughout the book is to obtain scientifically relevant information for parameters in the two populations, then incorporate that information into the model and ultimately make posterior and predictive inferences for scientific quantities of interest.

5.1   Comparing Proportions in Bernoulli Populations

Does smoking increase the probability of lung cancer? Would a new treatment better solve your medical problem than the conventional therapy? These questions involve comparing probabilities for two groups. Relevant data involve sampling individuals from each group and recording binary outcomes. More complex problems with binary data are examined in Chapter 8.

The basic model for the data involves two independent binomial samples. There are at least three versions of independent binomial sampling that we consider. The first involves sampling at a particular point in time to make inferences about the proportions of individuals in distinct populations that exhibit a particular characteristic; this is called *cross-sectional* sampling. For example, suppose there are two medical devices that can be used for a particular procedure. We wish to perform an experiment to compare the proportions of "successful" procedures under the two devices by randomly selecting one of the devices to use with each of a series of patients. We are interested in assessing which device has the better probability of being successful.

A second type of sampling is called *prospective cohort* sampling. In this instance, we could imagine fixed random samples of smokers and non-smokers who have all agreed to be followed over an extended but fixed period of time. We could then observe the number in each group that developed lung cancer during that period. Interest here focuses on comparing the proportion of smokers who develop cancer to the proportion of non-smokers who develop cancer. Using this type of sampling, it is possible to attribute whether or not the smoking has a causal effect on the occurrence of lung cancer.

In these two types of sampling, let the corresponding binomial proportions be θ_i, $i = 1, 2$. In these instances we assume data of the form

$$Y_1 \mid \theta_1 \sim Bin(n_1, \theta_1), \quad Y_2 \mid \theta_2 \sim Bin(n_2, \theta_2), \tag{5.1}$$

with the Y_i independent conditional on the parameters.

The third type of sampling is called a *case-control* design. Here, two distinct populations are again sampled but the Bernoulli responses do not correspond to the primary goals of the experiment. For example, suppose we obtained random samples of individuals known to have lung cancer and known to not have lung cancer at a particular fixed point in time. We then obtain information about each sampled individual as to whether they smoked or not. Here, the binomial proportions are the probabilities of smoking given lung cancer and the probability of smoking given no lung cancer. These are not the probabilities of primary interest. Nonetheless, we still have independent binomial sampling. It turns out that we are still able to directly address the question about whether or not smoking status is related to lung cancer occurrence. However, it is not possible to attribute causality to that effect. We explain this situation in greater detail later in this chapter.

Before analyzing data, we give an extensive discussion of how to specify priors for binomial proportions. A key feature is the elaboration on the selection of beta priors, but we also discuss the logit-normal prior. The logit-normal distribution also appears in two subsequent chapters as a model for random effects in the context of binary regression.

5.1.1   Prior Distributions for Binomial Proportions

We discuss prior distributions for binomial data. We have been using $Be(a, b)$ distributions in a number of examples already, but we provided little detail about how to get them. The beta family provides a flexible and convenient class of distributions for modeling uncertainty about probabilities. Different choices for the parameters a and b lead to a variety of density shapes, including U-shaped, J-shaped, L-shaped, unimodal symmetric, unimodal skewed right or left, and the uniform density on $(0, 1)$.

Finding a prior that agrees with expert information is far more important than the convenience of using a beta distribution. For example, if the expert's prior is bimodal, we would abandon beta distributions due to their unimodality.[1] We could accomplish bimodality by using a mixture of betas but do not discuss this possibility further, since we believe it would be rare that this was the case. In our experience the single beta works well.

We begin by discussing what we will call "reference" priors, if only because we have relatively little to say about them. A reference prior is meant to have

---

[1] Except with modes at 0 and 1, as with $a < 1, b < 1$.

minimal impact on the posterior. Whether or not a particular prior achieves this goal depends on the circumstances. Most of this subsection is devoted to methods for eliciting substantive information for use in a beta prior. The subsection closes with discussion of truncated beta priors and logit-normal priors.

5.1.1.1 Reference Priors

For a binomial random variable $Y \mid \theta \sim Bin(n, \theta)$, there is little agreement on how to choose a *reference* prior from among the three standard candidates: (1) the improper $Be(0, 0)$ distribution, (2) the Jeffreys prior $Be(0.5, 0.5)$, and (3) the $U(0, 1) = Be(1, 1)$ prior. We discuss what a Jeffreys prior is in the next chapter. The first two are U-shaped and place most of their probability on values very near 0 and 1, the improper prior $Be(0, 0)$ overwhelmingly so. In Chapter 6, where we discuss our general philosophy on priors, we argue that we would not use either of these priors for making inference in the absence of data in a scientific context. So in some sense, they are "silly." We have argued previously that the uniform prior would be silly if we were trying to model our uncertainty about the prevalence of a rare infection like HIV in a general population. Fortunately, these two priors tend to have little effect on the posterior when sample sizes are moderate and when the data do not concentrate near 0 or 1. So we call them "reference" priors.

The $Be(a, b)$ prior is a *data augmentation* prior in the sense that it can be viewed as adding a prior successes and b prior failures to the data. Thus the improper $Be(0, 0)$ prior adds no prior observations, while the Jeffreys prior adds one prior observation with half a success and half a failure, and the uniform adds two observations with one success and one failure.

When the data are all successes or all failures, these so-called reference priors can actually have a very large impact on the posterior, thus making clear that a particular prior may not be harmless, depending on the circumstances.

If no successes are observed in a large number of samples, the population probability of success is likely to be quite small. While it would not be appropriate to change the prior from whatever had been specified without a serious argument about flawed thinking when specifying that prior, we argue that if a success probability is very small, an expert would probably know that it was at least some order of small. It would thus be necessary to specify an appropriate prior that reflected that fact. We specifically discuss this issue in Example 5.1.

5.1.1.2 Informative Beta Priors

Suppose we are 95% sure that $\theta < 0.10$, and we believe that values of θ that are closer to 0 are more plausible than those that are not. Then a reasonable choice of prior is a beta distribution with a mode of 0 and 95% of the area under the density to the left of 0.10. If we pick $a = 1$ and $b > 1$, it is easy to see from the form of the beta density that the mode will be 0. (If $b = 1$ and $a > 1$, the mode is 1.)

With $a = 1$ and $b > 1$, simple calculus lets us solve for the b that gives $P(\theta < 0.10) = 0.95$. By the definition of the gamma function,

$$\Gamma(b + 1) = b\Gamma(b), \quad \Gamma(1) = 1.$$

Let $c = 0.10$ and

$$
\begin{aligned}
0.95 &= \int_0^c p(\theta)d\theta \\
&= \int_0^c \frac{\Gamma(1+b)}{\Gamma(1)\Gamma(b)}\theta^{1-1}(1-\theta)^{b-1}d\theta \\
&= \int_0^c b(1-\theta)^{b-1}d\theta \\
&= -(1-\theta)^b\Big|_0^c \\
&= 1 - (1-c)^b.
\end{aligned}
$$

Solving for b gives

$$
b = \frac{\log(1 - 0.95)}{\log(1 - c)},
$$

which is 28.43 for $c = 0.1$. A $Be(1, 28.43)$ agrees with our prior beliefs. If we take an arbitrary percentile α such that $\alpha = \int_0^c p(\theta)d\theta$, then $b = \log(1-\alpha)/\log(1-c)$.

Most often we obtain a prior on θ from an expert by eliciting two pieces of information:

- Give me your best scientifically based estimate for the probability.

- Give me the biggest value the probability could *reasonably* be, i.e., a value with only a 5% chance that the probability is bigger than it.

In essence, our elicitation involves the expert expressing available knowledge via a single value (best guess) for θ and providing a percentile (95th in the above statement) for the prior distribution for θ. We typically treat the best guess as the mode of the prior distribution. In some circumstances, we may ask for the smallest number the probability could reasonably be. In this case, we would be asking for, say, the 5th percentile. We might also change the percentiles (95th and 5th) themselves which are a quantification of what is meant by "reasonably" in the above bulleted statement. If the prior mode of θ is less than 0.5, we typically ask for an upper value that the expert is 95% or 99% sure θ falls below. If the prior mode is greater than 0.5, we typically ascertain a lower value that the expert thinks θ exceeds with high probability. These values must be elicited independently of the current data being analyzed. Priors are often elicited after the current data have been collected, which makes elicitation ignoring the current data more difficult. Rather than asking an expert, these inputs could be based on published values or historical data.

The application program BetaBuster[2] was designed to determine the parameters of the beta distribution given two such inputs. Here is a description of how Beta-Buster works. Suppose that our prior mode is θ_0. A beta distribution has mode

$$
\theta_0 = \frac{a-1}{a+b-2}
$$

---

[2]BetaBuster is available for free download at, for example, https://cadms.vetmed.ucdavis.edu/diagnostics/software under the heading "Prior Elicitation."

for $a, b \geq 1$, so solving yields

$$a(b) = \frac{1 + \theta_0(b-2)}{1 - \theta_0}. \tag{5.2}$$

Now we can find b by using information on a percentile, say a percentile c such that

$$\alpha = P(0 < \theta < c) = \int_0^c \frac{\Gamma(a(b) + b)}{\Gamma(a(b))\Gamma(b)} \theta^{a(b)-1}(1 - \theta)^{b-1} d\theta.$$

A simple computerized search procedure allows us to find a and b. Suppose $\theta_0 = 0.2$, $\alpha = 0.95$, and $c = 0.45$. We create a vector of possible b values, $\tilde{b} = (1, \ldots, 100)$ and corresponding $a(b)$ values. Then we find the 0.95 quantiles for all of these $Be(a(b), b)$ distributions, say qbeta(a(b),b) in R, and check the quantiles against the specified prior quantile $c = 0.45$. Suppose we find that $0.45 \in$ (qbeta(a(14),14),qbeta(a(15),15)). We create a new vector $\tilde{b}1 = 14 + (\tilde{b}/100)$, and repeat the process using $\tilde{b}1$ in place of $\tilde{b}$ until sufficient accuracy is achieved.

After inputting the mode and a quantile for the beta prior, BetaBuster computes a and b, reports summary characteristics of the distribution, and provides a graph of the density. The user can also specify a and b and then obtain summary characteristics and a density plot for that choice.

Example 5.1. *Prior for a Very Small Probability.* Tuyl et al. [335, 336] discuss the dangers of combining priors having $a < 1$ with data that are all failures (or $b < 1$ with all successes). Specifically, they consider data on bad reactions to a *new* radiological contrast agent. Let θ_N be the probability of a bad reaction using the *new* agent. The *standard* agent causes bad reactions about 15 times in 10,000, giving a prior estimate for θ_N of 0.0015. We consider two priors for this probability, both with mean 0.0015: a $Be(1, 666)$ and a $Be(0.05, 33.33)$. We think of the first prior as one bad reaction in 667 prior trials and the second as 0.05 bad trials in 33.38 prior trials. The number of prior trials indicates the amount of information in the prior. The *a priori* probabilities that $\theta_N \leq 0.0015$ are 0.63 and 0.88 for the two priors; the lower-information prior reflects a moderately strong belief that the new agent has fewer bad reactions. Now consider two sets of hypothetical data based on using the *new* agent, each with 100 trials, the first with no successes and the second with one success. Results for the various posterior probabilities that $\theta_N \leq 0.0015$ follow:

| | Prior parameters | |
Data	$(1, 666)$	$(0.05, 33.33)$
None	0.632	0.882
$(0/100)$	0.683	0.939
$(1/100)$	0.319	0.162

From the two posteriors, we see that the probability of $\theta_N \leq 0.0015$ is more affected by the data using the low-weight prior. Intuitively we would want a lot more than 100 observations (with no reactions) before we claimed that the new agent was better. Yet with the second prior, one is 94% sure that the new agent is better after only 100 good trials. It takes 1,330 trials without a reaction to be 95% sure that the new agent is better using the higher-weight $Be(1,666)$ prior, whereas only 145 good trials are needed with the $Be(0.05, 33.33)$ prior. Thus, it takes considerably less information to be convinced of the superiority of the new agent using the lower-information prior.

We actually want and need a very strong prior for this problem. To know that we are dealing with very small (or large) probabilities is to have a great deal of prior information, and we ignore or lessen that information at our peril. Imagine how much information we must have on the standard agent to be able to say with confidence that reactions occur about 15 times in 10,000. To change to the new agent, we should require data strong enough to make an impact on those very strong prior beliefs.

As a design issue, one would probably want to continue sampling until at least one reaction occurs. With the standard agent, we expect to see $667 = 1/0.0015$ trials before getting a reaction, so why would we be satisfied with 100 trials? Yet, even with the $Be(1,666)$ prior, the posterior gives more than a two-thirds chance that the new agent is better after 100 good trials. If anything, the $Be(1,666)$ prior is too weak. Fixing $a = 1$ in these situations is a way to force ourselves not to underestimate the prior information (too badly).

5.1.1.3 Other Priors

A prior that arises occasionally is restricted to a subset of $(0,1)$. For example, if θ is the proportion of blood donors that are infected with HIV, we could specify $\theta \sim U(0, 0.10)$, which is the same as a $Be(1,1)$ that is restricted to $(0, 0.10)$. We write this as $\theta \sim Be(1,1)I(0, 0.10)$. More generally, if we know that $\theta \in (s, t)$, we can consider a density

$$p(\theta) \propto \theta^{a-1}(1-\theta)^{b-1}I_{(s,t)}(\theta).$$

This distribution is a truncated beta expressed as $\theta \sim Be(a, b)I(s, t)$. The constant of integration is free of θ, so for most purposes we do not need to know it. Choosing $a = b = 1$ results in a $U(s, t)$ prior.

A viable alternative to the beta is the *logit-normal*(a, b^2) distribution. We say

$$\theta \sim \textit{logit-normal}(a, b^2) \Leftrightarrow \text{logit}(\theta) \sim N(a, b^2).$$

The logit function represents log odds, that is, $\text{logit}(\theta) = \ln(\theta/\{1-\theta\})$. The inverse of this function is called the *expit* function. It is easy to check that for $\beta = \text{logit}(\theta)$, we must have $\theta = e^\beta/\{1 + e^\beta\} = \text{expit}(\beta)$.

Since the logit function is monotone and increasing, and since the median of the $N(a, b^2)$ distribution is a, the median of the prior on θ is $\text{expit}(a)$. In fact, the α quantile of the prior on θ is $\text{expit}(a + z_\alpha b)$ where z_α is the α quantile of the standard normal distribution. Thus an *a priori* $1 - \alpha$ prior probability interval for θ under this prior is $\{\text{expit}(a + z_{\alpha/2}\, b), \text{expit}(a + z_{1-\alpha/2}\, b)\}$. When specifying an explicit logit-normal prior for θ, if θ_0 is our prior guess for θ, we have $\theta_0 = \text{expit}(a) \Leftrightarrow a = \text{logit}(\theta_0)$. If $\theta_0 < 0.5$, we specify a 95th percentile for θ, say c. Then we must have $c = \text{expit}(a + z_{0.95}\, b)$. Solving for b, after substituting $a = \text{logit}(\theta_0)$, we obtain

$$\text{logit}(c) = a + z_{0.95}\, b \Leftrightarrow b = \{\text{logit}(c) - \text{logit}(\theta_0)\}/z_{0.95}.$$

We do not pursue the analytical form of the posterior, since the logit-normal is not conjugate. However, the posterior is log-concave when using this prior, so that adaptive rejection sampling makes sampling easy. Of particular note is that the prior specification is easy, since we know the quantiles of the standard normal distribution and since the quantiles of the logit-normal distribution are so easily obtained using the expit function.

5.1.2 Effect Measures

With binary data, the main subject of interest is the probability of "success," θ. In biomedical sciences, θ is often referred to as a *risk*, which is a probability. For example, the proportion of smokers who develop lung cancer relates to the "risk" of lung cancer if one smokes. The word "risk" is used to connote both good and bad outcomes just as we call θ the probability of success even though θ may be the probability of death or failure.

A measure related to risk is the *odds*. The odds, Ω, are the ratio of the success probability to the failure probability,

$$\Omega = \theta/(1 - \theta).$$

Since, $0 < \theta < 1$, the odds are a positive number, $0 < \Omega < \infty$. The odds get larger as θ gets larger. Things that cannot happen have both probability 0 and odds of 0. Odds of 1 correspond to $\theta = 0.5$. The odds are infinite when the probability is 1, that is, the event is a sure thing.

Life gets more complicated and more interesting when we have two populations to compare. As discussed above, we can compare the probabilities of lung cancer for smokers, say θ_1, and non-smokers, θ_2. One comparison looks at their ratio, known as the *relative risk*,

$$RR \equiv \theta_1/\theta_2.$$

An RR of 3 means that the event of interest is three times more likely in the numerator group than in the other. RR is also sometimes called *risk ratio*.

For two populations we may also look at the *odds ratio*, defined as

$$OR = \Omega_1/\Omega_2 = \frac{\theta_1/(1 - \theta_1)}{\theta_2/(1 - \theta_2)}.$$

Why would anyone abandon a perfectly intuitive measure like risk ratios to discuss the odds ratio? Part of the reason is that it is embedded in the epidemiology literature and is convenient in many contexts. OR has a certain kind of simplicity that we will see in later chapters. Another reason is that it is not possible to estimate the RR with case-control data (Section 5.1.4), while it is possible to estimate the OR, as we shall soon see. Additionally, since probability cannot exceed 1, RR is capped at $1/\theta_2$, while OR is not limited in this way.

One issue with ORs is that there are many possible combinations of θ_1 and θ_2 that will give rise to the same OR but produce different RRs. For example, suppose $OR = 2$. That occurs when $\theta_1 = 1/2$ and $\theta_2 = 1/3$, which corresponds to $RR = 1.5$. It also occurs when $\theta_1 = 2/7$ and $\theta_2 = 1/6$, which corresponds to $RR = 12/7$. There can be a loss of information when only ORs are presented. However, if $\theta_1 = 0.002$ and $\theta_2 = 0.001$, $OR \doteq RR = 2$. In this latter case, we see that the risk ratio and the odds ratio are very similar numbers when both of the risks are small, as is the case in many epidemiology studies.

A third effect measure for two populations is the *risk difference*,

$$RD = \theta_1 - \theta_2,$$

also called the *attributable risk*. For smoking this is the difference between the proportion of smokers that get lung cancer and the proportion of non-smokers that get lung cancer.

Although odds and odds ratios are staples of medical research, RR and RD are easier to interpret, so preference should go to making statistical inferences about them when it is possible to do so. Point estimates and probability intervals for RD, RR, or OR are often readily available using a sample from the posterior. They can be used to assess both *statistical import* and *practical import* of differences between two probabilities. For example, if a 99% posterior interval for RR is $(9.9, 10.1)$, we are virtually certain that one risk is essentially ten times the other. This would be both practically and statistically important. On the other hand, if the 99% posterior interval was $(1.01, 1.02)$, we would be virtually certain that one risk was larger than the other, but would it be clinically important?

5.1.3 Cross-Sectional or Cohort Sampling

The model assumed here is the same as the one defined in equation (5.1). Assuming independent $Be(a_i, b_i)$ priors for θ_i, $i = 1, 2$, we obtain the posterior distribution

$$\theta_i \mid y_1, y_2 \overset{ind}{\sim} Be(y_i + a_i, n_i - y_i + b_i), \quad i = 1, 2. \tag{5.3}$$

This also means $p(\theta_1, \theta_2 \mid y_1, y_2) = p(\theta_1 \mid y_1)p(\theta_2 \mid y_2)$.

There will be many instances where a single population will be sampled either cross-sectionally or as a prospective cohort, and where *after* sampling, each individual is cross-classified as having had an event (*success*) or not, and whether they were from a particular subpopulation. We argue below that this sampling structure leads to the same posterior analysis as the structure that involves sampling n_i individuals from subpopulation i, and then observing the number of events or successful outcomes in each. The former type of sampling is termed *multinomial*, and the latter *product binomial*, since the likelihood function $Lik(\theta_1, \theta_2) = Lik(\theta_1)Lik(\theta_2)$

is the product of marginal likelihoods in that case. In the multinomial case, each individual can fall into one of four cells.

We consider multinomial sampling in the context of the lung cancer and smoking paradigm. We sample n individuals from a broad cohort, observe them over a specified period of time, and then at the end of that time observe whether they had acquired lung cancer (LC) or not, and also whether they smoked (Smoke) or not. The observed data would be in the form of a 2×2 table that is cross-classified according to counts of the number of individuals out of n that were observed to be in the categories (LC, Smoke), (LC, NoSmoke), (NoLC, Smoke), (NoLC, NoSmoke). The sum of these counts must be n, and the collection of the four counts would have a multinomial distribution. In this instance, we are interested in the probabilities of LC given Smoke and NoSmoke, respectively.

Let smoking categories be $i = 1$ for Smoke, and $i = 2$ for NoSmoke. It turns out that if we condition on the observed number of Smokers, say n_1, and the observed number of non-smokers, say n_2 ($n_1 + n_2 = n$), the counts for the numbers of lung cancers for these two cases are independent and $Bin(n_i, \theta_i)$ with $\theta_i = P(\text{LC} \mid \text{Smoke Category} = i)$, $i = 1, 2$. Thus even if the data are multinomial at the outset, and if they are cross-classified appropriately, we are able to use our two-sample binomial model to analyze the data. In statistical terms, the smoking status is called an explanatory *factor*, since we explore whether larger or smaller probabilities of lung cancer can be inferred to depend on smoking status. We proceed to illustrate using the **LE** data.

Example 5.2. Yen et al. [356] studied lymphedema (LE) in breast cancer patients as described in Example 1.2. We use data from the $n = 1{,}211$ women who were followed for 4 years with information available on LE status and the number of lymph nodes examined during breast cancer surgery.

After sampling, the 1,211 individuals were cross-classified into the 2×2 array of counts presented in Table 5.1. The rows correspond to high node counts (> 5) and low node counts (≤ 5), and the columns correspond to whether they had lymphedema or not (yes/no).

TABLE 5.1: LE data with number of nodes (high or low) examined

Nodes examined	Lymphedema Yes	No	
High (> 5)	126	351	477
Low (≤ 5)	53	681	734

Our interest focuses on ascertaining whether or not the probability of LE varies according to the number of nodes examined, so we condition on the high and low counts, which allows us to treat the number of lymphedema cases in the high and low categories as two independent binomial random variables (see Exercise 5.9). Here, θ_1 and θ_2 denote the probabilities of LE for high and low node counts, respectively.

The actual data are $n_1 = 477$, $n_2 = 734$, $y_1 = 126$, and $y_2 = 53$, where the n_i are viewed as fixed known numbers and the y_i are viewed as observations on random variables. The sample proportion of LE is 0.264 for high and 0.072 for low node counts.

In the absence of available prior information it is tempting to put independent $U(0,1)$ reference priors on the probabilities. However, literature in the field clearly indicated reasonable ranges for lymphedema probability after breast cancer surgery. The risk is about 2% per year and continues for many years. For a four-year period, we take 0.08 as the prior mode and specify 0.95 prior probability that LE risk is less than 0.3. Using BetaBuster, we obtain $a_1 = a_2 = 2.044$ and $b_1 = b_2 = 13.006$. This prior tacitly assumes that there is no prior belief that one of these probabilities would be larger than another. Using this information, the posteriors are

$$\theta_1 \mid y_1 \sim Be(128.044, 364.006) \quad indep. \quad \theta_2 \mid y_2 \sim Be(55.044, 694.006).$$

Summary information for these two distributions is listed in the top two rows of Table 5.2. The posterior means, medians, standard deviations (sds), and 95% probability intervals are shown. The clearly separated intervals show strong evidence of a higher risk of LE for the high exposure group. More directly, the last line of the table indicates virtual certainty that RD is positive. Other lines show similarly strong evidence that RR and OR are both greater than 1. Patients undergoing examination of more than five lymph nodes are estimated to be about 3.6 times more likely to develop lymphedema over 4 years compared to those having five or fewer nodes examined, with the true RR value in the interval $(2.68, 4.83)$ with probability 0.95.

TABLE 5.2: Posterior summaries for LE data

Parameter	mean	sd	2.5%	median	97.5%
θ_1	0.260	0.020	0.222	0.260	0.300
θ_2	0.073	0.010	0.056	0.073	0.093
RR	3.612	0.545	2.677	3.565	4.830
OR	4.543	0.789	3.204	4.472	6.300
RD	0.187	0.021	0.145	0.187	0.229

5.1.4 Case-Control Sampling

The type of data in the previous subsection involved sampling individuals from two distinct populations or classifying them into two distinct populations. As previously mentioned, we often refer to the population status as an explanatory factor. We are always interested in how the probabilities of a particular event that is of some consequence will vary as a function of the explanatory factor. However, in this section, we reverse the roles of explanatory factor and event of interest for practical reasons. In a case-control study, the investigators choose individuals based on case or control status and then examine exposure. With the type of data considered here, it is difficult to estimate $P(\text{LC} \mid \text{Smoke})$, for example. But we will be able to estimate the odds ratio

$$
\begin{aligned}
OR &= \frac{P(\text{LC} \mid \text{Smoke})/\{1 - P(\text{LC} \mid \text{Smoke})\}}{P(\text{LC} \mid \text{NoSmoke})/\{1 - P(\text{LC} \mid \text{NoSmoke})\}} \\
&\equiv \frac{\Omega(\text{LC} \mid \text{Smoke})}{\Omega(\text{LC} \mid \text{NoSmoke})},
\end{aligned}
$$

if the data are sampled as case-control data with cases corresponding to people with LC and controls corresponding to those with NoLC.

Prospective cohort sampling can often be very expensive if large samples of individuals have to be monitored over a considerable length of time, maybe decades. It is even more expensive when the event of interest is relatively rare, due to the necessity of taking larger sample sizes than might be needed otherwise. In addition, it is often difficult to sample certain populations based on the explanatory factor of interest.

Below, in Example 5.3, we consider Reye's syndrome (RS) in children where the factor of interest is whether or not children are given aspirin. RS is a rare but very serious condition. In order to obtain a prospective cohort sample, we would have to take a very large sample of children who were to be given aspirin, and a sample who were not to take aspirin, over an extended period of time. This would be an awkward experiment and, moreover, there would be no guarantee that we would see any or very many children with RS, even in a very large sample.

With case-control sampling, the event of interest itself is used to define populations to sample. In the RS example, n_1 known RS children would be sampled, and n_2 children known not to have RS would be sampled, independently. Then, for each group, the observed number of children who were given aspirin during appropriate windows of time would be obtained. More generally, independent samples are taken from each of the two levels of the "response variable." The sampled populations are called cases and controls, respectively. Then, for each group, there is a count for each of the two explanatory categories; for cases they add to n_1 and for controls they add to n_2, these numbers having been fixed by the design. We obtain two independent binomial samples, with success or failure corresponding to the two explanatory categories (often called "exposure levels").

In the RS example, we are only able to estimate $P(\text{Aspirin} \mid \text{RS})$ and $P(\text{Aspirin} \mid \text{NoRS})$, while the probabilities of interest, $P(\text{RS} \mid \text{Aspirin})$ and $P(\text{RS} \mid \text{NoAspirin})$, are not estimable using case-control data. Think about it. Since the number of individuals in the sample who have RS is fixed by design, the proportion of RS children in the combined sample is meaningless, since that proportion is determined in advance by the experimenters. However, as indicated above, we are able to estimate $OR = \Omega(\text{RS} \mid \text{Aspirin})/\Omega(\text{RS} \mid \text{NoAspirin})$.

This method of sampling is considerably less expensive than prospective cohort sampling. However, the price that is paid for the lower expense is that it is not possible to attribute causality to the explanatory factor, which is possible with prospective sampling. With case-control sampling, it is only possible to assert that there is an *association* between aspirin use and RS.

Example 5.3. Reye's Syndrome. In the late 1970s, it was observed that, in a sample of $n_1 = 7$ children with Reye's syndrome (RS), all seven of them were taking aspirin at the time they became sick. A second sample of size $n_2 = 16$ children known to be free of Reye's syndrome was also taken, and it was determined that eight of them were taking aspirin when sampled.

The sample fraction of children on aspirin in the RS group is 1 and the corresponding fraction in the non-RS group is 0.5. Based on these estimates, $\widehat{OR} = \infty$. Just for fun, we will see what happens if we had seen six aspirin takers with RS instead of the actual seven. The estimated OR would be $\widehat{OR} = [(6/7)/(1/7)]/[(1/2)/(1/2)] = 6$, which epidemiologists normally think of as quite large. But with the small sample sizes, is the result statistically important? More importantly, why would we care that children with RS are more likely to take aspirin? What we care about is whether children who take aspirin are more likely to get RS.

We introduce some notation in order to formally describe the situation we face. Consider a disease or infection or condition of interest, say D, with $D = 1$ indicating presence and $D = 0$ absence of the disease. Also consider an exposure variable, say E, with $E = 1$ indicating exposure and $E = 0$ no exposure. For example, if we were considering performing a case-control experiment to study the relationship between smoking and lung cancer, $E = 1$ would correspond to "smoker" and $E = 0$ to "non-smoker," while $D = 1$ would correspond to "lung cancer" and $D = 0$ to "no lung cancer." *Exposure status* is now the *explanatory factor*, in the language of epidemiology.

We are still primarily interested in determining the direct effect of E on the probability of D, namely $P(D \mid E)$. We want to compare $\theta_1 \equiv P(D = 1 \mid E = 1)$ and $\theta_2 \equiv P(D = 1 \mid E = 0)$. Ideally, we would like to make inferences about the risk ratio and risk difference,

$$RR = \theta_1/\theta_2, \quad RD = \theta_1 - \theta_2,$$

as we were able to do with prospective cohort data and cross-sectional data. But we well know at this stage that our study design does not allow us to estimate the θ_i, so it is also not possible to use the data alone to make inferences about RR or RD.

Now define $\tilde{\theta}_1 \equiv P(E = 1 \mid D = 1)$ and $\tilde{\theta}_2 \equiv P(E = 1 \mid D = 0)$. Let Y_i be the count of the number of individuals in sample i who have been exposed, for example, with $E = 1$. Then we have

$$Y_i \mid \tilde{\theta}_i \overset{ind}{\sim} Bin(n_i, \tilde{\theta}_i), \quad i = 1, 2.$$

Clearly we can estimate the $\tilde{\theta}_i$, and so we can also estimate the odds ratio

$$OR_1 = \frac{\Omega(E = 1 \mid D = 1)}{\Omega(E = 1 \mid D = 0)} = \frac{\tilde{\theta}_1/(1 - \tilde{\theta}_1)}{\tilde{\theta}_2/(1 - \tilde{\theta}_2)}.$$

The odds ratio that we are actually interested in is

$$OR_2 = \frac{\Omega(D = 1 \mid E = 1)}{\Omega(D = 1 \mid E = 0)} = \frac{\theta_1/(1-\theta_1)}{\theta_2/(1-\theta_2)}. \qquad (5.4)$$

It is left as an exercise to show that $OR_1 = OR_2 \equiv OR$. Then it is clear that we can obtain a data-based estimate of OR.

Recall our previous discussion about how there are generally multiple possible combinations of θ_1 and θ_2 that will give rise to the same value of OR. Thus, there is unavoidable information loss associated with case-control sampling. Nonetheless, we always know that

$$\theta_1 > \theta_2 \Leftrightarrow OR > 1.$$

Moreover,

$$OR = k \Leftrightarrow \Omega(D = 1 \mid E = 1) = k\,\Omega(D = 1 \mid E = 0).$$

So if $k = 10$, we say that the odds of disease for exposed individuals is 10 times the odds of disease for unexposed individuals, considerably higher than even odds. If $k = 3$, the odds are still high; if $k = 1.1$, not so much. Clearly we will be interested in obtaining $P(\theta_1 > \theta_2 \mid y) = P(OR > 1 \mid y)$ and more generally, $P(OR > k \mid y)$. If we are 98% certain that $OR > 3$, we have a clear statistical result. Such a probability is easily calculated from posterior samples.

As previously mentioned, with small probabilities, the odds ratio is a good approximation to the risk ratio. For example, if $OR = 10$, the odds of D in an exposed group would be 10 times that for the non-exposed group. If $P(D = 1 \mid E = 1) = 0.01$ and $P(D = 1 \mid E = 0) = 0.001$ we get $RR = 10 \doteq OR$. On the other hand, when the probabilities are not small, say if $P(D = 1 \mid E = 1) = 10/19 = 0.53$ and $P(D = 1 \mid E = 0) = 0.1$, $OR = 10$ but $RR = 5.3$, a big difference.

The analysis takes on different forms depending on how the prior information is specified. If the experts have prior information on $\tilde{\theta}_1 = P(E = 1 \mid D = 1)$ and $\tilde{\theta}_2 = P(E = 1 \mid D = 0)$, then simple independent beta priors on these may suffice and the analysis is just like the others illustrated in this section. The only caveat is that interest focuses almost entirely on the odds ratio. Here is pseudo-code borrowing from the BUGS syntax. One would supply the data (y[1],y[2]) and prior parameters for the group i beta prior distributions.

```
model{for (i in 1:2){
   y[i] ~ dbin(ttheta[i],n[i])
   ttheta[i] ~ dbeta(a[i],b[i])
   O[i] <- ttheta[i]/(1-ttheta[i]) }
   OR <- O[1]/O[2]
   prob <- step(OR -1)    #Posterior Pr(OR > 1)
   }
```

Another situation that can arise is where there is prior information about OR, perhaps based on a previous case-control study that is similar to the one at hand. We can place a prior on the parameters by placing, say, a normal prior on $\delta \equiv \log(OR)$

and an independent beta prior on $\tilde{\theta}_2$. These induce a prior on $(\tilde{\theta}_1, \tilde{\theta}_2)$. To apply this, we need to solve for $\tilde{\theta}_1$ in terms of δ and $\tilde{\theta}_2$. Some algebra gives

$$\tilde{\theta}_1 = \frac{e^\delta \tilde{\theta}_2}{1 - \tilde{\theta}_2(1 - e^\delta)}.$$

To elicit a prior on δ we think about OR. If our best guess is that $OR = 3$, then we take the mean of a prior normal distribution for δ to be $\log(3) = 1.1$. Moreover, if we are, say, 90% sure that the OR is at least 0.8, then we are also 90% sure that $\log(OR)$ is at least $\log(0.8) = -0.22$. We need to find a normal distribution with a mean of 1.1 and a 10th percentile of -0.22. We know (or can look up) that the 10th percentile of a normal is 1.28 standard deviations below the mean, so we set $1.1 - 1.28 \, \text{sd} = -0.22$ and solve for $\text{sd} = 1.03$. Our prior on δ is $N(1.1, (1.03)^2)$.

5.2   Comparing Normal Populations

Normal data are ubiquitous in the scientific world because they often arise from measurements. We have all been exposed to the "bell-shaped curve." Standardized test scores displayed in a histogram look like a bell. Data on how long people can hold their breath under water look like a bell. We already discussed how to handle one-sample normal data. Here, we move on to the comparison of two normal populations.

We consider the two-sample normal model:

$$Y_{i1}, \ldots, Y_{in_i} \mid \mu_i, \sigma_i^2 \overset{ind}{\sim} N(\mu_i, \sigma_i^2), \quad i = 1, 2.$$

We are often interested in making inferences about $\mu_1 - \mu_2$. This is perfectly sensible if $\sigma_1^2 \doteq \sigma_2^2$, but the issue becomes complicated if one variance is appreciably smaller than the other. We discuss this issue later in this section.

5.2.1   Priors for (μ_i, σ_i^2), $i = 1, 2$

Traditionally, Bayesians used either a reference prior or a conjugate prior. As we discussed previously in the one-sample case, the conjugate prior has limited practical utility for data analysis, since it is somewhat awkward to elicit expert information for the parameters, due to the dependence of the means on the variances. As in the one-sample case, we focus on priors with independent information on μ_i and σ_i^2. In fact, we assume

$$p(\mu_1, \sigma_1^2, \mu_2, \sigma_2^2) = p(\mu_1, \sigma_1^2)p(\mu_2, \sigma_2^2) = p(\mu_1)p(\sigma_1^2)p(\mu_2)p(\sigma_2^2).$$

5.2.1.1   Reference Priors

Let $\tau_i = 1/\sigma_i^2$ for $i = 1, 2$. Historically, the classic reference prior puts "independent" flat priors on both $\mu = (\mu_1, \mu_2)$ and $\gamma \equiv (\ln(\tau_1), \ln(\tau_2))$, that is, $p(\mu, \gamma) \propto 1$. This implies that

$$p(\mu, \tau) \propto \prod_{i=1}^{2} 1/\tau_i.$$

This is the obvious extension of the prior we used for the one-sample normal problem where results obtained were directly comparable to frequentist results, meaning that point, interval, and predictive inferences were numerically identical, except for their interpretations. If we were to assume that $\sigma_1^2 = \sigma_2^2 = \sigma^2$ here, with $p(\mu_1, \mu_2, \tau) \propto 1/\tau$, we would again obtain the standard frequentist point, interval, and prediction formulas. This is our *ideal* definition of a *reference* prior. However, we need to point out that these same priors rarely work for this purpose in other contexts, such as nonlinear modeling.

Using this improper reference prior, the joint posterior satisfies $p(\mu_1, \tau_1, \mu_2, \tau_2 \mid \boldsymbol{y}) = p(\mu_1, \tau_1 \mid \boldsymbol{y})p(\mu_2, \tau_2 \mid \boldsymbol{y})$, and the marginal posterior of μ_i is Student's $t(n_i - 1, \bar{y}_i, s_i^2/n_i)$, where $\bar{y}_i = \sum_j y_{ij}/n_i$ and $s_i^2 = \sum_j (y_{ij} - \bar{y}_i)^2/(n_i - 1)$, $i = 1, 2$. This result was derived in Chapter 3, except that now we have two independent samples resulting in two independent posteriors. The posteriors for the τ_i are independent and gamma. Nonetheless, there is no nice analytical result for the posterior of $\Delta = \mu_1 - \mu_2$.

A proper prior approximation to the improper reference prior is

$$\mu_i \stackrel{\text{ind}}{\sim} N(0, 10^6) \quad ind \quad \tau_i \stackrel{ind}{\sim} Ga(0.001, 0.001).$$

Since $\text{Var}(\mu_i) = 1{,}000{,}000$ and $\text{Var}(\tau_i) = 1{,}000$, the prior precisions for μ_i and τ_i are near zero, meaning that there is huge uncertainty involved in the prior specification. The posterior is largely "unaffected" by the prior in the normal data case; therefore, many are happy to regard this prior as "non-informative." However, no one would choose this prior to make inferences in the absence of data. We discuss this issue further in the next chapter. So in a sense, it is a "silly" prior, but since we all trust the frequentist formulas in this case, we are content to use it.

In BUGS, we can write the code:

```
model{
    for (i in 1:2){
        for (j in 1:n[i]){
        y[i,j] ~ dnorm(mu[i],tau[i])
    }
    mu[i] ~ dnorm(0,0.000001)
    tau[i] ~ dgamma(0.001, 0.001)}
    Delta <- mu[1] - mu[2]
    prob <- step(Delta) #Postprob(Delta > 0)
}
list(n = c(2,2))
  y[,1] y[,2]
  55.6   66.3
  45.8   59.7
  END
list(mu = c(0,0), tau = c(1,1))
```

This is a made-up data set with $n_1 = n_2 = 2$. The data are comprised of the first list, and the y_{ij} given in 2×2 array form. Two clicks of "load data" are needed to input the data before compiling. The second list gives initial values. An alternative to this code is to replace `dnorm(0,0.000001)` with `dflat()`, which replaces the normal prior on the means with the improper flat prior on them. Gibbs sampling is easily performed in BUGS, alternating between the normal and gamma full conditionals for μ_i and τ_i, respectively, for $i = 1, 2$, at each iteration, resulting in numerical approximations to full Bayesian inferences.

5.2.1.2 Informative Priors

We already discussed how to select a somewhat informative prior for the mean systolic blood pressure when we were discussing the one-sample normal case in Chapter 3. We continue the discussion here for a generic mean, μ, and we also discuss how to place a prior on the precision, τ. In general, we recommend specifying $\mu \sim N(\mu_0, \sigma_0^2)$. So μ_0 is a best guess for μ. As in the binomial proportion case, we pick a percentile of the prior, say μ_α (i.e., $P(\mu < \mu_\alpha) = \alpha$), so that

$$\alpha = P(\mu < \mu_\alpha) = P(\{\mu - \mu_0\}/\sigma_0 < \{\mu_\alpha - \mu_0\}/\sigma_0) \Rightarrow \{\mu_\alpha - \mu_0\}/\sigma_0 = z_\alpha$$

and thus

$$\sigma_0 = \{\mu_\alpha - \mu_0\}/z_\alpha.$$

Example 5.4. Consider blood serum sodium levels in a (new) population of interest. Assume that they are normally distributed and that we will collect a sample of individuals and make inferences about the average blood serum sodium levels in this population. On the web, we find that in the general population, "normal serum sodium levels are 135 to 145 mmol/L" (Wikipedia). Without any additional knowledge about whether the population of interest had a higher or lower average blood serum sodium, our best guess would be $\mu_0 = 140$. We assume that the (135, 145) range is a 95% prediction interval of some sort, meaning that it is expected that 95% of the general population would have sodium values inside this range. If we believe that the new population were similar to the general population, setting $\mu_{0.05} = 138$ mmol/L would be conservative if the prediction interval were to be believed. A considerably less informative prior would set $\mu_{0.05} = 135$ mmol/L.

An issue that requires serious consideration is that an individual with blood serum sodium < 135 mmol/L is considered to have hyponatremia, which is a serious condition that may result in hospitalization. So if $\mu = 135$, for example, half of the new population would be considered to have this condition. It is highly unlikely that this would go unnoticed. The main point of this example is that biology really matters when specifying a prior. For illustration, we set $\mu_{0.05} = 136$. Then we obtain $\sigma_0 = (140 - 136)/1.645 = 2.43$. Thus a 95% prior probability interval for μ would be (135.2, 144.7). If the new population is similar to the general population at all, this will be a very conservative prior, meaning that it is relatively quite diffuse.

In the two-population case, we proceed in the same way, regarding each population separately and independently. The case where we would regard means as dependent is discussed in the next chapter.

We now turn to specifying a mildly informative prior for the precision τ where we go to some effort to find an informative prior guess for it but otherwise allow for considerable uncertainty. Since it is not easy to think about τ, we think about the 90th percentile of the distribution of y values, $\gamma_{0.90}$. So $P(Y < \gamma_{0.90} \mid \mu, \sigma) = 0.90$. This means that 90% of the responses will be less than $\gamma_{0.90}$. Let u be a best guess for $\gamma_{0.9}$. Then, since

$$\gamma_{0.90} = \mu + 1.28\sqrt{1/\tau},$$

we can use our best guesses for μ and $\gamma_{0.90}$ to obtain a best guess for τ (τ_0) by solving

$$u = \mu_0 + 1.28\sqrt{1/\tau_0} \Leftrightarrow \tau_0 = 1.28/(u - \mu_0)^2.$$

We then specify the conditionally conjugate prior

$$\tau \sim Ga(c, d), \quad \frac{c-1}{d} = \tau_0,$$

so the mode is τ_0. We have $c = 1 + d\tau_0$. This prior will be diffuse for small d, since $Var(\tau) = (1 + d\tau_0)/d^2$. In Chapter 6, we consider how to specify a fully informative prior for σ^2. Of course in the two-population case, the same process applies to both sets of population parameters.

5.2.2   Posterior Inference for Comparing Populations

Under the assumption of independent priors for the means and variances or precisions, the joint posterior satisfies

$$p(\mu, \tau \mid \boldsymbol{y}) = p(\mu_1, \tau_1, \mu_2, \tau_2 \mid \boldsymbol{y}) = p(\mu_1, \tau_1 \mid \boldsymbol{y})p(\mu_2, \tau_2 \mid \boldsymbol{y}).$$

So inference procedures for the two sets of population parameters are identical to what they would be if we simply carried out posterior calculations for them separately. Either way, we can take Markov chain Monte Carlo iterates to make inferences about any function of the parameters, say $g(\mu, \tau)$.

Since we are comparing populations, particular interest will focus on $\Delta = \mu_2 - \mu_1$. This effect measure is most useful when σ_1 and σ_2 are not too different, since then the primary distinction between the two populations is characterized by Δ. For example, see Figure 5.1a where $\Delta = 1$.

When comparing two normal populations, it makes sense to first take a look at the ratio of standard deviations, $SDR \equiv \sigma_1/\sigma_2$. For example, if $P(SDR > 2 \mid \boldsymbol{y})$ is large, we need to think harder about what it means for $\mu_2 > \mu_1$, or vice versa. Figure 5.1b shows $N(0, 1)$ and $N(1, 0.25)$ pdfs where $\Delta = 1$, but the situation is quite different from the one with equal variances. It is obviously not enough to only focus on Δ.

In addition, it is possible that $\Delta \doteq 0$ and SDR is large. In this case, only focusing on Δ would lose sight of the fact that the distributions are quite different. Inference would require discussion of this type of difference in the context of the scientific background for the data.

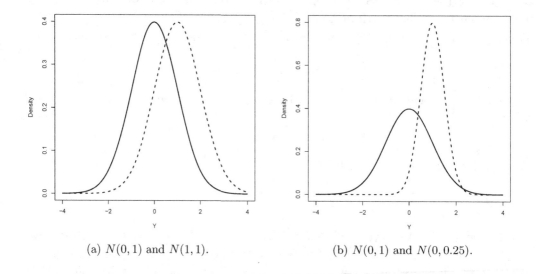

(a) $N(0,1)$ and $N(1,1)$.   (b) $N(0,1)$ and $N(0,0.25)$.

FIGURE 5.1: Graphs showing normal densities one may wish to compare and the effect of the variances on the comparisons. Panel (a) shows $N(0,1)$ (solid) and $N(1,1)$ (dashed) densities. Panel (b) shows $N(0,1)$ (solid) and $N(1,0.25)$ (dashed) densities.

Another quantity that may be of interest in comparing populations is the probability that a random value from population 2 would exceed a random value from population 1. Let us name it EPR for "exceedance in pairs rate," so that

$$EPR = P(Y_{21} > Y_{11} \mid \mu, \tau) = 1 - \Phi\left(\frac{-\Delta}{\sqrt{\sigma_1^2 + \sigma_2^2}}\right),$$

where $\Phi(\cdot)$ is the cdf for a standard normal variate. This probability equals 0.76 and 0.81 for the densities in Figure 5.1. As this value approaches 1, we know that the two pdfs approach complete separation, meaning virtually no overlap.

5.2.3   Prediction

Prediction is easy after we already have a random sample from the posterior (e.g., an MCMC sample) for the model parameters. Let $Z_i \mid \mu, \tau \perp\!\!\!\perp N(\mu_i, \tau_i)$, $i = 1, 2$, independently of the two-sample data, $\boldsymbol{y}$. The marginal predictive density for Z_i is

$$p(z_i \mid \boldsymbol{y}) = \int p(z_i \mid \mu_i, \tau_i) p(\mu_i, \tau_i \mid \boldsymbol{y}) d\mu_i d\tau_i, \quad i = 1, 2.$$

Because of the assumed independence, we have $p(z_1, z_2 \mid \boldsymbol{y}) = p(z_1 \mid \boldsymbol{y}) p(z_2 \mid \boldsymbol{y})$. These marginal predictive densities are identical to the ones we considered in the one-sample normal case: they are Student's t pdfs. However, for a variety of reasons, it is usually much easier to use MCMC sampling to make predictive and estimative inferences.

Suppose we are interested in the predictive probability that a future value from population 1 would be less than a future value from population 2. This is calculated as

$$P(Z_1 < Z_2 \mid \boldsymbol{y}) = \int_{-\infty}^{\infty} \int_{-\infty}^{z_2} p(z_1 \mid \boldsymbol{y}) p(z_2 \mid \boldsymbol{y}) dz_1 dz_2,$$

which is an intractable integral. But if we have a sample of iterates,

$$\{(\mu^{(t)}, \tau^{(t)}) : t = BI + 1, \ldots, M\},$$

we simply sample

$$Z_i^{(t)} \mid (\mu^{(t)}, \tau^{(t)}) \overset{ind}{\sim} N(\mu^{(t)}, 1/\tau^{(t)}), \quad i = 1, 2.$$

Then we approximate the above integral,

$$P(Z_1 < Z_2 \mid \boldsymbol{y}) \doteq \sum_{t=BI+1}^{M} I(z_1^{(t)} < z_2^{(t)})/(M - BI).$$

5.2.4 DiaSorin Data Analysis

Renal osteodystrophy is a bone disease that occurs when the kidneys fail to maintain proper levels of calcium and phosphorus in the blood. Monitoring patients with loss of kidney function for lower than normal bone turnover aids in managing the disease. A commercially available diagnostic assay, DiaSorin, was believed to have the potential to determine which patients have low versus normal bone turnover. A cross-section of 34 kidney patients from the bone registry at the University of Kentucky were identified as low or normal turnover by other means and then given the commercial assay to determine whether it could correctly identify them. From boxplots, a normal sampling model appears to be untenable, due to observable skewness; however, boxplots and quantile plots of the log-transformed data appear to be reasonably normal (see Figure 5.2).

Since data are on the log scale, we write $\log(Y) \mid \mu, \sigma^2 \sim N(\mu, \sigma^2)$. For analyzing the data, we could just take logs of all of the data and then treat them as normally distributed. The prior can be taken as $N(\mu_0, \sigma_0^2)$ for μ, and an independent $Ga(c, d)$ prior for $\tau = 1/\sigma^2$. This needs to be implemented for each of the two populations.

Prior Elicitation. We first consider eliciting prior information for μ. It is natural for us to specify such information on the original data scale instead of the log scale. We can then induce it onto the model parameter μ as follows.

Note that if m is the median of DiaSorin scores Y in a population, then $\log(m)$ is the median of $\log(Y)$ measurements in the population. This is because the logarithm is a monotone function. Now specify a best guess $\tilde{m}$ for the population median m of DiaSorin scores. Then we take $\mu_0 = \log(\tilde{m})$. Next specify a value, $\tilde{u}_{0.95}$, such that we are 95% percent certain that m cannot exceed it, namely $P(m < \tilde{u}_{0.95}) = 0.95$.

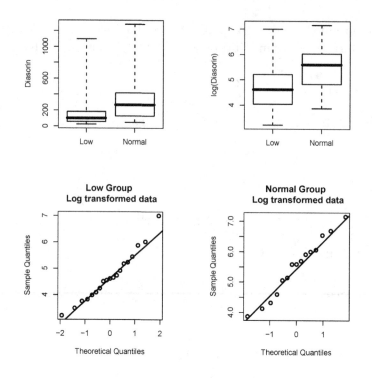

FIGURE 5.2: DiaSorin data.

This is equivalent to asserting $0.95 = P(\mu \leq \log(\tilde{u}_{0.95})) = P(\{\mu - \mu_0\}/\sigma_0 \leq \{\log(\tilde{u}_{0.95}) - \mu_0\}/\sigma_0)$, from which we get

$$\frac{\log(\tilde{u}_{0.95}) - \log(\tilde{m})}{\sigma_0} = 1.645 \Leftrightarrow \sigma_0 = \frac{\log(\tilde{u}_{0.95}) - \log(\tilde{m})}{1.645}.$$

Dr. Johann Herberth of the University of Kentucky gave his best guess of the median for the low bone turnover population as 130, and he was 95% sure that this median was less than 142 in this patient population. This results in $\mu_L \equiv \mu_1 \sim N(4.87, 0.00288)$. The corresponding values elicited from Dr. Herberth for the normal bone turnover population were 220 and 240, respectively. This led to $\mu_N \equiv \mu_2 \sim N(5.39, 0.00280)$.

Let us next consider the prior for τ. In general, we can ask the expert to think about the 100αth percentile, γ_α, of the distribution of Y values, with some comfortably high value of α such as 0.95. Let u be the value the expert specifies. Since the 100αth percentile of the $N(\mu, \tau)$ distribution is $\mu + z_\alpha/\sqrt{\tau}$, and since the log is a monotone increasing transformation, we must have $\gamma_\alpha = e^{\mu + z_\alpha/\sqrt{\tau}}$. Then our best prior guess for τ must satisfy $u = e^{\mu_0 + z_\alpha/\sqrt{\tau_0}} \Leftrightarrow \tau_0 = z_\alpha^2/\{\log(u) - \mu_0\}^2$. This can be taken for the prior mode for τ. Dr. Herberth provided his best guess for the 95th percentile of DiaSorin values in the low ($u = 170$) and normal ($u = 280$) bone turnover patient populations. Requiring gamma priors with modes $1.645^2/\{\log(170) - \log(130)\}^2 = 37.6$ and $1.645^2/\{\log(280) - \log(220)\}^2 = 46.53$,

TABLE 5.3: Posterior summaries for informative prior, log DiaSorin data

Parameter	mean	sd	2.5%	50%	97.5%
μ_1	4.860	0.052	4.757	4.860	4.961
μ_2	5.395	0.051	5.294	5.395	5.496
$\mu_2 - \mu_1$	0.536	0.073	0.392	0.536	0.679
τ_1	1.275	0.394	0.625	1.231	2.161
τ_2	1.285	0.439	0.576	1.236	2.274
τ_2/τ_1	1.114	0.555	0.387	1.003	2.495

and with large variances for τs specified by choosing $d_1 = d_2 = 0.001$, results in $\tau_1 \sim Ga(1.0376, 0.001)$ and $\tau_2 \sim Ga(1.04653, 0.001)$.

Inference on Log Scale. The analysis on the log scale with our informative prior begins with Table 5.3, which gives posterior summaries for the two groups. We glean from the table that a 95% probability interval for σ_1/σ_2 is $(\sqrt{0.387}, \sqrt{2.495}) = (0.62, 1.58)$, with posterior median 1.001. Thus there is no evidence that the standard deviations for the log data are different. Moreover, we are nearly 100% certain that $\Delta = \mu_N - \mu_L > 0$ (result not shown in Table 5.3) and we are 95% certain that $\Delta \in (0.39, 0.68)$. Thus we can conclude that $\Delta > 0$ and that we are 95% certain that μ_N is between 0.39 and 0.68 times larger than μ_L. We term this a highly statistically important result.

However, it is unclear what the practical import of the result is. We know for sure that "normal" DiaSorin scores tend to be higher than "low" DiaSorin scores, but we need to go further to address the question about whether or not DiaSorin scores can be used reliably to discriminate between individuals from the normal and low bone turnover populations.

Inference on Original Scale. Again using our informative prior, Table 5.4 gives results of the analysis on the untransformed scale. The posterior median and 95% probability interval for the median DiaSorin value among low bone turnover patients, e^{μ_L}, was 129 (116.4, 142.8), and the corresponding estimate and interval for the median among patients with normal bone turnover, e^{μ_N}, was 220.6 (199.1, 243.6). Inference for the relative median $e^{\mu_N}/e^{\mu_L} = e^{\mu_N - \mu_L}$ comparing the DiaSorin values of normal to low bone turnover patients was 1.71 (1.48, 1.97). We are thus 95% certain that the median of DiaSorin scores in the "normal" population is between about 1.5 and 2 times that for the "low" population. Prediction intervals for new values from both groups are also given. These intervals are substantially wide because of the small sample sizes ($n_1 = 19, n_2 = 15$). Code that generated these results is available on the book's webpage under Chapter 5 in files named `diasorin.bugs`.

Predictive Densities. Figure 5.3a gives predictive densities for a future log DiaSorin value from the low and normal groups. Note the similarity of the distributional

TABLE 5.4: Posterior summaries on original scale for DiaSorin data, informative prior

Inference target	mean	sd	2.5%	median	97.5%
Pred Dens L			20.1	128.0	821.7
Pred Dens N			34.4	219.9	1416.0
Med: e^{μ_L}	129.1	6.74	116.4	129.0	142.8
Med: e^{μ_N}	220.6	11.35	199.1	220.3	243.6
RelMed: $e^{\mu_N - \mu_L}$	1.71	0.13	1.48	1.71	1.97

shapes, which is due to the similarity of the precisions (see Table 5.3). With similar precisions, it becomes clear that the "normal" group has higher scores and that the means characterize the differences between the two distributions.

However, when we consider predictive distributions of DiaSorin scores on the original scale (Figure 5.3b) obtained by exponentiating samples from the predictive distribution on the log scale, we see that these densities are much more difficult to interpret relative to one another. In particular, it is not obvious that the difference in the means of the predictive distributions would be a good measure of how the two distributions differ.

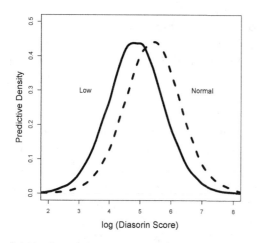 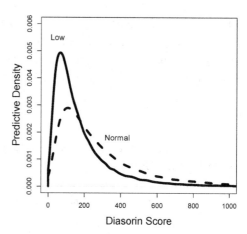

(a) Predictive densities for log(DiaSorin scores). (b) Predictive densities for raw DiaSorin scores.

FIGURE 5.3: Predictive distributions for the analyses of the DiaSorin data. (a) Predictive densities for analyses on the log scale. (b) Predictive densities for the analyses on the original scale.

Predictive Classification. We now address the question of whether a factor like DiaSorin can be used effectively to classify future patients as low or normal in bone turnover based on their DiaSorin score. Suppose, for example, we were to use the cutoff 164. This value is between the two estimated medians, 129 and 220. Our decision rule would assert that an individual had normal bone turnover if their score was greater than 164, and that they had low bone turnover if their score was less than 164. The predictive probability that someone from the "normal" population will score above this value is the area under the "normal" pdf in Figure 5.3b to the right of 164, here 0.63. The predictive probability that someone from the "low" group will score below 164 is the corresponding area under the "low" pdf in Figure 5.3b, here 0.61. These are the probabilities of making correct decisions. Correspondingly, the probabilities of making incorrect decisions are about 0.40 in each instance. This means that using 164 as a cutoff will result in about 40 out of every 100 "normal" individuals being misdiagnosed as "low," and about 40 out of every 100 "low" individuals being misdiagnosed as "normal." It should be clear due to the large overlap in the "normal" and "low" predictive pdfs that, regardless of the choice of cutoff, a substantial number of errors in diagnosis will result if DiaSorin score alone is used to make diagnoses.

5.3 Inferences for Rates

In this section we discuss the Poisson distribution for modeling two-sample data. As previously discussed, Poisson distributions are used to model counts. Examples include the number of emergency department admissions in a day, the number of fatal accidents in a geographic area over a specified period of time, and the number of individuals that become infected with particular virus over a specified geographic area and during a specified time window. With binomial data, we know that a count cannot exceed the fixed number of trials n. A Poisson variate has no obvious upper limit, but the magnitude of counts is usually associated with the length of time period or the size of geographic area.

The two-sample Poisson model has independent observations with

$$Y_i \overset{ind}{\sim} Po(\theta_i M_i), \quad i = 1, 2.$$

As in the one-sample case, M_i denotes a quantity related to the length of time sampling was performed or the size of a geographic area sampled, or the number of person-years sampled in the case of a longitudinal study with many individuals observed over time. θ_i is the rate of occurrence of the type of events that are under study. When events are observed over simple time, the rate is the number of event occurrences per unit time; when counts are observed over space, the rate is the number of events per unit area; and when events are observed in person-years, the rate is the number of events per person-year under study. Each particular situation actually dictates the units to be considered.

5.3.1 Reference Priors

We begin with a generic rate parameter, θ. The Jeffreys prior (Section 6.2) is

$$p(\theta) \propto 1/\sqrt{\theta},$$

which is equivalent to an improper $Ga(0.5, 0)$ distribution. An approximation with a proper gamma prior to the Jeffreys prior is $\theta \sim Ga(0.5, 0.001)$. The Jeffreys prior corresponds to a flat prior on $\gamma \equiv \sqrt{\theta}$. This follows by using the usual transformation technique, $p(\theta) = p_\gamma(\sqrt{\theta})\frac{\partial\sqrt{\theta}}{\partial\theta} \propto 1/\sqrt{\theta}$, since the prior on γ is constant. The Jeffreys prior for the two-sample problem is

$$p(\theta_1, \theta_2) \propto 1/\sqrt{\theta_1 \theta_2}.$$

It is well known that $\sqrt{Y} \mid \theta \stackrel{\cdot}{\sim} N(\sqrt{\theta}, 1/4)$, when θ is moderate to large ($\theta > 15$). This is shown using the delta method in conjunction with the fact that, for large θ, $Y \mid \theta \stackrel{\cdot}{\sim} N(\theta, \theta)$. Thus if we were analyzing Poisson counts that were themselves moderately large, indicating that θs were moderately large also, the usual reference prior for the mean of a normal distribution, in this case $\mu = \sqrt{\theta}$, would be a constant. This leads again to the choice $p(\theta) \propto 1/\sqrt{\theta}$ just as above when we let $\gamma = \sqrt{\theta}$. Arguing by analogy with placing a constant prior on the mean of a normal distribution, we expect posterior inferences to depend very little on this prior. We thus refer to it as a reference prior.

5.3.2 Informative Priors

For a generic rate θ, the conjugate prior is a $Ga(a_0, b_0)$. We again elicit a value for the prior mode θ_0, and for the α quantile, say c, for a chosen α. The mode of the $Ga(a_0, b_0)$ distribution is

$$\theta_0 = \frac{a_0 - 1}{b_0}, \quad a_0 \geq 1.$$

If $a_0 \leq 1$, the mode is 0. We solve to get a_0 as a function of b_0:

$$a_0(b_0) = 1 + b_0 \theta_0.$$

With specified mode θ_0, we thus have

$$\alpha = \int_0^c Ga(\theta \mid a_0, b_0)d\theta = \int_0^c Ga(\theta \mid 1 + b_0\theta_0, b_0)d\theta.$$

With a computer routine that gives the α quantile of a gamma distribution, we can find the values of b_0 by trial and error, which then determines a_0 as above. GammaBuster, which is a "shinyapp" that is analogous to BetaBuster, is available at https://gjones.shinyapps.io/priorapp/. For example, if we wanted a gamma prior with $\theta_0 = 30$ and with 95th percentile = 40, we find it quickly in GammaBuster to be approximately $Ga(34.16, 1.11)$. Alternatively, one can use the R function pgamma(alpha,1+b0*theta0,b0) iteratively with different choices of b0 until the result is close to α.

5.3.3 Nurses' Health Study Data Analysis

The Nurses' Health Study (Colditz et al. [83]) sought to estimate and compare the rates of breast cancer for 50–59-year-old postmenopausal women who were current users of estrogen replacement therapy (group 1) and those who were not (group 2). The data are given in Table 5.5.

TABLE 5.5: Breast cancer data

Group	Cases	Person-years
1—Hormone therapy	123	46,524
2—None	288	145,159

There were two cohorts of women who agreed to be in the study. The first cohort involved women who were on hormone therapy. During the course of the study, $M_1 = 46{,}524$ is the number of woman-years during which 123 women developed breast cancer. The second group involved women who were not using hormone therapy and $M_2 = 145{,}159$ is the number of woman-years during which 288 women developed breast cancer. The "size" of the group of women not on hormone therapy was on the order of three times the "size" of the group who were on hormone therapy, so one would expect three times as many cancers in that group compared to the hormone users on this basis alone.

We assume independent conjugate priors as discussed above. With

$$\theta_i \overset{ind}{\sim} Ga(a_i, b_i), \quad i = 1, 2,$$

we get independent posteriors

$$\theta_1 \mid y_1, M_1 \sim Ga(a_1 + y_1, b_1 + M_1),$$
$$\theta_2 \mid y_2, M_2 \sim Ga(a_2 + y_2, b_2 + M_2).$$

In addition to estimating the individual rates, θ_1 and θ_2, we also estimate the difference of rates (means) $RD = \theta_1 - \theta_2$, and the relative rate $RR = \theta_1/\theta_2$.

Prior elicitation from experts involves asking them to think about the θ_j independently and in whatever units with which they would be most familiar. We regard the θ_i as rates of breast cancers per 1,000 person-years at risk. Since we have no access to breast cancer experts, we use reference gamma priors on the incidence rates, $a_1 = b_1 = 0.5$, $a_2 = b_2 = 0.001$.

Based on this cohort, there was an estimated rate of 2.65 (2.21, 3.14) breast cancer cases per 1,000 person-years with hormone replacement therapy and 2.06 (1.83, 2.30) without. The 95% probability intervals have little overlap. The posterior median and 95% probability interval for the rate ratio comparing current hormone users to non-users are 1.28 (1.04, 1.58). Moreover, $P(\theta_1 > \theta_2 \mid y_1, y_2) > 0.9884$, so the incidence of breast cancer is higher for 50–59-year-old postmenopausal women who are current users of estrogen replacement therapy. Even knowing the exact posterior distribution, these numbers are easier to obtain by simulation.

We also used $Ga(0.001, 0.001)$ priors for the θs. Posterior inferences for the θs were 2.64 (2.20, 3.13) and 1.98 (1.76, 2.22), respectively. Rate ratio inferences were 1.33 (1.07, 1.64). Most of these are very close to the ones based on the Jeffreys prior, and all are close enough that there would be no practical import to their differences.

It is clear that these data suggest that the rate of breast cancers in the hormone replacement therapy group is greater than in the no-therapy group. We should add that there is considerable controversy about whether or not women should use hormone therapy during or after menopause. We are unaware of any definitive outcome of that controversy, which revolves around the fact that rates for other kinds of cancer have been found to be statistically lower in the hormone therapy group.

5.4   Recap and Readings

This chapter covered some aspects of Bayesian biostatistics and quantitative epidemiology. The sampling distributions that were discussed in the binomial comparisons section are important in epidemiology. Broemeling [55] parallels our own approach to Bayesian biostatistics, but from the point of view of epidemiology. We have emphasized the incorporation of prior information into Bayesian statistical analyses in the form of reference, informative, Jeffreys, and other prior distributions in this chapter. We see this as very important and also constructive. In thinking about what we know about scientifically relevant parameters, we are also forced to think about what are the scientific questions that we should be addressing in the analysis. Geisser [125] gives a full discussion of the relative merits of reference priors for binomial proportions. Tuyl et al. [335, 336] discuss unfortunate consequences associated with a possibly careless specification of priors for binomial proportions when they are very small, which we also discussed. We also addressed the important issue of how to analyze data that require transformation in order to satisfy model assumptions. The use of predictive distributions played a role in this analysis. Geisser was a major proponent of prediction for his entire professional life; details can be found in his monograph [127].

5.5   Exercises

EXERCISE 5.1.   Using calculus, find the mode and 5th percentile of a $Be(10, 1)$ distribution.

EXERCISE 5.2.   Using calculus, find a and b such that a $Be(a, b)$ distribution has a mode of 1 and a 5th percentile of 0.2.

EXERCISE 5.3.   Derive formula (5.2), including the formula for θ_0.

EXERCISE 5.4.   Use BetaBuster to find the $Be(a, b)$ priors for mode 0.75 and 5th percentile 0.60, and for mode 0.01 and 99th percentile 0.02. What is the beta prior when the mode is 1 and the first percentile is 0.80?

EXERCISE 5.5.   Show that $\theta \sim Be(1.6, 1)$ and $\theta \sim Be(1, 0.577)$ both have a mode of 1 and both have $P(\theta < 0.5) = 1/3$. Which of these two does BetaBuster give?

EXERCISE 5.6.   Find three sets of (θ_1, θ_2) values that correspond to $OR = 3$. Give the corresponding RR and RD values. Argue that $OR \doteq RR$ when the θs are close to zero.

EXERCISE 5.7.   Derive the result in equation (5.3).

*EXERCISE 5.8.   Let $X \equiv \{X_{ij} : i = 1, 2; j = 1, 2\}$ be a 2×2 table of counts that sum to n. Let $p \equiv \{p_{ij} : i = 1, 2; j = 1, 2\}$ be the corresponding 2×2 table of population probabilities for individuals falling into these cross-classified categories. Then we have

$$X \sim Mult_4(n, p).$$

Let $X_{i\cdot} = X_{i1} + X_{i2}$, $i = 1, 2$, be the row totals in the table and let $p_{i\cdot} = p_{i1} + p_{i2}$, $i = 1, 2$, be the corresponding row totals for the table of category probabilities. Then show that

$$X_{i1} \mid \{x_{1\cdot}, x_{2\cdot}\} \overset{ind}{\sim} Bin(x_{i\cdot}, p_{i1}/p_{i\cdot}), \quad i = 1, 2.$$

Note: The data in Table 5.1 of Example 5.2 are multinomial, and there we used the result of this exercise to analyze the data as two independent binomial samples.

EXERCISE 5.9.   Reproduce the results of Example 5.2. (We provide example BUGS code on the book's website. The file name is Lymphedema.bug.) Then perform a sensitivity analysis by changing the prior moderately and looking to see if results change enough that you would care.

EXERCISE 5.10.   Suppose we ignore the pre-data information available for the probability of LE and use the $U(0, 1)$ prior for θ_1 and θ_2 instead.

(a) Obtain the corresponding posterior summaries as in Table 5.2 and compare. In particular, notice the direction of change in the effect size measures. Does this agree with the usual intuition that the $U(0, 1)$ is a "less informative" prior?
(b) Write a program that you can use to look at the induced prior on RD, RR, and OR based on using uniform priors on the θs. Use summary information about the induced priors on these quantities to shed light on the obtained posterior results.

EXERCISE 5.11.   The following exercise applies independent logit-normal priors for the θ_i in the lymphedema analysis. Sample BUGS code is available on the book's website in a file named LogitNormalLE.bug. You may use this code or something similar in another language or program.

(a) Run your program for 11,000 iterations and obtain results with a 1,000 iteration burn-in. Observe that results are virtually identical to those obtained using independent $U(0, 1)$ priors.

(b) Now modify the code so that you can get plots of the induced priors on the θ_i. Try different values of d until the induced prior looks the closest to a $U(0, 1)$.

EXERCISE 5.12.   (a) Analyze the Reye's syndrome (RS) data using $U(0, 1)$ priors on $\tilde{\theta}_1$ and $\tilde{\theta}_2$.

(b) Discuss issues of causation and correlation for the RS data. For example, people with high blood pressure are more likely to take beta blocker drugs than people without high blood pressure. Can we conclude that using beta blockers causes high blood pressure?

EXERCISE 5.13.   An expert has no belief that there is or is not an effect of aspirin on the risk of Reye's syndrome (RS), but that if there is one, it will not be "huge" in either direction. They place a $N(0, 2)$ prior on δ, so their best guess for the OR is $e^0 = 1$. The prior also indicates that they are 95% sure that the OR is in the interval

$$\left(e^{(0-1.96*1.414)}, e^{(0+1.96*1.414)}\right) = (0.063, 16.0).$$

The interval is centered on 1 and allows for a broad range of possibilities in both directions. Place the Jeffreys $Be(0.5, 0.5)$ prior on θ_2.

(a) Analyze the RS data according to this expert's prior. (Example code in the BUGS language is available on the book's website. The file name is Reyes.bug.)

(b) Examine the sensitivity of the results to the choice of prior. Try a prior that reflects much more skepticism about any effect, and a prior that suggests that any effect will be a positive one. Also try a $Be(1, 1)$ prior for $\tilde{\theta}_2$ to see what impact that has on the results. Be sure to calculate the posterior probability that $OR > k$ for $k = 1, 2$.

EXERCISE 5.14.   Referring to the previous exercise, another possibility is to elicit prior information for

$$\theta_1 = P(D = 1 \mid E = 1), \quad \theta_2 = P(D = 1 \mid E = 0), \quad \gamma \equiv P(E = 1).$$

With priors on these three parameters, we can use the case-control likelihood to obtain posterior inferences for all parameters of interest, including the risk ratio of the θ_j. However, no matter how large are n_1 and n_2, the posterior for the θs will still have uncertainty that is commensurate with the uncertainty in the prior specification.

    Let θ_1, θ_2, and γ have independent beta priors. Write a program to handle case-control data. *Hint*: Since the model parameters are the $\tilde{\theta}$s and since the prior is on

$(\theta_1, \theta_2, \gamma)$, you will need to solve for the $\tilde{\theta}$s in terms of $(\theta_1, \theta_2, \gamma)$. You will also need to use Bayes' theorem.

EXERCISE 5.15. Let $\theta_i \stackrel{ind}{\sim} U(0,1)$ $i = 1, 2$. Simulate the induced prior on the corresponding odds ratio. Be sure to calculate the prior probability that OR exceeds several values, including 50. Comment.

EXERCISE 5.16. Using the fact $P(D = i, E = j) = P(E = j)P(D = i \mid E = j) = P(D = i)P(E = j \mid D = i)$, show $OR_1 = OR_2$ where the OR_i are defined in Equation 5.4 and just above.

EXERCISE 5.17. Use the approximate reference prior in this exercise.

(a) With possibly unequal variances, analyze the two-sample data that can be found on the book's website (Chapter 5, `dataforEx17.csv`).
(b) Repeat (a) under the assumption of equal variances.
(c) Obtain the predictive densities for the two populations and plot them on the same plot under model (a), and under model (b) on a separate plot. Compare the results. Give thoughts about whether the assumption of equal variances is tenable.

EXERCISE 5.18. It is possible to use the exact reference prior for the precision τ. Let $\gamma = \ln(\tau)$ and $p(\gamma) \propto 1$.

(a) Derive the induced (improper) pdf for γ.
(b) Write a program that uses the exact reference prior.
(c) Redo the analysis in part (a) of Exercise 5.17 using this prior for both precisions, and compare results.

EXERCISE 5.19. Let $\ln(Y_i) \equiv W_i \stackrel{ind}{\sim} N(\mu, \tau)$, $i = 1, \ldots, n$, namely $Y_i \mid \mu, \tau \stackrel{ind}{\sim} LN(\mu, 1/\tau)$.

(a) Derive the pdf for $Y_i \mid \mu, \tau$.
(b) Show that the independence prior with $\mu \sim N(\mu_0, \tau_0)$ and $\tau \sim Ga(c, d)$ results in conditional conjugacy for log-normal data. Give the full conditional distributions in precise form.

EXERCISE 5.20. (a) Perform an analysis for the DiaSorin data (on the book's website under Chapter 5 in `diasorin.csv`) on the original scale using the log-normal model of Exercise 5.19 with at least two different choices of prior. Comment.
(b) Analyze these data with the normal model (not log-normal) and consider inferences based on this *wrong model* assumption. Discuss.

EXERCISE 5.21. This problem will involve simulating two samples from normal distributions under several circumstances. Consider sample sizes $n_1 = n_2 = n$, means $\mu_1 = 20$, $\mu_2 = 20 + \Delta$, for $\Delta > 0$, and standard deviations $\sigma_1 = 5$, $\sigma_2 = 5 + \lambda$, for $\lambda > 0$.

(a) The first goal is to explore circumstances that make it easy or difficult to detect a statistically important difference in means when the standard deviations are equal (e.g., $\lambda = 0$).

(b) The second goal is to explore circumstances that make it easy or difficult to detect a statistically important difference in standard deviations. Explore with increasing sample sizes, $n = 10, 50, 100$, using several different combinations of (Δ, λ). Use independent reference prior approximations for all analyses. Make inferences for comparing means and standard deviations. A statistically important difference in means is defined to be a difference for which the posterior probability that $\lambda > 0$ is at least 0.95 or when the posterior probability that $SDR < 1$ is at least 0.95. To simulate normals in R, use the function `rnorm(n,mu,sigma)`, where n is the sample size, mu is the mean, and `sigma` is the desired standard deviation.

*EXERCISE 5.22.   Derive the Jeffreys prior for θ if $Y \mid \theta \sim Po(\theta)$.

EXERCISE 5.23.   Referring to Section 5.3.2, do a simple search to find b_0 for an example with $\theta_0 = 10$, $c = 30$, and $\alpha = 0.95$, using R. The resulting prior should be approximately $\theta \sim Ga(3.2, 0.22)$.

EXERCISE 5.24.   Differentiate the log of the $Ga(a_0, b_0)$ density and set it equal to 0 to solve for the mode of the distribution.

EXERCISE 5.25.   Reanalyze the breast cancer data using an informative prior where the modes for θ_1 and θ_2 are 3 and 1, respectively, and with 95th percentiles of 10 and 7, respectively. Are the results substantially different from those obtained in Section 5.3.3? (Example BUGS code is available on the book's website in a file named `NursesHealthStudy.bug`. You may want to modify that program or a similar one for this exercise.)

Since the M_i units are in the hundred thousands, the θ_i are rates per hundred thousand. If we changed $M_1 = 46.524$ and $M_2 = 145.159$, the rates would then be per 1,000, which is how we chose to interpret them. Care must be taken in the the analysis program to be sure that reported rates are in the correct units.

EXERCISE 5.26.   Reanalyze the breast cancer data (Section 5.3.3) using the reference prior but now change the data so that $M_1 = 93,000$ and $M_2 = 290,000$, that is, with about twice the amount of person-time. Compare results with those obtained earlier.

EXERCISE 5.27.   Suppose we have completely independent count data $Y = (Y_1, \ldots, Y_n)$ and $X = (X_1, \ldots, X_m)$ from two populations. The sampling model for the first population is $Y_i \mid \theta_1 \overset{iid}{\sim} Po(\theta_1)$ with prior $\theta_1 \sim Ga(a_1, b_1)$, and the sampling model for the second population is $X_j \mid \theta_2 \overset{iid}{\sim} Po(\theta_2)$ with prior $\theta_2 \sim Ga(a_2, b_2)$. Derive the analytical form of the joint posterior distribution for (θ_1, θ_2) and characterize it.

Chapter 6

Specifying Prior Distributions

The topics in this chapter are fundamental to the theory and application of Bayesian statistics at the intermediate and advanced levels. However, not all topics covered in this chapter are required for understanding much of the rest of the book. In a first reading, some may prefer to skip * sections and read them later as deemed necessary.

The specification of priors is extremely important in Bayesian statistics and is accordingly the main topic in this chapter. We have already introduced the topic in some examples in previous chapters, but we believe it deserves additional attention. The main reason is the great potential for misspecification of priors, which can easily lead to what has been termed *garbage in, garbage out*, in computer science and statistics.

In Section 1.3.4 the concept of the "prior" distribution was called an external knowledge distribution containing information outside the data being modeled and analyzed. The distribution is designed to capture such information as it reflects on the probability model for the data. While we have used this phrase "external knowledge distribution" to initially highlight the concept, much throughout the book we use the more traditional "prior distribution" as this terminology is nearly universal in the literature.

Advances in computational methods have made it fairly straightforward to apply Bayesian methods in many scientific contexts. A main goal of Section 6.3 is to emphasize the importance of incorporating scientifically relevant information into priors when it is available. These are called *informative* priors. We also focus on situations when this kind of information is not available, in which case there is obviously still a need to specify an appropriate prior in order to proceed with the Bayesian analysis. When information about scientifically relevant parameters is unavailable, we discuss the use of what we and others call *reference* priors, which are generally specified so as to have a minimal impact on the Bayesian analysis.

There are few general rules for developing priors in the absence of scientifically relevant information, and there are none that we know of that would apply across any broad range of statistical models. Thus, we have to be careful in each instance to study a candidate prior to make certain that it is sensible, not misleading or absurd.

By a reference prior[1] we mean any prior that is not chosen for the information that it models. Rather, it is chosen to provide a common base for people to evaluate

---

[1] We do not restrict our use of the term "reference prior" to the specific technical definition given by Bernardo (1979) [34].

data. Because their use avoids the inconvenience of specifying informative prior distributions, reference priors are sometimes called *convenience priors*.

Historically, there has been considerable effort spent on the development of so-called *non-informative* priors. The name stems from the fact that these priors are *meant* to have little influence on the posterior distribution. While attractive from a semantic point of view, we avoid this terminology. Although priors that have little effect on the posterior do exist, there is really no such thing as a *non*-informative prior. All priors express information about the parameters. Often, the information expressed by these priors is uniquely uninspired in the sense that *nobody would use them to make decisions in the absence of data*. Some may automatically believe from the name that a non-informative prior is genuinely not informative, since no scientific input has been applied. While there will be situations where priors that are so named would have little effect on the posterior, we will give examples of such priors that are in fact, *dis*informative, meaning that they convey a form of disinformation that is contrary to the scientific context. We will also argue that some are plainly silly from a subject-matter point of view.

6.1 Flat Priors

One sort of reference prior is called a flat prior. Consider $Y \mid \theta \sim Bin(n, \theta)$. Often people think that putting a uniform distribution on θ denotes ignorance of the value of θ. As argued by Raiffa, Schlaifer, and Pratt [264, 267], if you are ignorant about θ you should also be ignorant about θ^2, and you cannot find a distribution that is uniform on both θ and θ^2.

Nonetheless, people often use uniform priors for a univariate parameter θ that takes values on the entire real line. That is, they use $p(\theta) = c$, where c is a constant, as a prior. It really does not matter whether one uses $p(\theta) = 1$ or $p(\theta) = 123,456$. The point is that the prior is flat over the entire real line. The point is also that the prior is improper, because $\int p(\theta)d\theta = \infty$ regardless of the constant one chooses for the density. In fact, flat priors are inherently silly. Given any bounded set A and its complement A^c, the integral outside the set A is $\int_{A^c} p(\theta)d\theta = \infty$ whereas the integral inside is $\int_A p(\theta)d\theta < \infty$, so the prior belief is that virtually all weight goes to parameter values that are larger in absolute value than any number you can think of. Moreover, if you have a sampling distribution $p(y \mid \theta)$ and use a flat prior $p(\theta) = 1$, the marginal density for the data $p(y) = \int p(y \mid \theta)d\theta$ often does not exist.

The virtue of a flat prior is that it is often easily overwhelmed by the data. For example, using $p(\theta) = c$, Bayes' theorem gives

$$p(\theta \mid y) = \frac{Lik(\theta)p(\theta)}{\int Lik(\theta)p(\theta)d\theta} = \frac{Lik(\theta)c}{\int Lik(\theta)c\,d\theta} = \frac{Lik(\theta)}{\int Lik(\theta)d\theta}.$$

The posterior is simply a normalization of the likelihood into a density for θ. (Not all likelihoods can be normalized, because not all have finite integrals with respect to θ.)

Example 6.1. Normal Data. Assume independent normally distributed data with unknown mean θ, and known precision τ_0, namely

$$Y_1, \ldots, Y_n \mid \theta \overset{iid}{\sim} N(\theta, 1/\tau_0).$$

Then the likelihood is

$$Lik(\theta) \propto \exp\left[-\frac{\tau_0}{2} \sum_{i=1}^{n} (y_i - \theta)^2\right].$$

With $\bar{y} = (y_1 + \cdots + y_n)/n$ and recalling that $\sum_{i=1}^{n} (y_i - \theta)^2 = \sum_{i=1}^{n} (y_i - \bar{y})^2 + n(\bar{y} - \theta)^2$, we have

$$Lik(\theta) \propto \exp\left[-\frac{n\tau_0}{2} (\bar{y} - \theta)^2\right].$$

As a function of θ, this is proportional to a $N(\bar{y}, n\tau_0)$ density, so the normal distribution is the posterior under a flat prior. For example, with $\sigma_0 = 1/\sqrt{\tau_0}$, a 95% posterior interval with a flat prior is $\bar{y} \pm 1.96\sigma_0/\sqrt{n}$, which is numerically equivalent to, but philosophically vastly different from, the traditional 95% confidence interval for this problem.

Example 6.2. Suppose θ is a variance parameter. Then consider an improper prior on the positive real numbers

$$p(\theta) = \frac{1}{\theta}, \quad \theta > 0.$$

It is improper because $\int_0^\infty (1/\theta) d\theta = \infty$. We transform to $\gamma = \log(\theta) = g(\theta)$ and find the "density" using the usual transformation technique. Noting that $g^{-1}(\gamma) = e^\gamma$ and $de^\gamma/d\gamma = e^\gamma$, the density becomes

$$q(\gamma) = \frac{1}{e^\gamma} \mid e^\gamma \mid = 1, \quad \gamma \in (-\infty, \infty).$$

Thus, our initial prior corresponds to a flat prior on the transformed variate, $\log(\theta)$. Although the prior $p(\theta) = (1/\theta) I_{(0,\infty)}(\theta)$ may work well in the sense that it is not highly influenced by the data, one should never forget that in itself it implies silly things, namely that $p(\theta)$ is either huge if θ is close to 0 or essentially 0 when θ is large.

For

$$Y_1, \ldots, Y_n \mid \mu, \tau \overset{iid}{\sim} N(\mu, 1/\tau),$$

with μ and τ unknown, the traditional "flat" prior is

$$p(\mu, \tau) = \frac{1}{\tau}.$$

One can think of this as $p(\mu, \tau) = p(\mu)p(\tau)$ with $p(\mu) = 1$ and $p(\tau) = 1/\tau$. So in a sense we are taking independent flat priors on μ and $\log(\tau)$.

Example 6.3. Consider an improper prior on the unit interval for a probability θ:

$$p(\theta) = \theta^{-1}(1 - \theta)^{-1}, \quad \theta \in (0, 1).$$

It is improper because $\int_0^1 \theta^{-1}(1 - \theta)^{-1} d\theta = \infty$. We transform to the log odds, $\gamma = \log[\theta/(1 - \theta)] = g(\theta)$, and derive its density. Noting that $g^{-1}(\gamma) = e^{\gamma}/(1 + e^{\gamma})$ and $dg^{-1}(\gamma)/d\gamma = e^{\gamma}/[1 + e^{\gamma}]^2$, the density becomes

$$q(\gamma) = \left(\frac{e^{\gamma}}{1 + e^{\gamma}}\right)^{-1} \left(\frac{1}{1 + e^{\gamma}}\right)^{-1} \left|\frac{e^{\gamma}}{(1 + e^{\gamma})^2}\right| = 1, \quad \gamma \in (-\infty, \infty).$$

Thus, our initial prior corresponds to a flat prior on $\gamma = \log[\theta/(1 - \theta)]$. Although the prior $p(\theta) = \theta^{-1}(1 - \theta)^{-1} I_{(0,1)}(\theta)$ may work well in the sense that it is not highly influenced by the data, one should never forget that in itself it implies that θ is most likely to be essentially either 0 or 1.

The moral of this story is that a flat prior in one parameterization is not necessarily flat in another. So there is nothing intrinsically *non-informative* about a flat prior, at least according to what the negation of the English definition of the word "informative" would imply. However, we did find in Example 6.1 that, with the flat prior selected there, formulas for point and interval inferences were identical to standard frequentist formulas. Moreover, with unknown mean and precision, and with $p(\mu, \tau) \propto 1/\tau$, we also obtain identical formulas for posterior point and interval inferences to standard frequentist intervals based on the Student's t distribution. This was established in the remark on page 53 for the case with both mean and variance unknown, with jointly conjugate dependence prior in Section 3.2.2.

One of the definitions of a *reference* prior is that it leads to Bayesian (posterior) point and interval estimates, as well as predictive inferences, that are the same as a frequentist would obtain without a prior. In this sense, the selected prior is often deemed not to affect the posterior "adversely." We will see later that such reference priors are available for the linear model, so that corresponding Bayesian predictive inferences will again be identical to standard frequentist inferences, but with distinct interpretations of results.

6.2   *Jeffreys Priors

Jeffreys (1946) [177] proposed a class of non-subjective priors for Bayesian problems that can often be termed reference priors. A feature of the Jeffreys prior is that it is often improper, meaning that it does not integrate to 1. So it is often not probability based. However, it has a long history and it has been found to be useful in a number of instances. So we discuss it briefly here.

The Jeffreys prior is defined as

$$p(\theta) \propto \sqrt{I(\theta)},$$

where $I(\theta)$ is the Fisher expected information, which is the expected value of the negative second derivative of the log-likelihood. As mentioned above, this quantity will often integrate to infinity, resulting in an improper prior specification. To its credit, it is non-negative.

Jeffreys proposed it because it is invariant to monotone transformations. What does this mean? In words, it means that if we consider a reparameterization of the model, say $\eta = g(\theta)$, where $g(\cdot)$ is monotone over the domain of θ, then the Jeffreys prior for η is precisely the same as the induced prior that we would obtain for η using the transformation formula $p(\eta) = p(g^{-1}(\eta))|dg^{-1}(\eta)/d\theta|$. Proof of this fact is handled in an exercise.

Example 6.4. Normal Data. Suppose we have independent normal observations with known mean μ_0 and unknown variance σ^2:

$$Y_1, \ldots, Y_n \mid \sigma^2 \overset{\text{iid}}{\sim} N(\mu_0, \sigma^2).$$

With precision $\tau = 1/\sigma^2$, the likelihood for τ (up to a constant) is

$$Lik(\tau) \propto \prod_{i=1}^{n} \tau^{1/2} \exp\left\{ -\frac{\tau}{2}(y_i - \mu_0)^2 \right\} = \tau^{n/2} \exp\left\{ -\frac{\tau}{2} \sum_{i=1}^{n}(y_i - \mu_0)^2 \right\},$$

leading to

$$\log\{Lik(\tau)\} \propto \frac{n}{2}\log(\tau) + \left\{ -\frac{\tau}{2} \sum_{i=1}^{n}(y_i - \mu_0)^2 \right\}.$$

The derivative of the log-likelihood is

$$\frac{d}{d\tau}\log\{Lik(\tau)\} = \frac{n}{2}\tau^{-1} + \left\{ -\frac{1}{2} \sum_{i=1}^{n}(y_i - \mu_0)^2 \right\}$$

and the second derivative is

$$\frac{d^2}{d\tau^2}\log\{Lik(\tau)\} = -\frac{n}{2}\tau^{-2}.$$

So, Jeffreys prior for this problem is

$$p(\tau) \propto \sqrt{\frac{n}{2}\tau^{-2}} \propto \frac{1}{\tau}.$$

Example 6.5. Binomial Data. Let $Y \mid \theta \sim Bin(n, \theta)$, so

$$Lik(\theta) = \theta^y(1 - \theta)^{n-y}.$$

The log-likelihood is proportional to $y\log(\theta) + (n - y)\log(1 - \theta)$. The derivative is $(y/\theta) - (n - y)/(1 - \theta)$ and the negative of the second derivative is $(y/\theta^2) + (n - y)/(1 - \theta)^2$. The expected value of this under the binomial assumption is

$$\frac{n\theta}{\theta^2} + \frac{n - n\theta}{(1 - \theta)^2} = n\left\{ \frac{1}{\theta} + \frac{1}{(1 - \theta)} \right\} = \frac{n}{\theta(1 - \theta)}.$$

Then Jeffreys prior is

$$p(\theta) \propto \theta^{-1/2}(1-\theta)^{-1/2},$$

which is a proper $Be(0.5, 0.5)$ distribution. This is a U-shaped prior that favors values of θ close to 1 and 0 and thus would not be a likely candidate for a subjective prior. For example, it would be silly to say that we were equally ambivalent about whether the prevalence of HIV infection was near 1 or near 0, and that it was unlikely to be in the center range of θ.

Remark. Interestingly, the use of Jeffreys priors does not satisfy the *likelihood principle*. What does that mean? Loosely stated, the principle asserts that if two likelihoods are the same (up to a constant of proportionality), then inferences should be the same in the two cases. For example, suppose we randomly sample ten individuals from a population of students and we ask each of them if they have had the flu in the last year. Suppose three of them answer yes. Then with θ defined to be the proportion of students in this population who would say yes to this question, we have a binomial likelihood, $Lik_1(\theta) = \theta^3(1-\theta)^7$. Next, suppose we sample students from the same population until we observe the third student who had the flu in the last year. In this instance the random variable is the number of samples that it takes to observe the fixed number of successes. Suppose we observed the third student with the flu on the tenth try. Then we have observed a negative binomial response that results in the likelihood $Lik_2(\theta) = \theta^3(1-\theta)^7$, which is identical to the binomial likelihood. There are different constants that we ignore. According to the likelihood principle, we should obtain the same inferences for θ with the two distinct experiments.

The Jeffreys priors for binomial and negative binomial data are different, however, so the corresponding posterior pdfs are different as well, leading to distinct posterior inferences. This is true because, while finding the negative of the second derivative of the log-likelihood is equivalent in the two cases, the expected Fisher information involves taking an expected value under the two distinct model types. The expected values come out differently in the binomial and negative binomial cases.

6.3 Scientifically Informed Priors

In this section we discuss informative priors. We have previously discussed the importance of eliciting scientifically relevant information for parameters that are, well, scientifically relevant. When θ represents the probability of HIV infection in a population of interest, its relevance is automatic. When sampling a $Bin(n, \theta)$ model, θ is a model parameter, and it is often a scientifically relevant parameter at the same time. It is usually easy to imagine how to obtain information for it. We have already provided a number of examples. Our purpose here is to extend the conversation to more complex situations. In the previous chapter, we considered the two-sample binomial problem, with $Y_i \mid \theta_i \overset{ind}{\sim} Bin(n_i, \theta_i)$, $i = 1, 2$. Usually (but not always) both θ_i will be scientifically relevant. For example, θ_1 might be the proportion of men who survive at least 5 years after diagnosis with lung cancer, and θ_2 might be the corresponding proportion of women.

Before proceeding, we need to discuss the key assumption of prior independence between parameters. For example, with $N(\mu, \sigma^2)$ data, we usually assume independence of knowledge about these two parameters. Similarly with two binomial distributions, we usually assume independence of knowledge about population proportions. We make similar assumptions throughout the book. We now give an example of how to think about this assumption for the binomial case. The thought process is similar for other situations. This argument was made in Bedrick et al. [24], where they discuss priors for model parameters in binomial regression models that are induced from independent informative priors on scientifically relevant binomial proportions.

Example 6.6. Prior Independence for the Two-Sample Binomial Model.
Suppose we have specified prior information as

$$\theta_1 \sim Be(5, 5), \quad \theta_2 \sim Be(7, 3),$$

for which 95% prior probability intervals are $(0.21, 0.79)$ and $(0.40, 0.93)$, respectively. Consider the hypothetical situation in which we are informed that θ_1 is near its mode 0.5. Since this information is completely consistent with prior information, we would have no reason to alter the prior for θ_2. We argue that if we were informed that θ_1 was a particular value within most of the range of the above 95% interval for it, we would still choose not to revise the prior on θ_2. Consequently, since we would not think about revising the prior for θ_2 when informed in this way about θ_1, we are comfortable regarding these parameters independently.

A counterargument supposes that we are informed that $\theta_1 = 0.9$. Then, clearly, we would want to revise our prior for θ_2, and clearly we would not be thinking of knowledge being independent. Under this purely hypothetical scenario, it would be clear that our prior for θ_1 was poorly informed, which would likely lead us to believe that our prior on θ_2 was also bad.

In fact, under the prior on θ_1, $P(\theta_1 > 0.9) = 0.0009$, so knowing that θ_1 is so large is extremely unlikely under the given prior specification. Consequently, assuming we believe the prior specification, there is no point in considering hypotheticals that we do not consider to be relevant or plausible. Thus, if, after reflection, those situations that might cause concern about independence are believed unlikely, the independence assumption is reasonable.

An alternative situation would be one in which prior beliefs about the parameters were exchangeable, meaning that there was no reason to believe that $\theta_1 > \theta_2$, or vice versa, for example. By definition, such parameters cannot be regarded independently.

We now move on to consider a situation in which the model parameters and the scientifically relevant parameters are not the same. We do this in the context of a multinomial data example.

TABLE 6.1: Lung infection versus smoking

	S	NS			S	NS	
LI	y_{11}	y_{12}	$y_{1\cdot}$	LI	p_{11}	p_{12}	$p_{1\cdot}$
NLI	y_{21}	y_{22}	$y_{2\cdot}$	NLI	p_{21}	p_{22}	$p_{2\cdot}$
	$y_{\cdot 1}$	$y_{\cdot 2}$	n		$p_{\cdot 1}$	$p_{\cdot 2}$	1

Example 6.7. Multinomial Data. Suppose we randomly sample n individuals from a particular population of interest and observe them for a year. After the year, we ask each of them two questions: (i) Are you a smoker (S) or a non-smoker (NS)? (ii) Did you have any form of lung infection (LI) over the course of the year or not (NLI)? The data, $\{Y_{ij}\}$, form a 2×2 table of counts that follows a multinomial distribution with cell probabilities $\{p_{ij}\}$ (see Table 6.1). The model parameters are the p_{ij}. But note that this case is distinct from the sampling scheme discussed in Section 5.1, where independent binomial samples were considered. We now define the scientifically relevant parameters.

Let $\theta_1 = P(LI \mid S) = p_{11}/p_{\cdot 1}$, $\theta_2 = P(LI \mid NS) = p_{12}/p_{\cdot 2}$, and $\gamma = p_{\cdot 1} = P(S)$. Thus $p_{11} = \gamma\theta_1$, $p_{12} = (1 - \gamma)\theta_2$, $p_{21} = \gamma(1 - \theta_1)$, and $p_{22} = (1 - \gamma)(1 - \theta_2)$; observe that the cell probabilities sum to 1. Also note that we are unable to think directly about the p_{ij}, although with some effort we can find information for the scientifically relevant parameters $(\theta_1, \theta_2, \gamma)$. We place independent beta priors on them. Primary inferential interest would focus on the difference $\theta_1 - \theta_2$, or the ratio θ_1/θ_2. In the worst case, if absolutely nothing is known about $(\theta_1, \theta_2, \gamma)$, we could use uniform priors. But of course at a minimum, it would be easy to go on the web to obtain information about the proportion of smokers.

The next example illustrates a situation with two distinct parameterizations for the same model, where in the first instance the parameters are scientifically relevant, and in the second they are not. In general, it is important to know how to shift back and forth between different parameterizations. In the current instance, one version of the model considered is a special case of the well-known logistic regression model that we discuss in Chapter 8.

Example 6.8. The Two-Sample Binomial Revisited. We continue with the model

$$Y_i \mid \theta_i \stackrel{ind}{\sim} Bin(n_i, \theta_i), \quad i = 1, 2.$$

Consider the reparameterized model with

$$\theta_1 = \frac{e^{\beta_1}}{1 + e^{\beta_1}}, \quad \theta_2 = \frac{e^{\beta_1 + \beta_2}}{1 + e^{\beta_1 + \beta_2}}.$$

This is a one-to-one transformation, which means that we have precisely the same model as above, only with different meaning attached to the new parameters. For example, consider the odds ratio

$$OR = \frac{\theta_2/(1 - \theta_2)}{\theta_1/(1 - \theta_1)},$$

which was discussed in Chapter 5. Observing that $\theta_1/(1-\theta_1) = e^{\beta_1}$ and $\theta_2/(1-\theta_2) = e^{\beta_1 + \beta_2}$, we see that

$$OR = e^{\beta_2}, \quad \text{which implies } \beta_2 = \log(OR).$$

We also see that $\beta_1 = \log(\theta_1/(1 - \theta_1)) \equiv \text{logit}(\theta_1)$.

If the model were parameterized in terms of the vector $\beta = (\beta_1, \beta_2)'$, as above, it should be obvious that it would be difficult to directly think about β. It would be equally difficult to specify a prior for β. We would, of course, choose to directly place beta priors on the θs, as we have discussed in Chapter 5; or independent normal priors on $\beta_i = \text{logit}(\theta_i)$, $i = 1, 2$. This is the logit-normal model we discussed in Chapter 5 for the probability θ_i. If we were insistent on the parameterization in β, which we will be in the next chapter, we would then obtain the induced prior on β using the standard transformation technique that we now discuss.

As in Chapter 5, we regard the θs to be independent. Here we are able to display simple BUGS code that will generate the induced prior on β:

```
model{
 theta[1] ~ dbeta(a,b)
 theta[2] ~ dbeta(c,d)
 beta[1] <- logit(theta[1])
 beta[2] <- logit(theta[2]) - logit(theta[1])
}
```

Monitoring the βs, we can plot their induced prior pdfs via histograms.

The general principle that we apply throughout the book is that prior information should be elicited for scientifically relevant parameters to the extent possible, no matter how little may be available. A probability model that reflects the available information about these parameters is then specified. Inference is relatively straightforward if all model parameters are scientifically relevant. There are many details still to consider about placing priors on such parameters, both when information is available and when it is not. When model parameters are not scientifically relevant, we develop a prior for scientifically relevant quantities and then induce a prior on the model parameters. Bayesian inference follows directly by obtaining the corresponding posterior, most often using computational methods resulting in samples from the posterior.

Situations will commonly arise in which there are *many* parameters. It is generally difficult to specify information for many parameters in a coherent way, that is, in a way that does not violate the laws of probability. It would also be quite tiresome. In some instances we will be informative about a subset of scientifically relevant parameters, and we will look for priors on remaining parameters that will have a small impact on the analysis.

In what follows, we consider some simple situations in which more information is available for some parameters than for others. More complex examples are given as needed in subsequent chapters.

Example 6.9. Priors for Parameters of the Two-Sample Binomial Model, Continued. Suppose that scientific information is available for θ_1, but none is available for θ_2. Then we can place an informative beta prior on θ_1. If we believe all values of $\theta_2 \in (0,1)$ are equally plausible, then a $U(0,1)$ (i.e., $Be(1,1)$) prior is reasonable.

We now revisit the ubiquitous $N(\mu, \sigma^2)$ problem, where prior information is available for both parameters. This is followed by the situation where there is information for μ but not for σ.

Example 6.10. Priors for Parameters of the Normal Model, Continued.

Let $Y_1, \ldots, Y_n \mid \mu, \sigma^2 \overset{iid}{\sim} N(\mu, \sigma^2)$. We use an informative $N(\mu_0, 1/\tau_0)$ prior for μ, which is conditionally conjugate, meaning that the full conditional for μ is also normal. Recall that using a gamma prior for $\tau = 1/\sigma^2$ is also conditionally conjugate; however, τ is not easy to think about directly. It would be easier, but still somewhat difficult, to think about σ. At least the scale for σ is the same as for the data, and we can think about the actual support values for the data. For example, we know that ages cannot be very far above 100, thus we know that σ for age data would have to be less than 100, and would certainly be much less.

The 90th percentile of the $N(\mu, \sigma^2)$ distribution, $\gamma_{0.90} \equiv \mu + 1.28\sigma$, is a parameter that a scientist can think about. It is the value in the population that has 90% of all values below it and 10% above. If we also have information for μ (specifically the prior guess μ_0), we can think about the scientifically relevant parameter, $\gamma_{0.90}$, conditionally on $\mu = \mu_0$. As previously, we regard knowledge about μ and σ independently.

Suppose our best guess for $\gamma_{0.90}$ is m. Then our best guess for σ is $\sigma_0 = (m - \mu_0)/1.28$. Moreover, suppose that we are 95% certain that $\gamma_{0.9} < u$ for some $u > m$. Then

$$
\begin{aligned}
0.95 = P(\gamma_{0.9} < u \mid \mu = \mu_0) &= P(\sigma < (u - \mu_0)/1.28 \mid \mu = \mu_0) \\
&= P(\sigma < (u - \mu_0)/1.28).
\end{aligned}
$$

Thus $\sigma_{0.95} = (u - \mu_0)/1.28$ is the 95th percentile of the prior distribution of σ.

There are many possible choices of distribution for incorporating this prior knowledge, including the conditionally conjugate prior for $1/\sigma^2$. If we forget about conditional conjugacy, the gamma distribution for σ is a candidate since its support is $(0, \infty)$. We choose the log-normal distribution, since it is easier to find the precise prior distribution that has these characteristics. We remind the reader that specifying a prior is not rocket science. We are mainly interested in incorporating the prior scientific input in a reasonable way. We want the prior to cover a reasonable range of possible values for the parameter of interest. In the informative case, the precise form of the distribution is not expected to have a major impact on the posterior. Despite the lack of conditional conjugacy, modern computing methods often handle this issue with ease.

Specifying $\log(\sigma) \sim N(a, b^2)$, in other words a log-normal prior for σ or $\sigma \sim LN(a, b^2)$, we can easily find a and b values that result in the prior on σ having median σ_0 and 95th percentile $\sigma_{0.95}$. The median (and mode) of the

$LN(a, b)$ distribution is e^a, so we must have $a = \log(\sigma_0)$, since the log transformation is monotone and increasing. Moreover, the quantiles of the normal distribution transform directly, so the 95th percentile for σ is $\sigma_{0.95} = e^{a+1.645\,b}$. Thus we set $u = e^{\log(\sigma_0)+1.645\,b}$ to obtain $b = [\log(u) - \log(\sigma_0)]/1.645$.

Partially Informative Case. We continue with the same example. Some may find it difficult to specify u and/or m. The simplest solution in this case is to let $p(\tau) \propto 1/\tau$ while keeping the informative normal prior for μ. This is the Jeffreys prior for the known μ case. Packages for performing Bayesian analysis may not have this prior as an option. A solution is to observe that for a $Ga(a, b)$ prior on τ, we have $p(\tau) \propto \tau^{a-1}e^{-b\tau}$, which is approximately equal to $1/\tau$ for small a and b. This prior would not be used to make inference in the absence of data. However, with data, we expect little harm to come from its use as it is the standard diffuse reference prior for the normal model.

An alternative prior specification for σ that involves a little thought proceeds as follows. Suppose we still have a best guess for μ, namely μ_0. Also suppose that we would be incredulous that $\gamma_{0.9}$ could be larger than u^*. In this instance we get an upper bound for σ, $\sigma^* = (u^* - \mu_0)/1.28$. We could then place a $U(0, \sigma^*)$ prior on σ. For example, suppose we are looking at blood pressure data. If our best guess for the mean SBP is $\mu_0 = 130$, and we are 100% certain that $\gamma_{0.9}$ cannot be larger than $u^* = 190$, we have $\mu_0 + 1.28\sigma < 190$, which leaves us with $\sigma < (190 - 130)/1.28 = 47$, which is very conservative since two standard deviations is 94. It is interesting that a $Ga(0.001, 0.001)$ has prior probability 0.9975 that $\sigma < 47$ (using the `pgmama()` function in R).

Subsequent chapters present more examples of the basic principles that were presented here for prior elicitation and specification. The details may vary, but the basic approach is always the same. Specify priors on objects that you and/or an appropriate scientist can think about. Then convey that information through probability transformation onto the model parameters. Finally, obtain posterior inferences, having induced real prior information for those model parameters in a sensible way.

6.4 *Data Augmentation Priors

By definition, a data augmentation prior (DAP) has the same form as the likelihood. In other words, we base the prior for the parameters on "prior observations" that give rise to a likelihood that has the same form as the likelihood for our data. This results in a posterior that is also in the same form as the likelihood. With large sample sizes, standard software can be used in conjunction with a data file that is augmented by the "prior data observations." This results in large-sample posterior inferences corresponding to the specified DAP. The same software using only the observed data would result in large-sample MLE-based inferences.

We return to Example 6.8, which involved the reparameterization of the standard two-sample binomial model. With the independent beta priors that were assumed there, we establish that the induced prior on the β coefficients is a DAP.

Example 6.11. The Two-Sample Binomial, Continued. Recall that we have

$$Y_i \mid \theta_i \stackrel{ind}{\sim} Bin(n_i, \theta_i), \quad \text{logit}(\theta_1) = \beta_1, \quad \text{logit}(\theta_2) = \beta_1 + \beta_2.$$

We first show how this can be reframed as a regression model. Define covariate values $x_1 = 0$ and $x_2 = 1$. Then the observed data can be expressed as $\{(y_i, x_i) : i = 1, 2\}$ where the y_i are realizations of the random binomial variables above, and the x_i are regarded as fixed known covariates that are expected, in general, to be related to the y_i. We rewrite the model as

$$Y_i \mid x_i \stackrel{ind}{\sim} Bin(n_i, \theta_i), \quad \text{logit}(\theta_i) = \beta_1 + x_i \beta_2, \quad i = 1, 2.$$

This corresponds to

$$\theta_i = \frac{e^{\beta_1 + x_i \beta_2}}{1 + e^{\beta_1 + x_i \beta_2}}. \tag{6.1}$$

So we see that the probability of a success depends on whether x_i is 1 or 0, unless $\beta_2 = 0$. Thus $\theta_1 = \theta_2$ if and only if $\beta_2 = 0$ if and only if $OR = e^{\beta_2} = 1$.

The likelihood function is

$$Lik(\beta) = \prod_{i=1}^{2} \left\{ \frac{e^{\beta_1 + x_i \beta_2}}{1 + e^{\beta_1 + x_i \beta_2}} \right\}^{y_i} \left\{ \frac{1}{1 + e^{\beta_1 + x_i \beta_2}} \right\}^{n_i - y_i}. \tag{6.2}$$

Recall that $\beta_1 = \text{logit}(\theta_1)$ and $\beta_2 = \text{logit}(\theta_2) - \text{logit}(\theta_1)$. We write the transformation in vector notation, with $\theta = (\theta_1, \theta_2)$:

$$\beta = \begin{pmatrix} \beta_1 \\ \beta_2 \end{pmatrix} = \begin{pmatrix} \text{logit}(\theta_1) \\ \text{logit}(\theta_2) - \text{logit}(\theta_1) \end{pmatrix} = \begin{pmatrix} g_1(\theta) \\ g_2(\theta) \end{pmatrix} = g(\theta).$$

The inverse of this transformation is $g^{-1}(\beta) = \theta$, where the θ_i are given as functions of β in equation (6.1).

The standard transformation formula for obtaining the induced prior density function for β, $p(\beta)$, from the prior pdf $p(\theta)$ for θ, is

$$p(\beta) = p(\theta) \mid J \mid_+,$$

where θ in $p(\theta)$ are written as functions of β using (6.1), $| \cdot |_+$ denotes the absolute value of the determinant, and J is the 2×2 matrix of partial derivatives of $g^{-1}(\beta)$ with respect to β (i.e., the Jacobian). Using equation (6.1) again, we obtain

$$J = \begin{pmatrix} \theta_1(1 - \theta_1) & 0 \\ \theta_2(1 - \theta_2) & \theta_2(1 - \theta_2) \end{pmatrix},$$

where the θ_i are functions of β, again using equation (6.1). Thus

$$\mid J \mid_+ = \theta_1(1 - \theta_1)\theta_2(1 - \theta_2) = \prod_{i=1}^{2} \theta_i(1 - \theta_i).$$

We allow for the possibility of an informative prior by specifying $\theta_i \overset{ind}{\sim} Be(a_i, b_i)$. This specification leads to a posterior that is in the same form as the likelihood. It will be slightly easier to recognize this fact if we reparameterize to let $a_i = \tilde{y}_i$ and $b_i = \tilde{n}_i - \tilde{y}_i$. Thus $\tilde{n}_i = a_i + b_i$. We obtain

$$p(\beta) \propto \prod_{i=1}^{2} \theta_i^{\tilde{y}_i - 1}(1 - \theta_i)^{\tilde{n}_i - \tilde{y}_i - 1} \prod_{i=1}^{2} \theta_i(1 - \theta_i) = \prod_{i=1}^{2} \theta_i^{\tilde{y}_i}(1 - \theta_i)^{\tilde{n}_i - \tilde{y}_i}.$$

So we see that this is in exactly the same form as the likelihood function in equation (6.2), so it is a DAP. Now let $\tilde{x}_1 = 0$ and $\tilde{x}_2 = 1$. Since the posterior is proportional to the prior times the likelihood,

$$p(\beta \mid \boldsymbol{y}) \propto \left\{ \prod_{i=1}^{2} \left\{ \frac{e^{\beta_1 + x_i \beta_2}}{1 + e^{\beta_1 + x_i \beta_2}} \right\}^{y_i} \left\{ \frac{1}{1 + e^{\beta_1 + x_i \beta_2}} \right\}^{n_i - y_i} \right\}$$

$$\times \left\{ \frac{e^{\beta_1 + \tilde{x}_i \beta_2}}{1 + e^{\beta_1 + \tilde{x}_i \beta_2}} \right\}^{\tilde{y}_i} \left\{ \frac{1}{1 + e^{\beta_1 + \tilde{x}_i \beta_2}} \right\}^{\tilde{n}_i - \tilde{y}_i},$$

which is in the same form as the prior, resulting in a conjugate DAP.

6.5 Reference Priors

In this section we discuss a number of examples that illustrate the type of priors that we advocate in the absence of substantive scientific information. We hasten to point out that in virtually any modeling situation, there will be some background scientific information that should perhaps not be ignored. This section considers "diffuse" priors that are expected to have little impact on the posterior. At the same time, the process of examining whether we have achieved our goal of minimal impact will involve exploring the consequences of making particular choices. As previously indicated, there are no universal rules for selecting "reference" priors. The concept is illustrated in a series of examples.

Example 6.12. A reference prior for a binomial proportion, θ, would often be $U(0, 1)$. As previously indicated, however, a major goal of a reference prior is that it will have minimal impact on the posterior. If we have $Y \mid \theta \sim Bin(100,000, \theta)$, and if $y = 1$ is observed, the posterior mean is 2/100,002 while the usual frequentist estimate is 1/100,000, resulting in the Bayes estimate being double the usual frequentist estimate. The comparison is worse if $y = 0$, since the posterior mean is 1/100,002 and the frequentist estimate is 0. The problem is that the uniform prior contributes to the posterior information equivalent to a sample of size 2 from the population where there was one success and one failure. The uniform prior in this example corresponds to a data-augmentation prior. The posterior median or mode would be better choices than the posterior mean, but the problem of "arbitrarily" adding one success out of two trials remains.

If we are in a situation where the event being considered is extremely rare, it seems that someone would know that fact and consequently would not have regarded all values for θ as equally plausible. If scientists knew that the event under consideration was rare, it only seems fair that they should quantify that information using a prior.

Example 6.13. As another example, suppose one has just developed a new diagnostic test for a particular infection. (We discuss inference for diagnostic tests in greater detail in Chapter 15.) The quality of a diagnostic test, T, is determined by what are called the test *sensitivity* and *specificity*. Denote $I+$ and $I-$ as "infected" and "not infected," and $T+$ and $T-$ as test positive and negative, respectively. Then the sensitivity is $Se = P(T+ \mid I+)$ and the specificity is $Sp = P(T- \mid I-)$. Diagnostic tests are generally developed so that $Se > 0.5$ and $Sp > 0.5$; otherwise, we might just as well toss a coin to decide whether the individual being tested is positive or negative. At an absolute minimum, $Se + Sp > 1$ is required. Then, provided all possible values of Se and Sp are equally plausible, a possible choice of "flat" prior for each could be $U(0.5, 1)$. It is often the case that scientific information is available for either or both test accuracy measures, in which case independent beta priors are used (Branscum, Gardner, and Johnson [48]).

Example 6.14. Consider a situation, as we have discussed in Chapter 5, where we are interested in comparing two populations with respect to each one's average diastolic blood pressure. Let μ_1 and μ_2 denote these averages. In Chapter 5 we considered only conjugate and reference priors. Here, since we know with virtual certainty that these values must be between 40 and 200, we could place $U(40, 200)$ priors on them. With additional appropriate scientific information, we could further restrict the ranges of the uniform priors on the μs. And of course, we could place a subjective prior on one, and some form of "flat" $U(a, b)$ prior on the other, provided appropriate scientific information is used in choosing a and b.

Example 6.15. The Two-Sample Binomial (Example 6.8), Continued. A choice of diffuse prior for β_i, $i = 1, 2$, might be $\beta_i \sim N(0, 10^6)$. This prior has 95% of its area in the interval $(-2000, 2000)$. Specifying a prior in this way is clearly without any thought about scientific relevance; the scientifically relevant parameters are the θ_i. We have argued for specifying priors on these and then inducing the corresponding prior on the model parameters, β. Now we consider the reverse. Here, we have specified a diffuse prior for the model parameters, so now it is logical to consider the consequences of this choice by looking at the induced prior for the θs. We claimed earlier that the induced prior for each θ would be U-shaped with virtually all of the mass piled up near 0 and 1.

Note that $\beta_1 < -4$ if and only if $\theta_1 < 0.018$. Under this prior, we must have $0.4984 = P(\beta_1 < -4) = P(\theta_1 < 0.018)$. Similarly, $P(\theta_1 > 0.982) = 0.4984$. The induced prior on θ_1 has almost 50% of the probability on values less than about 0.02 and almost 50% of the probability on values greater than 0.98. We also have $P(0.018 < \theta_1 < 0.982) = 1 - 2 \times 0.4984 = 0.0032$. This is indeed a prior that no one would use by itself to make inferences about θ_1. This example illustrates the point that it is important to ascertain if a "diffuse" prior on model parameters induces a reasonable prior on scientifically relevant parameters.

We wrote R code to simulate the same results:

```
nSim = 10000
TH = matrix(NA, nrow=nSim, ncol=2)
b = sqrt(1000000)
beta = matrix(rnorm(2*nSim, 0, b), nrow=nSim,
                                  ncol=2, byrow=T)
TH[,1] = exp(beta[,1])/(1 + exp(beta[,1]))
TH[,2] = exp(beta[,1] + beta[,2])/(1 + exp(beta[,1]
                                  + beta[,2]))
```

Many of the generated values for `TH` are `NaN`. Thus, there are computer overflow problems when simulating the θs. (Think about calculating e^{β_1} for $\beta = 1,000$ or $2,000$.)

Example 6.16. Prior for Effect Size. We give an illustration of a "diffuse" prior that was selected with the intent for it to be "non-informative." The problem considered involves two independent normal samples with equal variances.

Let $Y_{ij} \overset{ind}{\sim} N(\mu_i, \sigma^2)$, $i = 1, 2$; $j = 1, \ldots, n_i$. A common focus in medical and psychology research is the effect size, $\Delta = (\mu_1 - \mu_2)/\sigma$. If $\Delta = 2$, we know that the difference in population means is two population standard deviations above zero. This is an extraordinary difference and exemplifies a difference that one could actually see. For example, the effect size for the difference between adult male and female heights in the U.S. is 2 (cf. Utts and Heckard [338, p. 541]). If one can actually see the difference, there may be no real need to conduct an expensive experiment to a forgone conclusion. In some literature, effect sizes between 0.2 and 0.5 are common and effect sizes larger than 0.8 are considered quite large.

There are a number of fairly recent Bayesian articles that propose different priors for Δ. See Gönen et al. [147] for a recent discussion. One particular choice of prior is Cauchy$(0, 1)$, that is, a Cauchy with location 0 and scale 1. The Cauchy is also a Student's t with one degree of freedom, so the mean and variance do not exist. The median is 0 and the tails of the pdf are "fat." Under this prior, $P(\Delta > k) \doteq (0.25, 0.15, 0.06, 0.03, 0.003)$ for $k = (1, 2, 5, 10, 100)$, respectively. If a scientist believes that the effect size cannot possibly be larger than 1 or 2, a standard Cauchy prior should be regarded as inappropriate. By considering a Cauchy$(0, b)$ with a small enough b, however, one can cover a more reasonable range of values, though it would still have relatively fat tails.

6.6 Recap and Readings

We have gone into some depth about how, and how not, to specify priors across a range of examples. The general principle is to think about parameters that scientists care about and understand, and to elicit information about these parameters that is independent of the observed data. The parameters that should be easiest to think about are the parameters that would be of most interest when having a discussion with colleagues or even the general public. For example, recall the reparameterization of the two-sample binomial problem in Example 6.8 where $\log(OR) = \beta_2$ was one of the model parameters. If θ_1 was the probability of living at least 5 years after diagnosis with cancer if a particular treatment regimen is used, and θ_2 was the same probability under a second regimen, it would be much more interesting to share the information that

$$P(0.8 < \theta_1 < 0.9 \mid y) = 0.95 \quad \text{and} \quad Pr(0.6 < \theta_2 < 0.7 \mid y) = 0.95,$$

which can be inferred from the information about the individual θ_i, than it would be to tell everyone that $P(0.54 < \log(OR) < 1.8 \mid y) = 0.95$. So thinking about the θ_i *a priori* and then inducing a prior on model parameters is purely logical.

On the other hand, if only a little information is available about the θ_i, it is still logical to specify diffuse priors for them and then to induce a prior onto model parameters. If one insists on placing diffuse priors on β_1 and β_2 in Example 6.8, say, then one should investigate the consequences by looking at the induced prior on the θ_i.

There are many articles in the literature that discuss how to elicit expert opinions that can expressed using probability distributions; see, for example, Kadane et al. [197], Garthwaite and Dickey [120], Kadane and Wolf [199], Ibrahim and Chen [170], Garthwaite, Kadane, and O'Hagan [121], Gill and Walker [144], and O'Hagan et al. [253]. The authors Kahneman and Tversky [200] famously discussed issues related to the quality of subjective determinations of the type involved in prior elicitation. The theory underpinning the types of priors discussed in Bedrick et al. [24] and their generalizations is discussed in Bedrick et al. [23]. Tools for actually finding prior distributions in a variety of families are given and illustrated in Jones and Johnson [191]. Seaman, Seaman, and Stamey [284] discuss a number of potential perils underlying the use of so-called "non-informative" priors.

6.7 Exercises

EXERCISE 6.1. (a) Find the Jeffreys prior and posterior for θ when $Y_1, \ldots, Y_n \mid \theta$ iid $Po(\theta)$.
(b) Now let $\eta = e^{-\theta}$, which is just the probability of no events under the Poisson model. Obtain the induced prior for η, and then obtain the Jeffreys prior for η by reparameterizing the log-likelihood and taking second derivatives of it with respect to η. You should get the same results.

EXERCISE 6.2. Find the Jeffreys prior for θ when $(Y_1, \ldots, Y_n) \mid \theta \overset{iid}{\sim} N(\theta, \tau)$ with known τ.

EXERCISE 6.3. Let $\eta = g(\theta)$ be a monotone transformation. Let $j_1(\theta)$ and $j_2(\eta)$ be the Jeffreys priors for θ and η, respectively.

(a) Derive $j_2(\eta)$ using the reparameterized likelihood, and using the definition of the Jeffreys prior.

(b) Obtain a formula for the induced prior on η, say $r(\eta)$, using the usual transformation technique.

(c) Argue that $r(\eta) = j_2(\eta)$, which means that the Jeffreys prior is invariant to monotone transformations.

EXERCISE 6.4.   Derive the Jacobian, J, given in Example 6.11.

EXERCISE 6.5.   Show that in Example 6.11, placing independent Jeffreys priors on the θs results in a DAP with $\tilde{y}_i = 0.5$ and $\tilde{n}_i = 1$ for $i = 1, 2$.

EXERCISE 6.6.   In Example 6.13, suppose that a random sample of 100 individuals has been taken from a population of interest and a test T applied to all. Let Y be the number that test positive and suppose that $y = 10$ is observed. Let $P(I+) = \pi$, the prevalence of infection in the sampled population.

(a) Using the above notation, give the likelihood function for (π, Se, Sp).

(b) What are the model parameters for this problem?

(c) What are the scientifically relevant parameters?

(d) What kinds of issues might you anticipate if all uniform priors were specified for (π, Se, Sp)?

EXERCISE 6.7.   (a) Run the R code at the end of Example 6.15 and obtain a density plot for θ_1 when $b = 100$. Use the iterates to approximate the prior probability $P(0.02 < \theta_1 < 0.98)$.

(b) Find a value of b that results in an induced pdf for θ_1 that looks crudely like the $U(0, 1)$ pdf.

EXERCISE 6.8.   Use R to verify the probabilities for the Cauchy distribution given in Example 6.16.

Chapter 7

Linear Regression

Regression models lie at the foundation of statistics and biostatistics. They play a major role in the analysis of data across many disciplines. These models are defined mathematically with a functional relationship between the mean of a response variable and one or more predictor variables (also called covariates). In addition, we must also specify a statistical model that describes the variation of individuals from the mean response.

For example, consider the **VetBP** data that was first introduced in Chapter 1 (Example 1.1). Suppose we want to model the baseline diastolic blood pressure (DBP) as a function of age. Here age is the predictor variable and DBP is the response variable. The regression function would describe how *average* diastolic blood pressure relates to age. If Y represents DBP and X represents age, then the regression of DBP on age is $E(Y \mid X)$. Regression models characterize this relationship through functions of predictor variables (or covariates) and parameters. The simplest functional relationship is no relationship—*average* DBP is the same regardless of age, $E(Y \mid X, \beta_0) = \beta_0$.

Next, we might consider a simple linear relationship between DBP and age, namely $E(Y \mid X, \beta_0, \beta_1) = \beta_0 + X\beta_1$. We might consider the effect of age on DBP by studying the difference in mean response for two distinct age groups of individuals who are d units in age apart. Taking the difference between the mean values for the older and younger individuals, we obtain $d \times \beta_1$, since β_0 cancels. If $d = 10$ and $\beta_1 = 0.5$, for example, the average DBP for individuals who are 10 years older would be 5 units (mm Hg) higher, regardless of their actual ages under this model. The value of d is often taken to be 1, but this difference in age may not be as interesting to interpret. Asserting that the one-year-older age group would have mean DBP response 0.5 units higher just does not seem as interesting or even practically important.

Nonetheless, a change in mean blood pressure corresponding to a single year's difference in ages is represented by the parameter β_1, which corresponds to the slope on a graph of mean DBP (y-axis) and age (x-axis). We apply the methods of linear regression to learn about the value of β_1, and $d \times \beta_1$ for appropriately chosen d. We also consider adding other predictor variables, as well as the possibility deleting any, including age, that may not be useful in predicting DBP. An important aspect of the development is to recognize that patients of the same age will not all have the same DBP. This requires a statistical model specifying how individual values of DBP distribute around the mean value given by the regression line for any age.

In regression modeling, it is important to distinguish two types of predictor variables: numerical and categorical. Examples of numerical predictors are age, weight, body mass index, number of nodes examined in breast cancer surgery, and number of children. Measurements here are numbers that are meaningful on an interval scale.

Alternatively, there are categorical predictors, such as smoking status (with categories: current, past, never) and marital status (married, divorced, never married). We would not want to label three categories with the numbers 1, 2, 3, and then treat them as if they were numerical. If we place a regression coefficient in front of such a variable, with only that variable in the model, the implication would be that the difference in mean response between the third and first categories would be twice the difference between the second and first categories. Thus the distinction between numerical and categorical variables is necessary to interpret the model parameters properly. We begin with the case of a single numerical predictor, then move on to categorical predictor(s) and to combining multiple predictors, introducing along the way various concepts arising in linear models.

Section 7.1 introduces the regression model and its basic analysis with one and multiple predictors. Section 7.2.1 introduces a matrix formulation for regression and discusses analytic posterior inference with flat priors. We then describe five different types of priors in Section 7.3. Interaction is introduced in Section 7.5. Section 7.6 presents analysis of variance from the Bayesian viewpoint, using the model formulation already discussed. The chapter concludes with a recap and further readings in Section 7.7.

7.1   The Linear Regression Model

Linear regression models generally presume that variation about the mean is normally distributed. The normal distribution was discussed in detail in previous chapters. Here we extend the normal model to involve data with a response and one or more predictor variables (sometimes called "covariates"). Generally, Y refers to the response or dependent variable, and X refers to the predictors (or covariates). We assume the data consist of sets of observations for each of n *units*, $\{(y_i, x_i) : i = 1, \ldots, n\}$, where the x_i may be vectors of covariates. Furthermore, we will assume that the outcomes that we observe vary randomly about a linear function of parameters and covariates that characterizes the outcome-specific expected values. The random deviation about the expected value follows a normal distribution in the linear regression model, with the variance of this normal distribution not changing with covariates. Mathematically, we write the statistical model in two parts:

$$Y_i \mid X_i, \beta \overset{\text{ind}}{\sim} N\left(E[Y_i \mid X_i, \beta], \sigma^2\right), \quad i = 1, \ldots, n, \tag{7.1}$$

$$E(Y_i \mid X_i, \beta) = \beta_0 + X_{i,1}\beta_1 + X_{i,2}\beta_2 + \ldots + X_{i,p}\beta_p. \tag{7.2}$$

As in previous chapters, we will also use the notation $\tau = 1/\sigma^2$ for precision as the reciprocal of variance.

Although the predictor variables often result from random sampling in practice, we *always* condition on them in this chapter; hence, we treat them as fixed, denoting them using lower-case letters as $(x_{i1}, \ldots, x_{ip})$. Covariate combinations can consist of continuous variables, categorical variables, or a mix of data types. The standard analysis of variance (ANOVA) model characterizes group-specific means and is a linear model with categorical covariates. Traditionally, the analysis of covariance (ANCOVA) is the special case in which there is a categorical and a continuous covariate. Both of these models are special cases of the linear regression model above.

7.1.1 Simple Linear Regression: Single Numeric Predictor

We first illustrate basic concepts by considering a simple linear regression. Simple linear regression predicts a continuous (measurement) response using only an intercept and one predictor variable. In this simple case, the likelihood is a function of the three parameters (β_0, β_1, τ).

Figure 7.1 shows what is called a scatter diagram of diastolic blood pressure versus age in the **VetBP** data introduced in Example 1.1. At each age there is appreciable variation in the blood pressure, and overall there is a downward trend as age values increase. A model that could lead to such data can be thought of in terms of the mean blood pressure being a deterministic function of age, with individual blood pressure values at any age scattered about that mean.

Using Y for the response variable (diastolic blood pressure), x for the predictor (age), and following equation (7.2), the conditional mean of Y given x—the deterministic part of the model—is

$$E(Y \mid x, \beta) = \beta_0 + \beta_1 x.$$

The model states that the relationship between average DBP and age is linear in age (x), with two regression coefficients: the intercept, β_0, and slope, β_1. Notice that the left-hand side in the above equation is the conditional expected value of Y given x and not an individual measurement. That is, we are modeling the conditional mean of Y as a linear function of the covariate x. The name *linear regression* comes from the model of the conditional mean of Y as a linear combination of regression coefficients times covariates.

To describe variation of individuals from this line, we need a statistical model as in equation (7.1), equivalently written as

$$Y = \beta_0 + \beta_1 x + \varepsilon, \quad \varepsilon \sim N(0, \sigma^2).$$

The model thus assumes that at each x, the distribution of deviations from the corresponding mean of Y is normal, with some variance σ^2. In practice, we need to model x and y values for several individuals, so we write

$$Y_i = \beta_0 + \beta_1 x_i + \varepsilon_i, \quad \varepsilon_i \overset{iid}{\sim} N(0, \sigma^2), \ i = 1, \ldots, n.$$

Now we have added two more assumptions: (1) the deviations from the mean,

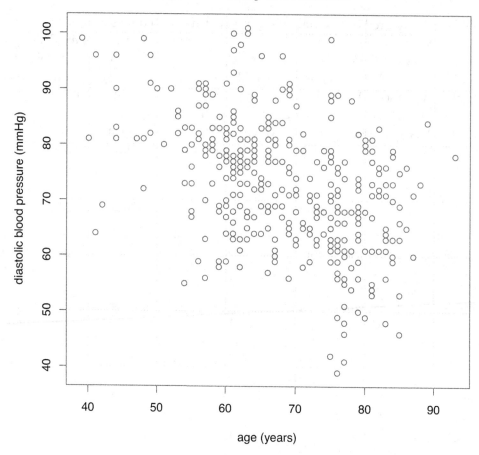

FIGURE 7.1: Scatter diagram of DBP versus age (**VetBP** data).

the ε_i, have the same scatter, no matter the value of the covariate; and (2) the ε_i $(i = 1, \ldots, n)$ are independent random variables. Figure 7.2 shows a stylistic picture of the model and the meaning of the parameters β_0 and β_1. The density curves centered on the regression should actually be drawn in the third dimension and aligned parallel to the y-axis, so that individual measurements Y generated from any given curve are all at the same value of x.

Combining equations (7.2) and (7.1), the model is

$$Y_1, \ldots, Y_n \mid \beta, \sigma^2 \overset{ind}{\sim} N(\beta_0 + \beta_1 x_i, \sigma^2),$$

which with $\tau = 1/\sigma^2$ leads to the likelihood

$$Lik(\beta_0, \beta_1, \tau) = p(y_1, \ldots, y_n \mid \beta_0, \beta_1, \sigma^2) \propto \prod_{i=1}^{n} \sqrt{\tau} e^{-\frac{\tau}{2}\{y_i - (\beta_0 + \beta_1 x_i)\}^2}.$$

With priors for the parameters β_0, β_1, and τ, we can proceed to sampling the posterior using MCMC methods.

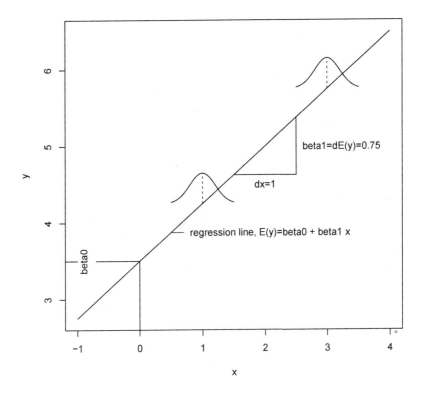

FIGURE 7.2: A depiction of the linear regression model with intercept $beta_0$ and slope $beta_1$.

7.1.2 From Model to Data Analysis

Adding priors to the sampling model, we can convey the linear regression model to Bayesian MCMC software (BUGS, JAGS, Stan, etc.); for example, in BUGS we use the model statements

```
model{
  for(i in 1:n){
    mu[i] <- beta0 + beta1 * x[i]
    y[i] ~ dnorm(mu[i],tau)
  }
  tau ~ dgamma(a,b)
  beta0 ~ dnorm(mubeta0,taubeta0)
  beta1 ~ dnorm(mubeta1,taubeta1)
}
```

The form of the priors used here should be familiar from Section 3.2.2 on normally distributed exchangeable data. It is like the independence prior there, which here, too, is conditionally conjugate for Gibbs sampling (see Section 7.3 below). Now we must choose the six parameters

```
(a, b, mubeta0, taubeta0, mubeta1, taubeta1).
```

With x[] containing the ages of the veterans in years, β_0 represents the mean

DBP for veterans of age 0. Clearly, this is not meaningful and only represents a mathematical abstraction. It is, therefore, not wise to express any knowledge about such a parameter directly. However, if we define the "centered" age variable $cx =$ Age $- 60 = cAge$, now with $cAge = 0$ we see that β_0 represents the mean DBP of 60-year-old veterans.[1] While this β_0 is unknown, a reasonable prior guess might be 75, so we could set `mubeta0 = 75`.

In the absence of additional real scientific knowledge, we could allow a considerable degree of uncertainty about it by taking the prior standard deviation for β_0 to be 10, say. This expresses the knowledge that the mean DBP of 60-year-old veterans can range from 55 to 95 with 95% probability. Notice that this interval is not for an individual's blood pressure; it is for the population mean. We can see that this is a very wide interval expressing very little information. A standard deviation of 10 is translated into precision as `taubeta0`$= 1/100 = 0.01$.

Next we must express our knowledge about the regression coefficient β_1. If we also have a prior guess for the mean DBP for 50-year-old veterans, say pg_{50}, then we can set $pg_{50} = \beta_0 - 10\beta_1$, from which we obtain prior guess for β_1, namely $(75 - pg_{50})/10$. If $pg_{50} = 70$, we would set `mubeta1`$= 0.5$. Suppose, on the other hand, that we are uncertain about whether mean DBP would increase or decrease from 75 for veterans who are older or younger than 60. In this case, we can take `mubeta1` $= 0$.

Next we need to specify `taubeta1`, which involves a little more effort. Suppose that we are virtually certain that, combining veterans of all ages in the age range of the data, the mean DBP is between 50 mm Hg and 100 mm Hg. This is a rather wide interval for such averages for DBP. Then using the prior guess for β_0, this information translates to $50 < 75 + cAge\,\beta_1 < 100$, or $-25 < cAge\,\beta_1 < 25$. Since the range of ages in the data is 35 to 85, or equivalently $-25 < cAge < 25$, we must have $-1 < \beta_1 < 1$. It is then reasonable to take a prior standard deviation for β_1 to be 0.5 as this gives 95% prior probability that β_1 is in this range, leading to `taubeta1`$= 1/0.25 = 4$.

The third unknown, τ, or equivalently σ, represents the variation in individual blood pressures at any fixed age. An extreme range would be about 60 mm Hg, implying $2\sigma = 30$, which translates to believing that $\sigma < 15$. Thus a prior guess for a lower bound for τ is $1/225 = 0.004$. For a low limit on σ, a tight range for individual DBPs at any fixed age would be 25. This leads to $2\sigma > 12.5$, or $\tau < 0.0256$. By trial and error using R functions `pgamma()` and `qgamma()`, we find that a $= 5$ and b $= 400$ yields a 95% interval for τ, $(0.0041, 0.0256)$. The corresponding interval for σ is $(6.25, 15.7)$, with a median of 9.25.

With these prior parameters, carrying out the analysis (using code on the book's webpage for Chapter 7 in files named `dbpage.R` and `dbpagemodel.txt`), we constructed Table 7.1 which shows posterior means, standard deviations, and 95% probability intervals for the three model parameters.

Taking the posterior means as our best estimates of corresponding parameters,

---

[1]We note that the mean age in the data is 68.18. Here, we have not centered age on the mean age.

TABLE 7.1: Posterior summary for **VetDP** analysis with one covariate

	Mean	sd	2.5%	97.5%
β_0	76.5	0.65	75.2	77.7
β_1	−0.49	0.05	−0.59	−0.39
σ	10.1	0.36	9.5	10.8

we can see that the estimated mean DBP among 60-year-olds is 76.5 mm Hg, and that this estimate decreases by about 0.5 mm Hg for each one-year increase in the age in such a population, or about 2.5mm Hg for each five-year increase in age. Of course, there are uncertainties associated with these estimates. These are quantified by the posterior standard deviations and probability intervals. It is quite unlikely, for example, that the population mean DBP at age 60 is higher than 78 mm Hg, and it is virtually certain that the slope of the regression line is negative (see the next two paragraphs!). We also know the variation in DBP from individual to individual up to a reasonable level of uncertainty. The standard deviation very likely is between 9.5 and 10.8 mm Hg.

It is important to point out a somewhat unexpected aspect of the above estimates and a possible explanation of it. For individuals in *this study*, inferences indicate that there is a negative association between age and mean DBP. Since the 95% probability interval for β_1 is well below zero, we are virtually certain that $\beta_1 < 0$. This result is contrary to what we all might believe, namely that as we age, average DBP would increase, not decrease.

We note that the measurements in Dr. Whittle's study were on *different* individuals in the same time-frame. This precludes making conclusions about the progression of DBP in those individuals as they get older. Even so, one might expect cross-sectional data by age to show an increasing trend. The explanation here lies in how the veterans were selected to be part of this study (see Example 1.1). They were asked, through veterans' organizations, to volunteer their participation. It is quite possible that older veterans participating in the activities of the organizations and who agreed to participate in this study were the healthier among their age cohorts. While this is an important point in interpreting the regression results, it has less relevance for Dr. Whittle's study, which aimed to distinguish between the effects of two interventions to lower blood pressure. He randomized the available subjects to the two interventions for that comparison. Randomization should lead to the same distribution of ages in the two treatment groups, so age-related effects on blood pressure should be balanced. Furthermore, one can adjust for the individuals' baseline DBPs, as we will see later in Section 7.1.3.

Limiting our conclusions to the population of those veterans who are active in some veterans' organizations and are inclined to participate in a blood pressure study, we can estimate the mean DBP at any age within the range of ages in the collected data, about 40 to 90 years. For example, at age 70, the posterior mean DBP is $76.5 - 0.49(70 - 60) = 71.6$. Posterior uncertainty is obtained for $\beta_0 + \beta_1(70 - 60)$ by using random samples from the joint posterior to obtain the corresponding approximate 95% posterior probability interval for this mean. With MCMC samples for regression coefficients, vectors beta0 and beta1 in R, we can summarize this posterior distribution by:

```
meandbpat70 <- beta0+beta1*(70-60)
summary(as.mcmc(meandbpat70))
```

We get a posterior mean DBP of 71.6 mm Hg, standard deviation 0.522 mm Hg and a 95% probability interval (70.6, 72.7). As expected, the estimated mean DBP is smaller at age 70 than at age 60. But note also that the standard deviation is smaller. The reason for this is more subtle. The information for the mean of the response variable is higher at values of the predictor that are closer to the mean predictor value in the data. In our case, the mean age is 68.15 years, where the information for estimating the mean response is the highest, or the variation the lowest. As we move away from this central age, the uncertainty of model-based estimates increases. By adding a couple of lines to the R code, you can verify that at age 90, the posterior mean for the mean DBP is 61.75 mm Hg, and the posterior standard deviation is 1.21 mm Hg with the corresponding 95% probability interval being wider, (59.5, 64.3).

We now turn to the prediction of DBP for a randomly chosen individual from the 70-year-old cohort in the population. While we have already seen that the uncertainty in $\beta_0 + \beta_1(70 - 60)$ is propagated from the uncertainty of the regression coefficients (β_0 and β_1), now there is additional variation from individual to individual, represented by σ. Moreover, σ itself is not completely known. As we have posterior samples at hand, we can easily account for all these sources of uncertainty or variation. With each posterior sample of the triplet (β_0, β_1, σ), we can simulate a normal random variate with mean $\beta_0 + \beta_1(70 - 60)$ and standard deviation σ. This yields samples from the *predictive distribution* that we want. Here is the R code:

```
preddbpat70 <- rnorm(length(beta0), beta0+beta1*(70-60), sigma)
summary(as.mcmc(preddbpat70))
```

Not surprisingly, we find the mean of the predictive distribution to be 71.1 (close to 71.6 above; they should be virtually identical up to MCMC error). The predictive standard deviation is 10.3 (considerably larger than mean estimation uncertainty 0.52), as it should be since $\sigma > 0$. The 95% prediction interval is $(51.8, 91.9)$, conditioning on the data and reflecting all remaining uncertainties in the model. We have plotted these in Figure 7.3 at 10-year age intervals from 40 to 90, with a slight offset from the decade points along the horizontal axis for clarity, and to emphasize the distinction between a probability interval for the population mean response and a prediction interval for an individual's response. A careful look also reveals how interval widths increase as one moves from the center of the data outward.

7.1.3   Multiple Covariates: Continuous and Categorical

We continue with the **VetBP** example to illustrate relationships between outcome and more than one predictor variable.

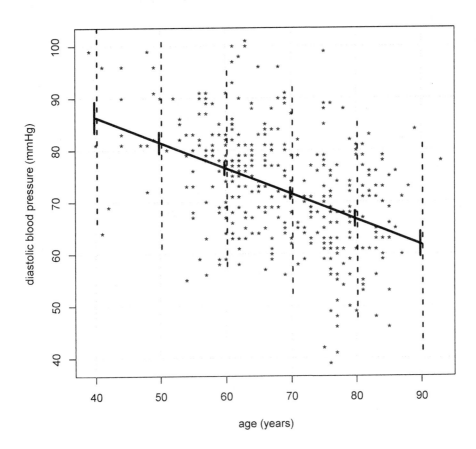

diastolic blood pressure (mmHg)

age (years)

FIGURE 7.3: Estimated regression line (solid sloped line), credible intervals for unknown line (solid vertical lines), and prediction intervals for individual response (dashed vertical lines), **VetBP** data.

Example 7.1. VetBP data. Recall from Example 1.1 that these data came from a randomized study evaluating two different methods of educating and encouraging hypertensive veterans to achieve better control of this condition. One method recruited and trained leaders from the veterans' organizations' posts (or local chapters), who then educated and encouraged their peers (treatment EP). The other method consisted of seminars given by health professionals at the posts (treatment EH). We take $DBP6$ (diastolic blood pressure in mm Hg) *six months after* the start of the educational program to be the outcome or response variable (y). We consider the following four covariates: x_1 = treatment (Trt), which takes the values 1 for EP and 2 for EH; x_2 = baseline DBP $(DBP0,$ mm Hg); x_3 = the participant's height in inches (Ht) at baseline; x_4 = the participant's weight in pounds (Wt) at baseline.

Figure 7.4 shows a scatterplot matrix of the continuous variables (y, x_2, x_3, x_4)

in order to visualize pairwise relationships with the response and between covariates. These plots illustrate that six-month diastolic BP is positively associated with baseline DBP, but the corresponding association with height and weight is less apparent.

The linear regression model for these data is expressed as

$$E(DBP6 \mid Trt, DBP0, Ht, Wt, \beta) = \beta_0 + (Trt - 1)\,\beta_1 + DBP0\,\beta_2 + Ht\,\beta_3 + Wt\,\beta_4,$$

which is a special case of equation (7.2). Why have we written $(Trt - 1)\,\beta_1$ instead of $Trt\,\beta_1$? If we did not subtract 1, $Trt \times \beta_1$ would equal β_1 under treatment 1 (EP) and $2\beta_1$ under treatment 2 (EH). If $\beta_1 > 0$, the implication would be that the added effect (added to β_0) of treatment 2 is assumed to be double the added effect of treatment 1 on the mean response. If $\beta_1 < 0$, the implication would be that the decline in mean DBP under treatment 2 is twice that of treatment 1. This assumption is unreasonable. With the treatment covariate being an indicator variable, coding it as 0 for one treatment and 1 for the other treatment, the regression coefficient is simply the effect of the treatment coded 1 over and above that of the one coded 0; $(Trt - 1)$ achieves this 0/1 coding from the original 1/2. Of course, the 0/1 coding could have been used in the original data to avoid subtracting 1 in the model.

We now turn to analyzing the data. To demonstrate a type of prior choice different from that in Section 7.1.2, we use flat priors on $\beta_0, \ldots, \beta_4$ and $\log(\sigma)$. This is a somewhat commonly used prior (sometimes called a reference prior) in the regression setting. We discuss it more in Section 7.3. Posterior results, using this flat prior, are given in Table 7.2. In addition to inferences for the βs, the table also includes predictive inferences for a new *future* observation y_f with covariates corresponding to a veteran randomized to the EH education program and whose baseline DBP is 84 mm Hg, height is 66 inches, and weight is 230 pounds at the start of the study (i.e., $Trt_f = 2, DBP0_f = 84, Ht_f = 66, Wt_f = 230$). These happen to be covariate values for the person with the highest six-month DBP in the data, 112 mm Hg.

TABLE 7.2: Results of regression of six-month DBP on treatment, baseline DBP, height and weight, with flat priors on the βs and $\log(\sigma)$

	Mean	sd	2.5%	97.5%
Const	9.30	8.53	−7.48	26.07
Trt	−0.86	0.84	−2.50	0.79
DBP0	0.62	0.038	0.55	0.70
Ht	0.24	0.13	−0.006	0.50
Wt	0.005	0.010	−0.015	0.025
$E(y_f)$	78.0	0.85	76.3	79.7
y_f	78.0	8.1	62.0	93.9

The output suggests that we are 95% sure a veteran who receives peer education (EP) will have a DBP, on average, between 2.5 mm Hg lower and 0.8 mm Hg higher

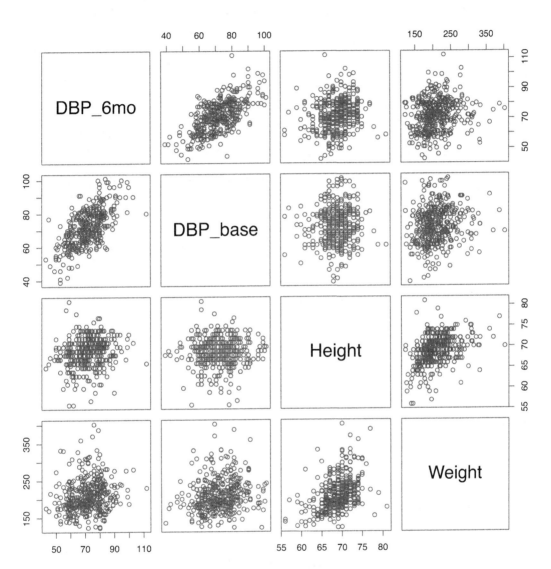

FIGURE 7.4: Pairwise scatterplots for continuous covariates and response.

than a veteran receiving eduction from a health professional (EH), both of them having the same baseline DBP, height, and weight. As this interval implies a possible decrease or increase, it is not clear which group is better off. In other words, with the estimated mean effect equaling -0.86, the interpretation would be that using the EP treatment would be associated with about 0.86 mm Hg lower mean DBP. However, because of the estimation uncertainty, we cannot be confident that EP is superior to EH in lowering DBP. We note also that the question unanswered by this analysis is whether either treatment would be helpful compared with no treatment, and whether the improvement would be clinically meaningful.

From the rest of the table, we can say that we are 95% sure that each additional 5 mm Hg diastolic blood pressure at baseline corresponds to an increased blood pressure after 6 months that is, on average, between 2.5 to 3.5 mm Hg higher, with other variables fixed. But there is a clear statistical import to this result since the 95% posterior probability interval is well above 0. This result does give some insight into within-individual change in DBP over a six-month period. Tempting as it may be, however, it is not possible to interpret this relationship as causal. Finally, the effect of Wt on the six-month DBP (in addition to the effect of baseline DBP) is unclear, based on the posterior distribution of β_4 (its regression coefficient). While the 95% two-sided probability interval for β_3 (coefficient of Ht) contains 0, there is substantial probability that $\beta_4 > 0$.

The future individual's DBP is predicted to be between 62.0 and 93.9 mm Hg with 95% assurance. Now the person in the sample with these covariates had DBP of 112 mm Hg at 6 months. While the wide interval indicates the prediction is not precise, it is still interesting that this veteran's six-month diastolic blood pressure is actually higher than the upper bound of the prediction interval. One possibility is that this veteran had some other health issues during the six months. Another is that the model we used is not appropriate for these data. The sampling model should always be validated using the standard array of regression diagnostics; we discuss these in Chapter 10.

7.1.4 Centering and Standardization of Covariates

In data analysis it is often useful to center and/or standardize (or rescale) continuous predictor variables. One reason for this is to improve convergence of MCMC sampling. Another is to make model parameters more easily interpretable, which can also help with prior specification. We saw an example of the latter in Section 7.1.2 where we created a centered covariate $cAge = \text{Age} - 60$. The centering value 60 was not exactly the average age in the data but was a convenient value near the average.

In this section we illustrate first centering, and then standardization, using the **VetBP** data again. There are three continuous covariates in those data: the baseline diastolic blood pressure ($DBP0$), height (Ht), and weight (Wt). There are $n = 383$ observations, and the sample means for these three covariates are 72.4 mm Hg, 68.9 inches, and 210.9 pounds, respectively. The treatment variable in the data, Trt, has levels 1 and 2. So we transform this variable into a 0/1 variable as $Trt - 1$, as discussed in Section 7.1.2. While it is possible to center such binary variables, we choose not to do this to keep the interpretation of its regression coefficient as the treatment effect. The model with centered continuous covariates is thus written as

$$E(DBP6 \mid x, \beta) = \beta_0 + (Trt - 1)\beta_1 + (DBP0 - 72.4)\beta_2$$
$$+ (Ht - 68.9)\beta_3 + (Wt - 205.9)\beta_4;$$

that is, β_0 is the expected $DBP6$ for vets of average height, weight and baseline DBP, and given treatment 1 ($Trt = 1$). Note that with some rearrangement of terms, this is the same as

$$E(DBP6 \mid x, \beta) = \beta_0^* + (Trt - 1)\beta_1 + DBP0\,\beta_2 + Ht\,\beta_3 + Wt\,\beta_4.$$

Now the intercept β_0^* in the model without centering, equaling $\beta_0 - 72.4\beta_2 - 68.9\beta_3 - 205.9\beta_4$, has a different interpretation from β_0 in the centered model. The predictor coefficients in the uncentered model, however, are exactly the same as in the centered model.

Standardizing covariates involves one more step. For example, with covariate DPB0, $sDBP0 = (DBP0 - \overline{DBP0})/\mathrm{sd}(DBP0)$, where $\overline{DBP0}$ and $\mathrm{sd}(DBP0)$ are the mean and standard deviation, respectively, of $DBP0$ in the data. As in the case of centering (at or around the mean), rescaling can be done by using a value other than the standard deviation (sd). However, the term "standardization" is generally reserved for centering at the mean and dividing by the sd. The model with the single standardized covariate, $sDBP0$, is

$$\begin{aligned} E(Y \mid DBP0, \beta) &= \beta_0^* + sDBP0\,\beta_1^* \\ &= \beta_0 + \{(DBP0 - \overline{DBP0})/\mathrm{sd}(DBP0)\}\beta_1. \end{aligned}$$

In this model, β_1 is interpreted as the effect on the mean response of a one standard deviation unit increase in $DBP0$. The sample mean and standard deviation of $DBP0$ are 71.8 mm Hg and 10.6 mm Hg, respectively. So $sDBP0 = (DBP0 - 71.8)/10.6 = 1$ implies $DBP0 = 71.8 + 10.6 = 82.4$, and β_2 is interpreted as the effect on the mean response of an increase in baseline diastolic blood pressure of 1 *standard* unit or 10.6 mm Hg from the average of 71.8.

Standardization (or centering and rescaling) of covariates can be easily done in data preparation before defining the model in any Bayesian MCMC software. Most such software will also allow new variable definitions for this purpose. For example, in a **BUGS** model the following statements do this:

```
DBP6[i] ~ dnorm(mu[i],tau)
mu[i] <- b0 + b1 * (DBP0[i] - mean(DBP0))/sd(DBP0)
```

Of course, the prior specification now must be relevant to **b0** and **b1** in this model.

7.2   Matrix Formulation and an Analytic Posterior Distribution

For algebraic and analytic simplicity, as well as for conceptual unity, it is useful to consider simultaneously the single (Section 7.1.1) and multiple (Section 7.1.3) predictor(s) cases. To do this, we introduce vector and matrix notation in Section 7.2.1. Then, in Section 7.2.2, we employ this notation and flat priors to derive the posterior distribution for the parameters in the linear model.

7.2.1   Matrix Notation

First, let us put the regression coefficients into a vector $\beta = (\beta_0, \beta_1, \ldots, \beta_p)'$ and, correspondingly, the covariate values for the ith individual into a vector $x_i = (1, x_{i1}, \ldots, x_{ip})'$. Notice that the first element of each x_i is 1 corresponding to the intercept β_0. Now this allows us to write equation (7.2) as

$$E(Y_i|\beta, x_i) = x_i'\beta.$$

Next, we represent the data for all n individuals: response variable values in the vector $Y = (Y_1, \ldots, Y_n)$ and covariate values in a matrix that stacks x_i', $i = 1, \ldots, n$, as rows. So we write the linear model for the data as

$$
\begin{bmatrix} Y_1 \\ Y_2 \\ \vdots \\ Y_n \end{bmatrix}
=
\begin{bmatrix}
1 & x_{11} & x_{12} & \cdots & x_{1p} \\
1 & x_{21} & x_{22} & \cdots & x_{2p} \\
\vdots & \vdots & \vdots & \ddots & \vdots \\
1 & x_{n1} & x_{n2} & \cdots & x_{np}
\end{bmatrix}
\begin{bmatrix} \beta_0 \\ \beta_1 \\ \vdots \\ \beta_p \end{bmatrix}
+
\begin{bmatrix} \varepsilon_1 \\ \varepsilon_2 \\ \vdots \\ \varepsilon_n \end{bmatrix}
$$

$$Y_{n \times 1} \quad = \quad X_{n \times (p+1)} \quad\quad \beta_{(p+1) \times 1} \quad + \quad \varepsilon_{n \times 1}$$

with

$$\varepsilon \mid \tau \sim N_n(0, \tau^{-1} I_n).$$

Succinctly, the multiple linear regression model is expressed as

$$Y = X\beta + \varepsilon, \quad \varepsilon \mid \tau \sim N_n(0, \tau^{-1} I_n). \tag{7.3}$$

It follows from simple rules, as in Appendix A, about expected values and covariances of linear transformations (Section A.3) that $E(Y) = X\beta$, $\mathrm{Cov}(Y) = \tau^{-1} I_n$. Therefore, the linear regression sampling model is also written

$$Y \mid \beta, \tau \sim N_n(X\beta, \tau^{-1} I_n). \tag{7.4}$$

The data (or sampling) distribution (or likelihood, see end of Section 7.1.1) is now, from the distribution table in Appendix B,

$$p(y \mid \beta, \tau, X) \propto \tau^{n/2} \exp\left\{ -\frac{\tau}{2}(y - X\beta)'(y - X\beta) \right\}. \tag{7.5}$$

7.2.2 Posterior Analysis using the Flat Prior

We begin with the flat prior: $p(\beta) \propto 1$ and $p(\log(\sigma)) \propto 1$. Using the method of transformations of random variables (Section A.2), it can be shown that this also means $p(\sigma) \propto 1/\sigma$, $p(\sigma^2) \propto 1/\sigma^2$ and $p(\tau) \propto 1/\tau$. We call this the flat prior, as in Sections 7.1.3 and 7.3. Assuming independence, we have the joint prior

$$p(\beta, \tau) \propto 1/\tau. \tag{7.6}$$

7.2.2.1 Deriving the Posterior with the Flat Prior

Multiplying the distributions in expressions (7.5) and (7.6), we can write the posterior as

$$p(\beta, \tau \mid data) \propto \tau^{n/2-1} \exp\left\{-\frac{1}{2}\tau(y - X\beta)'(y - X\beta)\right\}.$$

To recognize the form of this posterior, we note that the conditional distribution $p(\beta|\tau, data)$ is proportional to $\exp\{-\frac{1}{2}\tau \times$ a quadratic form in $\beta\}$, that is, a multivariate normal kernel. To identify the parameters of this distribution, we can expand out $(y - X\beta)'(y - X\beta)$ and collect terms to find coefficients of β and $\beta'\beta$ and compare to the $Nor_{p+1}(\cdot, \cdot)$ density in Appendix B. We can then proceed to convert the result to the $N_{p+1}(\cdot, \cdot)$ form. This approach is straightforward and we use it in Section 7.4. However, here it is algebraically a bit messy and lacking in insight. We now turn to a different simplification of $(y - X\beta)'(y - X\beta)$ using some introductory material from linear algebra, vector spaces, and orthogonal projections.

Consider the $n \times n$ matrix

$$\mathcal{P} = X(X'X)^{-1}X'.$$

Simple algebra reveals two interesting properties of $\mathcal{P}$: it is symmetric (i.e., $\mathcal{P}' = \mathcal{P}$) and idempotent (i.e., $\mathcal{PP} = \mathcal{P}$). As a mapping of the n-dimensional vector space $\mathbb{R}^n$, it orthogonally projects any vector $y \in \mathbb{R}^n$ onto $C(X)$, the vector space spanned by the columns of X. It is interesting and easy to see that $I_n - \mathcal{P}$ is also symmetric and idempotent, where I_n is the $n \times n$ identity matrix. Moreover, $I_n - \mathcal{P}$ maps $y \in \mathbb{R}^n$ onto the orthogonal complement of $C(X)$ in $\mathbb{R}^n$. Since $\mathcal{P}(I_n - \mathcal{P}) = 0$, vectors $\mathcal{P}y$ and $(I_n - \mathcal{P})y$ are orthogonal with inner product 0.

Returning to the quadratic form of interest, first write

$$
\begin{aligned}
y - X\beta &= y - \mathcal{P}y + \mathcal{P}y - X\beta \\
&= (I_n - \mathcal{P})y + X(X'X)^{-1}X'y - X\beta \\
&= (I_n - \mathcal{P})y + X(\hat{\beta} - \beta), \quad \hat{\beta} = (X'X)^{-1}X'y.
\end{aligned}
$$

This leads to

$$
\begin{aligned}
(y - X\beta)'(y - X\beta) &= \{y'(I_n - \mathcal{P})y + X(\hat{\beta} - \beta)\}' \\
&\quad \times \{(I_n - \mathcal{P})y + X(\hat{\beta} - \beta)\} \\
&= y'(I_n - \mathcal{P})y + (\beta - \hat{\beta})'X'X(\beta - \hat{\beta}),
\end{aligned}
$$

since $(I_n - \mathcal{P})X = 0$. Using this last expression for the quadratic form $(y - X\beta)'(y - X\beta)$, we have

$$p(\beta, \tau \mid data) \propto \tau^{n/2-1} \exp\left\{-\frac{1}{2}\tau y'(I_n - \mathcal{P})y\right\} \exp\left\{-\frac{1}{2}\tau(\beta - \hat{\beta})'X'X(\beta - \hat{\beta})\right\}.$$

As β here appears only in the third term, which is the kernel of a multivariate normal density, a simple comparison with the $No_{p+1}(\cdot, \cdot)$ entry in the table in Appendix B identifies the conditional posterior

$$\beta \mid \tau, data \; \sim \; No_{p+1}(\hat{\beta}, \tau X'X) \quad \text{or} \quad N_{p+1}(\hat{\beta}, \sigma^2(X'X)^{-1}).$$

Finally, to obtain $p(\tau|data)$, we can divide the expression for the kernel of $p(\beta, \tau|data)$ above by the conditional density of $\beta|\tau, data$ given by $No_{p+1}(\hat{\beta}, \tau X'X)$. We must be careful to account for the normalizing constant $|\tau X'X|^{-1/2} = \tau^{-(p+1)/2}|X'X|^{-1/2}$ in this density as the constant involves τ. Dividing and multiplying by $\tau^{-(p+1)/2}$, we get

$$p(\tau \mid data) \quad \propto \quad \tau^{n/2-1}\tau^{-(p+1)/2} \exp\left\{-\frac{1}{2}\tau y'(I_n - \mathcal{P})y\right\}$$

$$\propto \quad \tau^{(n-p-1)/2-1} \exp\left\{-\frac{1}{2}\tau y'(I_n - \mathcal{P})y\right\} \; \propto \; Ga(a, b),$$

where $a = (n - p - 1)/2$ and $b = y'(I_n - \mathcal{P})y/2$.

It is interesting here to note that $2b$ has a nice interpretation. Since $\mathcal{P}y = \hat{y}$, say, is the orthogonal projection of y, it is the "closest" point in $C(X)$ to the data y. Thus $(I_n - \mathcal{P})y$ is the error or residual in approximating y by $\hat{y}$, and $y'(I_n - \mathcal{P})y$ is the squared length of this error, namely, $\sum_{i=1}^{n}(y_i - \hat{y}_i)^2$. This squared error is typically denoted by SSE (sum of squares of errors). We also note that $\hat{\beta} = (X'X)^{-1}X'y$ is called the least squares estimate of β. It is also the MLE. Traditional regression methods emphasize $\hat{\beta}$, SSE, and related quantities. More details are available in many texts ([98],[351],[77]), especially in [79] as relates to the material here.

We summarize the posterior distribution as

$$\tau \mid y, x \sim Ga((n - p - 1)/2, SSE/2), \quad \beta \mid y, x, \tau \sim N_{p+1}(\hat{\beta}, \sigma^2 X'X^{-1}). \quad (7.7)$$

7.2.2.2 Inference with Flat Prior

The posterior in expression (7.7) is a multivariate version of the normal-gamma distribution ($NoGa$) from Appendix B. We have seen $NoGa(\cdot, \cdot, \cdot, \cdot)$ as the conjugate prior and posterior for exchangeable normal data in Section 3.2.2. To obtain posterior samples we do not need Markov chain methods and can do direct Monte Carlo. First simulate $\tau \mid data$ from the gamma distribution. Using the simulated τ, generate $\beta \mid \tau, data$ from a $(p + 1)$-dimensional multivariate normal by computing $\beta = \hat{\beta} + (1/\sqrt{\tau})Qz$, where Q is a matrix square root of $(X'X)^{-1}$, such that $QQ' = (X'X)^{-1}$, and z is a vector of $p + 1$ iid $N(0, 1)$ variables. The following stylistic R code will do this:

```
tau <- rgamma(1,shape=n-p-1,rate=SSE)
z <- rnorm(p+1)
XpX = t(X)%*%X
Q = chol(solve(XpX))
beta <- beta.hat + (diag(1/sqrt(tau)) %*% t(Q)%*%z)
```

In general, joint posterior samples of (β, τ) allow us to carry out Bayesian inference and prediction in linear regression. Of course, such functions of interest are closely tied to the scientific context. Even as posterior samples are versatile for general targets of inference, it is interesting to note that for linear combinations of the components of β we can get analytic posterior intervals without Monte Carlo sampling.

Such linear combinations of the regression coefficients, say $c'\beta$ for some vector of constants $c = (c_1, \ldots, c_{p+1})'$, are often of scientific interest. A vector c with all zeros except in the ith slot gives $c\beta = c_i\beta_i$. For example, if x_2 is the covariate for age measured in years, and we are interested in the effect of a five-year increase in age on the mean response, we would set $c = (0, 0, 5, 0, \ldots, 0)$, providing there are no interactions in the model.

Since linear combinations of multivariate normal variables are normal, namely $c'\beta \mid \sigma^2, y \sim N(c'\hat{\beta}, c'(X'X)^{-1}c\sigma^2)$, it follows that $(c'\beta, \tau)$ has the $NoGa(\hat{\beta}, (1/c'(X'X)^{-1}c), (n-p-1)/2, SSE/2)$ distribution. The marginal of $c'\beta \mid y$ is then a $t(n - p - 1, c'\hat{\beta}, \sqrt{(c'(X'X)^{-1}c)(SSE)/(n - p - 1)})$, similar to the derivation in Section 3.2.2. Thus,

$$\frac{c'\beta - c'\hat{\beta}}{\sqrt{MSE\, c'(X'X)^{-1}c}}\bigg| y \sim t_{n-p}, \quad MSE = SSE/(n - p - 1),$$

and the $1 - \alpha$ posterior probability interval is

$$c'\hat{\beta} \pm t_{\alpha/2}\sqrt{MSE\, c'(X'X)^{-1}c}. \tag{7.8}$$

This interval matches the $100(1 - \alpha)\%$ confidence interval from the frequentist perspective, providing a Bayesian interpretation for it that conditions on the data at hand. Of course, this agreement is under the flat prior.

Now consider setting $c = x_f$ so that the estimation interval $x_f'\hat{\beta} \pm t_{\alpha/2}\sqrt{MSE\, x_f'(X'X)^{-1}x_f}$ corresponds to estimating the mean response for all individuals with predictor variables x_f. It can be shown that the corresponding prediction interval is similar but with additional uncertainty: $x_f'\hat{\beta} \pm t_{\alpha/2}\sqrt{MSE\,(1 + x_f'(X'X)^{-1}x_f)}$. The estimation interval width depends on uncertainty about the parameters, while the prediction interval width also depends on variability among individuals. If β were known, the interval width for the mean response would of course be zero, while the prediction interval would still involve uncertainty resulting from individual variation in response, even though all such individuals have the same predictor combination x_f.

While these formulas are nice for shedding light on the frequentist intervals, they only work for one-at-a-time simple linear combinations of the components of β. There are many other inference targets that will not be tractable analytically. For example, let $p = 1$ and suppose x_1 is a binary indicator where $x_1 = 1$ corresponds to a particular treatment and $x_1 = 0$ corresponds to a placebo. Then, as in Chapter 5 but with different notation, the effect size for the treatment would be $\Delta = \beta_1/\sigma$. There is no simple formula for making inferences about Δ. Another example would involve inferences about the ratio of two mean responses, perhaps $(\beta_0 + \beta_1)/\beta_0 = 1 + \beta_1/\beta_0$. For Bayesian analysis, such inferences can be carried out by sampling $(\beta, \tau) \mid data$ as detailed above and computing these quantities from each sample.

Predictive inferences are also easily obtained using such posterior samples but with an additional step. For each iterate $(\beta^{(k)}, \tau^{(k)})$, sample $y_f^{(k)} \sim No(x_f\beta^{(k)}, \tau^{(k)})$, $k = 1, \ldots, m$, where m is the MCMC sample size. Then obtain the usual quantiles and smoothed histogram to approximate prediction intervals and predictive density estimates.

Example 7.2. VetBP, Continued. We discuss the **VetBP** data analysis from the formulaic point of view discussed in this section. Recall that the basic data analysis was performed in Section 7.1.3 using the flat prior. The basis for the analysis was the output given in Table 7.2. In the analysis, there were $n = 383$ observations in the data and four covariates, $(DBP0, Trt, Ht, Wt)$; the response was $DBP6$, diastolic blood pressure at 6 months. Under our assumptions, we have $\beta \mid y \sim t(378, \hat{\beta}, MSE\,(X'X)^{-1})$, where the degrees of freedom are $383 - 5 = 378$.

From Table 7.2, we see that $\hat{\beta}' = (9.30, -0.86, 0.62, 0.24, 0.005) = E(\beta' \mid y)$. It follows that $\beta_1 \mid y \sim t(378, -0.86, 0.84^2)$ and thus that a posterior 95% interval for β_1 is $\hat{\beta}_1 \pm t_{0.025}\,0.84 = (-2.5, 0.79)$, where $t_{0.025}$ based on 378 degrees of freedom is approximately 1.96. In addition, the posterior mean of $x_f'\beta = (1, 1, 84, 66, 230)\beta$ is $9.30 - 0.86 + 84 \times 0.62 + 66 \times 0.24 + 230 \times 0.005) \doteq 78$, etc. (there has been some rounding).

For inference about σ, we start with inference for τ. Using the fact that

$$\tau \mid y \sim \text{Gamma}(378/2, SSE/2),$$

where $SSE = 24{,}570.7$, we obtain

$$\hat{\tau} = E(\tau \mid y) = 378/SSE = 0.0154.$$

Since $\tau\,SSE \mid y \sim \chi^2_{378}$, we have

$$
\begin{aligned}
0.95 &= P(l < \tau\,SSE < u \mid y) = P(l/SSE < \tau < u/SSE \mid y) \\
&= P(\sqrt{SSE/u} < \sigma < \sqrt{SSE/l} \mid y),
\end{aligned}
$$

where $l = 326.03$ and $u = 433.76$ are the 0.025 and 0.975 quantiles of the χ^2_{378} distribution. Thus a 95% posterior probability interval for σ is $(7.53, 8.68)$.

7.3 Priors

We discuss five types of prior specifications for (β, τ) in the linear regression model in expression (7.4). These are: (i) the flat prior, which is the main prior we have been using up to now; (ii) a proper prior approximation to the flat prior; (iii) a conditionally conjugate independence prior, including its informative elicitation via the conditional means prior (CMP) for β, with β and τ independent; (iv) a partially informative CMP; and (v) the conjugate normal-gamma prior. The Zellner (1986) g-prior is discussed as an important special case of the conjugate normal-gamma prior. [361].

7.3.1 Flat Prior

The flat prior for linear regression analysis is defined by

$$p(\beta, \tau) \propto 1/\tau.$$

Its integral is not finite and hence it is an improper prior. The prior results from taking independent flat priors on the components of β, and an independent flat prior on $\log(\sigma)$.[2]

Although improper, we noted in Section 7.2.2.2 that this prior results in nice formulas for point and interval inference that are the same formulas as one finds in frequentist presentations of linear regression. In particular, the posterior mean of β is the least-squares estimate which, with normally distributed εs, is also the maximum likelihood estimate, $\hat{\beta}$. Even with the nice formulas for basic inference for model parameters, we note it is still necessary to obtain posterior samples to make inferences for nonlinear functions of the parameters.

7.3.2 A Proper Approximation to the Flat Prior

A commonly used proper prior is

$$\beta_j \overset{\text{iid}}{\sim} N(0, b), \quad \tau \sim Ga(c, c), \ \tau \text{ independent of the } \beta_j.$$

With b large and c small, this prior approximates the flat prior, since the kernel of a $Gamma(c, c)$ is $\tau^{c-1} e^{-\tau c}$, so if c is a small number, we have $p(\tau) \overset{.}{\propto} 1/\tau$. Similarly, $p(\beta)$ is approximately uniform over any realistic finite range when b is large (cf. Exercise 7.13). The actual values of b and c in the normal and gamma distributions should be selected depending on the scale of the measurements being considered. This prior can be used when very little information is available or for sensitivity analysis when an informative prior is available. The posterior requires MCMC simulation. The conditionals for Gibbs sampling are conveniently conjugate in this case. Results typically are very similar to those from the flat prior.

7.3.3 Conditionally Conjugate Independence Prior

This section presents the priors that we use most often in practice. We again assume prior independence of β and τ, that is, $p(\beta, \tau) = p(\beta)p(\tau)$. We write it as

$$\beta \sim N_p(b_0, C_0), \quad \tau \sim Ga(a, b), \ \tau \text{ independent of } \beta. \tag{7.9}$$

---

[2]Using the method of transformations of random variables (Section A.2), it can be shown that this also means $p(\sigma) \propto 1/\sigma$, $p(\sigma^2) \propto 1/\sigma^2$, and $p(\tau) \propto 1/\tau$.

Notice that, unlike with the flat prior and its proper prior approximation, the components of β are not necessarily independent or identically distributed; β has a multivariate normal distribution. Our task is to determine values a, b, b_0, and C_0 that accurately reflect available prior information. We address this in Sections 7.3.3.1 and 7.3.3.2 below and focus on the conditional conjugacy of the prior here.

*Conditional Conjugacy. The prior in expression (7.9) translates to

$$p(\beta, \tau) \propto \exp\{-(\beta - b_0)'C_0^{-1}(\beta - b_0)/2\}\tau^{a-1}\exp\{-\tau b\}.$$

Multiplying this by the data sampling distribution (or likelihood) in expression (7.5) and expanding the terms in the exponent, we obtain

$$p(\beta, \tau \mid data) \propto \tau^{a+n/2-1}\exp\{-\tau(b + y'y/2)\}$$
$$\times \exp\left\{-\frac{\tau}{2}(\beta'X'X\beta - 2y'X\beta) + (\beta - b_0)'C_0^{-1}(\beta - b_0)\right\}$$
$$\propto \tau^{a+n/2-1}\exp\{-\tau(b + y'y/2)\}$$
$$\times \exp\left\{-\frac{1}{2}(\beta'(\tau X'X + C_0^{-1})\beta - 2(\tau y'X + b_0'C_0^{-1})\beta\right\}.$$

From the last expression, we can write

$$p(\beta \mid \tau, data) \propto \exp\left\{-\frac{1}{2}(\beta'(\tau X'X + C_0^{-1})\beta - 2(\tau y'X + b_0'C_0^{-1})\beta\right\},$$
$$p(\tau \mid \beta, data) \propto \tau^{a+n/2-1}\exp\{-\tau(b + (y'y + \beta'X'X\beta - 2y'X\beta)/2)\}.$$

We now recognize these as

$$\beta \mid \tau, data \sim Nor_{p+1}\left(\tau X'X + C_0^{-1}, (\tau X'y + C_0^{-1}b_0)'\right),$$
$$\tau \mid \beta, data \sim Ga\left(a + n/2, b + (y'y + \beta'X'X\beta - 2y'X\beta)/2\right).$$

By using the multivariate normal mean and covariance on the Nor line of the Distributions Table in Appendix B, we can also write the posterior of $\beta \mid \tau$ in the more familiar $N_{p+1}(\mu_{\beta|\tau,data}, \Sigma_{\beta|\tau,data})$ form as

$$\beta \mid \tau, data \sim N_{p+1}\left(\{\tau X'X + C_0^{-1}\}^{-1}\{\tau X'y + C_0^{-1}b_0\}, \{\tau X'X + C_0^{-1}\}^{-1}\right).$$

For posterior simulation, we can simulate $\beta \mid \tau, data$ and $\tau \mid \beta, data$ from these distributions in a cycle of a Gibbs sampler, using their most recently generated values for conditioning. Notice that three statistics (compact data description quantities) can be computed before entering the Gibbs iteration: $y'y$, $X'X$, $X'y$—a scalar, a $(p + 1) \times (p + 1)$ matrix, and a $(p + 1)$-dimensional vector, respectively.

It is also possible, and perhaps comforting to those who have seen traditional regression methods, that the parameters for the posterior conditionals can be put in terms of the least squares and maximum likelihood estimates $\hat{\beta} = (X'X)^{-1}X'y$ and $SSE = (y - X\hat{\beta})'(y - X\hat{\beta})$. For example,

$$E(\beta|\tau, data) = \mu_{\beta|\tau, data} = \{\tau X'X + C_0^{-1}\}^{-1}\{\tau X'X\hat{\beta} + C_0^{-1}b_0\}$$

by noting $X'y = X'X(X'X)^{-1}X'y = X'X\hat{\beta}$. Observe that this is a linear combination of the MLE and the prior guess. Similarly, the second parameter in the gamma distribution for $\tau \mid \beta, data$ can be written as

$$b + \left(SSE + (\beta - \hat{\beta})'X'X(\beta - \hat{\beta})\right)/2.$$

In this form, the three statistics $\hat{\beta}, SSE$, and $X'X$ can be computed outside the Gibbs loop.

7.3.3.1 Conditional Means Prior for β

To implement the conditionally conjugate independence prior, we now turn to the task of determining values for b_0, C_0, a, and b. Since it is not straightforward to think about β, the regression coefficients, we think about the *mean values of potential observables*. We elicit a prior for the mean response at a particular set of values of predictor variables. Thus we elicit priors on conditional means

$$\tilde{\mu}_i \equiv E(Y \mid \tilde{x}_i) = \tilde{x}_i'\beta$$

for $p + 1$ subpopulations defined by different predictor vectors $\tilde{x}_i$, $i = 1, \ldots, p+1$. That is, we specify a knowledge-based prior for

$$E(Y \mid \tilde{X}, \beta) \equiv \tilde{\mu} = \tilde{X}\beta,$$

where $\tilde{X}$ consists of the $p + 1$ rows of predictor variable combinations, x_i', that correspond to types of individuals that an expert can easily think about. The x_i are chosen so that the matrix $\tilde{X}$ is non-singular. We specify prior uncertainty about $\tilde{\mu}$ as

$$\tilde{\mu} \sim N_{p+1}(\tilde{m}, D(\tilde{w})), \quad \text{i.e.,} \quad \tilde{\mu}_i \overset{ind}{\sim} N(\tilde{m}_i, \tilde{w}_i), \quad i = 1, \ldots, p+1, \qquad (7.10)$$

with a knowledge-based $(p + 1)$-vector $\tilde{m}$, and diagonal matrix $D(\tilde{w})$. The induced prior on β is obtained by noting $\beta = \tilde{X}^{-1}\tilde{\mu}$ and using the well-known fact about multivariate normal distributions that such linear transformations of them are also multivariate normal. For example if $V \sim N_k(\mu, \Sigma)$ and A is an $r \times k$ matrix of constants, then $AV \sim N_r(A\mu, A\Sigma A')$. Thus

$$\beta \sim N_{p+1}\left[\tilde{X}^{-1}\tilde{m}, \tilde{X}^{-1}D(\tilde{w})(\tilde{X}^{-1})'\right]. \qquad (7.11)$$

This is the method of informative prior specification described in Bedrick et al. [23] that is termed the conditional means prior, since the prior specification is on the conditional mean. Our goal is not to find the perfect prior to characterize someone's beliefs but to find a sensible prior that incorporates some basic scientific, experiential or historical knowledge. We now illustrate the method.

Remark. While the narrative here is in the form of communicating with a subject-matter expert, the elicited quantities could be calculated from historical data if available.

Example 7.3. FEV Data. Rosner (2006) [272] provides a data set on pulmonary function (lung capacity) in adolescents. The response y is forced expiratory volume (FEV), which measures the air in liters expelled in 1 second of a forceful breath. Lung function is expected to increase during adolescence, but smoking may slow its progression. The association between smoking and lung capacity in adolescents is investigated using data from $n = 345$ adolescents between the ages of 10 and 19. The predictor variables include *Age* in years (x_1); a 0/1 indicator variable for smoking status, *Smoke* (x_2); and the interaction term $x_3 = x_1 x_2$. Adding an interaction to the model implies a belief that the effect of smoking status on FEV is different for different ages. Interactions are discussed in Section 7.5. A predictor vector is $x' = (1, x_1, x_2, x_3)$. The data are in the file named `FEVdata.txt` on the book's website under Chapter 7.

With four regression parameters, we select four covariate combinations $\tilde{x}_i$, $i = 1, 2, 3, 4$, corresponding to circumstances that the expert can assess independently. In particular, we use prior experience to specify information about the subpopulation of 11-year-old non-smokers, $\tilde{x}_1' = (1, 11, 0, 0)$; 13-year-old smokers, $\tilde{x}_2' = (1, 13, 1, 13)$; 16-year-old non-smokers, $\tilde{x}_3' = (1, 16, 0, 0)$; and 18-year-old smokers, $\tilde{x}_4' = (1, 18, 1, 18)$. In matrix form we have

$$\tilde{X} = \begin{bmatrix} 1 & 11 & 0 & 0 \\ 1 & 13 & 1 & 13 \\ 1 & 16 & 0 & 0 \\ 1 & 18 & 1 & 18 \end{bmatrix} = \begin{bmatrix} \tilde{x}_1' \\ \tilde{x}_2' \\ \tilde{x}_3' \\ \tilde{x}_4' \end{bmatrix}.$$

It is important to choose the $\tilde{x}_i$ so that, during elicitation, the $\tilde{\mu}_i$ can be each regarded separately and independently of the others.

Although FEV values display variability, even within subpopulations, first we are interested in the mean FEV value $\tilde{\mu}_i$ for the four circumstances $\tilde{x}_1$, $\tilde{x}_2$, $\tilde{x}_3$, and $\tilde{x}_4$. The elicitation process mimics that for the one- and two-sample normal cases discussed in Chapter 5, only here we are eliciting information about four groups.

To illustrate, suppose that our medical collaborator expects the average FEV among all 18-year-old smokers in the sampled population to be 3.3, and is 99% sure that the mean FEV is less than 4.0 in this group. Thus we take $\tilde{m}_4 = 3.3$ and, with $\tilde{w}_4$ denoting the prior uncertainty about $\tilde{\mu}$ (in the form of variance), the 99th percentile of $\tilde{\mu}_4$ satisfies $4.0 = 3.3 + 2.33\sqrt{\tilde{w}_4}$. This gives $\tilde{w}_4 = (4.0 - 3.3)^2 / 2.33^2 = 0.09$, so that

$$\tilde{\mu}_4 \sim N(3.3, 0.09).$$

Similar steps are used to construct normal priors for $\tilde{\mu}_1$, $\tilde{\mu}_2$, and $\tilde{\mu}_3$; suppose they yield

$$\tilde{\mu}_1 \sim N(2.8, 0.04), \quad \tilde{\mu}_2 \sim N(3.0, 0.04), \quad \tilde{\mu}_3 \sim N(4.0, 0.04).$$

In matrix form, we have

$$\tilde{X}\beta \equiv \tilde{m} = \begin{bmatrix} \tilde{m}_1 \\ \tilde{m}_2 \\ \tilde{m}_3 \\ \tilde{m}_4 \end{bmatrix} \sim N \left(\begin{bmatrix} 2.8 \\ 3.0 \\ 4.0 \\ 3.3 \end{bmatrix}, \begin{bmatrix} 0.04 & 0 & 0 & 0 \\ 0 & 0.04 & 0 & 0 \\ 0 & 0 & 0.04 & 0 \\ 0 & 0 & 0 & 0.09 \end{bmatrix} \right),$$

leading to the induced prior on β,

$$\beta = \tilde{X}^{-1} \begin{bmatrix} \tilde{\mu}_1 \\ \tilde{\mu}_2 \\ \tilde{\mu}_3 \\ \tilde{\mu}_4 \end{bmatrix} \sim N \left(\tilde{X}^{-1} \begin{bmatrix} 2.8 \\ 3.0 \\ 4.0 \\ 3.3 \end{bmatrix}, \tilde{X}^{-1} \begin{bmatrix} 0.04 & 0 & 0 & 0 \\ 0 & 0.04 & 0 & 0 \\ 0 & 0 & 0.04 & 0 \\ 0 & 0 & 0 & 0.09 \end{bmatrix} \tilde{X}^{-1\prime} \right),$$

where

$$\tilde{X}^{-1} = \begin{bmatrix} 3.2 & 0 & -2.2 & 0 \\ -0.2 & 0 & 0.2 & 0 \\ -3.2 & 3.6 & 2.2 & -2.6 \\ 0.2 & -0.2 & -0.2 & 0.2 \end{bmatrix}$$

is easily obtained in R using the command `solve(tildeX)` after defining `tildeX`.
So

$$\beta \sim N \left(\begin{bmatrix} 0.16 \\ 0.24 \\ 2.06 \\ -0.18 \end{bmatrix}, \begin{bmatrix} 0.603 & -0.043 & -0.603 & 0.043 \\ -0.043 & 0.003 & 0.043 & -0.003 \\ -0.603 & 0.043 & 1.73 & -0.119 \\ 0.043 & -0.003 & -0.119 & 0.008 \end{bmatrix} \right),$$

which is also easily accomplished in R. It is important to remember that this method obviously requires that $\tilde{X}$ be invertible. If it is not, then perhaps the partial prior specification in the next section would be the easiest solution. Alternatively, one can replace one or more of the $\tilde{x}_i$ to obtain a non-singular matrix.

7.3.3.2   An Informative Prior for τ and σ

To construct an informative $Ga(a, b)$ prior for τ, we ask an expert to think about a percentile for the response values in the population of individuals corresponding to a particular predictor vector, say $\tilde{x}$. To be specific, the $1 - \alpha$ quantile equals $\tilde{x}\beta + z_{1-\alpha}\sigma$. We elicit a best guess for this quantile, conditional on the best guess for $\tilde{x}\beta$ from the elicitation in Section 7.3.3.1. Setting this elicited value to $\tilde{x}\beta + z_{1-\alpha}\sigma$ leads to a best guess for σ, and subsequently to one for $\tau = 1/\sqrt{\sigma}$. While this can be used to specify a central value for the prior distribution, we need additional information to express uncertainty about the best guess for τ. We illustrate using the **FEV** data.

Example 7.4. FEV Data, Continued. To choose a and b for a $Ga(a, b)$ prior on τ, we again consider 18-year-old smokers, $\tilde{x}_4' = (1, 18, 1, 18)$. Given the expert's best guess for the mean FEV for this population, $\tilde{m}_4 = 3.3$, we ask the expert what would be a large value for an *individual FEV observation* that s/he would expect to see from this group that could be considered as the 95th percentile. We then set this value equal to $\tilde{m}_4 + 1.645\sigma$, where $z_{0.95} = 1.645$ is the 95th percentile of the $N(0, 1)$ distribution. Suppose the expert's best guess for the 95th percentile is 5. Since $\tilde{m}_4 = 3.3$, our best guess for σ, say σ_0, satisfies $5 = 3.3 + 1.645\sigma_0$. So $\sigma_0 = 1.7/1.645 = 1.03$, and $\tau_0 = (1.645/1.7)^2 = 0.94$ is the best guess for τ. We take τ_0 to be the mode of the gamma prior for τ, that is,

$$0.94 = \frac{a-1}{b} \quad \text{or} \quad a = 0.94b + 1.$$

We complete the specification of the gamma prior by eliciting a measure of uncertainty about the 95th percentile. In addition to a best guess (5 above) for the 95th percentile, we ask for a lower bound on this guess, looking for the 95th percentile of the best guess. Suppose the expert gives the value 4. It follows that

$$\begin{aligned} 0.95 &= P\left(3.3 + 1.645\sigma > 4\right) = P\left(1.645\sigma > 0.7\right) \\ &= P\left(\tau < (1.645/0.7)^2\right) = P(\tau < 5.52). \end{aligned}$$

So we want a and b such that $a = 0.94b + 1$ and the 95th percentile of $G(a, b)$ equals 5.52; equivalently, b such that the 95th percentile of $G(0.94b + 1, b)$ equals 5.52. We can solve this equation in b numerically by using, for example, `pgamma` or `qgamma` functions in R. A solution can be obtained by trial and error or, more systematically, with a method such as the golden search (see Exercise 7.5).

These specifications, combined with the model, have implications worth pointing out. For example, suppose we consider 11-year-old non-smokers with the specified conditional mean FEV of $\tilde{m}_1 = 2.8$ instead of $\tilde{m}_4 = 3.3$ for 18-year-old smokers. The corresponding 95th percentile should be about $2.8 + 1.7 = 4.5$. According to the model and being consistent with the first information, the 95th percentile should be about $1.645\sigma_0 = 1.7$ units above the mean FEV, regardless of the values of the predictor variables x_2, x_3, and x_4. The expert should be made aware of this to see if these implications are numerically reasonable. If not, some changes, perhaps to the model, should be considered.

7.3.4   Partial Information Prior

In practice, it may often be the case that the available information is insufficient to specify a complete conditional means prior (as in Section 7.3.3.1) for the regression coefficients, especially when p is moderate or large. Eliciting real prior information can be time-consuming. In this section we discuss how to place a partial prior on regression coefficients when we are only able to specify information for $p_1 < p + 1$ mean values, corresponding to a subset of p_1 predictor vectors $\tilde{x}_i$, as opposed to $p + 1$ as necessary for CMP.

The simplest case corresponds to $p_1 = 1$, that is, when prior information is available at only one setting of the p predictor variables. For models with an intercept, consider an individual whose dichotomous predictor variables were all equal to 0, with all the continuous covariate values set to their sample mean from the data. If the continuous variates are standardized or centered, then we simply set

$\tilde{x}_1 = (1, 0, \ldots, 0)'$. In this case, $\tilde{\mu}_1 = \beta_0$, the intercept. We place an informative prior normal distribution on $\tilde{\mu}_1$ as we have previously discussed. We now require some kind of a reference prior to be placed on $(\beta_1, \ldots, \beta_p)$. We either select an improper flat prior for these coefficients or a set of independent normal priors with mean 0 and large variances.

If an additional elicitation is made for $\tilde{\mu}_2$ corresponding to predictor vector $\tilde{x}_2 = (1, 1, 0, \ldots, 0)$, then independent normal distributions are placed on the $\tilde{\mu}_i$, which induces a joint normal distribution on β_0 and β_1 via

$$\begin{pmatrix} \tilde{\mu}_1 \\ \tilde{\mu}_2 \end{pmatrix} = \begin{bmatrix} 1 & 0 \\ 1 & 1 \end{bmatrix} \begin{pmatrix} \beta_0 \\ \beta_1 \end{pmatrix} \equiv \tilde{X}\beta.$$

A reference prior can be placed on the remaining β_j. In this case of two equations in two unknowns, we can solve them to get $\beta_0 = \tilde{\mu}_1$ and $\beta_1 = \tilde{m}_2 - \tilde{m}_1$. Using such explicit transformations, a prior for (β_0, β_1) is easily specified in software such as BUGS, JAGS, or Stan: we specify the independent normal priors for μ_1, μ_2 with means $\tilde{m}_1, \tilde{m}_2$ and variances w_1, w_2, and define β_0, β_1 as explicit deterministic functions of μ_1, μ_2. An example of this is in the file `partialinfopriorcode.txt` on the book's webpage under Chapter 7.

More generally, let $\tilde{X}$ be a $(p_1 + 1) \times (p + 1)$ matrix containing the row vectors $\tilde{x}_i'$, and let $\tilde{\mu} = \tilde{X}\beta$ be the $(p_1 + 1) \times 1$ vector of mean responses that correspond to $\tilde{X}$. We would generally pick $\tilde{X}$ so that $\tilde{\mu}$ only depends on the same p_1 predictor coefficients and no others (although this is not strictly necessary; see Christensen et al. [79] for details). This can be done using $\tilde{X} = (\tilde{X}_1, \tilde{X}_2) = (\tilde{X}_1, 0)$, where $\tilde{X}_1$ is $(p_1 + 1) \times (p_1 + 1)$. We have rearranged the columns of $\tilde{X}$ so that the first $p_1 + 1$ correspond to the $p_1 + 1$ components of β. We denote this "shortened" β by $\tilde{\beta}$. The rows of $\tilde{X}$ must be linearly independent, as was the case with the full CMP, so $\tilde{X}_1$ must be non-singular. Write $\tilde{\mu}_0 = \tilde{X}_1\tilde{\beta} = (\beta_0, \ldots, \beta_{p_1})'$ as the corresponding "shortened" version of $\tilde{\mu}$.

We then specify $\tilde{\mu} = \tilde{X}_1\tilde{\beta} \sim N_{p_1}(\tilde{m}_0, D(w))$ as in the CMP (Section 7.3.3.1), $\tilde{X}_1$ being a non-singular $p_1 \times p_1$ matrix. Thus the same argument applies to obtain the result given in equation (7.11), with $\tilde{X}_1$ replacing $\tilde{X}$, and p_1 replacing $p + 1$.

Using a technical argument, Christensen et al. (Section 8.4.5 in [79]) suggest that it is reasonable under these circumstances to place independent $N(0, b)$ priors on the remaining β_is, namely for $i = p_1 + 1, \ldots, p + 1$, with b large.

Example 7.5. FEV Data, Continued. There are two additional predictor variables available for the FEV data: height and sex. In the expanded regression problem, we can use the CMP prior as a partial information prior in conjunction with flat priors on the two additional regression coefficients. This presumes that the earlier elicitation applies to children in the four subpopulations with, say, the same average height and the same sex. This may be unrealistic in that adding knowledge of a person's sex would probably change one's opinions about 18-year-old smokers' mean FEV. In any case, the parameterization of the model requires height to be standardized and that the selected sex correspond to a predictor value of 0.

7.4 *Conjugate Priors

For exchangeable normal observations in Section 3.2.2, we introduced a jointly conjugate dependence prior. Here we have a similar situation, except that β is a vector, while in Chapter 3 μ is a scalar. Thus we will use a multivariate normal prior for β here, but again conditioning on τ as there. We first discuss a generic conjugate prior and then an important special case of it.

7.4.1   Generic Normal-Gamma Prior

The conjugate prior for linear regression specifies a normal-gamma distribution for β, τ via a gamma marginal for τ and a normal for β conditional on τ. Specifically,

$$\tau \sim Ga(a, b), \quad \beta \mid \tau \sim No_{p+1}(\beta_0, k_0 \tau T_0). \tag{7.12}$$

The parameters here are a, b, β_0, k_0, and T_0, with a and b as before, β_0 a $(p+1)$-dimensional vector,[3] T_0 a $(p+1) \times (p+1)$ symmetric non-singular matrix, and $k_0 > 0$. This is not as convenient as the independence prior used in the CMP for prior parameter elicitation. The difference is that the expert needs to think about β conditional on knowing the value of τ. Nonetheless, the mathematical results are pretty, and they have historical as well as practical significance, especially as building blocks in Bayesian nonparametric analysis involving Dirichlet process mixture models. With sampling distribution

$$Y \mid \beta, \tau \sim No_n(X\beta, \tau I_n)$$

we can write the posterior as

$$
\begin{aligned}
p(\beta, \tau \mid y) &\propto \tau^{a-1} \exp\{-b\tau\} \tau^{(p+1)/2} \exp\left\{ -\frac{k_0 \tau}{2}(\beta - \beta_0)' T_0 (\beta - \beta_0) \right\} \\
&\quad \times \tau^{n/2} \exp\left\{ -\frac{\tau}{2}(y - X\beta)'(y - X\beta) \right\} \\
&\propto \tau^{(a+n/2)-1} \exp\left\{ -\left(b + \frac{1}{2}(y'y + k_0 \beta_0' T_0 \beta_0) \right) \tau \right\} \\
&\quad \times \tau^{(p+1)/2} \exp\left\{ -\frac{\tau}{2}\{\beta'(k_0 T_0 + X'X)\beta - 2(y'X + k_0 \beta_0' T_0)\beta\} \right\}.
\end{aligned}
$$

Recognizing this as a product of a gamma kernel in τ and a normal kernel (in $Nor_{p+1}(A, B)$ form) for β conditional on τ, we conclude that this posterior is again normal-gamma, hence conjugate. To identify the parameters, we observe $A = \tau(k_0 T_0 + X'X)$, $B = \tau(X'y + k_0 T_0 \beta_0)$, note that A and B involve τ, and so does the normalizing constant $(2\pi)^{p/2}|A|^{-1/2}e^{(1/2)B'A^{-1}B}$.

---

[3]Here we use β_0 to denote a vector that is a prior guess for β, even though we have used β_0 as the scalar first component of β. We rely on context to recognize its meaning.

To see how τ appears in this, we write

$$|A|^{-1/2} = |\tau(k_0 T_0 + X'X)|^{-1/2} \propto \tau^{-(p+1)/2},$$

$$\begin{aligned} B'A^{-1}B &= \tau(y'X + k_0\beta_0'T_0)(\tau(k_0T_0 + X'X))^{-1}\tau(X'y + k_0T_0\beta_0) \\ &= \tau(y'X + k_0\beta_0'T_0)(k_0T_0 + X'X)^{-1}(X'y + k_0T_0\beta_0) \\ &= \tau c, \quad \text{say.} \end{aligned}$$

Thus, as a function of τ, the normalizing constant is proportional to $\tau^{-(p+1)/2}\exp\{(1/2)\tau c\}$ (see the *Nor* line for multivariate normal distribution in Appendix B). Dividing and multiplying by $e^{(1/2)c}$ as $\tau^{-(p+1)/2}$ is included in the last expression for $p(\beta, \tau \mid data)$ above, we get

$$\beta \mid \tau, y \sim N_{p+1}\left((k_0T_0 + X'X)^{-1}(X'y + k_0T_0\beta_0), \tau^{-1}(k_0T_0 + X'X)^{-1}\right),$$

$$\tau \mid y \sim Ga\left(a + n/2, b + \frac{1}{2}(y'y + k_0\beta_0'T_0\beta_0 - c)\right). \tag{7.13}$$

It is interesting to note that by formally setting $a = b = k_0 = 0$ you can almost recover the normal-gamma posterior in Section 7.2.2 when using flat priors. This follows since, with these choices, we have

$$y'y - c = y'I_n y - y'X(X'X)^{-1}X'y = y'I_n y - y'\mathcal{P}y = y'(I_n - \mathcal{P})y = SSE.$$

The only difference is in the first parameter of the gamma: $n/2$ here and $(n-p-1)/2$ there in expression (7.7). As we noted there, posterior samples in this case can be obtained without Markov chain methods by sampling τ from its posterior gamma marginal, followed by $\beta|\tau$ from the multivariate normal. The gamma parameters, the covariance matrix of the normal, and its mean up to the multiplier τ^{-1} can be computed before entering the sampling loop.

If we elicit priors as in the previous section, we would specify

$$\tilde{X}\beta \mid \tau \sim N_{p+1}(\tilde{m}, (1/\tau)D(w)),$$

with known $(p+1) \times (p+1)$ matrix $\tilde{X}$, $p+1$ vector $\tilde{m}$, and diagonal matrix $D(w)$. The induced prior for β is

$$\beta \mid \tau \sim N_p(\tilde{X}^{-1}\tilde{m}, (1/\tau)\tilde{X}^{-1}D(w)\tilde{X}^{-1\prime}).$$

Thus we have

$$\beta_0 = \tilde{X}^{-1}\tilde{m}, \quad T_0 = \tilde{X}'[D(w)]^{-1}\tilde{X}, \quad k_0 = 1,$$

and the posterior is given by

$$\beta \mid \tau, y \sim N_p\left(E(\beta \mid \tau, y), \frac{1}{\tau}\left\{X'X + \tilde{X}'D^{-1}(w)\tilde{X}\right\}^{-1}\right),$$

where

$$E(\beta \mid \tau, y) = \left\{X'X + \tilde{X}'D^{-1}(w)\tilde{X}\right\}^{-1}\left\{X'y + \tilde{X}'D^{-1}(\tilde{w})\tilde{m}\right\},$$

$$\tau \mid y \sim Ga\left(a + n/2, b + \frac{1}{2}(y'y + \tilde{m}\tilde{X}^{-1}\tilde{X}'\{D(w)\}^{-1}\tilde{X}\tilde{X}^{-1}\tilde{m} - C)\right).$$

7.4.2   Zellner's g-Prior

Zellner (1986) [361] recommended the prior

$$p(\tau) \propto \frac{1}{\tau}, \quad \beta \mid \tau \sim N_{p+1}(\beta_0, g\,\tau^{-1}\,(X'X)^{-1}), \tag{7.14}$$

where g is a fixed (tuning parameter) constant. This is known as Zellner's g-prior. Model (7.14) is almost a special case of the conjugate prior in expression (7.12) with $T_0 = X'X$, $k_0 = 1/g$, but with flat prior on $\log(\tau)$ (or $\log(\sigma)$) which could be represented by formally taking $a = b = 0$. With some care, we can use the normal-gamma posteriors in expressions (7.13) and (7.7). As we noted immediately after expression (7.13), the first parameter in the gamma posterior for τ should be $(n - p - 1)/2$, in place of $n/2$. Moreover, the choice of $T_0 = X'X$, $k_0 = 1/g$ in expression (7.14) leads to considerable simplifications. In the posterior conditional N_{p+1} distribution for β in expression (7.13), the covariance matrix reduces to

$$\Sigma_{\beta \mid \tau, data} = \frac{\sigma^2 g}{1 + g}(X'X)^{-1}$$

and the expectation to

$$\mu_{\beta \mid \tau, data} = \frac{g}{1+g}(X'X)^{-1}\left(X'y + \frac{1}{g}X'X\beta_0\right) = \frac{g}{1+g}\hat{\beta} + \frac{1}{1+g}\beta_0,$$

since $X'y = X'X(X'X)^{-1}X'y = X'X\hat{\beta}$. While it is possible similarly to obtain an expression for the second parameter in the gamma posterior for τ in (7.13), it is algebraically simpler to follow the pattern of derivation in the conjugate prior case that led to the posterior. In either case we obtain

$$\tau \mid y \sim Ga\left(\frac{n-p-1}{2}, \frac{1}{2}\left\{SSE + \frac{1}{1+g}(\hat{\beta} - \beta_0)'X'X(\hat{\beta} - \beta_0)\right\}\right),$$

$$\beta \mid \tau, y \sim N_p\left(\frac{g}{1+g}\hat{\beta} + \frac{1}{1+g}\beta_0, \ \tau^{-1}\frac{g}{1+g}(X'X)^{-1}\right). \tag{7.15}$$

This posterior has some interesting properties. Since it is normal-gamma, as in the flat and conjugate prior cases, Markov chain sampling is not needed; independent Monte Carlo samples can be drawn. As g becomes indefinitely large, it agrees with the flat prior inference in expression (7.7). With $g = 1$, the posterior mean for β gives equal weights to the maximum likelihood estimate $\hat{\beta}$ and the prior mean β_0. The choice $g = n$ corresponds to assigning a weight to the prior comparable to a single observation. For this reason, setting $g = n$ is sometimes called a "unit information prior." Several other choices of g, including suitable priors on it, have also been developed (see Section 7.7).

7.5 Beyond Additivity: Interaction (Effect Modification)

Here we discuss the situation where a treatment may have a different effect on an outcome depending on which subgroup of individuals the treatment may be applied to. For example, suppose that a well-established drug is known to improve survival time after diagnosis for individuals who have been diagnosed with a certain cancer. However, suppose that the drug can be safely applied at a low dose and also at a high dose. It is of interest to study if dose level affects the degree of survival outcome. As the study endpoint, let us use the median survival after diagnosis. The comparison of median survival times at high versus low levels of the drug is thought of as the "dose effect." This comparison can be made, for example, by a ratio of these two medians or the difference. Now, as the drug can be used for women as well as men, the comparison of median survival between women and men is then the "sex effect." Now suppose that the median survival time for women on the low dose is 10 years, and with a high dose is 5 years; for men, the low dose results in a median survival of 4 years under the low dose, and 10 years under the high dose. This artificial example is made to illustrate an exaggerated instance of an interaction between the drug's dose effect and its sex effect. Women benefit from the low dose over high; but men benefit from the high dose over low. Conversely, we can say that at low dose, women derive a greater benefit than men, but at the high dose, men have a greater benefit. In both cases, the effect of one factor is modified by the levels of the other factor. In most practical examples, such "directional reversal" is rare. Typically, the size of the effect changes with level of the other factor but the direction (or sign) remains the same.

To be specific, let us use the relative median as a means of comparison or a measure of effect size. This relative median for women to men is, at the low dose, $10/4 = 2.25$; and at the high dose it is $5/10 = 1/2$. If there had been no effect modification, the relative medians would have been the same for both doses. On the other hand, the relative median for comparing low to high dose is $10/5 = 2$ for women; and $4/10$ for men. Here again we see that women have double the median survival under the low dose than under the high dose, and men have less than half the median survival under the low dose than under the high dose.

The effect modification does not have to be opposite as in the hypothetical above. It could be that the dose effect on median survival is non-existent for men, that is, if the relative median comparing low to high dose for men was 1 (in this case it would not matter if men took the high or the low dose); but that it was appreciable for women, that is, the relative median was 2 as above (in this case women would be encouraged to take the low dose). Another scenario could be a positive effect of taking the low dose for both men and for women (longer survival on the low dose than for the high dose), but that the effect is appreciably stronger for women than it is for men (e.g., the relative medians above were 2 for women and 1.5 for men). For all of these situations, effect modification is modeled by including a cross-product (or interaction) term in the model.

In general, a predictor x_1 is an effect modifier of a predictor x_2 if the effect of x_2 depends on the value of x_1. Note that x_1 and x_2 can both be continuous, both categorical, or a mixture of both. The hypothetical example above involved both being binary. In general, the model written in regression notation is

$$E(Y \mid x_1, x_2) = \beta_0 + \beta_1 x_1 + \beta_2 x_2 + \beta_3 x_1 x_2. \qquad (7.16)$$

For the two binary predictors case, if we let $E(Y \mid x_1 = i, x_2 = j) = \mu_{ij}$, $i, j = 0, 1$, then we have

$$\mu_{00} = \beta_0, \quad \mu_{10} = \beta_0 + \beta_1, \quad \mu_{01} = \beta_0 + \beta_2, \quad \mu_{11} = \beta_0 + \beta_1 + \beta_2 + \beta_3.$$

In this instance, we would define the effect of x_1 when $x_2 = 1$ to be $\mu_{11} - \mu_{01} = \beta_1 + \beta_3$, and the effect of x_1 when $x_2 = 0$ to be $\mu_{10} - \mu_{00} = \beta_1$. So the model allows these effects to be different, provided $\beta_3 \neq 0$. With a non-zero value, the sign of β_3 can take the effect modification in either direction. Depending on the values of $\beta_1, \beta_2, \beta_3$, an effect reversal as in the above hypothetical example is possible. Symmetrically, we could have discussed the effect of x_2 for different levels of x_1.

Next, we consider the case with x_1 binary, taking the values 0 or 1, and with x_2 continuous. The model is again expressed as equation (7.16). We can easily see that if $\beta_3 = 0$ and if $x_1 = 0$, this is just a simple linear regression model in x_2 with intercept β_0 and slope β_2. And if $x_1 = 1$, it is again a simple linear regression model in x_2, but now with intercept $\beta_0 + \beta_1$ and slope β_2. So the model allows two regression lines, but forces them to be parallel. The effect of the predictor x_1 is measured as

$$E(Y \mid x_1 = 1, x_2) - E(Y \mid x_1 = 0, x_2) = \beta_2$$

for all values of x_2. This is a special case of the so-called analysis of covariance model. With $\beta_3 = 0$, there is no interaction; the effects of x_1 and x_2 are *additive*. If $\beta_1 \neq 0$ and $\beta_2 \neq 0$, both x_1 and x_2 modify the *response*, but neither modifies the other's *effect*.

So what happens when $\beta_3 \neq 0$? We still have two lines, but now the slopes are different. The slope when $x_1 = 0$ is β_2 as before, but when $x_1 = 1$, it is $\beta_2 + \beta_3$. The effect modification is no longer as simple to explain. First, suppose that the two lines cross, say somewhere in the middle. And for concreteness, suppose that x_2 is age and x_1 is sex, with $x_1 = 1$ corresponding to females. Also assume that $\beta_2 < 0$ and $\beta_2 + \beta_3 > 0$. So the mean response is increasing in age for females and decreasing in age for males. This is clear-cut effect modification. If $\beta_3 = 0$, the effect of age (i.e., how response *varies with age*) is the same for males and for females. If any slopes are 0, there is no corresponding age effect. If $\beta_2 = 0$ and $\beta_3 \neq 0$, then there is no effect of age for men, but there is for women.

Example 7.6. FEV Data Analysis. We now analyze the FEV data that were described in Example 7.3, and discussed there and in Example 7.4 with an informative prior specification. The model was

$$E(FEV \mid Smoke, Age) = \beta_0 + Smoke\,\beta_1 + Age\,\beta_2 + Smoke \times Age\,\beta_3,$$

where $Smoke = 1$ denotes smoker status and 0 denotes non-smoker status, and *Age* represents ages between 11 and 19 treated as a continuous variable. We did not previously discuss the interaction term ,so we do so now.

We ran this model in BUGS using a proper prior approximation to the reference prior $p(\beta, \tau) \propto 1/\tau$ and obtained the output in Table 7.3. In a model with an

TABLE 7.3: Posterior summary for **FEV** analysis with predictors *Smoke*, *Age* and *Smoke* × *Age*

Predictor	Reg. coef.	2.5%	50%	97.5%
Intercept	β_0	0.43	1.09	1.75
Smoke	β_1	0.13	0.18	0.23
Age	β_2	0.0022	1.29	2.67
Interaction	β_3	-0.21	-0.11	-0.018
	σ	0.64	0.70	1.72

interaction term, it does not make sense to attempt to interpret the regression coefficients for the variables, in this case *Age* and *Smoke*, by themselves. This is because we know that the effect of *Smoke* may be different for different ages, and conversely, the regression line of *FEV* on *Age* itself depends on the level of *Smoke*. The one regression coefficient that we can discuss is β_3. Since the 95% probability interval for β_3 is $(-0.21, -0.018)$, we are at least 97.5% certain that it is less than zero. We thus assert that the interaction is statistically important.

The two regression lines for smokers and for non-smokers respectively are

$$E(FEV \mid Smoke = 1, Age) = \beta_0 + \beta_1 + Age(\beta_2 + \beta_3),$$
$$E(FEV \mid Smoke = 0, Age) = \beta_0 + Age\,\beta_2.$$

The posterior means (not shown in Table 7.3) for the regression coefficients are virtually identical to the posterior medians, so it can be seen from the table that the posterior estimates of β_2 and $\beta_2 + \beta_3$ are positive. Thus both estimated regression lines show an increasing trend in expected FEV as a function of age or lung power is increasing with age in both cases. However, since the estimate of $\beta_3 < 0$, the slope of the line for smokers, is estimated to be attenuated by about -0.11. While FEV capacity is increasing with age, the rate of increase is diminished somewhat for smokers relative to non-smokers. Since $P(\beta_3 < 0 \mid y) > 0.975$, this effect has *statistical importance*.

A definition of the effect of smoking on the mean FEV response for a particular age is the difference

$$E(FEV \mid Smoke = 1, Age) - E(FEV \mid Smoke = 0, Age) = \beta_1 + \beta_3 Age.$$

If there were no interaction in the model, the effect of smoking would be the same, β_1, for all ages. Another definition might be the ratio of the two means, but we prefer the difference for this example.

In order to ascertain if there is any *practical* import to this observation, we can make more explicit the effect of *Smoke* on the FEV response. Posterior inferences for the mean FEV responses for smokers and non-smokers for three different ages are shown in Table 7.4. It is clear that there is not a statistically important dif-

TABLE 7.4: Posterior inferences for mean FEV values for smokers and non-smokers, and their differences, for ages 11, 15, and 19

	Mean response/difference	2.5%	50%	97.5%
Smoker, age 11	$\beta_0 + \beta_1 + 11(\beta_2 + \beta_3)$	2.96	3.19	3.43
Non-Smoker, age 11	$\beta_0 + 11\beta_2$	2.94	3.07	3.19
Difference	$\beta_1 + 11\beta_3$	−0.26	0.06	0.40
Smoker, age 15	$\beta_0 + \beta_1 + 15(\beta_2 + \beta_3)$	3.19	3.39	3.59
Non-Smoker, age 15	$\beta_0 + 15\beta_2$	3.62	3.78	3.95
Difference	$\beta_1 + 15\beta_3$	−0.66	−0.39	−0.14
Smoker, age 19	$\beta_0 + \beta_1 + 19(\beta_2 + \beta_3)$	3.19	3.66	4.11
Non-Smoker, age 19	$\beta_0 + 19\beta_2$	4.15	4.50	4.86
Difference	$\beta_1 + 19\beta_3$	−1.46	−0.85	−0.28

ference in the mean FEV values for smokers versus non-smokers for 11-year-olds, but the differences for 15- and for 19-year-olds are statistically important. In fact, the posterior probabilities that these mean differences are negative are 0.35, 0.9985 and 0.9977, respectively. So, because of the interaction, while we see that younger smokers have similar expected FEV values to younger non-smokers, there is an obvious deterioration in expected FEV values for older smokers compared to older non-smokers. In 15-year-olds we see a reduction in FEV for smokers of about 0.4, and in 19-year-olds it is about 0.85. While we suspect that these differences are of practical import, we would have to rely on the expertise of a qualified physician to know for sure. Presumably, the team that collected these data involved precisely such an expert.

One question that arises at this stage is whether the assumption of a linear relationship in age for smokers and for non-smokers is appropriate. Perhaps the relationship is nonlinear for smokers and linear for non-smokers, or vice versa. We leave it as an exercise for readers to address this question.

There will often be more than two predictor variables, and, consequently, there could be more than one pair of them that one might expect to be effect modifiers. One may be tempted to simply add multiple or perhaps even all possible pairwise interaction terms in a model. If the number of original predictors is large, this would create many additional predictors in the model. For example, if there were five predictors and all possible pairs of interactions were included in the model, there would then be an intercept, five so-called main effects, and ten interaction terms. The number grows quickly as the number of predictors grows. Models with many interactions are difficult to interpret, and in some instances, the number of parameters involved might exceed the amount of information in the data that would be available to estimate them. Data analysis is almost always an endeavor involving some well-informed judgments. While it would be important not to ignore an obvious interaction when choosing a model, it would also be important not to fit an overabundance of terms. Parsimony is a general principle in data analysis, meaning that smaller models have a general tendency to be better for prediction than larger models. Interpretability of models is also very important, and smaller models are surely easier to interpret than larger ones. The exercises as the end of the chapter will involve analyzing data with interactions, including the full FEV data, which has a total for four predictor variables.

A Note Regarding Measurement and Absence of Interaction. A subtle and seldom emphasized aspect of effect modification or interaction is that its very definition depends on how we define the effect of a treatment (or any covariate or predictor or regressor). Two things matter:

1. The measure of response or outcome (e.g., population mean, population median, probability or odds of success).

2. The definition of effect (i.e., the function used for comparison of response measure at two levels of a covariate). Examples are difference (in means, medians, probabilities, etc.), ratio (of means, medians, probabilities, odds, etc.), and percent change.

The answer to whether or not an interaction is present depends on each of these. To illustrate the second consideration, we return to the example at the beginning of this section, with survival time medians at two dose levels for women and men. Consider the scenario in the following table, albeit numerically very different from the original:

	Low dose	High dose	Difference	Ratio
Women	8	4	4	2.00
Men	10	6	4	1.67

Comparison by differences shows no effect modification by sex. However, if we use ratios for dose-level comparisons (i.e., effects), sex is an effect modifier.

An instance where the response measure matters (first point in the list above) is for a binary outcome as in Chapters 5 and 8. Using probability or odds will influence the existence of an interaction.

Typically, the *absence* of effect modification or interaction is considered desirable, as this situation leads to a simpler explanation of the regression relationship. This note is intended as a caution that such simplicity is limited to the chosen measure of the response and the function used to compare responses at two levels.

7.6   ANOVA

The methods from Chapter 5 for analyzing two-sample normal data can be extended to compare three or more populations. Treatment of such data was pioneered by the famed early twentieth-century statistician Sir Ronald Fisher and termed *analysis of variance* (ANOVA). Fisher also made many other seminal advances in statistical theory and methods, including likelihood-based inference and design of agricultural experiments that led to the green revolution in agricultural productivity of the twentieth century that is widely credited with alleviating world-wide food shortages. Now ANOVA has come to mean the special case of linear models in which only categorical predictor variables are used. One-way ANOVA involves a single multilevel factor, two-way ANOVA has two categorical predictors (and possibly their interaction), etc. Such multilevel factor variables must be transformed into a series of group indicator variables to include as predictors in a linear model. A related model is the analysis of covariance (ANCOVA), which also falls within the framework of the linear model. The simplest ANCOVA model has one continuous and one categorical predictor but no interaction. The analysis of FEV data in Section 7.5 is an example of this.

Suppose we have one categorical variable called Factor A with levels $1, 2, \ldots, k$. Such levels often correspond to distinct groups or populations of patients; for example, patients with a certain condition that are untreated or treated by one of several possible drugs. Suppose there are n_j response observations $y_{1j}, \ldots, y_{n_j j}$ in the jth group (or level or population) with $n = \sum_{j=1}^{k} n_j$ being the total sample size. For $j = 1, \ldots, k$, let μ_j and σ_j denote the mean and standard deviation of the response in the jth population. Then we can write the model as

$$Y_{ij} \overset{ind}{\sim} N(\mu_j, \sigma^2), \quad i = 1, \ldots, n_j; \; j = 1, \ldots, k. \tag{7.17}$$

This is a straightforward extension of the normally distributed two-population comparison in Chapter 5. In this model, means are allowed to differ among populations but the variance is constant.

To put this in the linear model framework, we first label the response values with a single subscript as $y_1, \ldots, y_n$. We then construct k binary indicator variables $x_i = (x_{i1}, \ldots, x_{ik})'$ for each subject, with $x_{ij} = 1$ if the observation of response y_i is at level j of Factor A, and 0 otherwise. Clearly, we must have $\sum_{j=1}^{k} x_{ij} = 1$ for each i. For observations $y_1, \ldots, y_n$, we can then write

$$Y_i \mid x_i, \mu \overset{ind}{\sim} N(x_i'\mu, \sigma^2), \quad i = 1, \ldots, n, \tag{7.18}$$

where $\mu = (\mu_1, \ldots, \mu_k)$. Note that for each y_i the value of one and only one predictor, say the jth one, equals 1, the rest being 0; and $x_i'\mu$ picks off the jth component of μ. We also note that, unlike in expression (7.2), there is no intercept here, and the symbol β is replaced by μ because of the context. Stacking the y_i into a vector and the x_i' into a matrix, we can also write this model as

$$Y \mid \mu, \sigma^2 \sim N_n(X\mu, \sigma^2 I_n).$$

Finally, from a Bayesian modeling viewpoint it is simple to allow the variances to differ from population to population. In the model, σ^2 simply acquires the subscript j. But then, a separate prior must be specified for each variance (or precision τ_j). The MCMC sampling structure remains essentially intact with some changes in details of parameters for the full conditionals. If using Bayesian software, the code changes minimally.

We now illustrate one-way ANOVA by an extension of the DiaSorin data example of Section 5.2.4.

Example 7.7. DiaSorin Data. We compared DiaSorin levels of chronic kidney disease patients with low bone turnover to those with normal turnover using a two-group normal analysis. In addition, there is a third group of $n_3 \equiv n_H = 50$ patients with high bone turnover. It is useful to distinguish low bone turnover patients, so that they can be properly treated. It is also important to identify patients with high turnover, because a different course of treatment is given to them.

In Section 5.2.4, we transformed DiaSorin scores (y) to achieve approximate normality. Using the prior information provided by Dr. Herberth (on the scale of the scores), we carefully specified the priors for means of $\log(y)$ as $\mu_L \equiv \mu_1 \sim N(4.87, 0.00288)$ and $\mu_N \equiv \mu_2 \sim N(5.39, 0.00280)$. Similar methods to those described there also led to the informative prior $\mu_3 \equiv \mu_H \sim N(6.40, 0.006)$. To show another possibility, we also employ here independent flat priors on μ_1, μ_2, μ_3.

A standard assumption in traditional ANOVA is that variances are the same in the separate populations. In Section 5.2.4 we made no such assumption. Instead, we elicited distinct but diffuse priors for (τ_1, τ_2): $\tau_1 \sim Ga(1.0376, d)$, $\tau_2 \sim Ga(1.04653, d)$, with $d = 0.001$. However, to mimic traditional ANOVA, we make the equal variance assumption and model uncertainty about the resulting common precision as $\tau \sim Ga(0.001, 0.001)$. We combine this prior for τ with two different prior specifications for the means: (a) informative priors on the μs as above; and (b) flat priors on the μs.

The one-way ANOVA consists of the factor "turnover group" having three levels: low, normal, and high. The primary scientific issue is whether DiaSorin can discriminate among the three groups. As a first step, the data analysis looks for evidence that $\mu_1 < \mu_2 < \mu_3$. While the inferences we made on the means of $\log(y)$ can be reinterpreted on the original measurement scale as inferences for medians (we did this in Section 5.2.4), we do not need to do this to address the primary inference target $P(\mu_1 < \mu_2 < \mu_3 \mid data)$.

Basic posterior inference is shown in Table 7.5 under both the informative and the flat priors. Posterior location summaries (means and medians) of the μs increase from low to normal to high turnover groups in both analyses. Notice, however, that for the high-turnover group, these location summaries are considerably larger under prior (a). Moreover, all of the posterior standard deviations for the μs are appreciably smaller under prior (a) than under prior (b). As is often the case, the informative prior yields less posterior uncertainty and tighter probability intervals for the μs.

While not included in Table 7.5, it is easy to approximate $P(\mu_1 < \mu_2 < \mu_3 \mid data)$ with posterior MCMC samples by simply computing the fraction of samples

TABLE 7.5: Posterior summaries from ANOVA of the DiaSorin data

Parameter	(a) Informative Prior on μs				
	Mean	sd	2.5%	Median	97.5%
μ_L	4.86	0.05	4.76	4.86	4.96
μ_N	5.40	0.05	5.29	5.40	5.50
μ_H	6.26	0.07	6.12	6.26	6.39
τ	1.20	0.19	0.85	1.19	1.60
	(b) Approximate Flat Prior on μs				
	Mean	sd	2.5%	Median	97.5%
μ_L	4.70	0.20	4.31	4.71	5.10
μ_N	5.49	0.23	5.05	5.49	5.94
μ_H	5.85	0.12	5.61	5.85	6.10
τ	1.32	0.21	0.95	1.31	1.76

that show $\mu_1 < \mu_2 < \mu_3$. Under both priors, at least 90% of the samples satisfy this inequality. So we are quite certain that the median in the high group is larger than the median in the normal group, which is larger than the median in the low group. The posterior probability $P(\mu_1 < \mu_2 < \mu_3 \mid data)$ equals 1 under prior (a), and equals 0.91 under prior (b). With prior (b), the 95% probability interval for $\mu_H - \mu_N$ includes 0, but the posterior probability that μ_H is larger than μ_N is 0.92.

Figure 7.5 shows predictive densities using prior (a) for all three groups on the log scale. While these predictive pdfs appear to be somewhat different from each other, they show substantial overlap. Note, as always, that predictive distributions have larger variances than the corresponding posterior distributions of the μs (not shown). The diagnostic potential of DiaSorin to distinguish among bone turnover groups will depend more on how different the predictive distributions are from each other than on clear separation of the posterior distributions of the μs.

For inference on the original DiaSorin score scale, we transformed the MCMC samples summarized in Table 7.5, exponentiated each μ in each sample, and summarized these in Table 7.6. We note that the inference targets are now the population medians of DiaSorin scores, and for comparing low, normal, and high bone turnover groups the targets are median ratios. With informative prior (a), just as the 95% probability intervals for $\mu_i - \mu_j$ all excluded 0 on the log scale, the intervals for the relative medians on the original scale all exclude 1. Thus for any two medians, we are quite sure that they differ. In addition, we are 97.5% sure that the median in the high group is at least 3.41 times that for the low group. The posterior means of the group medians are 129.0, 220.2, and 520.5 for the low, normal, and high categories, respectively. The analysis for prior (b) is similar but with greater posterior uncertainty.

Relevant files for this analysis are on the book's webpage under Chapter 7 as `diasorinANOVA.txt`.

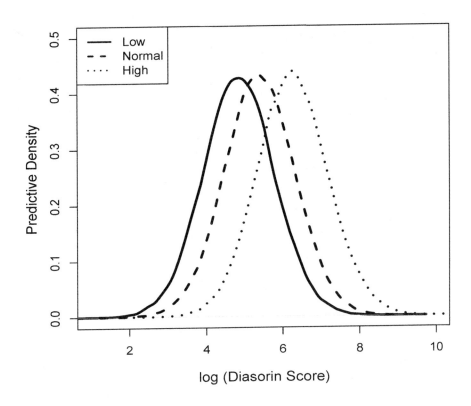

FIGURE 7.5: Predictive densities for log DiaSorin scores.

A Note on Traditional ANOVA. In this book nearly all data analysis techniques begin with a probability model for the data to be observed—a conceptualization of the mechanisms by which the data are thought to arise (i.e., data sampling model or distribution; sometimes called the likelihood). Then we express knowledge (via a prior distribution) about certain numerical characteristics of the sampled population and induce this prior information onto the parameters of the model. Next we use Bayes' theorem to update our knowledge in light of the data (posterior distribution). Finally, all inference flows from this data-informed knowledge distribution. Prediction is accomplished using this distribution and the model.

Notice that the data aspects (descriptions and summaries such as mean, median, range, standard deviation) themselves do not directly play any role. In traditional statistics, on the other hand, one often begins with such functions of data (in fact, these are called *statistics*!) that are contextually useful. Then one tries to address the question of how the particular value of the statistic fits into the possible values that would be obtained if the data collection were repeated a very large number of times under the data sampling mechanism, *regardless* of the values of the unknowns in this mechanism.

This traditional approach to data analysis has proved very successful in pro-

TABLE 7.6: Posterior summaries from ANOVA of the DiaSorin data, original scale

(a) Informative prior on μs					
Inference target	Mean	sd	2.5%	Median	97.5%
Med_L	129.2	6.72	116.5	129.0	142.8
Med_N	220.5	11.36	199.1	220.2	243.7
Med_H	522.0	36.03	455.5	520.5	596.8
$\text{Med}_N/\text{Med}_L$	1.71	0.13	1.48	1.71	1.97
$\text{Med}_H/\text{Med}_L$	4.05	0.35	3.41	4.04	4.78
$\text{Med}_H/\text{Med}_N$	2.37	0.20	2.00	2.36	2.80
(b) Approximate flat prior on μs					
	Mean	sd	2.5%	Median	97.5%
Med_L	112.7	22.98	74.32	110.50	164.10
Med_N	248.40	57.12	155.30	242.10	377.90
Med_H	349.80	43.84	272.10	347.10	444.10
$\text{Med}_N/\text{Med}_L$	2.30	0.72	1.21	2.19	3.99
$\text{Med}_H/\text{Med}_L$	3.23	0.78	1.97	3.14	4.99
$\text{Med}_H/\text{Med}_N$	1.48	0.39	0.86	1.43	2.38

viding scientists and researchers with many tools to carry out inference (drawing conclusions from data), especially over the past century. Early examples of these are the ubiquitous "t test" and, of course, ANOVA. We take this opportunity to explain ANOVA from this Fisherian approach. It might also shed light on why it is called analysis of "variance" when the main goal is to detect whether several *means* are all equal or not.

To keep notational simplicity, let us consider samples of equal sizes n from three populations for a total sample size of $3n$. The individual observations in the first group are denoted $y_{11}, y_{12}, \ldots, y_{1n}$, using 1 as the first subscript. This subscript order is reversed from that used in our previous notation (e.g., in expression 7.18) to keep it consistent with common practice. The previous notation was designed to fit into the general linear regression model. Similarly denoting observations from the other groups, we write the observations as y_{ij}, $i = 1, 2, 3$; $j = 1, \ldots, n$. This extends easily to more groups.

Now we would like to construct a single statistic that will measure the degree of discrepancy in the three group means. A clear separation of the means will result if distances *between group means* much exceed the sizes of distances of observations *within groups*. A convenient single number summary of distances between numbers in a set is the *variance* of the numbers. So, we should compare the between-group variance to the within-group variance.

Recall that, in general, the variance of numbers $z_1, \ldots, z_n$ is $s_z^2 = \frac{1}{n-1} \sum_{k=1}^n (z_k - \bar{z})^2$. Applying this to group means $\bar{y}_1, \bar{y}_2, \bar{y}_3$, we get the between-group variance $\frac{1}{2} \sum_{i=1}^3 (\bar{y}_i - \bar{y})^2$, where $\bar{y}_i = \frac{1}{n} \sum_{j=1}^n y_{ij}$ is the mean of ith group, and

$\bar{y} = \frac{1}{3n} \sum_{i=1}^{3} \sum_{j=1}^{n} y_{ij}$ is the overall mean of all $3n$ observations. The within-group variance should, clearly, use the squared deviation $(y_{ij} - \bar{y}_i)^2$ of an individual observation from the mean of the group to which it belongs. All such squared deviations are to be added and divided by $3n - 3$, as 3 distinct means are used as centers for deviations,[4] resulting in $\frac{1}{3n-3} \sum_{i=1}^{3} \sum_{j=1}^{n} (y_{ij} - \bar{y}_i)^2$. Extending to I groups of equal sizes n, we thus arrive at the single statistic we set out to define, called the *F statistic* in honor of Fisher:[5]

$$ F = \frac{\frac{1}{I-1} \sum_{i=1}^{I} (\bar{y}_i - \bar{y})^2}{\frac{1}{nI-I} \sum_{i=1}^{I} \sum_{j=1}^{n} (y_{ij} - \bar{y}_i)^2}, \quad i = 1, \ldots, I; \ j = 1, \ldots, n. $$

Setting aside the divisors $I-1$ and $nI-I$, a closer look at the sum of squares (SS) in the numerator and denominator reveals a very interesting (and by now fundamental) equality of statistics: these two SSs add up to the *total* SS, $\sum_{i=1}^{I} \sum_{j=1}^{n} (y_{ij} - \bar{y})^2$, which ignores the groups and treats the data as arising from a single population. We now see why Fisher termed it *analysis* of *variance*; the total sum of squares is broken down into a between-group SS and a within-group SS. A rescaled ratio of these two pieces is the statistic we were looking for. This brilliant construction, from the data up, played a ubiquitous role in many sciences and engineering where experimentation is common, especially in the pre-computer-age twentieth century. Of course, it continues to be quite useful in many contexts. The Bayesian formulation and analysis described earlier, using computer-age posterior sampling techniques, allows us to make inferences more readily for a much richer variety of targets than the basic and important detection of differences in population means.

7.7 Recap and Readings

Regression, that is, modeling the relationship between the expected value of an outcome and potentially explanatory variables, is a basic and fundamental method for statistical inference. Most scientific endeavors seek to understand associations and relationships. Linear regression is, perhaps, the simplest form of regression, particularly since it often involves inference on the scale of measurement without requiring a transformation. As we indicated, the topic of linear regression includes ANOVA and ANCOVA models. The differences relate to the covariates' data types. Historically, though, the ability to derive answers analytically contributed to the separate development of these models.

We have introduced the topic of linear regression and developed it from the Bayesian viewpoint for students who may or may not have previous experience with it. Two early classic books that concerned models we have discussed in this

---

[4]The mathematical reason for this $n - 3$ divisor is subtle, having to do with the expected value of the statistic over conceptually repeated experiments.

[5]This definition is for equal-sized groups.

chapter are the book on ANOVA by Scheffé [280], originally published in 1959, and the 1971 book on linear models by Searle [285]. These books base inference on frequentist statistics. An early Bayesian book on linear models is by Broemeling [54].

As Bayesian statisticians, we consider the regression coefficients as unknowns about which we wish to learn more than just a single value—which values may be more likely and which less likely? We characterize the entire distribution of the coefficients' values via probability distributions that incorporate the data and, possibly, other sources of information. Classical regression books consider probability distributions for the estimates of the regression coefficients, because they are functions of the data. The classical development does not consider variation coming from uncertainty regarding the coefficients themselves or from other sources. An early exception is the case of random effects in regression models. The motivation for adding random effects (as opposed to so-called fixed effects, which are the usual regression coefficients) seems to have arisen in agricultural applications. Analyses of studies in animals often appeared to exhibit more variation than one may have anticipated. Adding a random herd effect, for example, or some other source of variation as a coefficient with a probability distribution often improved model fit. These random effects in the regression models were essentially treated as nuisance parameters in the sense that they were not the focus of the inference. Instead of estimating the contribution of these coefficients, the methods integrated over them, thereby adding more variation. This methodology is developed in the book by Searle et al. [286]. These random effects do have some relationship with Bayesian regression modeling. It is not a great leap to see that "extra variation" in terms of deviation of observations from expected values and "uncertainty" in the regression model may be related.

Attempts to improve efficiency and reduce mean squared error in frequentist estimation led to two topics that are closely related. James–Stein and ridge regression estimators are two methodologies that lead to shrinkage estimators that are more efficient than regular estimation in ANOVA and general regression settings, respectively [152]. The ridge estimator in linear regression is $\hat{\beta} = (X'X + kI)^{-1} X'Y$, where k is a positive constant. If we look closely at the ridge estimator and compare it to the posterior mean in the case of known (or conditioning on) residual variance, we see that these two quantities are quite similar. From Section 7.3.3 and with the prior of β being $N(0, I)$, $E[\beta \mid \tau, y_1, \ldots, y_n] = (\tau X'X + I)^{-1}(\tau X'y) = (X'X + \sigma^2 I)^{-1}(X'y)$. That is, the ridge estimator is the posterior mean of the regression coefficients when the prior mean of the coefficients is 0 and the prior variance is the identity matrix. We discussed posterior means as shrinkage estimators in Chapter 2. In particular, the case of univariate normal exchangeable models showed that the posterior mean is a precision-weighted average of the prior mean and the sample mean, conditional on the residual variance (see expression (3.6)). This notion of the posterior mean being a weighted combination carries over to the multivariate case, as we can see in the development in Section 7.3.3.

An important part of building regression models is selecting the covariates that matter in the regression. In regression, one will likely start with a set of covariates and then decide whether or not each should stay in the model. We talked about looking at individual regression coefficients' posterior distributions in this chapter to help make this decision. An approach that several researchers have chosen for regression modeling is the so-called spike-and-slab prior for the regression coefficients. Initially proposed for linear regression [243], the spike-and-slab prior assigns to each regression coefficient β_j for the jth covariate (x_j) the following prior distribution: $p(\beta_j = 0) = \pi_{0j}$ and $p(\beta_j \in [-w_j, w_j], \beta_j \neq 0) = 2w_j\pi_{1j} = (1 - \pi_{0j})$. This prior distribution for β_j consists of a *spike* of height π_{0j} at zero and a *slab* of width $2w_j$ centered at zero with height π_{1j}. Each of the 2^p possible models from the p covariates has a prior probability that is a product of the $1 - \pi_{0j}$ for the covariates that are included in the model and a product of the π_{0j} for those covariates that are left out of the model. The spike-and-slab prior and variants are easy to program via MCMC and also lend themselves to posterior averaging across multiple models (Bayesian model averaging [165]). Further details may be found in George and Mc-Cullogh (1993, 1997) [139, 140]. Statistical research continues to provide extensions and variations of the spike-and-slab prior

Assessing the fit of different models includes more than just deciding whether or not to include a covariate, of course. We discuss model comparison in Chapter 10. The Zellner g-prior is especially useful for Bayesian hypothesis testing using Bayes factors (see Chapter 10). With this prior, the Bayes factor is available in closed form for testing a coefficient having value 0 [352]. This approach was used in a pharmacogenomics study to screen through single nucleotide polymorphisms' associations with a drug's pharmacokinetics [274].

The mathematical derivation of the distribution of the regression coefficients used many techniques from linear algebra. The multivariate normal model finds itself used very often across several Bayesian models. An important paper that presents many results for the multivariate normal distribution is by Lindley and Smith [228]. In fact, the ideas in that paper form the basis for analysis of so-called multilevel or hierarchical models (Chapter 14).

Many of the remaining chapters of this book build on the concepts we have presented for linear regression. Although the mathematical formulations of the models differ according to the sampling distribution of the observed outcome or response, the basic idea of a regression and a conditional mean being a linear function of coefficients and covariates is fundamental.

7.8 Exercises

EXERCISE 7.1. Refer to the **VetBP data** analysis in Section 7.1.2 for this exercise. Using "flat" priors, or proper approximations to them, do the following:

(a) Obtain inferences (posterior median, 95% probability intervals) and comment on them for:

(i) the mean DBP for 50-, 60-, and 70-year-old veterans;

(ii) the three pairwise differences in these means.

(b) Compute the posterior probabilities of:

(i) $\beta_1 < 0$;   (ii) $\beta_0 < 78$.

(c) Obtain predictive inferences for 50-, 60-, and 70-year-old patients.

(d) Obtain the predictive probability that a randomly chosen 50-year-old veteran will have a higher DBP than a randomly chosen 70-year-old veteran.

EXERCISE 7.2.   Refer to Example 7.1 and posterior results that were given in Table 7.2. Write your own code to obtain inferences for the model after *centering* the continuous covariates $DBP0$, Ht and Wt.

(a) Assess convergence of your Markov chains.

(b) Construct a table similar to Table 7.2; compare results and discuss.

(c) Using posterior samples, obtain appropriate quantities to interpret the effect of an increase in 10 mm Hg of the baseline DBP ($DBP0$) on the six-month DBP for populations of veterans under treatment 1, and under treatment 2. Discuss.

(d) Rerun your MCMC sampling code, this time using original *uncentered* variables. Discuss how well the MCMC procedure is converging under this parameterization.

*EXERCISE 7.3.   Define $\hat{\beta} = (X'X)^{-1}X'y$, $SSE = (y - X\hat{\beta})'(y - X\hat{\beta})$ as in Section 7.3.3, just before Section 7.3.3.1.

(a) Show that

$$(y - X\beta)'(y - X\beta) = y'y + \beta'X'X\beta - 2y'X\beta.$$

(b) Then use the result in (a) to show that

$$(y - X\beta)'(y - X\beta) = SSE + (\beta - \hat{\beta})'X'X(\beta - \hat{\beta}).$$

(c) Argue that the minimizer of this quantity is $\beta = \hat{\beta}$, and consequently argue that the MLE for β is just $\hat{\beta}$. The first of these is a classic result from traditional linear models theory, which is the essence of the Gauss–Markov theorem.

*(d) Defining $\mathcal{P}$ as in Section 7.2.2, using its properties from that section, and using that fact that

$$(y - X\beta)'(y - X\beta) = (y - \mathcal{P}y + \mathcal{P}y + X\beta)'(y - \mathcal{P}y + \mathcal{P}y + X\beta),$$

prove the result in part (b); this is obviously a different approach than was used in part (b).

EXERCISE 7.4.   Consider the FEV data and CMP prior specified for β that was discussed in Example 7.3. There, $\tilde{m}' = (2.8, 3.0, 4.0, 3.3)$ is the vector of prior guesses for the mean FEV values for the predictor combinations specified in the matrix $\tilde{X}$ in the example.

(a) If you believe that smoking might affect lung capacity over time, is the prior specification in this example reasonable? Explain in words what the prior is suggesting in terms of the effects of smoking and age on the FEV response.

(b) Now consider an alternative prior specification with $\tilde{m}' = (2.8, 2.5, 4.0, 3.5)$. How are these prior beliefs different from those in the example?

(c) Simulate the induced marginal prior distributions for the components of β using both priors discussed above; discuss similarities and differences between the corresponding induced priors.

(d) Analyze the FEV data using both priors discussed above. Discuss. The data can be found on the book's website (Chapter 7, `FEVdata.txt`).

(e) Analyze the FEV data using the standard reference prior (flat prior from Section 7.2.2), $p(\beta, \tau) \propto 1/\tau$, or a proper prior approximation to it. Compare results with those obtained in part (d).

EXERCISE 7.5. *FEV data.* Consider Example 7.4, where we discussed the elicitation of a $Ga(a, b)$ prior for τ.

(a) Complete the trial and error needed to obtain values of a and b. Plot this gamma density.

(b) Simulate 5,000 samples of τ from this gamma density and plot a histogram of corresponding σs.

(c) How well does the plot in (b) satisfy the prior input?

(d) Obtain posterior inferences for regression coefficients for the FEV data using a flat prior for β and with prior for τ:

(i) $Ga(a, b)$ from part (a); and (ii) $Ga(0.001, 0.001)$.

Compare results. The data can be found on the book's website (Chapter 7, `FEVdata.txt`).

EXERCISE 7.6. *FEV data.* Consider Example 7.4 where we discussed the elicitation of a $Ga(a, b)$ prior for τ.

(a) Place a $Ga(a', b')$ prior on σ (instead of τ) using the same prior information that was given in the example. Find the (a', b') pair that best satisfies the given prior information.

(b) Simulate 5,000 samples of $\sigma \sim Ga(a', b')$ and plot a histogram of the corresponding σs.

(c) How well does the plot satisfy the specified prior input?

(d) If you did Exercise 7.5, compare the two histograms for σ. Are they nearly the same? Which is more consistent with the elicitation information in Example 7.4?

EXERCISE 7.7. With FEV data from the book's website (Chapter 7, `FEVdata,txt`), obtain posterior inferences using the CMP prior in Section 7.3.3.1 on β and a $Ga(a', b')$ prior on σ.

(a) Select the prior on σ to satisfy the prior information specified in Example 7.4. If you did Exercise 7.6(b), you already know (a', b').

(b) Discuss convergence of your Markov chains.

(c) Compute posterior probability intervals for

(i) $E(FEV \mid Age = c, Smoke = 1, \beta) - E(FEV \mid Age = c, Smoke = 0, \beta)$ for $c = 13$ and $c = 18$

(ii) $E(FEV \mid Age = 18, Smoke = 1, \beta) - E(FEV \mid Age = 13, Smoke = 0, \beta)$

(iii) the β_i

and obtain

(iv) numerical approximations to $P(\beta_i > 0 \mid data)$, for all β_i.

(d) Give a brief one- or two-paragraph summary of the most salient conclusions that can be made based on your output. Explain in terms that would be clear to a medical professional. Make distinctions between statistical and practical import.

EXERCISE 7.8. *Head circumference and gestational age.* Consider fitting a simple linear regression model for the average head circumference (in centimeters) at birth as a linear function of the newborn's gestational age (in weeks). We elicit a prior for $\tilde{\mu}_1$, the average head circumference for male infants at 40 weeks' gestation, based on tables for boys from the World Health Organization (WHO) available at

`www.who.int/childgrowth/standards/second_set/chts_hcfa_boys_z/en/`

The tables list the average head circumferences at birth (and at various ages *after* birth).

Average human gestation is 40 weeks (280 days). We use here the head circumference at birth from the WHO table (downloaded 7/28/2018) as the prior mean for a boy baby's head circumference at birth after 40 weeks' gestation. The WHO table ("Head circumference-for-age: Birth to 13 weeks") gave the median head circumference for boys at birth to be 34.5 cm, and 97.5th percentile 37.0 cm. We thus take the prior mean $\tilde{m}_1 = 34.5$. For the standard deviation, we equate $34.5 + 2\sigma = 37.0$ and solve $\sigma = (37.0 - 34.5)/2 = 1.25$ cm, assuming that the head circumferences are roughly normally distributed with standard deviation σ. Note that this represents variation from infant to infant. We can, quite conservatively, take this as the upper limit on our prior uncertainty about $\tilde{\mu}_1$.

Now consider $\tilde{\mu}_2$, mean head circumference corresponding to a birth at 36 weeks of gestation. For illustrative purposes, we specify that the average boy baby's head circumference at 36 weeks is a centimeter smaller, $\tilde{m}_2 = 33.5$ cm. To compensate for this assumption, we allow for greater uncertainty by doubling the standard deviation for the mean head circumference at birth after 40 weeks' gestation. In other words, we are 97.5% certain that the head circumference of a baby boy born at 36 weeks' gestation is less than 38.5 cm $(= 33.5 + (2 \times 2.5))$. We note that the greater uncertainty for a boy born at 36 weeks leads to a larger upper bound than the corresponding upper bound for a 40-week gestational period, even though the 40-week mean is larger than the 36-week mean.

(a) Derive the induced CMP for β and give 95% prior probability intervals for β_0 and β_1 using normal distributions

(b) Simulate from the induced prior on β by first simulating $\tilde{\mu}$ and then solving for β in terms of $\tilde{\mu}$. Then obtain exact 95% prior probability intervals using the results in part (a). Compare the simulated results with the exact ones.

(c) Place independent uniform priors on the two mean head circumferences, say $\tilde{\mu}_1 \sim U(32, 37)$ and $\tilde{\mu}_2 \sim U(28.5, 38.5)$. Simulate from the new induced prior on β and compare intervals with the previous results.

EXERCISE 7.9. *Head circumference and gestational age, continued.* Consider the problem described in Exercise 7.8. Suppose that, independently of the data, the best estimate of the 90th percentile of head circumferences among baby boys born at 36 weeks was 32.0 cm. Moreover, with 95% certainty assume that the 90th percentile of the head circumferences of these babies is believed to be at least 35.0 cm.

(a) Using any additional needed prior information from the description in Exercise 7.8, derive an appropriate gamma prior for τ given this information. Plot the prior. Then obtain the induced prior for σ using the usual transformation technique and plot it. Comment.

(b) Now assume, with 95% certainty, that the 90th percentile of the head circumferences of these babies is believed to be at most 38.0 cm. Find an appropriate $Ga(a, b)$ prior for σ. Plot it.

EXERCISE 7.10. *Head circumference and gestational age, continued from Exercises 7.8 and 7.9.* Now suppose that there is a second predictor variable for the head circumference data, say the baby's weight. Assume that the prior information collected in Exercise 7.8 can be regarded as if it was for babies that were of an average weight of 3.4 kg.

(a) Using the CMP prior developed in Exercise 7.8(a), construct a partial information prior for regressing head circumference on both gestational age and weight. (*Hint*: Consider reparameterizing the model by using the centered covariates, *cAge* and *cWeight*. It is then easier to obtain the precise induced prior on the "new" parameters.)

(b) Simulate from your partial information prior and induce a prior on mean head circumference corresponding to four newborns as follows:

(i) Two babies born after 37 weeks' gestation: one baby weighs 2.7 kg, and the other baby weighs 3.5 kg.

(ii) Two babies born at 41 weeks: one baby weighs 3.4 kg, and the other baby weighs 4.5 kg. Comment.

EXERCISE 7.11 Consider a situation with $p = 4$ covariates and suppose the first covariate is *Sex*, which takes the value 1 for females and 0 for males, and the second covariate is *Long*, which takes the value 1 if there is "good longevity" in their close family and 0 if not. Let the third covariate be centered *cAge*, and the fourth be centered diastolic blood pressure, *cDBP* (centered meaning that their means in the data have been subtracted). Suppose that individuals under study all have high-quality insurance and that the response is the total cost of medical treatment over a five-year period. Also suppose that cost information is available for two types of individuals. The first is a male with *Long* = 0 and of average age and DBP ($cAge = 0$, $cDBP = 0$). The second is the same as the first, except that their $cDBP = 15$. The two $\tilde{m}_i$ are $25,000$ and $30,000$, respectively; and both $\tilde{w}_i$

equal \$5,000. Give an appropriate partial information prior for the five-dimensional β.

EXERCISE 7.12. *Full FEV data.*   Recall the FEV data from Example 7.6. We now consider the full data set, which includes two additional predictor variables, height and weight. The data now include predictor variables smoking status (S), age (A), height (H), and sex as an indicator of being male (M); (see the book's website, Chapter 7, `FEVdata-full.csv`). We consider the model with sex and centered age and height, namely

$$E(FEV|S, cA, cH, M) = \beta_0 + \beta_1 cA + \beta_2 S + \beta_3 S \times cA + \beta_4 cH + \beta_5 M.$$

Assume a normal linear model with constant variance, $\sigma^2 = 1/\tau$.

(a) Analyze the data using a flat prior $(p(\beta, \tau) \propto 1/\tau)$, or a proper diffuse approximation to it.

(b) Interpret the interaction effect in terms of practical and statistical import.

(c) Compare inferences for the full model to inferences for the model without height or weight. Do they change appreciably, and if so how? If they do change, what might that mean from a scientific vantage point?

EXERCISE 7.13. *Full FEV data, continued.*   Recall the FEV data from Example 7.6. We consider the full data set, which includes predictor variables $(Age, Hgt, Male, Smoke)$; (see the book's website, Chapter 7, `FEVdata-full.csv`). We consider the same model as in Exercise 7.12 with centered age and height.

   We construct a partially informative prior for β based on the prior of Example 7.3. We specify a normal prior on two expected FEV values that correspond to two predictor combinations, $\tilde{\mu}_i$, $i = 1, 2$. These will correspond to an 11-year-old and a 16-year-old female, both non-smokers and both of average height. Recall in Example 7.3, where we only had age and smoking status as predictors, we specified a CMP that included specifications for 11- and 16-year-old non-smokers. If we regard those two children as having average height, then the prior specifications made there will be precisely the same here (ignoring differences in average heights for male and female children in this age range). One difference is that here we have centered the continuous covariates. For convenience, center age at 16, so that the 16 in the $\tilde{X}$ matrix in Example 7.3 becomes 0 and the 11 becomes -5. Now we have $\tilde{x}'_1 = (1, -5, 0, 0, 0, 0)$ and $\tilde{x}'_2 = (1, 0, 0, 0, 0, 0)$. Using the prior specified in Example 7.3, we have $\tilde{\mu}_1 \sim N(2.8, 0.04)$ and $\tilde{\mu}_2 \sim N(4.0, 0.04)$, independently. This will induce a prior on β_0 and β_1. Specify a flat prior on the remaining parameters, namely $p(\beta_2, \beta_3, \beta_4, \beta_5, \tau) \propto 1/\tau$, or a proper diffuse approximation to it.

(a) Obtain posterior inferences using this prior. If you did Exercise 7.12, compare inferences.

(b) Repeat (a) using a partial prior that uses only the specification for $\tilde{\mu}_2$. Compare results with those in (a).

(c) Now extend the partial prior in (a), so that it includes an additional normal prior for $\tilde{\mu}_3$, which corresponds to $\tilde{x}'_3 = (1, 0, 0, 0, 1, 0)$. Assume that there is no reason to believe that being one standard deviation above the mean in height will result in a higher or lower mean FEV value. You may be more uncertain about this than we were in the previous example for the corresponding situation. Then again, using the prior information given in Example 7.3, obtain the induced partial information prior for $(\beta_0, \beta_1, \beta_4)$. You can do this analytically by obtaining the exact trivariate normal distribution, or by simulating the marginal prior distributions for these three regression coefficients.

EXERCISE 7.14. *Blood versus breath alcohol project.* Most governments impose an upper limit on blood alcohol levels of drivers as a way to reduce the risk of accidents caused by driving impairment. It is easier for law enforcement agents to collect a sample of the alcohol level by measuring the alcohol concentration in the driver's breath than by drawing a blood sample on the side of the highway. The research question was whether one can estimate a person's blood alcohol concentration by measuring the concentration of alcohol in the breath.

Austrian researchers sought to answer this question. They assembled a group of 59 Austrian volunteers (27 women and 32 men) to participate in this experiment. The volunteers' ages ranged from 20 years to 40 years. After verifying that each participant was sober at the start of the experiment, the experimenters allowed the participants to drink alcoholic beverages of their choice over a two-hour period. The average alcohol consumption for the volunteers was 1.07 ± 0.23 g/kg body weight. The experimenters then measured the alcohol concentration in the individual's breath every 30 minutes, starting 30 minutes after the volunteer finished drinking. Blood alcohol measurements occurred at the same time. Breath and blood sampling continued up to five hours after the individual finished drinking or until the breath alcohol concentration was ≤ 0.1 mg/L. Volunteers could eat sandwiches and drink water during the measurement phase.

The data, available on the book's website under Chapter 7 in file named `breathalcohol.csv`, consist of an identification number for each participant, whether the participant was male (0) or female (1), the breath alcohol concentration (mg/L), and the concentration of alcohol in the blood (g/L). We wish to predict y (blood alcohol level) based on x (breath alcohol concentration level). We also wish to know if the relationship between these two alcohol elimination rates differs for men and women.

(a) Make a scatterplot of blood alcohol versus breath alcohol with different symbols or colors representing males and females. Comment.

(b) Model the data using a linear model that allows for two distinct lines. Superimpose a plot of the two fitted lines on the scatterplot of the data from part (a). Comment on the plot. Do the data suggest the possibility of fitting the model with parallel lines?

(c) Interpret the model that was fit in part (b). Then fit the model with parallel lines and decide if the simpler model might be preferable. Discuss.

(d) For your chosen model in part (c), plot the estimated mean response as a function of the measured alcohol level in breath over a grid, and also plot 95%

probability interval values (upper and lower) for each grid point. Then repeat giving 95% prediction curves.

(e) To interpret the association between x and y, present posterior inferences for parameters and predictions in an appropriately designed table. Give a brief narrative with the table, addressing the association.

EXERCISE 7.15. *FEV data.*   For the two-predictor version of the FEV data (see the book's website, Chapter 7, FEVdata.txt), analyze the data with the goal of assessing whether or not the square of age should be added to the model that has linear terms in age for smokers and non-smokers. It could be that there is a quadratic trend in age for smokers or for non-smokers or both. You may wish to start by plotting FEV values versus age for smokers and for non-smokers on the same plot with different colors or symbols for smokers and non-smokers. Justify your conclusions based on an appropriate data analysis. You may use flat priors or proper prior approximations to them.

*EXERCISE 7.16 *Marginal posterior for* β.*   With the flat (or reference) prior $p(\beta, \tau) \propto 1/\tau$, and referring to Section 7.2.2 for background and notation, show that

$$\beta \mid y \sim T_{p+1}\left(n - p - 1, \hat{\beta}, MSE(X'X)^{-1}\right),$$

the multivariate T distribution with dimension $p + 1$, location $\hat{\beta}$ and dispersion matrix $MSE(X'X)^{-1}$; the general form is given in Appendix B.

*EXERCISE 7.17. *Marginal posterior for* $c'\beta$.*   Under the same conditions as Exercise 7.16, show that

$$c'\beta \mid y \sim T_1\left(n - p - 1, c'\hat{\beta}, MSE\, c'(X'X)^{-1}c\right).$$

(*Hint:* First obtain the distributional result for $c'\beta \mid \tau, y$ and then obtain the kernel of the marginal density for $c'\beta \mid y$ by integrating the density for $(c'\beta, \tau) \mid y$ with respect to τ.)

*EXERCISE 7.18. *Prediction of* y_f.*   Assume the same conditions as in Exercise 7.16.

(a) Derive the predictive density for a future response, y_f, for an individual with a known predictor combination x_f, that is, show that

$$y_f \mid x_f, y \sim T_1\left(n - p - 1, x_f'\hat{\beta}, MSE\left(1 + x_f'(X'X)^{-1}x_f\right)\right).$$

(b) Find an expression for a 95% predictive probability interval for y_f.

Chapter 8

Binary Response Regression

As we saw in Chapter 7, linear regression involves modeling the average of a numeric and continuous response variable Y as depending on a vector of predictors (or covariates), say x, via a linear function of x and the regression coefficients. In this chapter, we consider binary (or dichotomous) Y responses that take on one of two possible values (typically, 0 or 1). In particular, we introduce logistic regression and some other forms of binary regression models.

As one example, we analyze the data on lymphedema (LE), a possible consequence of surgical treatment of breast cancer that results in arm swelling that can lead to decreased functioning, skin breakdown, and chronic infections if left untreated. The goal is to ascertain whether the probability of LE depends on the number of lymph nodes examined during breast cancer surgery, whether cancer was found in one or more of the nodes (lymph node metastasis), and the age of the patient. We also analyze a second data set that has not yet been introduced. Here we have records of whether patients admitted to the University of New Mexico Trauma Center were discharged alive or died prior to discharge. The goal is to model the probability of death as a function of a number of potential predictors, such as age; nature of the injury that brought them to the center, classified as blunt or penetrating; and a measure that reflects injury severity.

Section 8.1 introduces the logistic regression model and its basic analysis for Bernoulli as well as grouped binomial data. Section 8.2 discusses interaction between predictors. Section, 8.3, tackles inference for functions of model parameters. Section 8.4 considers priors, and Section 8.5 considers prediction. Section 8.6 briefly treats the probit and complementary log-log links.

8.1 Logistic Regression Model

Binary and binomial data were discussed in detail in Chapters 3 and 5. To model such data when the outcome (or response) probability is thought to possibly depend on predictors (or covariates), we begin with data denoted $\{(y_i, x_i) : i = 1, \ldots, n\}$, where the y_i are the Bernoulli outcomes and x_i are the covariate vectors. To begin with, let us denote the unknown probability of the conditional event $Y_i = 1 \mid x_i$ by θ_i so that $Y_i \mid x_i, \theta_i \sim Ber(\theta_i)$. Now we wish to specify a model for θ_i to depend on x_i. Looking to linear regression for guidance and noting $E(Y_i \mid x_i, \theta_i) = \theta_i$, we might think of modeling the θ_i as a linear function of the covariates and suitable regression parameters. However, since the θ_i are probabilities, they must be restricted to the interval $[0, 1]$. Linear functions, without cumbersome side conditions, do not have such a limited range. We thus turn to transforming probability to a logit (the log of the odds, first defined in Section 5.1.1.3), which has range $(-\infty, \infty)$. Then $\text{logit}(\theta_i)$ can be modeled as a linear function of regression coefficients, namely,

$$\text{logit}(\theta_i) = \beta_0 + \beta_1 x_{i1} + \cdots + \beta_p x_{ip}$$

following notation from Chapter 7 on the right-hand side. Moreover, using vector notation as in linear regression, we also write this as

$$\text{logit}(\theta_i) = x_i'\beta,$$

where $x_i = (1, x_{i1}, \ldots, x_{ip})'$ is the vector with first element equal to 1 for the intercept and the rest corresponding to the p covariate values for the ith observation. The data model can now be written as

$$Y_1, \ldots, Y_n \mid \theta_1, \ldots, \theta_n \overset{\text{ind}}{\sim} Ber(\theta_i), \quad \text{logit}(\theta_i) = x_i'\beta. \tag{8.1}$$

To see explicitly how θ_i, the probability that $Y_i = 1 | x_i, \beta$, relates to the regression coefficients, we invert the linear logit function as

$$\text{logit}(\theta_i) = \log\left(\frac{\theta_i}{1 - \theta_i}\right) = x_i'\beta \Rightarrow \frac{\theta_i}{1 - \theta_i} = e^{x_i'\beta} \Rightarrow \theta_i = \frac{e^{x_i'\beta}}{1 + e^{x_i'\beta}}.$$

The last expression is the inverse of the logit function. We formalize it with the name *expit* as

$$\text{expit}(a) = \frac{e^a}{1 + e^a}, \quad a \in (-\infty, \infty),$$

which is also known to be the cdf of the standard logistic distribution. From the above two displays, it follows that $1 - \theta_i = 1/(1 + e^{x_i'\beta})$ and the odds of $Y_i = 1 | x_i, \beta$ equal $e^{x_i'\beta}$.

To complete the Bayesian model, we need priors for the intercept and the regression coefficients in β. Unlike in previous chapters (where data model and scientifically meaningful priors are discussed before data analysis), for simplicity, we proceed here from the data model directly to analysis. We do this initially using (improper) flat priors on the regression parameters. The intent here is to emphasize tools of inference and prediction first. A detailed discussion of more suitable priors is given in Section 8.4.

Another point of departure from our development of the linear regression model is that we will move from this model specification to computation using Bayesian software, such as BUGS, JAGS or Stan, without first "deriving" the posterior distribution. The reason for this is twofold. First, the derivation does not lead to any familiar family of distributions for $\beta \mid data$, that is, conjugate or other analytically tractable priors are not available. Second, most current Bayesian data analysis software allows one to specify the model and priors in the language of random quantities and their distributions. Then, given data, the software automatically generates posterior samples using appropriate techniques from Chapter 4 by means of symbol manipulation to generate code. It is, however, quite possible (and very useful for students intending to develop new models for data) to start from first principles, namely, write down densities for the data model and priors, and proceed to develop MCMC sampling algorithms, writing code in R, C++, Python, etc. It turns out that with log-concave priors, posterior samples can be generated using Gibbs sampling and log-concave simulation. It is possible also to employ other techniques, such as the Metropolis–Hastings algorithm or Hamiltonian Monte Carlo. In this chapter we avoid this first-principles effort, except in some optional exercises.

Finally, before turning to examples, we briefly discuss the binomial regression model, closely related to the Bernoulli specification above and useful when appropriate. When data arise in groups, it is convenient to use counts of observations in each group. Let n_i, $i = 1, \ldots, g$, be the number of individuals (or experimental units) in each group, and the number of "successes" (typically coded 1 in the Bernoulli formulation) be y_i, $i = 1, \ldots, g$. The number of observations here can be seen as g with each observation having a binomial distribution, $Y_i \mid \theta_i \overset{\text{ind}}{\sim} Bin(n_i, \theta_i)$. Thus, we can write

$$Y_1, \ldots, Y_g \mid \theta_1, \ldots, \theta_g \overset{\text{ind}}{\sim} Bin(n_i, \theta_i), \quad \text{logit}(\theta_g) = x_i' \beta. \tag{8.2}$$

For this formulation, all observations within a group have identical predictor values. This situation typically arises when all covariates are categorical in nature and the data can be represented as cross-tabulated counts. Our first example below considers a simple case: one covariate with two categories. Thus $g = 2$ is the number of observations in the data set. For an equivalent Bernoulli model as in expression (8.1), there would need to be $n = \sum_{i=1}^{g} n_i$ Bernoulli observations in the next data set ($n = 1{,}211$ in the example).

Example 8.1. Analyzing Grouped LE Data Using a Logistic Regression Model for Binomial Observations. We return to the study of lymphedema (LE) in breast cancer patients described in Example 1.2 and further discussed in Example 5.2. Recall that there were $n = 1{,}211$ women who were followed for up to 4 years. We will consider the LE status as the outcome and the number of lymph nodes examined during breast cancer surgery as the covariate. We set $Y = 1$ if LE is present and 0 otherwise. As previously, we dichotomize the number of nodes examined. The covariate $High = 1$ if the number of lymph nodes is greater than 5, and $High = 0$ if the count is 5 or less. We note from Table 5.2 that for $\theta_1 = P(Y_1 = 1 \mid High = 1)$ and $\theta_2 = P(Y_2 \mid High = 0)$, the posterior medians were 0.26 and 0.073, respectively, indicating a large difference. We now revisit this problem using a regression approach. We are summarizing the data set of 1,211 women as data for two groups. In effect, then, this example's data set has outcome observations (number of women with LE) for two groups with $n_1 = 477$ for $High_1 = 1$ and $n_2 = 734$ for $High_2 = 0$, not 1,211 individual observations. Thus, the data in Table 5.1 are represented here as $\{(y_1 = 126, High_1 = 1), (y_2 = 53, High_2 = 0)\}$, with $Y_1 \mid High_1, \theta_1 \sim Bin(477, \theta_1)$ and $Y_2 \mid High_2, \theta_2 \sim Bin(734, \theta_2)$. The linear logit relationship in expression (8.2) is then written as

$$\text{logit}(\theta_i) = \beta_0 + \beta_1 \, High_i, \quad i = 1, 2.$$

where

$$\theta_1 = \frac{e^{\beta_0 + \beta_1}}{1 + e^{\beta_0 + \beta_1}}, \quad \theta_2 = \frac{e^{\beta_0}}{1 + e^{\beta_0}}.$$

The odds ratio comparing odds of LE for a woman with a high count of nodes examined to one with a low count is $OR = \frac{\theta_1}{1-\theta_1} / \frac{\theta_2}{1-\theta_2} = e^{\beta_1}$.

In Chapter 5, we used an informative prior for θ_1 and θ_2. Here, we consider flat (and thus improper) priors for the β_i, which could be used if there really was no scientific information available. The model and data can then be conveyed to software such as WinBUGS, OpenBUGS, JAGS, Stan, etc. For example, BUGS code is on the book's website for Chapter 8 in file `example8-1.txt`. Using this code, inferences given in Table 8.1 are close to those given in Table 5.2, indicating that the somewhat informative prior used there had little impact on the analysis due to the large sample size. The posterior probability that $OR > 1$ is effectively 1.

TABLE 8.1: Posterior summaries for LE data using the logistic regression model

Parameter	mean	sd	2.5%	median	97.5%
θ_1	0.26	0.02	0.23	0.26	0.30
θ_2	0.072	0.01	0.055	0.072	0.092
RR	3.72	0.58	2.74	3.68	4.99
OR	4.72	0.84	3.30	4.64	6.68
RD	0.19	0.022	0.15	0.19	0.24

The next example involves three covariates.

Example 8.2. Consider the LE data again, with the same covariate $High$ as before and two more covariates: Met, taking the value 1 if there was metastasis found in any examined nodes and 0 otherwise; and Age, the patient's age in years as of 2003.

Using the subset of 1,210 patients with complete information on these three covariates, we represent the data as

$$\{(y_i, High_i, Met_i, Age_i) : i = 1, \ldots, 1210\}.$$

With $x_i = (1, High_i, Met_i, Age_i)'$ and following expression (8.1), the data are modeled as conditionally independent Bernoulli observations $Y_i \mid x_i, \theta_i \sim Ber(\theta_i)$, with

$$\text{logit}(\theta_i) = \beta_0 + High_i \, \beta_1 + Met_i \, \beta_2 + Age_i \, \beta_3 = x_i' \beta \tag{8.3}$$

where $\beta = (\beta_0, \ldots, \beta_3)'$.

It is often useful in regression problems to standardize (center and scale) *continuous* covariates to improve interpretation and computational performance. Here we standardize the covariate Age by subtracting the mean age (72.7 years) in the data and dividing by the sample standard deviation of ages (5.6 years), defining a new variable $sAge = (Age - 72.7)/5.6$ for the standardized Age. Now the model is

$$\text{logit}(\theta_i) = \beta_0^* + High_i\,\beta_1 + Met_i\,\beta_2 + sAge_i\,\beta_3^*. \tag{8.4}$$

While this model for the *data* is equivalent to the model in equation (8.3), the meanings of the starred first and fourth βs are different. The intercept's interpretation changes because of centering and the regression coefficient for the age variables is different, because of the change in units of age from 1 year to 5.6 years. In particular, β_0 has the awkward interpretation that a woman of *age zero* (and $High = 0, Met = 0$) has LE probability $\text{logit}^{-1}(\beta_0)$, while $\text{logit}^{-1}(\beta_0^*)$ is the probability of LE for a woman of average age (here 72.7 years) with $High = 0$ and $Met = 0$.

Now let us look at the regression coefficients β_3 and β_3^*. In (8.3), the odds ratio comparing the odds of LE for a woman who is $a + 1$ years old to the odds of LE for a woman who is a years old (other covariates being equal for the two) is $e^{(a+1)\beta_3}/e^{a\beta_3} = e^{\beta_3}$. A neat fact is that this odds ratio is free of a. Now the effect of a single year in age on the odds of LE might be less useful to report than, perhaps, the effect of a five-year difference. In this case, we get the odds ratio $e^{5\beta_3}$. In (8.4), $e^{\beta_3^*}$ is the ratio of LE odds for a woman one standard unit above the mean age (or above any other age a) to a woman who is of average age (or age a). In years, these two women would be 5.6 years apart in age.

One can go back and forth between the βs and the β^*s using the relationships

$$\beta_3 = \frac{1}{s}\beta_3^*, \quad \beta_0 = \beta_0^* - \frac{m}{s}\beta_3*; \quad \beta_3^* = s\beta_3, \quad \beta_0^* = \beta_0 + m\beta_3.$$

where m and s, respectively, are the mean and standard deviation of the original variable. From here on, we will write models with standardized and unstandardized covariates using the same notation, namely, $\text{logit}(\theta_i) = x_i'\beta$, with the understanding that coefficients must be interpreted appropriately as illustrated above.

For inference, we will mainly focus on the relative risks (RRs), odds ratios (ORs), risk differences (RDs), and the risks (θ_i) themselves rather than on the β_i, which are on a peculiar scale and thus are more difficult to interpret.

Results using flat priors on the βs, standardized age, and code (available on the book's webpage under Chapter 8 code in the file `example8-2.txt`) are given in Table 8.2. The inferential targets considered are:

Notation	Interpretation
OR_1	e^{β_1}, odds ratio, high to low node exam count
OR_2	e^{β_2}, odds ratio, with to without metastasis
OR_3	e^{β_3}, odds ratio, standardized age $a_{st} + 1$ to age a_{st}
RR_1	risk ratio, high to low node exam count
	(age 72.7 years, $Met = 1$)

RR_2 risk ratio, high to low node exam count
(age 72.7 years, $Met = 0$)

RR_3 risk ratio, high to low node exam count
(age 78.3 years, $Met = 1$)

RR_4 risk ratio, high to low node exam count
(age 78.3 years, $Met = 0$)

Note: The sample mean age is 72.7 years, and the standard deviation is 5.6 years.

Observe that posterior means and medians are very similar, indicating that the posterior distributions are roughly symmetric. We, therefore, focus on means in our analysis. If they were noticeably different, we would focus on medians. The estimated OR_1 is 3.80 with an interval that is far above 1. The posterior probability that $OR_1 > 1$ is very close to 1. The interpretation is that the odds of LE for a woman with a high node count are estimated to be between about 2.5 and 5.5 times greater than for a woman with a low node count, other covariate values being equal. Moreover, this interpretation remains the same regardless of the particular values of the other covariates, as long as they are equal for the two women in the comparison. This last property is a feature of odds ratios in the particular regression model we used. It is an additive (or no-interaction) logistic regression model. It leads to simplicity of interpretation but involves the no-interaction assumption. We also note that even in this case, relative risks do not have this property of being free of the other covariate values.

TABLE 8.2: Posterior summary for LE data using three covariates

	Mean	sd	2.5%	Median	97.5%
OR_1	3.80	0.74	2.57	3.73	5.46
OR_2	1.98	0.39	1.32	1.95	2.85
OR_3	0.83	0.07	0.69	0.83	0.98
RR_1	2.84	0.48	2.04	2.79	3.91
RR_2	3.20	0.54	2.28	3.15	4.38
RR_3	2.95	0.52	2.10	2.90	4.11
RR_4	3.28	0.57	2.32	3.23	4.54

Turning to relative risks, $\widehat{RR_1} = 2.84$ is the estimated relative risk of LE comparing women with high node counts to women with low node counts (i.e., $High = 1$ vs. $High = 0$) for women with a metastasis and of age 72.7 years. Comparing two women who are 78.3 years old and have a metastasis, the one who has a high count is estimated to be 2.95 ($\widehat{RR_3}$) times as likely to acquire LE as the one with a low count. Similarly, $\widehat{RR_2} = 3.20$ involves the same type of comparison of two 72.7-year-old women who did not have metastases; and $\widehat{RR_4} = 3.28$ involves the comparison of 78.3-year-old women who did not have metastases. First observe that none of these RR estimates is the same as OR_1, although they are all in the same direction. All estimate the "effect" of the number of nodes tested on the risk of acquiring LE, each on its own terms. Since all intervals are considerably above 1, there is a strong indication that the number of nodes is strongly associated with the risk of acquiring LE, regardless of whether there was a metastasis or whether the woman was younger or older.

The estimated odds ratio $\widehat{OR}_2 = 1.98$ estimates the effect of having a metastasis or not on the odds of LE, and similarly, the estimate $\widehat{OR}_3 = 0.83$ estimates the effect of being 5.6 years older on the odds of LE. So, having a metastasis is positively associated, and being older in negatively associated, with acquiring LE. The posterior probability that $OR_2 > 1$ is again effectively 1, and the corresponding probability that $OR_3 < 1$ is 0.986. These last two probabilities are not shown in the table, but the code on the book webpage shows how these can be calculated. We could also obtain relative risks corresponding to these risk factors if we wished. All effects here are statistically important and appear to have practical import as well.

Table 8.3 gives estimates of the eight probabilities of LE corresponding to the eight combinations of the covariates: *High* (1 or 0), *Met* (1 or 0), *Age* (78.3 years or 72.7 years). This table provides what are perhaps the most interesting outcomes of the analysis. We know we have statistically important predictors in the model. Now by simply looking at this table, we can see if those differences are practically meaningful. Comparing high versus low node counts for older women with metastases, the estimates are 0.3 and 0.10. Not only do we know that the relative risk is about 3, we also know the actual estimated probabilities of LE for these women with high counts and with low counts. These could be used in a large population of women to estimate, for instance, the added population-wide burden of examining more than five nodes. We can also see, looking at the same ratios across all combinations of presence of metastasis and age, that the relative risks are about 3. In addition, we can look at the effect of metastasis by comparing 0.30 to 0.18, 0.10 to 0.06, 0.34 to 0.21, and 0.12 to 0.068. All the corresponding ratios are in a neighborhood of 1.6. Similarly, we can look at the effect of age. The highest estimated probability of LE in the table, 0.34, is for a woman with a high count, with a metastasis, and who is younger. The lowest estimated probability, 0.06, is for a woman with a low number of examined nodes, no metastasis, and who is older. Recall that when we only considered the effect of the number of nodes (more than 5 vs. 5 or fewer) on LE, as in Example 8.1 and Table 8.1, the risk estimates were 0.26 versus 0.072. Clearly there is a more nuanced message to be told when adjusting for age and metastasis.

TABLE 8.3: Estimated probabilities of LE across *High* (1 or 0), *Met* (1 or 0), and *Age* (78.3 years or 72.7 years); posterior medians and 95% probability intervals

	Age = 78.3		Age = 72.7	
High	*Met* = 1	*Met* = 0	*Met* = 1	*Met* = 0
1	0.30 (0.23, 0.38)	0.18 (0.14, 0.23)	0.34 (0.28, 0.41)	0.21 (0.17, 0.26)
0	0.10 (0.07, 0.16)	0.06 (0.04, 0.08)	0.12 (0.08, 0.18)	0.068 (0.050, 0.09)

8.2   Logistic Regression Model with Interaction

While the logistic regression model as expressed in expression (8.1) is general enough
to contain the models presented in this section, the notion of interaction was not
included explicitly there and also not included in the examples. In fact, the models
in those examples are additive logit models in which each predictive variable (e.g.,
age, metastasis, node count status) contributes only an additive piece to the logit of
the probability being modeled. Possible effect modification is not allowed. However,
this additivity assumption led to simpler interpretations. For instance, in Example
8.2 the effect of metastasis, as measured by the odds ratio, is captured in a single
odds ratio regardless of age. This may not be appropriate. If so, we can use the
device of including an interaction term in the model discussed in Section 7.5 for
linear regression. There, additivity (or its violation) was on the scale of the response
means. Here, it is on the scale of *logits* of probabilities of an event. While conclusions
about interactions on this scale often translate to the probability axis, this is not
guaranteed (see the note at the end of Section 7.5). We turn to an example to
illustrate interaction in the context of logistic regression.

Example 8.3. Trauma Data. Dr. Turner Osler, a trauma surgeon and former
head of the Burn Unit at the University of New Mexico Trauma Center, provided
data on survival of patients admitted to the Trauma Center between 1991 and 1994.
The predictor variables are injury severity score (ISS), revised trauma score (RTS),
age, and type of injury (TI). TI is either blunt ($TI = 0$, e.g., the result of a car
crash), or penetrating ($TI = 1$, e.g., a gunshot or stab wound). The ISS is an overall
index of a patient's injuries based on the approximately 1,300 injuries catalogued
in the Abbreviated Injury Scale. The ISS takes on values from 0 for a patient with
no injuries to 75 for a patient with severe injuries in three or more body areas. The
RTS is an index of physiologic status derived from the Glasgow Coma Scale. It is
a weighted average of a number of measurements on an incoming patient, such as
systolic blood pressure and respiratory rate. The RTS takes on values from 0 for a
patient with no vital signs to 7.84 for a patient with normal vital signs. We used a
randomly selected subset of 300 observations. Bedrick et al. [24], Christensen [76],
and Christensen et al. [79] provide similar analyses to that given here. The data
are contained in the file `trauma.csv` on the book's website.

Dr. Osler proposed a logistic regression model to estimate the probability of
a patient's death using an intercept; the predictors ISS, RTS, age, and TI; and
an interaction between age and TI. Age is viewed as a surrogate for a patient's
physiologic reserve, that is, their ability to withstand trauma. With θ_i standing
for the ith patient's probability of death given his or her covariate values and the
regression coefficients, the model can be written as

$$\text{logit}(\theta_i) = \beta_0 + \beta_1 ISS_i + \beta_2 RTS_i + \beta_3 AGE_i + \beta_4 TI_i + \beta_5 (AGE \times TI)_i \quad (8.5)$$

or, using the generic x notation for covariates, as

$$\text{logit}(\theta_i) = \beta_0 + \beta_1 x_{i1} + \beta_2 x_{i2} + \beta_3 x_{i3} + \beta_4 x_{i4} + \beta_5 x_{i5}, \quad x_{i5} = x_{i3} x_{i4}.$$

So what is the point of including an interaction term in the model? It is to allow the possibility that the effect of the type of injury on the odds of dying (i.e., the difference in the logit of death for penetrating versus blunt injury) may depend on age. In fact, Dr. Osler anticipated that there will be little difference in risk by type of injury for older patients, because of their lack of "reserve." For younger patients, on the other hand, this difference in the risk of death by injury type is expected to be substantial.

Including a regression term with a product of covariates as an added covariate is a means of allowing the effect of one covariate to depend on the level of another. But the added regression coefficient has a direct meaning only on the scale chosen for the response variable side of the regression equation. The effect difference, say d, in our example is

$$
\begin{aligned}
d &\equiv \; \text{logit}(\text{Death} \mid \beta, ISS, RTS, TI = 1, AGE) \\
&\quad - \text{logit}(\text{Death} \mid \beta, ISS, RTS, TI = 0, AGE) \\
&= \; \beta_0 + \beta_1\, ISS + \beta_2\, RTS + \beta_3\, AGE + \beta_4\,(1) + \beta_5\,(1) \times AGE \\
&\quad - \beta_0 + \beta_1\, ISS + \beta_2\, RTS + \beta_3\, AGE + \beta_4\,(0) + \beta_5\, AGE \\
&= \; \beta_5\, AGE.
\end{aligned}
$$

To interpret this more readily, we can convert this to the odds scale. In particular, the odds of "death" for a patient with a penetrating injury equal

$$
e^{\beta_0 + \beta_1\, ISS + \beta_2\, RTS + \beta_4 + (\beta_3 + \beta_5)\, AGE},
$$

and for the same type of patient with a blunt injury the odds equal

$$
e^{\beta_0 + \beta_1\, ISS + \beta_2\, RTS + \beta_3\, AGE}.
$$

Thus the odds ratio is $e^{\beta_4 + \beta_5\, AGE} = e^d$. The dependence of the effect of TI on age, as measured by the odds ratio, is now clearly expressed as a function of age. Of course, this odds ratio is β_4 if $\beta_5 = 0$, in which case the effect of TI does not depend on age. In the next section on inference, we discuss what the data tell us about this.

8.3 Inference for Regression Coefficients and Their Functions

As usual, to carry out inference we need to compute the posterior distribution for β or, more usefully, obtain samples from this posterior. We do this by conveying the model and data to appropriate software, such as BUGS, JAGS, or Stan. Until we discuss informative priors in Section 8.4, we continue to use independent flat priors on components of the vector β. Example code is provided on the book's website.

The model is stated in terms of regression coefficients, so the posterior samples of these are generated by the Bayesian software you use. Inference for these is straightforward: make summaries, histograms, density plots, probability statements, etc.,

TABLE 8.4: Trauma data: Posterior summaries with flat prior

Variable	Flat Prior				
	mean	sd	2.5%	median	97.5%
Intercept	−2.71	1.71	−6.04	−2.71	0.66
ISS	0.085	0.029	0.029	0.085	0.142
RTS	−0.60	0.18	−0.96	−0.59	−0.26
AGE	0.056	0.017	0.024	0.055	0.091
TI	1.41	1.42	−1.43	1.42	4.17
AGE × *TI*	−0.008	0.035	−0.081	−0.007	0.057

from the samples. As we have seen in the previous sections, these regression coefficients are generally less interesting in logistic regression, because they are on the log odds or logit scale. Nonetheless, sometimes it is important to address whether they are zero or not. If a 95% interval for a regression coefficient excludes zero, we can be at least 95% certain that the coefficient is either positive, or negative, depending on the placement of the interval. Suppose we find $P(\beta_j > c \mid \text{data}) = 0.95$ for some positive $c > 0$. Then we can say that the corresponding variable x_j is *statistically important*. Because the phrase *statistically significant* has been used extensively to indicate a specific repeated-data frequency related to a "null hypothesis," it is not appropriate to use that phrase in a Bayesian context.

Our probability statement is conditional on the data at hand. It does not refer to a frequency in conceptual replications of such data. It quantifies the updated certainty about β_j in light of the data at hand, updating it from our initial (prior) certainty. Even so, we emphasize that a statistically important variable may have little practical import, the latter depending on the magnitude of c. Conversely, statistical importance may not be achieved in light of a particular data set even when the variable may be of *potentially* practical importance. Typically, this happens when the data set does not contain sufficient information about β_j, such as when the sample size is relatively small.

Example 8.4. Trauma Data (Example 8.3, Continued). Table 8.4 presents means, standard deviations, and percentiles of posterior samples of the β_j of the trauma data model. When an interaction is included in the model, its statistical importance should be considered first. If it is important, the interpretation of coefficients of covariates that constitute the interaction is substantially affected (as we saw in Section 7.5 for the linear model). On the other hand, these coefficients have simpler interpretations if the interaction is judged not statistically important. In Table 8.4, the interval for the $TI \times AGE$ interaction coefficient includes 0, so the interaction is judged not statistically important. In other words, the effect of TI, if any, does not appear to depend on age.

The coefficient of TI can now be interpreted directly from the row for TI in Table 8.4. We see that 0 is well within the 95% interval. Type of injury does not appear to affect the probability of death. As for RTS, low values are bad for the patient, so the tendency of the RTS coefficient to be negative is reasonable. The 95% probability interval for this coefficient is entirely below zero, so RTS is counted as a statistically important variable. Similarly, the intervals for ISS and AGE are entirely above 0, so they are also statistically important predictors of death. Higher RTS is associated with smaller probabilities, and higher ISS and AGE are associated with larger probabilities.

It would be possible now to consider reducing the number of terms in the model by removing TI and $AGE{\times}TI$. Such decisions can be guided by methods introduced in Chapter 10. Here we choose not to do that, keeping all variables suggested by Dr. Osler in the model. For more discussion of this interaction, see Example 8.10.

8.3.1 Inference for Lethal Dose α

An interesting target of inference has its origins in the field of toxicology where logistic regression was used in its early days. It involves the dose of an insecticide at which a specified percentage of an insect population would be killed. This percentile relating to the lethality of the chemical to $100\alpha\%$ of the population is called the LD_α for *lethal dose* in bioassay problems. In general, the dose at which $100\alpha\%$ of subjects would have some form of event is of interest. For example, a pharmaceutical company might be interested to know the dose of a drug at which a certain percentage of a population of patients, perhaps 95%, would be cured. In this context, such a dose would be denoted ED95 for *effective dose*; we denote it ED_α, $\alpha = 0.95$.

ED_α is obtained by solving $\alpha = P(Event \mid \beta_0, \beta_1, x_1) = \text{logit}^{-1}(\beta_0 + d_\alpha \beta_1)$ for dose d_α. This means $\text{logit}(\alpha) = \beta_0 + d_\alpha \beta_1$ so that $d_\alpha = \{\text{logit}(\alpha) - \beta_0\}/\beta_1$. If β_1 is near zero, posterior samples of d_α can be highly variable and unstable. Summaries of the posterior distribution should be based on percentiles, such as the median and quartiles, *not the mean and standard deviation*. Of course, if β_1 is small, the drug or insecticide does not much affect the probability of the event and is not of much interest to the scientist, nor is ED_α.

Example 8.5. Snake Bite Data. Parveen et al. (2017) [257] studied the effect on survival of mice after injection with different types of snake venom. We consider their data involving the saw-scaled viper. Four distinct doses were applied to eight rats each. The doses were $(32, 16, 8, 4)$ μg. To stabilize the analysis, we standardized dose by subtracting 8 and dividing by 4. So, $sDose = (Dose - 8)/4$, and the observed standardized doses were $(6, 2, 0, -1)$. The observed binomial death counts were $(y_1 = 8, y_2 = 5, y_3 = 3, y_4 = 0)$, each out of 8 mice. Coding this as a logistic regression model for binomial data with "flat" priors (code on the book's website under Chapter 8 in the file `example8-5.txt`), we obtained posterior samples of β_0 and β_1. From each such sample, we then calculated, in addition to $LD_{0.5}$, the probabilities of death (denoted $p[1], p[2], p[3], p[4]$) at the experimental dose levels $(sDose = 6, 2, 0, -1)$, respectively. Results are shown in Table 8.5.

The estimated probabilities of death are $(0.91, 0.77, 0.10, 0.007)$ for doses $(32, 16, 8, 4)$, respectively, based on the medians of the MCMC samples. The estimated $LD_{0.5}$ is $sDose = 1.19$, which corresponds to a dose od $8 + 4 \times 1.18 = 12.7$ μg;

TABLE 8.5: Snake bite data: Posterior summaries

	Percentiles		
	2.5%	50%	97.5%
$LD_{0.5}$	0.27	1.19	2.31
$p[1]$	0.70	0.91	0.98
$p[2]$	0.56	0.77	0.92
$p[3]$	0.10	0.31	0.56
$p[4]$	0.0001	0.007	0.118

we are 95% certain that it is in the interval $(8 + 4 \times 0.027, 8 + 4 \times 2.31) = (9.1, 17.2)$ μg, which is quite wide. More dose values and larger numbers of mice would be required to have better precision.

8.4   Prior Distributions

Thus far in this chapter we have used flat priors on regression coefficients. It is not a practice we recommend. We used flat priors only as a device to postpone discussion of priors and focus on different aspects of the logistic regression model and to demonstrate the types of inference possible. We now turn to more appropriate priors, informative as well as low-information omnibus priors that work well when context-specific prior information is not available or one wishes to keep such information out of the analysis in an attempt to "let the data speak for themselves."

8.4.1   Conditional Means Priors

As was pointed out in the linear regression case in Section 7.3.3.1, regression parameters are difficult targets for direct quantification of prior information. So we again turn to the conditional expectation of the observable $Y \mid x$ for some chosen covariate vectors x that are convenient for elicitation of prior information. For binary regression, Y has the Bernoulli distribution so $E(Y|x) = P(Y = 1|x)$. This is much more meaningful to subject-matter experts than the regression coefficients. The prior information specified for these conditional means is then induced on the regression parameters. The development parallels that in Section 7.3.3.1. We first illustrate with a simple example, then state the method in general, followed by another example.

Example 8.6. Conditional Means Priors for Lymphedema Data. In Example 5.2 we considered the LE data with one covariate. In particular, although we were dealing with data on 1,211 women, we considered it as a grouped logistic regression analysis with only two binomial observations. Specifically, we had

$$Y_i | \theta_i, High_i \stackrel{\text{ind}}{\sim} Bin(n_i, \theta_i), \quad \text{logit}(\theta_i) = \beta_0 + \beta_1 High_i, \quad i = 1, 2,$$

with $n_1 = 734, n_2 = 477$ as known constants that correspond to subscript $i = 1$ for the $High = 0$ (i.e., the low count) group (see Table 5.1). Here, we take the informative prior from Example 5.2 to induce an informative prior for β. Recall that available information in the literature on LE rates after surgical treatment of breast cancer led to representing this knowledge by a $Be(2.044, 13.006)$ distribution for the probability of LE without knowing the number of nodes examined. Desiring *a priori* not to enforce a particular direction for this probability (increase or decrease) with the number of nodes examined, we take identical independent priors for both θ_i:

$$\theta_i \stackrel{\text{ind}}{\sim} Be(2.044, 13.006), \quad i = 1, 2.$$

Since $\text{logit}(\theta_1) = \beta_0$ and $\text{logit}(\theta_2) = \beta_0 + \beta_1$, we must have $\beta_0 = \text{logit}(\theta_1)$ and $\beta_1 = \text{logit}(\theta_2) - \beta_0$. To "see" the prior on the β_i, we can take advantage of a feature of most Bayesian MCMC software (e.g., BUGS, JAGS, Stan) that allows us to simulate from a prior (i.e., without data). We can then transform the simulated values. In fact, in the analysis code itself we can include these steps to define the prior for the transformed parameters (see Example 8.7 below). For simulating the prior, see the BUGS code on the book's website under Chapter 8 in the file example8-6.txt. The corresponding R code is also in this file.

Running such code and summarizing the samples, we find that the induced prior on β_0 has median and 95% probability interval -2.00 $(-3.96, -0.65)$, and the prior on β_1 has median and 95% interval 0.0036 $(-2.36, 2.35)$. Observe that the prior inference for "slope" (or effect size β_1) is neutral in terms of whether the slope might be positive or negative, as we wanted. The two βs are also correlated in the induced joint prior as expected. Interestingly, β_1 has an approximately normal distribution with mean 0 and a standard deviation about 1.2. The analysis involving the two probabilities will be identical, up to Monte Carlo error, to the analysis that was performed in Example 5.2.

The induced prior construction in the above example can be stated in general similar to the discussion in the linear regression case (see Section 7.3.3.1). As there, we begin with a $(p + 1) \times (p + 1)$ matrix $\tilde{X}$ with rows corresponding to $(p + 1)$ covariate vectors chosen for convenience in eliciting prior and such that $\tilde{X}$ is of full rank. Then we equate $\tilde{X}\beta$ to a vector, θ_i, whose ith component is $\text{logit}(\tilde{\theta}_i)$ where $\tilde{\theta}_i = P(Y_i = 1 \mid \tilde{x}_i')$ for $i = 1, \ldots, p + 1$. Since $\tilde{\theta}$ is more directly interpretable than β, we elicit a prior on $\tilde{\theta}$ that induces a prior on $\beta = \tilde{X}^{-1}\text{logit}(\tilde{\theta})$, with the logit function applied componentwise to $\tilde{\theta}$. Typically we take independent $Be(a_i, b_i)$ priors on $\tilde{\theta}_i$. As in Chapter 7, rows of $\tilde{X}$ should be chosen so that the independence of priors on the components of $\tilde{\theta}$ is reasonable.

Reframing Example 8.6, let $\text{logit}(\tilde{\theta}_1) = \beta_0$ and $\text{logit}(\tilde{\theta}_2) = \beta_0 + \beta_1$. We thus have $\text{logit}(\tilde{\theta}_i) = \tilde{x}_i'\beta$, with $\tilde{x}_1' = (1, 0)$ and $\tilde{x}_2 = (1, 1)$. So

$$\tilde{X} = \begin{pmatrix} 1 & 0 \\ 1 & 1 \end{pmatrix}, \quad \tilde{X}^{-1} = \begin{pmatrix} 1 & 0 \\ -1 & 1 \end{pmatrix}, \quad \begin{pmatrix} \beta_0 \\ \beta_1 \end{pmatrix} = \tilde{X}^{-1} \begin{pmatrix} \text{logit}(\tilde{\theta}_1) \\ \text{logit}(\tilde{\theta}_2) \end{pmatrix}.$$

TABLE 8.6: Trauma data: prior specification

j	Design for prior $\tilde{x}'_j$						$Be(a_j, b_j)$ a_j	b_j	Prior median
1	1	25	7.84	60	0	0	1.1	8.5	0.09
2	1	25	3.34	10	0	0	3.0	11.0	0.20
3	1	41	3.34	60	1	60	5.9	1.7	0.80
4	1	41	7.84	10	1	10	1.3	12.0	0.07
5	1	33	5.74	35	0	0	1.1	4.9	0.15
6	1	33	5.74	35	1	35	1.5	5.5	0.19

The solution, as before, is $\beta_0 = \text{logit}(\tilde{\theta}_1)$ and $\beta_1 = \text{logit}(\tilde{\theta}_2) - \beta_1$. We now illustrate the CMP with $p = 5$ predictors so that β is a six-dimensional vector, including the intercept.

Example 8.7. Trauma Data. For these data as analyzed in Example 8.3, $p+1 = 6$. To induce a CMP on β, we require a joint distribution on death probabilities for six sets of conditions $\tilde{x}'_j = (1, ISS_j, RTS_j, AGE_j, TI_j, AGE_j \times TI_j)$. We now describe the process that led to the selected covariate conditions and the resulting informative priors on $\tilde{\theta}$ listed in Table 8.6.

With four distinct predictor variables, our expert Dr. Osler selected four "comfortable" covariate combinations. The idea was to select values of the variables that were sufficiently different within the data range but still had substantial probabilities for both success and failure. Dr. Osler had relatively little difficulty specifying priors for these first four combinations in Table 8.6. The first setting for eliciting $\tilde{\theta}_1$ corresponds to an individual who "has good physiology, is 'not badly hurt,' does not have a lot of reserve," and for whom there is "added uncertainty due to age." Following elicitation methods for a prior on a probability that were detailed in Section 5.1.1.2, and using the key values supplied by Dr. Osler, we determined that the $Be(1.1, 8.5)$ distribution suitably reflects his uncertainty about $\tilde{\theta}_1$. The median of his prior is around 0.09. The second type of individual "has bad physiology, is very ill, but is young and resilient and is not so badly hurt." The prior for $\tilde{\theta}_2$ is $Be(3, 11)$, with median around 0.20. Incidentally, "bad physiology" and "very ill" refer to poor RTS scores, while how badly hurt one is relates to ISS. The third individual has "bad physiology, a pretty bad injury, and there is much more uncertainty here due to the age factor." The prior is $Be(5.9, 1.7)$ with median around 0.8. Prior individual four "is young, resilient, and has a big injury." The prior is $Be(1.3, 12)$ with a median of around 0.07.

Since our logistic regression model in Example 8.3 also included an intercept and an interaction, we needed $p + 1 = 6$ combinations to specify a full prior. The last two rows were constructed to keep $\tilde{X}$ non-singular and satisfy some design principles (beyond the scope of this book) by the authors of [23, 24]. Admittedly, Dr. Osler had more difficulty with these fifth and sixth types of individuals, because

TABLE 8.7: Trauma data: posterior summaries with informative prior

| Variable | Informative prior | | | | |
	mean	sd	2.5%	median	97.5%
Intercept	−1.76	1.15	−4.00	−1.76	0.49
ISS	0.065	0.021	0.024	0.065	0.106
RTS	−0.60	0.15	−0.90	−0.60	−0.33
AGE	0.047	0.014	0.021	0.047	0.075
TI	1.10	1.09	−1.23	1.10	3.24
$AGE \times TI$	−0.017	0.028	−0.072	−0.016	0.037

their conditions were less extreme than those already considered, and, presumably, because he did not select them. Nonetheless, the resulting priors for $\tilde{\theta}_5$ and $\tilde{\theta}_6$ are, respectively, $Be(1.1, 4.9)$ with median 0.15, and $Be(1.5, 5.5)$ with median 0.19.

Since inducing these priors shown in Table 8.6 onto the regression coefficients requires inverting a matrix, we provide a combination of R and BUGS or JAGS code on the book's website under Chapter 8 in the file `example8-7.txt`. The process consists of converting the data in Table 8.6 to the object `Xtilde`, converting it to a 6×6 matrix, and inverting it, all in R. This inverse is then read into BUGS by a somewhat manual process by printing and copying. Running the BUGS code generated the results in Table 8.7.

Comparing these results in Table 8.7 with flat-prior results in Table 8.4, we see that they are qualitatively the same. However, intervals in Table 8.7 for ISS, RTS, and AGE are more narrow than they were in Table 8.4. The estimated coefficient for the interaction is a bit more negative than before but is still not statistically important. We discuss this further in Example 8.10.

8.4.2 Partial Prior Information

As we saw in Chapter 7, specifying a prior distribution for a regression model with several predictor variables can be daunting. For logistic regression, priors that are partially CMP and partially diffuse follow in much the same way as for linear regression in Chapter 7. There are two cases: (i) we can specify $p + 1$ linearly independent covariate vectors $\tilde{x}$ but can get priors on $\tilde{\theta}$s elicited for only $r < p + 1$ vectors; or (ii) $p + 1$ is too large to even consider specifying that many conditions, so we settle for $r \leq p$ $\tilde{x}$s. Strategies in these two cases and their examples follow.

In case (i) we put informative priors on some $\tilde{\theta}_i$ and flat $U(0, 1)$ or Jeffreys invariant $Be(0.5, 0.5)$ priors on the rest. The approach is presented and justified in Christensen et al. [79].

In case (ii), specifying fewer than $r \leq p$ vectors, we choose the $\{\tilde{x}_j : j = 1, \ldots, r\}$ so that the corresponding $\tilde{\theta}_j$ only induce information on a subset of r regression coefficients. We accomplish this by choosing the $\tilde{x}_j$ so that the predictor variables associated with the remaining $p - r$ coefficients are fixed at the same values, often 0 for standardized continuous covariates (standardization as discussed

TABLE 8.8: Trauma data: partial prior specification with standardized ISS, RTS, and AGE

	Design for prior						$Be(a_j, b_j)$		
i			$\tilde{x}_i'$				a_i	b_i	Prior mode
1	1	0	0	0	0	0	2.06	21.2	0.05
2	1	1	0	0	0	0	2.70	10.66	0.15
3	1	1	−2	0	0	0	1.9	3.7	0.25

in Section 7.1.4) and at a reference category, 0, for categorical covariates. We then place independent appropriate $N(0, b)$ priors on the corresponding $p - r$ regression coefficients. The choice $b = 1$ provides a relatively diffuse prior for coefficients of categorical as well as standardized continuous covariates.

Example 8.8. Grouped LE Data. Assume that $P(LE \mid High = 0) = \tilde{\theta}_1 \sim Be(2.044, 13.006)$, but that there is now no information for $P(LE \mid High = 1) = \tilde{\theta}_2$. As in Example 8.6, $\beta_0 = \text{logit}(\tilde{\theta}_1)$, so the informative prior on θ_1 induces an informative prior on β_0. The other regression parameter is $\beta_1 = \text{logit}(\tilde{\theta}_2) - \beta_0$. At this point, we have two choices. Our preference is for a reference prior on the probability $\tilde{\theta}_1$, such as a uniform or Jeffreys prior. This induces a diffuse prior on β_1. Alternatively, we can put a flat or large-variance, mean-zero normal prior directly on β_1. The latter type of choice will be much simpler when p is large, since then we do not have to specify so many appropriate $\tilde{x}_i$ vectors.

Example 8.9. Trauma Data. We use the model from Example 8.3, but now with standardized covariates (see Section 7.1.4). We will assume that our expert was only willing to specify three $\tilde{x}_j$ and three corresponding probabilities. We take as "baseline" conditions a patient who has the average values (mean(ISS) = 14.3, mean(RTS) = 7.29, and mean(AGE) = 31.4, these corresponding to 0s on the standardized covariates) and has a blunt injury (mean$TI = 0$). Let $\tilde{x}_1 = (1, 0, 0, 0, 0, 0)$ correspond to the baseline patient. This $\tilde{x}_1$ implies that $\text{logit}(\tilde{\theta}_1) = \beta_0$. Next, let $\tilde{x}_2 = (1, 1, 0, 0, 0, 0)$, which corresponds to a baseline patient except with an ISS score that is one standard deviation *above* the mean. From $\tilde{x}_2$ we have $\text{logit}(\tilde{\theta}_2) = \beta_0 + \beta_1$. Finally, let $\tilde{x}_3 = (1, 1, -2, 0, 0, 0)$, which corresponds to a hypothetical patient who is the same as the second patient except that this patient's RTS is two standard deviations *below* the mean. Then $\text{logit}(\tilde{\theta}_3) = \beta_0 + \beta_1 - 2\beta_2$. We place independent $Be(a_i, b_i)$ priors on these parameters with (a_i, b_i) given in Table 8.8, along with the prior modes for each probability. These choices were made by the authors based in the information that was provided by Dr. Osler for the six probabilities of death discussed earlier.

Clearly, the prior information involves only β_0, β_1, and β_2. More importantly, since AGE, TI, and $AGE \times TI$ never varied from their baseline values, it is reasonable to treat the information on β_0, β_1, and β_2 as independent of β_3, β_4, and β_5. These parameters only affect how probabilities *change* as AGE, TI, and $AGE \times TI$

change from the baseline case. Finally, we complete the prior by taking independent $\beta_j \sim N(0, b)$ with large $b \approx 1$ for $j = 4, 5, 6$.

8.4.3 Low-Information Omnibus Priors

We consider the ability of Bayesian analysis to include all available information, suitably quantified via informative priors, to be the central feature of this approach to statistical inference and prediction. While we have emphasized this throughout the book, there are situations when such inclusion of information external to the data is not feasible. Resource availability is often the limitation. In biostatistical practice, it is often desirable to keep the external information away from the analysis to convince those who may not agree with its value or to carry out a "what if" analysis. Bayesian researchers pursuing so-called objective priors have long sought to create coherent analyses without any (or much) extra-data information. We have already come across such priors, namely, flat, reference, information invariant (Jeffreys), and approximately flat. Most of these are improper priors and should be used with care, as we have pointed out.

Here, we describe proper priors that are designed to be of weak or low information and work well in almost any data situation in practice. Gelman et al. [136] introduced such priors for logistic regression with the following observations: "We recommend this prior distribution as a default choice for routine applied use. It has the advantage of always giving answers, even when there is complete separation in logistic regression (a common problem, even when the sample size is large and the number of predictors is small), and also automatically applying more shrinkage to higher-order interactions. This can be useful in routine data analysis as well as in automated procedures such as chained equations for missing-data imputation." Recently, Shi et al. [296], using a similar viewpoint, constructed what they termed "low-information omnibus" (LIO) priors for a popular Bayesian nonparametric model. In their words: "Gelman et al. (2008) suggested specific scaling and a low information prior that is 'vague enough to be used as a default in routine applied work' instead of aiming for a no-information prior. The latter pursuit can be challenging both theoretically and computationally." We now summarize Gelman's LIO prior for logistic regression.

The prior requires standardization of predictor variables in a specific manner. Binary variables are centered to have a mean 0 and to differ by "1" in their lower and upper levels. If the two levels are originally coded as 0 and 1, simply subtracting the mean achieves the required standardization. Continuous variables are centered to have a mean 0 and standard deviation 0.5. Subtracting the original mean and dividing by *twice* the standard deviation meets the requirement. The motivation for this standardization is to better align the continuous covariate case with the binary one (which has a range of 1), so that the same prior specification (see below) can work for regression coefficients of both types of covariates.

With this standardization, independent Cauchy priors are used for $\beta_0, \beta_1, \ldots, \beta_p$. For β_0, the prior has median 0 and scale 10. The prior for each of $\beta_1, \ldots, \beta_p$ has median 0 and scale 2.5. Some Bayesian model specification software may not offer the Cauchy distribution as a choice. One can use a combination of normal and gamma, or the t-distribution to circumvent this. In particular (and in notational agreement with BUGS),

$$\beta_0 \mid \tau \sim No(0,\tau), \ \tau \sim Ga(0.5,50) \quad \text{or} \quad \beta_0 \sim St(0,0.01,1)$$

and

$$\beta_1 \mid \tau \sim No(0,\tau), \ \tau \sim Ga(0.5,3.125) \quad \text{or} \quad \beta_1 \sim St(0,0.16,1)$$

are alternate specifications that result in the appropriate Cauchy marginals for the βs.

This prior assigns approximately 0.7 probability to odds ratios between e^{-5} and $e^5 \approx 150$ for one standard deviation unit change in any predictor. This wide spread easily covers almost any practical situation. Any covariate effects greater than these 70% limits would be dramatically obvious from the scientific point of view, perhaps without the need for statistical models. Nonetheless, use of the Cauchy distribution allows for occasionally extreme values too. At the mean setting for all predictors, the success odds are between 10^{-9} and 10^9 with approximate probability 0.7. These choices align with the intended low-information nature of the prior while maintaining good Markov chain convergence and numerical stability for almost any practical application in biostatistics.

8.5 Prediction

In the context of logistic regression, we are interested in predicting binary outcomes, so the focus is on a probability for a certain type of patient. For example, what is the probability that a cancer patient will survive 5 years after diagnosis given the patient's characteristics as measured by the covariates and the data we analyzed? Or what is the probability that a treatment will be effective, conditioned on the data and the patient's covariates? Given our data and analysis, what is the probability that a particular patient who has been admitted to the emergency department will survive?

We have denoted logistic regression data by $\{(y_i, x_i) : i = 1, \ldots, n\}$, where y_i is an indicator of an event. In the sampling model, the predictive probability of the event for a new patient with known covariate vector x_f is

$$P(Y_f = 1 \mid data) = \int \frac{e^{x'_f \beta}}{1 + e^{x'_f \beta}} \, p(\beta \mid data) \, d\beta.$$

The Monte Carlo approximation with a random sample $\beta^{(1)}, \ldots, \beta^{(M)}$ from the posterior distribution of β is

$$P(y_f = 1 \mid x_f, data) \doteq \frac{1}{M} \sum_{j=1}^{M} \frac{e^{x'_f \beta^{(j)}}}{1 + e^{x'_f \beta^{(j)}}}. \tag{8.6}$$

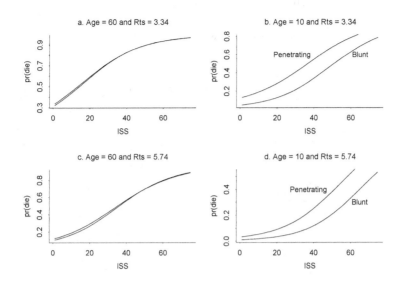

FIGURE 8.1: Trauma data: predictive probabilities of death.

As in other prediction formulas we have encountered before, equation (8.6) has a direct interpretation as the predictive probability that the next trial will be a success, without reference to the regression coefficients, as they have been integrated out. It also has a secondary interpretation as the posterior mean of the parameter, $e^{x'_f\beta}/(1 + e^{x'_f\beta})$, which is the proportion of future patients that we expect to have the event. With the second interpretation, one may be interested in interval estimates. A 95% probability interval, say, is approximated by finding the appropriate percentiles of $\{(e^{x'_f\beta^{(j)}})/(1 + e^{x'_f\beta^{(j)}}) : j = 1, \ldots, M\}$.

Example 8.10. Trauma Data (Examples 8.3 and 8.7, Continued). We return to our discussion of the trauma data where the outcome is death, and the covariates in our analysis are injury severity score (ISS), revised trauma score (RTS), age of the patient (AGE), and type of injury (TI). Using the posterior samples from our informative prior analysis from Table 8.7, we computed (with equation (8.6)) predictive probabilities of death for various specifications of x_f. Figure 8.1 presents predictive probabilities of death as a function of ISS for blunt and penetrating injuries. The four graphs are for two values each of RTS and AGE. The general effect of ISS is obvious, as the probability of death increases dramatically with increasing values, regardless of the values of RTS and AGE. The effect of RTS is observed by comparing top plots to bottom plots in each column, and the effect of AGE is noted by comparing row plots from left to right. There are clear and dramatic effects for all three of these predictors, a visual confirmation of the results in Table 8.7.

Also note that for 60-year-old individuals, there is essentially no difference in the probability of death due to blunt or penetrating injury, while for 10-year-olds, the probability of death is higher for a penetrating injury than for an blunt injury type. Thus, the effect of TI, as reflected by the difference in plots of predictive probabilities of death for penetrating and blunt injuries, appears to depend on AGE. In Table 8.7, however, the regression coefficient for the $AGE \times TI$ interaction was not seen to be statistically different from 0. It is important to recognize that interaction in the logistic regression model speaks to non-additivity of the *log odds*, but the plots in Figure 8.1 are on the probability scale. In addition, the figure does not show any uncertainty measure, such as posterior probability intervals. Nonetheless, including the interaction (cross-product) term allows for quantifying what is termed "effect modification" in the epidemiology literature. If the interaction term were left out, the model would dictate that whatever effect TI might have would be the same regardless of the value of AGE. Similarly, the effect of age on the risk of death would be the same for each TI type.

Careful inspection of Figure 8.1 allows us to visualize the statistically important effects of RTS, ISS, and AGE in terms of probabilities. It also allows us to ascertain whether these effects are of practical import (they clearly are), and whether there is any potential practical importance for the variable TI. It appears to us that indeed there is, but the importance may differ by age. TI affects the probability of death for a younger patient, but clearly not for an older one. It is this difference in potential effect that is so effectively portrayed in this figure.

It is important here to point out that the interaction effect may be due to the influence of the prior specification by Dr. Osler. We prefer to include the interaction in the model, in part since it nicely illustrates the concept of effect modification. In addition, it illustrates a situation where scientific judgment is needed, perhaps with additional data, to determine if this interaction is statistically and scientifically important.

8.6 Alternatives to Logistic Regression: Other Link Functions

The logistic regression model is actually a special case within a general class of models for binary regression. With data $y_i \mid x_i, \beta \sim Ber(\theta_x)$, independent for each i, we can generalize the logistic regression model by considering other possible ways to specify $\theta_x \equiv P(Y = 1 \mid x, \beta)$. The logistic regression model specifies this as $\theta_x = e^{x'\beta}/(1 + e^{x'\beta}) = \mathrm{expit}(x'\beta)$. Restricting to linear functions of β, we can look for other functions of the linear combination $x'\beta$ that could work. The main requirement for such a function is that θ_x be a probability (i.e., between 0 and 1) with domain $(-\infty, \infty)$. We also want it to be an increasing function for simplicity in interpreting the regression relationship. The above expit function is actually the cdf of the logistic distribution, $F(w) = e^w/(1 + e^w)$, $-\infty < w < \infty$. This indicates that for any cdf corresponding to a random variable with support $(-\infty, \infty)$, we can specify a new binary regression model.

Here we only consider two alternative choices for $F(\cdot)$. First, consider the natural choice, $F(w) = \Phi(w)$, where $\Phi(\cdot)$ is the standard normal cdf. Second, consider the choice $F(w) = 1 - e^{-e^w}$ which is the cdf of what is called the extreme-value distribution. So the general form for such models is $\theta_x = F(x'\beta)$. In the theory of generalized linear models, which we have not discussed up to now, the relationship is described in the reverse form

$$F^{-1}(\theta) = x'\beta, \quad \text{so that } F(x'\beta) = \theta_x = P(Y = 1 \mid x, \beta).$$

The model is described as having as link function F^{-1}, since this is the function that links the probability of an event to the linear form $x'\beta$.

Thus when we solve for $x'\beta$ in terms of θ, we have $\text{logit}(\theta) = x'\beta$ when we use the logistic cdf; we have $\Phi^{-1}(\theta) = x'\beta$ in the case of the normal cdf; and we have $\log(-\log(1 - \theta)) = x'\beta$ for the extreme-value cdf. These three link functions are called logit, probit, and complementary log-log, respectively.

The reason why the logit link is preferred in applications over the others is that it is the only link function for which the odds ratio simplifies interpretation. In particular, with one covariate in a model, the odds ratio for the response is e^{β_1} for predictor value $x + 1$ versus x, regardless of the particular value of x. With other links, the odds ratio is a complicated function of the covariate, and β_1 does not have a simple interpretation. Moreover, there is no other simple way to describe how the probability at covariate value $x + 1$ relates to the probability when the covariate value is x such that the description is free of x.

We discuss link functions and generalized linear models further in Chapter 9. In Chapter 10, we discuss the choice of link function based on certain criteria. Of course, simple interpretation is not a great excuse for the choice of the logit link if one of the other models provides a better fit to the data or, more importantly, better predictions.

In general, with a link function F^{-1} (i.e., with $\theta_i = F(x_i'\beta)$), we have the model

$$Y_i \mid x_i, \theta_i \overset{\text{ind}}{\sim} Ber(\theta_i), \quad i = 1, \ldots, n.$$

The sampling distribution (likelihood function) is

$$Lik(\beta) \propto p(y \mid X, \beta) = \prod_{i=1}^{n} [F(x_i'\beta)]^{y_i} [1 - F(x_i'\beta)]^{1-y_i}.$$

For Bayesian analysis, these models are fit and estimated in much the same manner as with the logistic regression model. Software we have referenced throughout the book (BUGS, JAGS, and Stan) can accommodate different link functions very nicely. For example, if one wants to carry out probit regression in BUGS, one simply specifies Φ as PHI. For the complementary log-log model, one must specify the extreme-value cdf directly using the exponential function. The rest of the code for these alternatives is identical to that for logistic regression to obtain posterior samples of β. Processing these samples for suitable inference targets (functions of β) is, however, distinct for each link function.

Finally, we need to comment on the important topic of priors. One choice is to simply use an improper flat prior. Another is to use a CMP or a partially informative version of it. A nice feature of the CMP is that the scientific information is elicited for event probabilities no matter which link function is being used. The induction of the prior information onto the regression coefficients is different due to solving different equations for β in terms of θ_x. This is straightforward to do, however. In the case of a flat prior, using it for regression coefficients with one link function is not the same as a flat prior for the coefficients with another link function. So there are issues with comparing models with different links, due to lack of comparability in the prior specifications. The LIO prior, too, is not the same as for logistic regression. It requires separate development for each link function.

8.7 Recap and Readings

Binary regression is one of the more important topics in biostatistics. We have attempted to provide a fully Bayesian approach that allows for the use of informative priors through collaboration of scientists and statisticians. Since the sample sizes for our main two illustrations were quite large, external information was less important than it would have been with smaller sample sizes. We have also emphasized the importance of attempting to provide sensible diffuse priors on regression coefficients. Placing uniform priors on probabilities to induce diffuse priors on β can be reasonable, provided there really is no information about event probabilities of interest, which is seldom the case. When prior information about one or more event probabilities is available, we recommend a partial prior that induces scientific information onto some of the components of β. We encourage looking at the induced prior on event probabilities for any choice of diffuse prior on β to make sure that misinformation or disinformation is not being conveyed.

Since logistic regression models logits, it is particularly useful to summarize posterior inference in terms of probabilities that are more readily interpreted. Presence or absence of interactions is readily understood for linear regression but, as we saw in the section on prediction, it is more subtle for logistic regression. Transforming inference to understandable targets is important in practice, and this requires special attention when more complex models are used.

We discuss link functions and generalized linear models again in Section 9.3, where we provide some of the theory of these models. McCullagh and Nelder [239] provided the first complete development of generalized linear models (GLMs), albeit from a non-Bayesian perspective. Ibrahim and Laud showed why Jeffreys priors are better than uniform priors for the coefficients in GLMs [172]. Zeger and Karim [359] applied Gibbs sampling to carry out inference in GLMs that include random effects by capitalizing on the similarity with Bayesian models. Other notable publications expanded the use of MCMC algorithms for inference in Bayesian GLMs, such as Dellaportas and Smith [93] and Gamerman [119]. Dey, Ghosh, and Mallick published an edited volume that discusses carrying out Bayesian inference with generalized linear models [96].

8.8 Exercises

EXERCISE 8.1. Refer to the LE data and analysis in Example 8.1 using a logistic regression model and the flat prior, with results given in Table 8.1. Recall that θ_1 and θ_2 were probabilities of LE corresponding to high- and low-count groups, respectively, and that the model specified $\text{logit}(\theta_2) = \beta_0$ and $\text{logit}(\theta_1) = \beta_0 + \beta_1$.

(a) Using the flat prior, write code to reproduce the results in Table 8.1. Be sure to be careful about convergence. Comment.

(b) Now analyze the data using a CMP prior on the βs induced by iid $Be(2.044, 13.006)$ priors on probabilities θ_1 and θ_2 for the high- and low-count groups, respectively. Comment on the information conveyed by the priors. Then compare results of your analysis with your results in part (a).

(c) Now use a partially informative prior by using the prior information about θ_2 in part (b), and a $U(0,1)$ prior on θ_1. Compare results again.

(d) Now use a different partially informative prior by using the prior information about θ_2 in part (b) and an improper uniform prior on β_1. Compare results again.

(e) Finally, use a low-information omnibus prior on β. Compare results again.

EXERCISE 8.2. Refer to Example 8.2. Let $\theta_1 = P(LE \mid High = 0, Met = 0, sAge = 0)$, $\theta_2 = P(LE \mid High = 1, Met = 0, sAge = 0)$, $\theta_3 = P(LE \mid High = 0, Met = 1, sAge = 0)$, $\theta_4 = P(LE \mid High = 0, Met = 0, sAge = 1)$.

(a) Using a flat prior, provide a table of posterior inferences for all regression coefficients as well as the odds ratios given in Table 8.2. Be sure to check convergence of chains. Discuss.

(b) Now regard the covariate combinations in the probability specifications as $\tilde{x}_i$. Write down the corresponding matrix $\tilde{X}$. Is it non-singular? Solve for each β_i in terms of the θ_i. Then write this in matrix form using $\tilde{X}$. Find the explicit solution by simply solving four equations in four unknowns. Then solve using the matrix formulation. Observe that you get the same results.

(c) Write a program to analyze the data using the implied CMP prior that uses the predictor combinations discussed in part (b) and that has independent uniform priors on the θ_i. Provide a table of posterior inferences for all regression coefficients as well as the odds ratios given in Table 8.2. Compare results with those in part (a). Be sure to check convergence of chains. Discuss.

EXERCISE 8.3. In Example 8.2, we considered the LE data with three covariates: $High$ (0/1), Met (0/1), and $sAge$ (standardized age). There were $p + 1 = 4$ regression coefficients and we used flat priors on the β.

(a) Consider specifying independent beta priors on the two probabilities of LE corresponding to $\tilde{x}_1 = (1, 1, 0, 0)$ and $\tilde{x}_2 = (1, 0, 0, 0)$. Define corresponding probabilities of LE, $\tilde{\theta}_2$ and $\tilde{\theta}_1$, respectively. Use the independent priors specified in Exercise 8.1(b) for these and flat priors for the remaining coefficients. Analyze the data.

(b) With $\tilde{\theta}_1$, $\tilde{\theta}_2$, and priors for these as in part (a), use independent $N(0,1)$ priors on coefficients of standardized versions of the remaining covariates. Analyze the data and compare the results with those obtained in part (a). This situation is in the framework of Section 8.4.2.

(c) Now extend the partial prior to a full CMP for all four regression coefficients. Select two more $\tilde{x}$s appropriately to obtain $\tilde{X}$. Then solve for β algebraically and by numerically inverting $\tilde{X}$.

(d) Now place $U(0,1)$ priors on $\tilde{\theta}_3$ and $\tilde{\theta}_4$ and write code to analyze the data using this prior. You may either just obtain the analytically induced prior on β or specify the prior on $\tilde{\theta}$ and then induce the prior on β in a program. Compare results with those in Table 8.2.

EXERCISE 8.4.   Refer to the trauma data in Examples 8.3 and 8.7. Table 8.4 gives results with a flat prior on β.

(a) Analyze the data and check your results with Table 8.4.

(b) Obtain the predictive probabilities of death for the covariate vectors

$$(ISS, RTS, AGE, TI) = \begin{array}{ll} (25, 5, 20, 1), & (25, 3, 20, 1), \\ (25, 5, 50, 1), & (25, 3, 50, 1), \\ (50, 5, 20, 1), & (50, 3, 20, 1), \\ (50, 5, 50, 1), & (50, 5, 50, 1). \end{array}$$

(c) Make a $2 \times 2 \times 2$ table of estimated probabilities of death under these circumstances and discuss it in terms of practical import. You may want to look up ISS and RTS on the web to ascertain what these values mean on those scales.

EXERCISE 8.5.   Give a full analysis of the trauma data using (i) flat priors and (ii) low information omnibus priors. Be sure to monitor convergence. With each, include:

(a) assessment of posterior probabilities that regression coefficients are positive (or negative).

(b) estimates of probabilities of "death on the table" for the 16 possible combinations of (ISS, RTS, AGE, TI) corresponding to $ISS = 20, 40$; $RTS = 3.34, 5.74$; $AGE = 10, 60$; and $TI = 0, 1$. As part of your analysis, create a table of entries that includes the median and a 95% probability interval for each combination. Inferences are for the proportions of deaths in the populations of trauma patients that fall into these 16 categories.

(c) Compare with results obtained using priors (i) and (ii) with those in Figure 8.1.

EXERCISE 8.6.   Repeat Exercise 8.5 using standardized continuous covariates. (There is no need to repeat analyses with the LIO prior for parts (a) and (b), as this prior is only defined with standardized covariates.) Comment on statistical versus practical import in the words of the problem as relevant below.

(a) Compare your estimates of the 16 probabilities. They should be nearly the same if everything was done correctly, since this is just a reparameterization of the model used there. Be sure to monitor convergence. Was convergence better than, worse than, or about the same as it was in Exercise 8.5?

(b) Obtain and interpret (in the words of the problem) estimated odds ratios for the effect of TI for $AGE = 60$ and then for $AGE = 10$.

(c) Obtain and interpret estimated odds ratios for the effect of ISS, comparing $ISS = 41$ to 25, and for RTS, comparing $RTS = 3.34$ to 7.84. Be sure to interpret the results in the words of the problem.

EXERCISE 8.7.   Refer to the snake bite data in Example 8.5. Table 8.5 shows results with an improper uniform prior on β.

(a) Use $U(0, 1)$ priors on the death probabilities at dose 8 and 16 to induce a prior on β. Analyze the data with this prior and carry out inference for components of β.

(b) With your posterior MCMC samples, make a table corresponding to Table 8.5 and compare.

(c) Obtain inferences for the dose at which 90% of mice would die using this prior.

(d) Change the prior to uniforms on probabilities at dose 32 and 4. Repeat parts (a), (b), and (c). Compare. *Note:* These would be stupid priors, since it is doubtful that the experimenters would believe in a prior that was equivalent to adding one success and one failure for an imaginary rat that was given a dose of 32 and also for such a rat at a dose of 4. They would surely believe there would be a smaller probability of death for the much lower dose than for the higher one. However, they could think of this prior information as being quite neutral and that sufficient data would be needed to overwhelm the information that was contrary to their true prior beliefs.

EXERCISE 8.8.   Consider two independent binomial samples with probabilities θ_1 and θ_2. Define $\beta_1 = \text{logit}(\theta_1)$ and $\beta_2 = \text{logit}(\theta_2) - \text{logit}(\theta_1)$.

(a) For independent $\beta_j \sim N(0, 10^3)$, $j = 1, 2$, simulate the induced prior distributions on θ_1, θ_2, and $OR = [\theta_1/(1 - \theta_1)]/[\theta_2/(1 - \theta_2)]$. Note that the densities for the θ_js are concentrated near 0 and 1, and the density for OR will be widely dispersed.

(b) Place independent $N(0, b)$ priors on the β_j and, by trial and error, find a value of b that induces reasonably spread-out (ideally, close to uniform) priors on the θ_j.

(c) Place independent $N(0, c)$ priors on the β_j and, by trial and error, find a value of c that induces a prior on OR that has about 95% of its probability concentrated between -10 and 10. In our experience, estimated ORs tend to be relatively small, perhaps in this range.

(d) Now let $\theta_j \sim U(0, 1)$. Plot histograms of the induced distributions for the β_j. Do they resemble the $N(0, b)$ prior you found in part (b)?

EXERCISE 8.9.   Use a flat prior to reanalyze the LE data with the single covariate *High* that was discussed in Example 8.1.

(a) Using the probit link, compare estimates of the two probabilities of LE with those using the logit link presented in the example. How was convergence?

(b) Using the complementary log-log link, compare estimates of the two probabilities of LE with those using the probit and logit links. How was convergence?

EXERCISE 8.10.   Write code, using links specified in parts below, to analyze the trauma data using the full model but with standardized continuous covariates. Using a flat prior, obtain the usual table of inferences for all regression coefficients. Also obtain a plot of the probabilities of death for individuals with $IS = 1$, $sAge = 0$, $sRTS = 0$, and over a suitable grid of $sISS$ scores that range from the smallest to the largest values in the data.

(a) Use the logit link.
(b) Use the probit link.
(c) Use the complimentary log-log link.
(d) Discuss any qualitative and/or appreciable quantitative differences in the results from the analysis with these three links and give all three plots on the same graph.

EXERCISE 8.11.   Consider the binary regression model with two predictor variables and with no interaction. Fix the second predictor at the value c and obtain the odds ratio comparing the odds of an event for an individual with value $a + 1$ to the odds for an individual with value a for the first predictor. Show this for all three links discussed in this chapter.

EXERCISE 8.12.   Consider the binary regression model with one predictor variable.
(a) Describe how to implement a CMP prior for the two regression coefficients if you have elicited information for two distinct covariate combinations (i) in the probit link case and (ii) in the complementary log-log case. One way to do this is to write the code that is necessary for inducing the CMP onto the regression coefficients.
(b) Write the analytical form for the two induced priors for β. Are either of them data augmentation priors?

Chapter 9

Poisson and Nonlinear Regression

In this chapter we first consider regression models for Poisson data. In binary regression we related appropriately transformed success probabilities—via logit, probit and complementary log-log functions—to linear combinations of covariates. Here, we relate log-transformed rates of Poisson events, $\log E(Y_i)$, to linear combinations of covariates.

This chapter also includes the extension to the problem of overdispersion and its resolution by considering continuous mixtures of Poisson regression models. An additional extension is to the common problem where considerably more zeros occur than are expected under either of these two Poisson models. This leads to the introduction of the zero-inflated Poisson regression model. We also briefly discuss how these and other like models fit into a broader framework of models called generalized linear models.

Finally, we introduce nonlinear regression models via one particular model where the data are considered to be normally distributed but the mean response has a nonlinear structure.

9.1 The Basic Poisson Regression Model

We discussed exchangeable Poisson distributed observations in Chapter 3. Poisson data are counts of events where there is no specified upper limit for the number of events that could occur over time or in space. There are four basic assumptions required for count data to be Poisson distributed (Ross, 2014; [275]). The first assumption is that events are "rare" in the sense that the chance that there would be two or more events in a small interval of time, or a small region in space, would tend to zero very quickly as the interval or region becomes small. Second, event occurrence is stationary in the sense that the probability of a specified number of events in an interval of fixed length (or a region of fixed size) is the same regardless of where the interval appears on the time line (or where the region is located in space). Third, counts in non-overlapping intervals of time (or regions in space) are mutually independent. This is referred to as "independent increments." The final assumption is that the probability of a single event in a small interval (or region) is proportional to the length (or size) of the interval (or region). Under these circumstances, the number of events counted in any fixed time interval (or region) is a Poisson random variable with mean equal to the constant rate λ multiplied by the length of the time interval (or size of the region). What is new in this chapter is that the time-constant or space-constant rate at which events occur depends on covariates. As the rate λ is a *positive* number, we use the log link here, so the linear combination of covariates can be any *real* number.

Let the response data $y = (y_1, \ldots, y_n)$ constitute a vector of Poisson counts, and let $x_i' = (1, x_{i1}, \ldots, x_{ip})$ where $x_{i1}, \ldots, x_{ip}$ are p predictor variables for individual i, $i = 1, \ldots, n$. For example, we could have randomly sampled n children from a population of interest and over the course of several years counted the number of colds each child caught over a period of time. Possible predictor variables are age, number of family members, family income, race and ethnicity. The basic model for Poisson regression is

$$Y_i \mid x_i, \lambda_i \stackrel{ind}{\sim} Po(\lambda_i), \quad \log(\lambda_i) = x_i'\beta, \quad \beta = (\beta_0, \ldots, \beta_p)', \; i = 1, \ldots, n. \quad (9.1)$$

We observe some similarities between this and the logistic regression model in expression (8.1). Here,[1] $E(Y_i) = \lambda_i$ and $\log(E(Y_i))$ is related to covariates via a linear function. In logistic regression, $E(Y_i) = P(Y_i = 1)$ and $\text{logit}(E(Y_i))$ is a linear function of covariates. In linear regression for normally distributed data, $E(Y_i)$ itself is a linear function of the covariates, that is, the link function is the identity function.

Example 9.1. Epilepsy Data. We analyze a simplified version of a data set that was discussed in Thall and Vail (1990) [321] and which was subsequently analyzed in Breslow and Clayton (1993) [52]. The data are seizure counts over a fixed period of time (four two-week intervals post-randomization) in a randomized trial of anti-convulsant therapy for epilepsy. The counts are for 59 patients, and covariates are treatment (Trt: $0, 1$), eight-week baseline seizure count ($Base$), and age in years (Age). Counts range from 0 to 302, with a median of 16; ages range from 18 to 42, with a median of 28; baseline counts ranged from 6 to 151, with a median of 22; and 31 individuals were treated out of the 59. BUGS code and programs for JAGS and Stan may be found on the book's website for Chapter 9. The data and program files include "epilepsy" in their names.

Since the data on *Age* and *Base* are clearly skewed to the right, we use the logarithms of these variables. We also standardize them by subtracting their respective means and dividing by their standard deviations. While standardization is not strictly necessary, it will often stabilize the implementation of statistical inferences. We have found that placing independent standard normal priors on the regression coefficients for standardized and dichotomous predictors to be a reasonable reference prior.

In the following regression model, we denote the standardized logarithm of the baseline seizure count as $slogBase_i$ for patient i and this patient's standardized age by $sAge_i$. The model is

$$\log(\lambda_i) = \beta_0 + \beta_1 \, slogBase_i + \beta_2 \, Trt_i + \beta_3 \, slogBase_i \times Trt_i + \beta_4 sAge_i,$$

---

[1] All observations are initially assumed to be on an interval of unit length (or region of unit size). We address other situations later, through examples.

TABLE 9.1: Model parameter inferences for epilepsy data

Predictor	Med	95% PI
$slogBase$	0.68	$(0.62, 0.74)$
Trt	-0.31	$(-0.42, -0.19)$
$slogBase \times Trt$	0.40	$(0.31, 0.49)$
$sAge$	0.20	$(0.15, 0.25)$

where we include an interaction between the treatment and the standardized logarithm of the base count, since it was anticipated that the effect of the treatment could vary with age. The original data were obtained longitudinally where counts were obtained over four distinct time periods. Our version of the data simply takes the total over the four periods, since we have not discussed how to handle longitudinal outcomes at this stage in the book. Those methods are discussed in Chapter 14.

Since all predictors are standardized or are binary, we use independent $N(0, 1)$ priors on the βs. As an alternative, we also use independent improper flat priors on the βs. (dflat() in BUGS or Stan's facility for allowing improper priors). Posterior results using this latter prior are virtually identical to those presented in Table 9.1, where we used the $N(0, 1)$ priors. We see that all of the regression coefficients are clearly statistically important, including the coefficient for the interaction.

Because the interaction is important, it is not easy to interpret results directly from Table 9.1. Therefore, we include Table 9.2 in which we present inferences that show how the effect of the treatment varies as we vary the baseline seizure count ($Base$) for fixed ages. The table shows posterior median seizure rates for $Trt = 1$ and $Trt = 0$ for individuals with $Base = 22$ and Age taking values $(22, 28, 35)$, and then again with $Base = 50$. We also show inferences for the differences in rates for $Trt = 1$ versus $Trt = 0$ in Table 9.2 to highlight how the effect of treatment varies across all of these conditions. We did this by monitoring the posterior samples of rates

$$\lambda_{Trt} = \exp(\beta_0 + \beta_1 \, slogBase + \beta_2 \, Trt + \beta_3 \, slogBase \times Trt + \beta_4 \, sAge) \quad (9.2)$$

for all of these combinations of covariates and for the rate differences, $\lambda_1 - \lambda_0$, for each sample.

Observe that the first three posterior median rate differences in Table 9.2 are -5.6, -7.6, and -9.2, respectively, while the bottom three are 3.4, 4.6, and 5.6. The implication is that there is an appreciably lower rate of seizures for treated than for non-treated individuals who have average baseline seizure counts ($Base = 22$), while there is an appreciably greater rate for treated versus non-treated individuals who have baseline seizure counts of 50. Moreover, these estimated effects become more pronounced with increasing age. Thus, with average baseline counts, the estimated treatment effect improves with age, and with $Base = 50$, the negative effect of

TABLE 9.2: Inferences for seizure rates (λ) according to *Age*, *Base*, and *Trt*

	Trt = 1		*Trt = 0*		Difference	
	Med	95% PI	Med	95% PI	Med	95% PI
Age	*Base = 22*					
22	12.4	$(10.9, 14.0)$	18.0	$(16.0, 20.3)$	-5.6	$(-7.7, -3.7)$
28	16.7	$(15.2, 18.3)$	24.3,	$(22.3, 26.4)$	-7.6	$(-10.1, -5.1)$
35	20.4	$(18.4, 22.5)$	29.6	$(27.0, 32.4)$	-9.2	$(-12.4, -6.2)$;
Age	*Base = 50*					
22	42.8	$(39.4, 46.4)$	39.4	$(35.2, 43.9)$	3.4	$(-0.6, 7.3)$
28	57.7	$(53.9, 61.7)$	53.1	$(49.6, 56.8)$	4.6	$(-0.8, 10.1)$
35	70.4	$(63.7, 77.5)$	64.7	$(60.0, 69.9)$	5.6	$(-0.9, 12.6)$

treatment also increases. The modeled interaction effect is clearly appreciable and of both statistical and practical import.

Finally, observe that the effect of increasing the baseline seizure count (*Base*) is quite substantial; the estimated rates for those with higher *Base* values are all considerably larger than their counterparts with smaller *Base* values. It is not surprising that individuals with higher baseline seizure counts would also have higher estimated counts during the study than would individuals with lower baseline counts. It may be surprising, however, that the treatment works well for individuals with smaller baseline counts but is evidently detrimental for individuals with high baseline counts.

Another summary, besides rate difference, that is often used to compare two treatments in Poisson regression is the relative rate (*RR*) of occurrence of seizures under the two conditions, defined by

$$\frac{\lambda \mid Trt = 1}{\lambda \mid Trt = 0} = \frac{\exp\{\beta_0 + \beta_1 slogBase + \beta_2 + \beta_3 slogBase + \beta_4 Age\}}{\exp\{\beta_0 + \beta_1 slogBase + \beta_4 Age\}}$$

$$= e^{\beta_2 + \beta_3 slogBase}.$$

This formula makes clear that the treatment effect is modified by the value for *Base*. For these data, the estimated value for β_2 is -0.31 and for β_3 is 0.40. So we anticipate that the relative rate of seizures will be smaller (and less than 1) when the *Base* rate is relatively small and that the relative rate will be larger (and greater than 1) when the *Base* rate is relatively high. This is precisely what we can glean from Table 9.2 by visually comparing rates with and without treatment for the situations with low and high *Base* rates.

To elaborate further, if $slogBase = 0$, the treatment effect is measured as e^{β_2}; while if $slogBase = 1$, the treatment effect is measured as $e^{\beta_2 + \beta_3}$; $slogBase = 0$ corresponds to $Base \doteq 25$, and $slogBase = 1$ corresponds to $Base \doteq 51$. These values are obtained by transforming $slogBase$ values back to *Base* using the average and standard deviation of the $logBase$ values, 3.21 and 0.72, respectively. The posterior inference for the treatment effect *RR* at $Base \doteq 25$ is $e^{-0.31} \left(e^{-0.42}, e^{-0.19} \right) =$

TABLE 9.3: Predicted seizure counts for an individual according to *Age*, *Base*, and *Trt*

	$Trt = 1$		$Trt = 0$	
	Med	95% PI	Med	95% PI
Age	*Base* = 22			
22	12	(6, 20)	18	(10, 27)
28	17	(9, 25)	24	(15, 35)
35	20	(12, 30)	30	(19, 41)
Age	*Base* = 50			
22	43	(30, 57)	39	(27, 53)
28	58	(43, 74)	53	(39, 68)
35	70	(53, 89)	65	(49, 82)

0.73 (0.66, 0.83). At $Base = 51$, the median $RR = e^{-0.31+0.40} = 1.20$. The probability interval, however, is not available from Table 9.1. The interval could be easily obtained by monitoring $\beta_2 + \beta_3$ if posterior samples of β were available. It turns out that this interval is entirely above 1. As the RR is below 1 for $Base \doteq 25$, we infer that the two measured effects are statistically different from 1 and in opposite directions. Thus again, from a different quantification, we reach the same conclusion that the treatment appears to be effective for patients with average baseline rates of seizures, but harmful for patients with high baseline rates.

We conclude the example by showing prediction results in Table 9.3 that are parallel to the estimation results in Table 9.2. Observe how the point predictions are directly comparable to the corresponding rate estimates in Table 9.2, while the corresponding intervals are considerably wider here, as they should be.

Next we consider the common situation in which one carries out long-term studies on patient populations. The studies seek to address major health issues, such as the effect of smoking on eventual acquisition of lung cancer or the effect of obesity, smoking, and other factors on the eventual acquisition of coronary heart disease. Such studies are generally quite large, take many years to complete, and are expensive. We have two small versions of such data that we analyze below. Our intent here is to illustrate methodology.

Example 9.2. Framingham Heart Study. The Framingham Heart Study was initiated in 1948 with the primary goal of identifying common factors or characteristics that contribute to cardiovascular disease [236]. The data involve 4,699 subjects collectively contributing 103,710 person-years of follow-up. While there are a number of outcomes and predictors that are considered in the study, we use a small version of the data on the web that involved counts of coronary heart disease (CHD) for men and for women for specified person-years of exposure. In particular, there were 823 men who experienced CHD over the course of 42,259 person-years of follow-up, and there were 650 women who experienced CHD over a total of 61,451 person-years of follow-up.

When fitting a Poisson regression model, we input the person-years of follow-up as what is called an "offset variable." The reason is that the rate parameter gives the expected number of events per unit time. If the total amount of time is M person-years, then the expected number of events is $\lambda \times M$, which is the rate parameter for the corresponding Poisson sampling distribution. (A similar argument applies when one is modeling occurrences over space, with the offset corresponding to the size of the space in appropriate units.) Offset variables are treated as fixed and are used so that the rates corresponding to all Poisson counts will be comparable in terms of units. For example, the raw estimate of rate of CHD occurrence for men is $823/42{,}259 = 0.0195$ events per person-year and for women is $650/61{,}451 = 0.0106$ events per person-year. If we divide person-years by 1,000, then we obtain 19.5 and 10.6 events per 1,000 person-years, respectively, which is easier to think about.

A feature of this example, distinct from the epilepsy example, is that, all other factors being the same, we would expect larger counts in the group that had the larger number of person-years of exposure. In the epilepsy example, each individual was observed over the same length of time, so the number of person-years was the same for each of the sets of conditions considered. Differences in follow-up times did not play a role in the analysis. Here we write a model to accommodate varying exposure time as follows.

As we wish to study differences by sex, we first think of the model

$$Y_i|\lambda_i \sim Po(\lambda_i), \quad \log(\lambda_i) = \beta_0 + \beta_1 \, Sex_i, \quad i = 1, 2,$$

where observations correspond to the two groups $Sex_1 = 0$ for men and $Sex_2 = 1$ for women. However, this does not account for different exposure times for the two groups. We therefore write, with M_i equal to the total exposure in group i,

$$Y_i|\lambda_i \sim Po(M_i\lambda_i), \quad \log(\lambda_i) = \beta_0 + \beta_1 \, Sex_i, \quad i = 1, 2.$$

In this model, $E(Y_i)$ is not λ_i, but $M_i\lambda_i$. Alternatively, we can write the model as

$$Y_i|\lambda_i^* \sim Po(\lambda_i^*), \quad log(\lambda_i^*) = log(M_i) + \beta_0 + \beta_1 \, Sex_i, \ i = 1, 2.$$

With $M_1 = 42{,}259$ and $M_2 = 61{,}451$, $\beta' = (\beta_0, \beta_1)$, and $x_1' = (1, 0)$ and $x_2' = (1, 1)$, we can write the model in vector form as

$$Y_i|\lambda_i^* \sim Po(\lambda_i^*), \quad \log(\lambda_i^*) = \log(M_i) + x_i'\beta, \quad i = 1, 2.$$

For our analysis, we specify independent standard normal priors for β_0 and β_1. The relative rate comparing males to females with offsets set to be equal is $RR = \lambda_1/\lambda_2 = \exp(-\beta_1)$ with $\lambda_i = \lambda_i^*/M_i$, $i = 1, 2$.

Fitting this model, we obtained the posterior median for the rate of CHD among men as 19.5 events per 1,000 person-years with a 95% posterior probability interval of $(18.2, 20.8)$ events per 1,000 person-years. (Data and code for fitting the data have a name that includes "CHD" on the book's website for Chapter 9.) For women, the corresponding results were 10.6 (9.8, 11.4). The rate ratio of CHD for men relative to women was estimated to be 1.84 (1.66, 2.04). Thus men are estimated to experience CHD at between 66% and 104% higher rate compared to women.

Of course these results do not account for potential person-level covariates that might be relevant, for example, age at the beginning of the study, or any behavior patterns like alcohol consumption and smoking. Other factors such as blood pressure and body mass index might even be of greater interest than sex as predictors of CHD. We address such a situation next.

Example 9.2 used a grouped data model that, when appropriate, can condense the data considerably. While there are $n = 4{,}699$ individuals contributing $42{,}259 + 61{,}451 = 103{,}710$ person-years of follow-up, the data for the model consisted of only two observations! On the other hand, perhaps important individual-level information was ignored in the analysis. The following model can correct the situation:

$$Y_i \mid \lambda_i \overset{iid}{\sim} Po(\lambda_i), \quad \log(\lambda_i) = \log(M_i) + x_i'\beta, \quad i = 1, \dots, n.$$

As in regression models of Chapters 7 and 8, here $\beta' = (\beta_0, \dots, \beta_p)$ is the vector of regression coefficients, including the intercept β_0, and x_i is the corresponding $(p+1) \times 1$ vector of covariates for individual i with first element set to 1. In addition, M_i is the number of years over which individual i was in the study (exposure time). As before, if we wish to express event rates per 1,000 person-years, we would use $M_i^* = M_i/1{,}000$ as the offset; alternatively, rates obtained with M_i can be multiplied by 1,000. The next example illustrates an analysis with such a model.

Example 9.3. British Doctors Study. Christensen et al. (2010) analyzed data from a historic study on the effects of smoking [79]. Table 9.4 presents the data. The participants were male British doctors surveyed in 1951. The data consist of age and whether the respondent smoked tobacco. Ten years later the investigators determined the number of deaths from CHD and the number of person-years on study in each group defined by initial smoking status. We compare death rates for smokers and non-smokers, controlling for age.

TABLE 9.4: Ten-year mortalities from CHD and empirical rate ratios by age categories

	Smoker		Non-smoker		
Age	y	M	y	M	Observed rate ratio
35–44	32	52,407	2	18,790	5.7
45–54	104	43,248	12	10,673	2.1
55–64	206	28,612	28	5,710	1.5
65–74	186	12,663	28	2,585	1.4
75–84	102	5,317	31	1,462	0.9

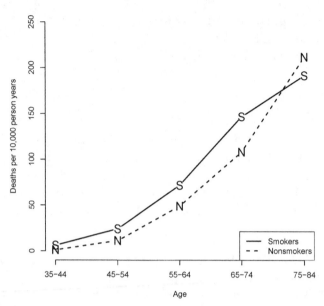

FIGURE 9.1: Empirical death rates from CHD for smokers and non-smokers.

Before carrying out model-based inference, we describe the sample data consisting of five age groups. Figure 9.1 plots these death rates for smokers and nonsmokers. With the exception of the 75–84 age range, the empirical (or sample or raw) mortality rates from CHD are higher in smokers than non-smokers, and the differences increase with age, with one exception: the 75–84 range shows non-smokers with a higher empirical rate of death than for smokers. It is also noticeable that the death rates increase at an increasing pace rather than at a constant or linear pace in age. Table 9.4 displays calculations from the sample, including rate ratios comparing smokers to non-smokers, which decrease from over 5 for the youngest group to about 1 for the eldest group. This decline indicates that the magnitude of the smoking effect may diminish with age, in spite of the fact that death rates themselves and even the differences in death rates for smokers and non-smokers increase with age, except for the difference in the eldest group.

While these are good summaries of the data, they do not contain measures of variability in these rates, differences, and rate ratios. Variability assessment is essential to draw conclusions from the data. To this end we propose some models for the data. Let $(y_1, \ldots, y_5)$ be the mortality counts for smokers and $(y_6, \ldots, y_{10})$ be the corresponding mortality counts for non-smokers in each of the five age categories. Also let $(M_1, \ldots, M_5)$ and $(M_6, \ldots, M_{10})$ be the corresponding numbers of person-years of observation.

We have a number of choices for a model. Christensen et al. (2010) [79] treated categorical age groups as numerical. Thus, as a covariate in the model, *Age* took on the values $1, \ldots, 5$; and of course *Smoke* is binary. An issue we need to address, however, is the fact that *Age* in these data is categorical. If we let *Age* take the values $1, \ldots, 5$, there is a presumption that the rate difference (on the logarithmic scale) between $Age = 1$ and $Age = 2$ equals that between $Age = 2$ and $Age = 3$. In general, it is not a good idea to treat a categorical variable as numerical. For example, think about what it would mean if the categories were colors, a situation in which it would make no sense to think that the response difference in the color blue and the color red equals that between the red and white. Even so, age being numerical in nature and the categories being equally spaced lessen this concern assuming, of course, that log(rate) is a linear function of age.

To account for the shape of the empirical curves displayed in Figure 9.1, Christensen et al. [79] included both a linear and a quadratic term for *Age*. They also included an interaction between *Age* and *Smoke*, and between Age^2 and *Smoke*, so that distinct nonlinear curves could be modeled for smokers and for non-smokers. In our version of the model, we standardize *Age* and use the square of $(Age - mean(Age))/sd(Age)$. The regression model is

$$\log(\lambda_i) = \beta_0 + \beta_1 Smoke_i + \beta_2 sA_i + \beta_3 sA_i^2 + \beta_4 Smoke_i sA_i + \beta_5 Smoke_i\, sA_i^2, \quad (9.3)$$

where $Smoke_i$ is smoker status (1 for smoker, 0 for non-smoker), A_i is age, $sA_i = (A_i - mean(Age))/sd(Age)$, and $sA_i^2 = [(Age_i - mean(Age))/sd(Age)]^2$, for groups $i = 1, \ldots, 10$. With these standardizations, if $A_i = mean(Age) = 3$, then $sA_i = sA_i^2 = 0$. This will allow us to easily specify a conditional means prior (CMP), or at least a partially informative CMP, as we shall see.

For our initial analysis of the data, we let $\beta_i \overset{iid}{\sim} U(-10, 10)$, which is a proper prior that gives virtually the same results as $p(\beta) \propto c$ for any constant c. In the analysis, we divided all of the person-years at risk by 10,000. This means that risk is to be interpreted as expected number of deaths per 10,000 person-years at risk. (BUGS and **Stan** code can be found on the course website, under Chapter 9, in the file with name that starts "British".) Results for regression coefficients are given in Table 9.5. Observe that all coefficients except β_5 are statistically important, since

TABLE 9.5: Inference for regression coefficients, model equation (9.3)

Coef.	Med	95% PI
β_0	3.81	$(3.52, 4.08)$
β_1	0.47	$(0.18, 0.77)$
β_2	1.85	$(1.54, 2.21)$
β_3	-0.55	$(-0.91, -0.23)$
β_4	-0.53	$(-0.92, -0.21)$
β_5	0.12	$(-0.22, 0.50)$

the corresponding 95% posterior probability intervals exclude zero. The effects of *Age* and *Smoke* are nuanced, because the model includes an interaction between them. These effects are discussed next. Clearly β_5 is not statistically important. We leave it as an exercise to compare this model to the one without β_5, as well as to consider a model that treats *Age* as a factor rather than as a quantitative variable.

We also estimated death rates for smokers and for non-smokers, the rate differences (RD), and the relative rates (RR). Results are given in Tables 9.6 and 9.7. Clearly, fitted rates increase with age for smokers and for non-smokers. For the first three age categories, there is no overlap for smoker and non-smoker intervals (see Table 9.6); consequently, results for these rate differences and relative rates show clear statistical import (see also Table 9.7).

TABLE 9.6: Ten-year posterior mortality rates, model equation (9.3)

Flat prior				
	Smokers		Non-smokers	
Age	Med	95% PI	Med	95% PI
35–44	5.7	(4.3, 7.6)	1.4	(0.5, 3.1)
45–54	24.7	(21.7, 27.9)	10.2	(6.7, 14.5)
55–64	72.2	(65.1, 80.1)	45.1	(33.7, 59.1)
65–74	143.4	(130.3158.4)	121.6	(94.6, 154.6)
75–84	194.0	(162.9, 230.1)	199.4	(138.5, 278.3)

Observe that interval widths increase with age, because the number of person-years at risk decreases with age for both smokers and non-smokers. For any given age cohort, intervals are wider for non-smokers since there are fewer person-years for them than there are for smokers.

TABLE 9.7: Ten-year posterior mortality rate differences and relative rates, model equation (9.3)

Flat Prior				
	Smokers		Non-smokers	
	RD		RR	
Age	Med	95% PI	Med	95% PI
35–44	4.3	(2.1, 6.4)	4.1	(1.7, 11.5)
45–54	14.5	(9.2, 19.2)	2.4	(1.7, 3.7)
55–64	27.0	(11.5, 40.8)	1.6	(1.2, 2.2)
65–74	21.8	(−13.4, 52.3)	1.2	(0.9, 1.5)
75–84	−5.5	(−90.1, 65.6)	0.97	(0.67, 1.5)
Partially informative prior				
35–44	4.3	(2.1, 6.4)	4.2	(1.7, 11.8)
45–54	14.5	(9.1, 19.3)	2.4	(1.6, 3.8)
55–64	26.6	(12.4, 40.2)	1.6	(1.2, 2.1)
65–74	21.3	(−12.6, 51.8)	1.2	(0.9, 1.5)
75–84	−4.5	(−89.3, 66.8)	0.98	(0.67, 1.46)

Next we consider a partially informative CMP by specifying independent, informative log-normal distributions for two scientifically relevant rates, which then induces informative distributions on two regression coefficients. We specify diffuse distributions on the remaining coefficients. While we could use gamma distributions, the log-normal is slightly more convenient to specify as a prior distribution because there are simple formulas for the median and a quantile of the log-normal. With extra effort, the gamma can be used as well.

The first specified mortality rate, $\tilde{\lambda}_1$, corresponds to a doctor who is in the middle age category and is a non-smoker. The second specified rate, $\tilde{\lambda}_2$, corresponds to a doctor who is also in the third age category but is a smoker. From equation (9.3), we obtain

$$\tilde{\lambda}_1 = e^{\beta_1}, \quad \tilde{\lambda}_2 = e^{\beta_1 + \beta_2}.$$

Specifying the prior as

$$\log(\tilde{\lambda}_i) \overset{ind}{\sim} LN(b_{i0}, \sigma_{i0}^2), \quad i = 1, 2,$$

we can induce the prior on (β_1, β_2) by specifying the relationship as

$$\beta_1 = \log(\tilde{\lambda}_1), \quad \beta_2 = \log(\tilde{\lambda}_2) - \beta_1. \tag{9.4}$$

In this way, we would use scientifically relevant information to induce a prior for the model parameters (β_1, β_2). For the remaining regression coefficients, we specify independent diffuse priors: $\beta_i \overset{ind}{\sim} U(-10, 10)$, $i = 3, \ldots, 6$. With these steps, we will have induced some real prior information into the model. We could of course have focused on a single rate, or more than two rates, and accordingly modify this prior induction process.

How do we specify the parameters in the log-normal priors? We have done this before in previous chapters. We first specify a guess for the rate corresponding to individuals in the middle age cohort who do not smoke. We might think that the rate is 50 deaths per 10,000 person-years. For the smoker in the same age cohort, we hypothesize that the rate might be 80 deaths per 10,000 person-years. (We cheated and looked at the data, so our exercise here is purely illustrative of the technique.) We then specify the 95th percentile of the prior for the rates to be 100 and 150, respectively; we are 95% certain that the mortality rate per 10,000 person-years for smokers is less than 100, among non-smoker doctors in the middle age cohort, and that for smokers it is less than 150.

Generically, if $\tilde{\lambda} \sim LN(b_0, \sigma_0^2)$, the corresponding α quantile is

$$\tilde{\lambda}_\alpha = e^{b_0 + z_\alpha \sigma_0}.$$

Thus, if our best guess for $\tilde{\lambda}$ is λ_0 and we let λ_u be the user-specified value that satisfies $P(\tilde{\lambda} < \lambda_u) = 0.95$, then we have $\lambda_0 = e^{b_0}$ and $\lambda_u = e^{b_0 + 1.645 \sigma_0}$, which results in $b_0 = \log(\lambda_0)$ and $\sigma_0 = (\log(\lambda_u) - \log(\lambda_0))/1.645$. Then for our specific problem, we have $b_{10} = \log(50)$, $\sigma_{10} = (\log(100) - \log(50))/1.645$, $b_{20} = \log(80)$, $\sigma_{20} = (\log(150) - \log(80))/1.645$.

Results for rate differences and ratios using this partially informative prior are given in Table 9.7. They are remarkably similar to those using the flat prior. The similarity may be in part because of the large number of person-years involved in the study.

9.2   Poisson-Based More General Models for Count Data

We now discuss two models that address typical violations of the basic Poisson model frequently seen in practice. Both still use the Poisson distribution but extend the model in interesting ways to account for its shortcomings in the basic form. The first addresses higher variation than indicated by the Poisson distribution, and the second addresses higher frequency of zero counts.

9.2.1   Overdispersion

We know that the Poisson distribution imposes the restriction that its variance equals its mean, $Y \sim Po(\lambda) \Rightarrow E(Y) = \text{Var}(Y) = \lambda$ (see distribution table in Appendix B). In many instances with data, y_i, that have been assumed to be, say $Po(\lambda_i)$, it can be empirically verified that $\text{Var}(Y_i \mid \lambda_i) > E(Y_i \mid \lambda_i)$. Since the mean and variance must be the same if the data are actually Poisson distributed, this is termed "extra-Poisson variation." If the data indicate extra variation, a common solution is to use a model that employs a mixture of Poisson distributions. It is generally the case that mixtures of distributions will have larger variances than the components in the mixture. This is shown using the iterated variance formula, which we demonstrate here for a continuous mixture of Poisson distributions.

Take $Y \sim Po(\lambda)$ and let $\lambda \sim Ga(\alpha, \gamma)$ be the mixing distribution where α and γ are unknown parameters. The resulting mixture model will have (α, γ) as its unknown parameters. We observe that

$$
\begin{aligned}
E(Y \mid \alpha, \gamma) &= E(E(Y \mid \lambda, \alpha, \gamma)) = E(\lambda \mid \alpha, \gamma) = \alpha/\gamma, \\
\text{Var}(Y \mid \alpha, \gamma) &= \text{Var}(E(Y \mid \lambda, \alpha, \gamma)) + E(\text{Var}(Y \mid \lambda, \alpha, \gamma)) \\
&= \text{Var}(\lambda \mid \alpha, \gamma) + E(\lambda \mid \alpha, \gamma) = \alpha/\gamma^2 + \alpha/\gamma > \alpha/\gamma.
\end{aligned}
$$

We can also derive the mixture distribution as

$$
\begin{aligned}
p(y \mid \alpha, \gamma) &= \int_0^\infty p(y \mid \lambda) p(\lambda \mid \alpha, \gamma) d\lambda \\
&= \int_0^\infty \frac{\lambda^y e^{-\lambda}}{y!} \frac{\gamma^\alpha \lambda^{\alpha-1} e^{-\lambda\gamma}}{\Gamma(\alpha)} d\lambda \\
&= \frac{\gamma^\alpha}{y!\Gamma(\alpha)} \int_0^\infty \lambda^{\alpha+y-1} e^{-\lambda(1+\gamma)} d\lambda \\
&= \frac{\gamma^\alpha \Gamma(\alpha+y)}{y!(1+\gamma)^{\alpha+y}\Gamma(\alpha)} \\
&= \left(\frac{\gamma}{1+\gamma}\right)^\alpha \left(\frac{1}{1+\gamma}\right)^y \frac{\Gamma(\alpha+y)}{y!\Gamma(\alpha)}.
\end{aligned}
$$

This is a negative binomial distribution.

We can now model multiple counts as independent gamma mixtures of Poisson random variables, resulting in a model that allows for variances to be larger than the means. An alternative mixture distribution places a log-normal distribution on λ, which will also generate overdispersion.

We first consider grouped data of the form $y = \{y_{ij} : i = 1, \ldots, k; j = 1, \ldots, n_i\}$. This is to allow for the possibility of easily checking the assumption of equal variances. Later, we go back to the case with $n_i = 1$. We have k groups of data. Let M_{ij} be the offset for the jth individual in group i and let $M_i = \sum_j M_{ij}$. We also assume a common covariate vector, x_i, for each group. Our regression model that allows for overdispersion is

$$Y_{ij} \mid \lambda_i \overset{\text{ind}}{\sim} Po(M_i \lambda_i), \quad j = 1, \ldots, n_i,$$
$$\log(\lambda_i) \overset{\text{ind}}{\sim} N(x_i' \beta, \sigma_u^2), \quad i = 1, \ldots, k. \tag{9.5}$$

This parameterization is termed "centered," since the mean of $\log(\lambda_i)$ is $x_i'\beta$, in contrast to the standard parameterization below. If σ_u^2 is very small, the model reduces to regular Poisson regression for grouped data. If n_i are all 1 and σ_u^2 is small, it is just Poisson regression as we have discussed it in the previous section. We observe that there is only one additional parameter from the standard Poisson regression model.

The model in expression (9.5) is equivalent to the model

$$Y_{ij} \mid \lambda_i \overset{\text{ind}}{\sim} Po(M_i \lambda_i), \quad i = 1, \ldots k; j = 1, \ldots, n_i,$$
$$\log(\lambda_i) = x_i'\beta + U_i, \tag{9.6}$$
$$U_i \overset{\text{iid}}{\sim} N(0, \sigma_u^2).$$

This version of the model is termed the "standard parameterization" and is obviously structurally equivalent to the centered version. The standard version is often used in more traditional non-Bayesian analysis. Motivation for the centered version is that the corresponding Markov chains may have better convergence properties than those in the standard version.

With grouped data, it is possible to directly check the assumption that the mean equals the variance. Assume for the moment that the Poisson model holds. Since, for each i, the observations $\{y_{ij} : j = 1, \ldots, n_i\}$ constitute a random sample with mean λ_i, then the sample mean for group i, $\bar{y}_i = \sum_j y_{ij}/n_i$, is a reasonable estimate of the Poisson mean. Moreover, the sample variance, $s_i^2 = \sum_j (y_{ij} - \bar{y}_i)^2/(n_i - 1)$, can also be used as an estimate of λ_i, the Poisson variance for the model. Then we could order the $\bar{y}_i$ from smallest to largest and subsequently plot these ordered values versus their corresponding s_i^2. We would expect to see something resembling a 45-degree straight line if the Poisson assumption was correct. On the other hand, if we see a pattern of variances that are above the 45-degree line, we might suspect overdispersion. When we suspect overdispersion, we can turn to models in expressions (9.5) or (9.6) as alternatives.

Example 9.4. British Doctors Study with Overdispersion. We modified the code used in Example 9.3 to allow for overdispersion using both parameterizations discussed above. We used $\sigma_u \sim U(0,1)$ and we have $n_i = 1$ for all i. We found

Markov chains to be much better behaved using the version in expression (9.5) than with the version corresponding to expression (9.6). MCMC with the latter model was somewhat ill-behaved at the outset, but the chains did eventually converge. Inference for σ_u was 0.06 (0.002, 0.33), so the point estimate was not particularly large. Our decision to stick with the regular Poisson regression model over this one was because of the fact that inferences were not appreciably different from those in Table 9.6, which led us to believe that overdispersion was not a concern.

9.2.2   Zero-Inflated Poisson Data

Count data sometimes exhibit more zeros than expected under a Poisson sampling model. This is due to the fact that $e^{-\lambda}$ may not be large enough to account for excess zero values. The expected number of zero counts, $ne^{-\lambda}$, will be too small and the expected values for a number of non-zero counts will be too large compared to actual count data. We now define a model that can be used when it is anticipated that there will be more zeros than allowed under a standard Poisson model. The basic problem of having excess zeros has been termed "zero-inflation." This model is a mixture of a point mass at zero for the excess zeros and a Poisson regression model. The probability of zero is modeled as a logistic regression.

We assume data $\{y_1, \ldots, y_n\}$, with covariate vectors $\{x_1, \ldots, x_n\}$. For brevity, we ignore the possibility that there are offsets, M_i, but the model is easily adapted to that situation. Each of the Y_i is modeled as its own zero-inflated Poisson (ZIP) as follows:

$$
\begin{aligned}
Y_i \mid z_i, \lambda_i &\overset{\text{ind}}{\sim} Po(z_i \times 0 + (1 - z_i) \times \lambda_i), \\
Z_i \mid \pi_i &\overset{\text{ind}}{\sim} Ber(\pi_i), \quad \text{logit}(\pi_i) = x_i'\gamma, \\
\log(\lambda_i) &= x_i'\beta.
\end{aligned}
\tag{9.7}
$$

A Poisson with a rate of zero is just zero with probability 1. Thus the model specifies point mass at zero of probability π_i, and a Poisson count with probability $1 - \pi_i$, allowing the possibility that a zero count can come from the point mass or the Poisson. The expected proportion of zeros in the ZIP is $\pi_i + (1 - \pi_i)e^{-\lambda_i}$, and the proportion in excess of what would be observed using the ZIP model over the basic Poisson regression model is $\pi_i + (1 - \pi_i)e^{-\lambda_i} - e^{-\lambda_i} = \pi_i(1 - e^{-\lambda_i})$.

We would not necessarily expect exactly the same covariates to be related to the binary and Poisson counts. A subset of x can be used for the binary regression and a different subset for the non-zero Poisson regression. Li (2012) has shown that the model is identifiable [222], which means that the parameters of the model can be estimated. There are many models that lack identifiability, so this is an important issue in order to avoid nonsense inferences for non-identifiable parameters in the model. In general, lack of parameter identifiability does not mean the model is invalid for all inferences. In fact, there often exist useful and identifiable targets for inference even when some parameters are not identifiable.[2]

---

[2] In some cases, it is even useful to include non-identifiable model parameters; an example, while not treated there, is a version of the ANOVA model of Section 7.6.

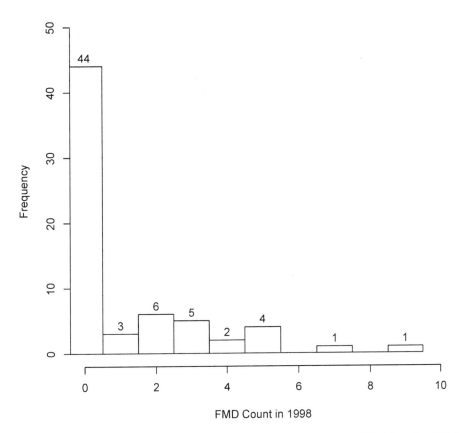

FIGURE 9.2: Histogram of FMD in 66 provinces of Turkey in 1998.

Example 9.5. Foot-and-Mouth Disease. Branscum et al. (2008) [51] analyzed data on reported cases of foot-and-mouth disease (FMD) in each province of Turkey over the eight years from 1996 to 2003. We consider data from 1998, with the goal of assessing the difference in FMD incidence between the eastern and western regions of the country. The histogram in Figure 9.2 shows that the majority of provinces (44 out of 66) had no reported FMD cases in 1998.

We consider both ordinary and zero-inflated Poisson regression models using *Region* (1 = eastern, 0 = western) and standardized cattle population size, $sSize = (Size - \text{mean}(Size))/\text{sd}(Size)$, for each province as covariates. We used uniform priors for the regression coefficients.

We immediately suspect that there are far too many zeros for the standard Poisson regression model to be reasonable. For the purpose of illustration, we ran this model using $U(-5, 5)$ priors for the regression coefficients. (**BUGS**, **JAGS**, and **Stan** code are on the book's website in files with names that contain "FMD".) We obtained virtually identical results with $U(-2, 2)$ priors. History or trace plots were very well behaved with these diffuse priors. Inferences for β_1 (eastern versus western) and β_2 (*sSize*) are -0.14 ($-0.65, 0.35$) and 0.46 ($0.29, 0.62$), respectively. Under this standard analysis, there is no statistical import for the difference in eastern versus western rates of FMD, but the size of the cattle population (*Size*) is clearly important. The larger the population, the larger the rate of FMD. Of course the latter result is no surprise, since we know that FMD is endemic in Turkey; FMD rates would necessarily increase with population size.

In our analysis we also obtained a Bayesian version of the Pearson goodness-of-fit statistic and the corresponding Pearson residuals. In addition, we obtained the expected number of zeros if the standard Poisson model were valid. The standard Pearson goodness of fit measure is

$$PGOF = \sum_i \frac{(y_i - \lambda_i)^2}{\lambda_i}, \tag{9.8}$$

where of course $E(Y_i \mid \lambda_i) = \lambda_i$. In most non-Bayesian analyses, the MLE would be substituted for λ_i. Here, we use the posterior median of the PGOF. We do not have a direct way to calibrate this median for how large is large in our approach. We could use probabilities from the posterior distribution for PGOF. In what follows, we take a simpler route and compare the magnitude of the median PGOF for a standard Poisson regression to the median PGOF for the ZIP model. The posterior median PGOF is 183.6 for the standard Poisson regression model, and 50.9 for the ZIP model.

The Bayesian version of a Pearson residual is simply the posterior median of

$$PR_i = (y_i - \lambda_i)/\sqrt{\lambda_i}.$$

Note that PGOF is just the sum of squares of the PR_i. A plot of these residuals gives some indication of which observations in the data might be contributing to a large PGOF. The usual rule of thumb is to look for values for which $|PR| > 2$. By analogy with normal theory, we might expect 5% of these to be larger than 2. We give an index plot of the Pearson residuals in Figure 9.3. While we would expect about half of the residuals (33) to be below zero, there are 46 that are negative. We might expect 66/20, or about three or four, to be above 2 in absolute value, but there are 10 that actually exceed 2 and none that are below -2. These results indicate the failure of the standard Poisson model. Moreover, the expected number of zeros in the data set is $\sum_i e^{-\lambda_i}$, with a posterior median of 26. We have observed 44 zeros and we expect 26 under the Poisson model. We are justifiably concerned about the validity of our assumptions.

We proceed to consider the ZIP model. (Code is available on the book's website for Chapter 9 in files that include "FMD-ZIP" in the name.) We regressed non-zero FMD counts and the probability of zero counts on both *Region* and *Size*. Inferences for regression coefficients are given in Table 9.8. We see that *Size* is statistically important regarding both the logistic probability of a zero count (the larger is *Size*, the smaller the probability of a zero), and the Poisson rates of FMD (the larger the *Size*, the larger the expected count). The effect of region is not statistically important in the logistic model of a zero count or for the rate of

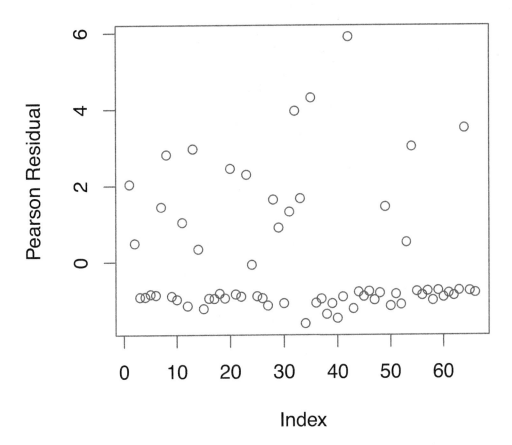

FIGURE 9.3: Pearson residuals for FMD data using the standard Poisson regression model.

FMD. The estimated coefficient for γ_1 is 0.16, which seems negligible. However, the regression coefficient for region in the binary regression model has posterior probability 0.86 of being positive. The estimated coefficient is 0.62, which seems non-negligible.

We obtained posterior inferences for the excess probability of zero counts, comparing ZIP and standard regression models, for West versus East when *Size* was equal to its average value. The posterior medians were 0.72 and 0.59, respectively. The posterior probability for the difference being positive is 0.87, giving some evidence that there may be more zero counts in the West than in the East.

The Pearson goodness-of-fit measure for this model was 50.9, which is much smaller than 183.6, its value for the standard Poisson model. The corresponding residuals are given in Figure 9.4. They also look better than the ones in Figure 9.3. In summary, there is not a definitive case for a difference in rates between eastern and western Turkey.

TABLE 9.8: Inferences for regression coefficients for ZIP model (9.7)

Coef.	Med	95% PI	$P(\beta > 0 \mid y)$
β_0	1.07	$(0.76, 1.36)$	
Region	0.16	$(-0.48, 0.71)$	0.69
Size	0.15	$(-0.04, 0.34)$	0.94
			$P(\gamma > 0 \mid y)$
γ_0	0.52	$(-0.14, 1.20)$	
Region	0.62	$(-0.50, 1.84)$	0.86
Size	-0.52	$(-1.12, 0.02)$	0.03

9.3   Overview of Generalized Linear Model Regression

The generalized linear model (GLM) includes a fairly broad class of regression models, including many we have discussed already, such as binary regression, linear regression, and Poisson regression. The class of GLMs was introduced by Nelder and Wedderburn (1972) [249], and has been discussed by many authors since. We do not study this class in detail, but we introduce it so that readers can have a bigger picture of how they fit together.

What GLMs do is tie together models in which the response variable has a distribution in what is called the *exponential class* of families of distributions. In addition, these models relate a linear combination of covariates, $x'\beta$, to the mean $E(Y \mid x, \beta)$, through what is called a *link* function. We came across link functions for binary regression in Section 8.6. Recall the notation $g(x'\beta) = E(Y \mid x, \beta)$, or equivalently,

$$g^{-1}[E(Y \mid x, \beta)] = x'\beta.$$

So, for GLMs the first assumption is that the response distribution family is in the exponential class, and the second is that the expectation of the response is a known function of a linear combination of the covariates. The link function is defined to be $g^{-1}(\cdot)$, as we have seen. The first assumption requires that the model for the data, y, satisfies

$$p(y \mid \theta_x) = h(y, \sigma) e^{[T(y)b(\theta_x) - q(\theta_x)]/\sigma^2},$$

where the support for y is free of θ_x. In the formula, $T(y)$ is some function of the data only, $b(\cdot)$ and $q(\cdot)$ are functions of θ_x only, and $h(\cdot, \cdot)$ is a function of the data and σ only; σ is a scale parameter. The only situation that we have considered so far where σ could play a role is when we considered the normal linear model; it plays no role in binary or Poisson regression.

If $b(\theta) = \theta_x$, the exponential family is said to be in *canonical form*. If $T(y) = y$, then θ_x is called the *canonical* or *natural* parameter. The exponential family is usually introduced in non-regression settings but, being in the regression context, we have used the notation θ_x.

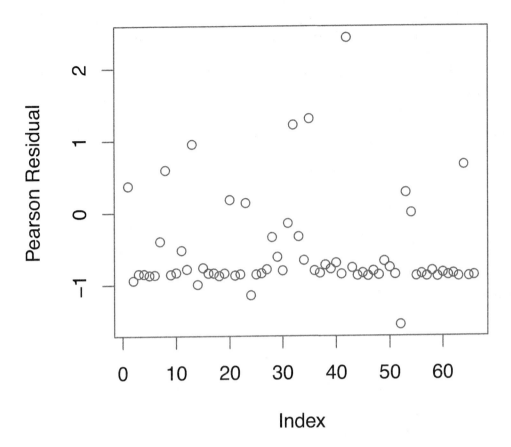

FIGURE 9.4: Pearson residuals for FMD data using the ZIP regression model.

Perhaps the main feature of this description is that it covers a broad class of models, including almost all of those discussed so far[3] and many more. It turns out that making large-sample maximum-likelihood-based inferences within this framework is straightforward. This has made it possible for traditional statistical packages to handle many GLMs; all that is needed is to specify the appropriate family of distributions and the link function. Easy access to such packages has made them very popular. This, however, is not of advantage for the Bayesian approach. So we conclude this section with a couple of illustrations.

Example 9.6. Binomial Regression. If $Y \mid \theta_x \sim Bin(n, \theta_x)$, we have

$$p(y \mid \theta_x) = \binom{n}{y} e^{[y\text{logit}(\theta_x) - (-n \log(1 - \theta_x))]},$$

so we have

$$T(y) = y, \quad b(\theta_x) = \text{logit}(\theta_x), \quad q(\theta_x) = -n \log(1 - \theta_x), \quad h(y) = \binom{n}{y}.$$

---

[3]Exceptions are the ZIP and the nonlinear models.

Thus it turns out that if we were to choose the logit link, $\text{logit}(\theta_x) = x'\beta$, it would be termed the canonical link. This is related to the fact that, if we had reparameterized to $\gamma_x = \text{logit}(\theta_x)$, then it would be the case that γ_x was the canonical parameter of the model. If we had chosen the probit link, $\Phi^{\theta_x} = x'\beta$, the specification would correspond to probit regression. Similarly for the complementary log-log link that was discussed in Chapter 8.

Example 9.7. Poisson Regression. For $Y \mid \theta_x \sim Po(\lambda_x)$, we have

$$p(y \mid \theta_x) = \frac{e^{y \log(\lambda_x) - \lambda_x}}{y!},$$

so we have

$$T(y) = y, \quad b(\lambda_x) = \log(\lambda_x), \quad q(\lambda_x) = \lambda_x, \quad h(y) = 1/y!.$$

In this instance it turns out that, since $T(y) = y$, $b(\theta_x) = \log(\lambda_x) = x'\beta$ is the canonical link. We are not aware of other links that are actually used in Poisson regression data analysis.

9.4 *Nonlinear Regression

All of our regression models up to now have been of the form $g(E(Y \mid x, \beta)) = x'\beta$, where $g(\cdot)$ is a link function. In the case of a linear model, g was the identity; for binary regression, it was a logit, probit, or complementary log-log link; and for Poisson, it was a log link. In this section we depart from that structure and allow an even more general form for the regression function. Our treatment here parallels that of Christensen et al. (2010) [79]. We consider the nonlinear form

$$E(Y|x, \beta) = m(x; \beta),$$

where $m(x; \beta)$ is a known (nonlinear) function of x and β; x is observed but β is a vector of unknown parameters. For data $y = (y_1, \ldots, y_n)$, with covariate vectors $(x_1, \ldots, x_n)$, we further assume that observations deviate from the mean response according to a normal distribution. Then the model can be written as

$$Y_i \mid \beta, \tau \stackrel{\text{ind}}{\sim} N(\lambda_i, 1/\tau), \quad \lambda_i = m(x_i; \beta).$$

Before going into more detail, we emphasize an important notational point for this section. In all regression models thus far, all being linear in β, we have denoted the components of the $(p+1)$-dimensional regression parameter vector β by $\beta_0, \beta_1, \ldots, \beta_p$. The first component β_0 stood for the intercept and the rest were coefficients of covariates. We make a change in this section. We let β stand for a generic q-dimensional parameter vector of components $\beta_1, \ldots, \beta_q$. It is important to recognize that with nonlinear functions, these βs may not be multiplying coefficients; they are just parameters in the function $m(x; \beta)$. Hence the change in notation. The following example and discussion related to it will help to clarify.

Example 9.8. Carlin and Gelfand (1991) [61] reported data from a growth study by Ratkowsky (1983) [268] on length y and age x measurements collected on 27 dugongs, large marine mammals. Carlin and Gelfand consider a growth curve model that is similar to

$$\lambda_i = \beta_1 - e^{\beta_2 + \beta_3 Age_i}.$$

There are no new issues as far as making statistical inferences is concerned. As we have seen and already used, there are programs available (such as BUGS, JAGS, or Stan) that use Markov chain Monte Carlo for posterior inference even in cases where full conditionals are not in familiar mathematical forms. Readers can of course write their own code to do this as an exercise; but with the availability of easy-to-use programs, we prefer to focus on the specification of the prior and the analysis of the data.

We proceed as always by placing a prior on quantities that a scientist can think about directly. For the dugong data, the dimension of β is 3, so we choose three covariate vectors of convenient pseudo-observations $\tilde{x}_i$ and write

$$\tilde{m}_i \equiv m_i(\beta) \equiv m(\tilde{x}_i; \beta), \quad i = 1, 2, 3. \tag{9.9}$$

We can write this in matrix and vector notation as $\tilde{m} = m(\tilde{X}; \beta)$, where $\tilde{X} = (\tilde{x}_1, \tilde{x}_2, \tilde{x}_3)'$. For the dugong data, $\tilde{X} = (\tilde{Age}_1, \tilde{Age}_2, \tilde{Age}_3)'$ is a 3×1 vector of ages that will be selected for eliciting information for the mean lengths for three large groups of hypothetical dugongs of corresponding ages. A conditional means prior is obtained by eliciting

$$\tilde{m} \sim N_3(\tilde{m}_0, D(\tilde{w})). \tag{9.10}$$

So the components of $\tilde{m}_0$ are our expert's best specifications of mean dugong length for the three chosen age values, and the $\sqrt{\tilde{w}_i}$ are elicited by specifying something like the 95th percentile of the prior distribution for $\tilde{m}_i$, as we have done many times before.

Our standard protocol involves inducing the prior on β from the prior on $\tilde{m}$. This is slightly trickier here than it was with the linear structure. We need to solve for β in terms of $\tilde{m}$, as we did in Chapters 7 and 8, only now there is no general explicit solution. Assuming $\tilde{m}(\beta)$ is a one-to-one mapping, we let h be its inverse satisfying $\beta = h(\tilde{m})$. Obviously, $m(h(\tilde{m})) = m(\beta) = \tilde{m}$, by definition.

As usual, we standardize the ages to get $sAge_i$ and let the standardized version be $\tilde{X} = (0, 1, -1)'$, which corresponds to a hypothetical dugong of average age, another that is one standard deviation above the average age, and a third that is one standard deviation below average age. We would then like to solve

$$\begin{pmatrix} \tilde{m}_1 \\ \tilde{m}_2 \\ \tilde{m}_3 \end{pmatrix} = \begin{pmatrix} \beta_1 - e^{\beta_2} \\ \beta_1 - e^{\beta_2 + \beta_3} \\ \beta_1 - e^{\beta_2 - \beta_3} \end{pmatrix} \tag{9.11}$$

for β. When there is no obvious solution, as in this case, we obtain a linear approximation to the nonlinear model that does have an explicit solution. This is done using a standard Taylor series approximation. Given the linear approximation, our approach results in an approximate CMP, since we are able solve the corresponding linear equations for β. To elaborate, we now describe the process.

First, find β_0 that satisfies $\tilde{m}_0 = m(\beta_0)$, where $\tilde{m}_0$ is our vector of prior estimates of the $\tilde{m}_i$. If we know the mapping function $h(\cdot)$, the solution is easy: $\beta_0 = h(\tilde{m}_0)$. Since we usually will not know h in any closed form, we need to find a solution by using an iterative scheme. This approach requires the matrix of partial derivatives of $m(\beta)$,

$$\dot{m}(\beta) = \left\{ \frac{\partial m(\tilde{x}_i; \beta)}{\partial \beta_j} : i, j = 1, 2, 3 \right\},$$

which are obtained by taking each row on the right-hand side of equation (9.11) and differentiating with respect to β_1, β_2, and β_3, forming a matrix in which each row is a vector of partial derivatives. In our example, we obtain

$$\dot{m}(\beta) = \begin{pmatrix} 1 & -e^{\beta_2} & 0 \\ 1 & -e^{\beta_2+\beta_3} & -e^{\beta_2+\beta_3} \\ 1 & -e^{\beta_2-\beta_3} & e^{\beta_2-\beta_3} \end{pmatrix}. \tag{9.12}$$

Now the first-order expansion about an arbitrary value β^* is

$$m(\beta) \doteq m(\beta^*) + \dot{m}(\beta^*)(\beta - \beta^*),$$

with $\dot{m}(\beta^*)$ defined as in equation (9.12). We find an approximate solution of $\tilde{m}_0 = m(\beta_0)$ by writing

$$m(\beta_0) = \tilde{m}_0 \doteq m(\beta^*) + \dot{m}(\beta^*)(\beta_0 - \beta^*),$$

and solving for β_0, obtaining

$$\beta_0 \doteq \beta^* + [\dot{m}(\beta^*)]^{-1} (\tilde{m}_0 - m(\beta^*)). \tag{9.13}$$

Note that we need the matrix $\dot{m}(\beta^*)$ to be non-singular. We also need to specify a value for β^* as an initial value for the procedure. Let $\beta^{(0)}$ denote this initial value. A standard first try might be $\beta_0^{(0)} = 0$. A better choice would be the maximum likelihood estimate (MLE). Rewriting equation (9.13) as

$$\beta_0^{(1)} = \beta^{(0)} + \left[\dot{m}(\beta^{(0)}) \right]^{-1} \left(\tilde{m}_0 - m(\beta^{(0)}) \right),$$

we repeat this process k times to obtain $\beta^{(k)}$. If m is well behaved, $\beta^{(k)}$ will converge to the solution β_0.

At every iteration, the value $\beta^{(j)}$ must result in a non-singular matrix $\dot{m}$. In our example, $\beta = 0$ gives a singular matrix in equation (9.12). It is easy to show, however, that as long as $\beta_3^{(0)} \neq 0$, the matrix will be non-singular. One way to decide when $\beta^{(k+1)}$ is close enough to $\beta^{(k)}$ to stop is to continue until $\sum_j |\beta_j^{(k+1)} - \beta_j^{(k)}| \leq \delta$ for some value of k, where δ is a small value, perhaps 0.001.

We resume our quest for an induced normal prior for β. We have the prior mean, β_0. Since the Taylor expansion worked so well for finding β_0, we use it again for obtaining an approximation to the full distribution. Since $\beta = h(\tilde{m})$, we can take a first-order approximation to this equality by expanding about $\tilde{m}_0$,

$$\beta = h(\tilde{m}) \doteq h(\tilde{m}_0) + \dot{h}(\tilde{m}_0)(\tilde{m} - \tilde{m}_0) = \beta_0 + \dot{h}(\tilde{m}_0)(\tilde{m} - \tilde{m}_0).$$

Now, β is approximated by a linear function of $\tilde{m}$. Since we have placed a normal prior on $\tilde{m}$ in equation (9.10), we obtain an approximate induced normal prior for β, namely

$$\beta \sim N(\beta_0, \dot{h}(\tilde{m}_0)D(\tilde{w})\dot{h}(\tilde{m}_0)'), \tag{9.14}$$

by using the usual formula for a linear transformation of normals.

We still need $\dot{h}(\tilde{m}_0)$, the derivative of h evaluated at $\tilde{m}_0$. We assumed the existence of h, but it is generally only implicitly defined. Since $m(h(\tilde{m})) = \tilde{m}$, differentiating both sides gives $\dot{m}(h(\tilde{m}))\dot{h}(\tilde{m}) = I$, which is equivalent to $\dot{h}(\tilde{m}) = [\dot{m}(h(\tilde{m}))]^{-1}$. This equality implies that $\dot{h}(\tilde{m}_0) = [\dot{m}(h(\tilde{m}_0))]^{-1} = [\dot{m}(\beta_0))]^{-1}$. Thus, from equation (9.14) we have the final computable result,

$$\beta \sim N(\beta_0, [\dot{m}(\beta_0)]^{-1}D(\tilde{w})[\dot{m}(\beta_0)]^{-1'}).$$

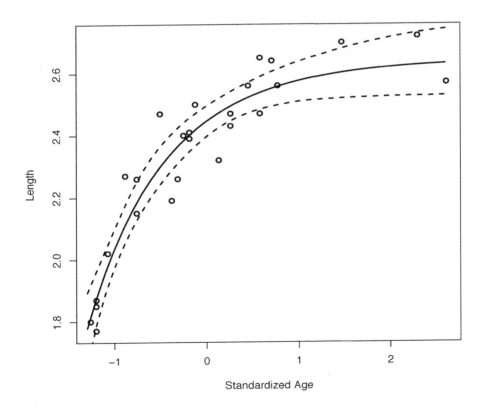

FIGURE 9.5: Dugong growth curve: posterior mean (solid) and 95% pointwise posterior band (dashed).

One can obtain a diffuse prior by specifying a maximum range of values for the $\tilde{m}$s and selecting normal distributions for the $\tilde{m}_i$ that cover those ranges with sufficient probability.

Finally, a word of warning. It can be difficult to get convergence in the MCMC algorithms for nonlinear regression. You may need to run very long chains, and it might help to reparameterize the problem.

Example 9.9. Dugong Growth Study, Continued. For the dugong growth study, primary interest lies in the mean length as a function of age. Figure 9.5 plots posterior medians of expected lengths and the corresponding 95% PIs across standardized ages of -1.3 (*Age* 0.7), $-1.2, \ldots, 2.6$ (*Age* 31.4). Clearly, mean length increases with a plateau around 1 (*Age* 19).

We obtained β_0 and the prior precision matrix in R. We used $\tilde{X} = (0, 1, -1)'$, $\tilde{m}_0 = (2.4, 2.6, 2.0)$, $D(\tilde{w}) = \text{diag}(25, 25, 25)$, and tolerance $\delta = 0.001$, with $Ga(0.001, 0.001)$ prior for τ. The induced prior on β is

$$\beta \sim N \left(\begin{bmatrix} 2.8 \\ -0.9 \\ -0.7 \end{bmatrix}, \begin{bmatrix} 825.0 & 2312.5 & 1312.5 \\ 2312.5 & 6562.5 & 3750.0 \\ 1312.5 & 3750.0 & 2187.5 \end{bmatrix} \right).$$

9.5 Recap and Readings

We covered the highlights of basic Poisson regression modeling, and its complements that attempt to cope with overdispersion and too many zeros. There are many papers that discuss these issues; we are guessing that the majority of them are non-Bayesian. Much of the material in this chapter is similar to that presented in Christensen et al. (2010) [79]. We have revised and/or expanded some of their analyses and added new ones. The dugong analysis is effectively theirs, and the section on nonlinear modeling parallels their section on this material quite closely.

The material discussed here should find considerable utility for those performing long-term studies that involve counts per person-year. Extensions to spatial and spatial-temporal count data are beyond the scope of this book. The book by Banerjee, Carlin, and Gelfand (2015) [15] is an important reference and provides the right background for diving into this important area. GeoBUGS is an add-on to WinBUGS that uses conditionally autoregressive models for spatial data. Barker et al. (2010) [16] used GeoBUGS in WinBUGS to model spatio-temporal mosquito count data. These are just a few places to begin a study of this area.

We note that the Hurdle model (Mullahy, 1986; [244]) is a competitor for the ZIP model. This model specifies a logistic regression for the zeros, as in the ZIP model, but then specifies a zero-truncated Poisson model for the non-negative counts. Thus the probability of a zero count is just π_i using our notation, and the probabilities for all non-zero counts are obtained as zero-truncated Poisson(λ_i). The zero-truncated Poisson can be found most easily on Wikipedia.

9.6   Exercises

EXERCISE 9.1. *Re-examining the epilepsy data (Example 9.1).*   The data and some code are available on the book's website for Chapter 9 with file names that include "Epilepsy". Observe that the data include 12 NAs (indicating missing data) at the end of the Poisson counts y. Also, for each of the covariates, there are 12 additional records in the data set beyond the 59 values that correspond to actual data. Adding these 12 pseudo-observations is a trick we used for obtaining the inferences in Table 9.2. For example, the first three of the 12 added records have Trt values equal to 1, followed by three that are 0, followed by three that are 1, and three more that are 0. The first six values of $Base$ for the 12 pseudo-observations are 22, and the last six are 50. Finally, the pseudo-observations' values for the variable Age are listed as 22, 28, and 35 repeated four times. In this way, the program that generates the posterior samples via MCMC for the Bayesian model also estimates the corresponding predicted risks for these 12 sets of covariates, $(\lambda_{60}, \ldots, \lambda_{71})$, using posterior samples for the model parameters to obtain predictions for the unobserved $(Y_{60}, \ldots, Y_{71})$. These posterior risks and predictions are summarized in Tables 9.2 and 9.3, respectively.

(a) Using any method of your choosing and $N(0,1)$ priors for the regression co-efficients, write code to reproduce the results in Example 9.1 for all rates, RDs, and RRs. Also obtain the posterior probabilities that the RRs are greater than 1. Compare your results with those in the example.

(b) Repeat part (a) using the specified partially informative prior discussed in the example. Compare results.

(c) Rerun your code using a flat reference prior as a default prior for the regression coefficients and assess the effect of this choice of prior compared to using $N(0,1)$ priors for the regression coefficients (i.e., compare to results from part (a)).

(d) Rerun the model from the example without the interaction effect using any of the above priors. Compare inferences with those obtained in part (a) and in the example. Comment.

EXERCISE 9.2   Revise the model from Example 9.1 to simply involve $\log(Base)$ instead of standardized $\log(Base)$, keeping everything else the same. Modify your code in Exercise 9.1 to handle this reparameterization of that model. Run the code and compare results with those in the example. Are there any convergence issues when performing this analysis? If not, compare inferences to those in the example. Except for regression coefficients, the results should be the same, namely RRs and RDs corresponding to the same specifications of predictors should be the same up to Monte Carlo error. Explain as precisely as you can why this would be the case.

EXERCISE 9.3   Refer to the Framingham Study and Example 9.2.

(a) Using your preferred programming language, write a program that you can use to specify a generic conditional means prior. Use the program to induce the corresponding prior for β in a Poisson regression model with two regression coefficients: an intercept and a coefficient for a dichotomous variable, such as a treatment indicator. Use independent gamma priors for the two means and induce the prior for $\beta = (\beta_0, \beta_1)$.

(b) Suppose your best guesses for the rate of CHD for men and women are 25 and 20, respectively, and that you are 95% certain that these rates are less than 50 and 45, respectively. Obtain specific gamma priors that reflect this information.

(c) Using this prior, obtain the induced prior for β using your code from part (a) and plot the corresponding induced priors.

(d) Now write code that can be used to analyze the Framingham Study data using this specific prior. Analyze the data and compare your results with the means for men and women and the corresponding rate ratio given in Example 9.2.

(e) Now write code to reanalyze the data using the gamma priors in part (b) directly, the way you would have in Section 5.3. Compare results from part (d). They should be identical up to Monte Carlo error.

EXERCISE 9.4   Repeat Exercise 9.3 replacing gamma priors with log-normal priors.

EXERCISE 9.5.   Consider the British Doctors Study in Example 9.3 using BUGS. The data and some code are on the book's website for Chapter 9, with a file name that includes "British". In the data, A is age, S is smoking status, and y and M give the Poisson counts and offsets, respectively.

(a) Write your own code to analyze the data using the flat prior that was specified in Example 9.3 (i.e., $\beta_i \overset{iid}{\sim} U(-10, 10)$). Run the code, and then modify and run it using an improper flat prior for β (or substantially increase the limits of the uniform prior if you are using JAGS). Compare with results in Tables 9.5 and 9.6. Comment.

(b) Now modify the code in part (a) to handle the model without β_5 and compare inferences with those obtained in part (a) for the risks and for RR and RD. Do inferences change appreciably? If they do, how?

(c) Now treat the variable A (age) as a factor with five categories, which means you will have a reference category, perhaps the middle age group, and then four variables that take values of 0 or 1 to indicate the other four age categories. There will be no opportunity for linear and quadratic terms, but you will need to include an interaction between A and S (smoking status) that will involve these four terms. Interpret the results and compare them with those from parts (a) and (b).

(d) For the three models discussed above, plot posterior median estimates of the death rate per 10,000 person years as a function of age group (i) for smokers and (ii) for non-smokers. Include the empirical rates on the same plot (i) for smokers and (ii) for non-smokers. Comment.

*EXERCISE 9.6.   Suppose you have three independent Poisson counts, (y_1, y_2, y_3) with rates $(\lambda_1, \lambda_2, \lambda_3)$ where

$$\log(\lambda_1) = \beta_1, \quad \log(\lambda_2) = \beta_1 + \beta_2, \quad \log(\lambda_3) = \beta_1 + \beta_3.$$

(a) Assume that prior information about the rates can be expressed as $\lambda_i \overset{\text{ind}}{\sim} Ga(a_i, b_i)$. Show that this prior is a data augmentation prior; in other words, using the usual transformation technique, obtain $p(\beta)$ from the known joint pdf for the rates.

(b) Now assume $\lambda_i \overset{\text{ind}}{\sim} LN(c_i, d_i)$. Obtain the joint pdf, $p(\beta)$, and argue that it is not a data augmentation prior.

(c) Write code, with comments, for obtaining the induced prior for β in parts (a) and (b) above.

(d) Now just consider one rate, say, $\lambda = e^\beta$. Let $(a - 1)/b = 5$ and $c = \log(5)$ so that both priors have mode $= 5$. Obtain b and d such that each prior has a 95th percentile of around 20. Plot the two priors for λ and compare.

(e) Now obtain the induced prior for β in each case in part (d) and compare.

EXERCISE 9.7.   Modify and run two versions of the code in Exercise 9.1 to extend the Poisson regression model to allow for overdispersion in the epilepsy data using the parameterizations in expressions (9.5) and (9.6), respectively. Check for convergence in each case and compare the Markov chain behavior for the two parameterizations. Compare inferences in Example 9.1 with those obtained here. Are they sufficiently different to raise concerns about overdispersion?

EXERCISE 9.8.   Modify and run the code in Exercise 5 (British Doctors Data) to extend the Poisson regression model to allow for overdispersion using the parameterizations in expressions (9.5) and (9.6). Check for convergence in each case and compare the Markov chain behavior for the two parameterizations. Compare inferences with those obtained in Example 9.3. Are they sufficiently different to be concerned about overdispersion?

EXERCISE 9.9.   Refer to the foot-and-mouth disease data in Example 9.5.

(a) Either run your own program or use code available on the book's website for Chapter 9 (files with "FMD" in their names) to analyze these data using the priors that were specified in the example. Then try different priors, including normal and an improper flat prior, to see what effect these other priors have on the results. Obtain inferences for the relative rate, comparing the eastern and western regions, which are of the same size.

(b) It might have seemed unusual not to think of the region's size as an offset for this problem. Now revise your model to use the actual size (which is given in the data as the variable $Size$) as an offset rather than as a covariate. Using this model, check on the assumptions as we did in Example 9.5. Compare inferences for the eastern and western regions with those obtained in the example.

EXERCISE 9.10.   Code and data for analyzing the FMD data using the zero-inflated Poisson regression model in Example 9.5 are on the book's website in files with "FMD-ZIP" in their names.

(a) Run the code from the website or write your own program to analyze the data using a zero-inflated Poisson model with the priors that were specified in the example. Then try different priors, including a normal prior and an improper flat prior, to see what effect they have on the results. Obtain inferences for the relative rate comparing the two regions (East and West) that are of the same size.
(b) Compare the probabilities of zero counts for East and West for a couple of same-size regions.
(c) Redo the analysis after revising your program to treat the variable *Size* as an offset rather than a covariate for this problem. Actual size is given in the data. Using this model, check on the assumptions as we did in the example in the text. Compare inferences for East and West.

EXERCISE 9.11.   In our analysis of the FMD data using the zero-inflated Poisson regression model, we also obtained a Bayesian version of the Pearson goodness-of-fit statistic and corresponding Pearson residuals in equation (9.8). Explain why the Pearson residuals and the Pearson goodness-of-fit measure are sensible. Give an explicit formula using mathematical notation for the PGOF for the zero-inflated model.

*EXERCISE 9.12.   Prove that the matrix in equation (9.12) is singular if $\beta = 0$ and is non-singular as long as $\beta_3 \neq 0$. *Hint*: Use the standard formula for finding the determinant of a 3×3 matrix.

*EXERCISE 9.13.   The dugong data are available in the Chapter 9 directory of the book's website. Write your own program or use code from the website to analyze the dugong data. Use the prior development in Section 9.4 and prior inputs given in Example 9.9, in conjunction with R, to obtain the approximate induced prior for the three regression coefficients. Then run the code and report results. Also obtain a plot that is similar to the one in Figure 9.5. Perform a sensitivity analysis by using at least one other prior to see how the results might change.

Chapter 10

Model Assessment

Until now, our primary inferential goals have been estimation and prediction, and we have generally assumed one model for each data set. For the most part, we have not explored the possibility that there could or would be very many alternative models for consideration. Moreover, thus far we have generally assumed that fitted models were reasonable for the data without making checks.

In this chapter we consider the topics of model selection and model checking, which are special cases of model assessment. Model selection is a big topic and has been studied by researchers over many years. See Kadane and Lazar (2004) [198] for a review from Bayesian and frequentist perspectives. We discuss how to choose among a finite number possible known models.

One approach to model selection is to obtain posterior probabilities that each model is "correct." Often, the model with the largest posterior probability is selected. In simple cases, this could be choosing among logit, probit or complementary log-log links for binomial regression data (see Chapter 8); or choosing between models with and without interaction between two selected covariates; or deciding whether or not to include a particular covariate in the model. We discuss this approach based on posterior model probabilities in Section 10.1.

Another approach, addressed in Section 10.2, involves the consideration of prediction-based criteria for model selection. Such methods are also termed "information criteria," and they involve selecting models that satisfy a form of goodness of fit that is penalized in different ways for overfitting. The criteria involve the sum of a measure of goodness of fit and a penalty. There is an obvious tradeoff between the two competing factors, namely, goodness of fit and too good a fit to the current data. For example, it is often easy to get a good fit to data in simple linear regression modeling if the model includes a large number of polynomial terms in the covariates. More generally, model fit is always improved by fitting additional covariates, so adding more covariates will appear to fit the data better in terms of goodness of fit. Unfortunately, such models will rarely be useful for making predictions about future observations. Moreover, estimates of parameters will be biased. Adding a penalty for overfitting improves this situation considerably.

We also discuss hypothesis testing in this chapter, which is a special case of model selection. Bayesian hypothesis testing involves a formal decision-making process to choose between two (or more) hypotheses. The process begins with a model for each hypothesis, priors on the model parameters, and prior probabilities of hypotheses being considered. This is followed by the calculation of posterior probabilities of hypotheses given the data. At the simplest level, the model or hypothesis with the highest posterior probability might be selected. At a more general level not considered here, one would specify a loss function, and the Bayes decision would correspond to minimizing the posterior expected loss.

Once we have selected a model (or models) by one or more criteria, we need to assess whether it (they) is (are) reasonable. Goodness-of-fit criteria play a major role in this endeavor, with the understanding that models that are overfit may be problematic. On the other hand, if the "best" model according to a particular criterion does not fit the data well, additional modeling is usually necessary. We also give an introductory discussion of model diagnostics (model checking), a rather large topic, in Section 10.3.

A considerable amount of model selection involves variable selection in regression. For example, if a regression model has age and body mass index in it, it may be the case that the simpler model with just age in it would suffice. So the corresponding two models can be compared according to the above criteria for selection and for model fit.

Finally, we note that a major aspect of model selection involves the consideration of science in the process. Medical researchers will often be concerned with the attendant biology involved in a statistical analysis to the extent that they require that certain variables be included in a model, no matter what the statistical criteria appear to dictate. This aspect of model selection cannot be ignored.

10.1   Model Selection Based on Posterior Probabilities and Bayes Factors

With a fixed number of models, and when proper priors are used, the most straightforward Bayesian approach simply selects the model associated with the largest posterior probability. We will see that the Bayes factor (BF), which is a ratio of two marginal densities for the data under different models, plays an integral role in the expression for these posterior probabilities. In fact, Bayes factors are often used by themselves for model selection. They are, however, often difficult to compute, can be quite sensitive to prior specification, and are undefined when improper priors are used. Nonetheless, in this section we will define, discuss, and use Bayes factors, pointing out as needed how care must be taken in their use.

10.1.1   Choice between Two Models

Suppose we have two competing models for data, y. Model M_0 has a sampling density $p_0(y \mid \theta_0)$, and the competing model is M_1 with sampling density $p_1(y \mid \theta_1)$. For clarity, we will often also use the somewhat redundant notation $p_j(y \mid \theta_j) = p_j(y \mid \theta_j, M_j)$ to make clear that the subscript refers to model M_j. We wish to distinguish the functional form of the sampling density under model M_j, namely, $p_j(\cdot \mid \theta_j)$, from the fact that we are assuming model M_j. For example, one model might be a log-normal sampling distribution for the data ($M_0 : y \sim LN(\mu, \sigma^2)$), and the alternative model might be a Weibull distribution for the data ($M_1 : y \sim Weib(\alpha, \lambda)$). Then $p_0(\cdot \mid \theta_0)$ is the log-normal density, $p_1(\cdot \mid \theta_1)$ is the Weibull density, and we can write $y \mid M_j \sim p_j(y \mid \theta_j, M_j)$, $j = 0, 1$.

The parameters for the models and the model-specific distributional families may be quite distinct as indicated above. Alternatively, for two models relating to distributions that are in the same family, the parameters in θ_0 could be a subset of the parameters in θ_1, in which case we would say that the model M_0 is nested in model M_1.

We place prior distributions on θ_0 and θ_1, namely, $p_0(\theta_0)$ and $p_1(\theta_1)$, and we have prior probabilities on the two models, $q_0 = P(M_0)$ and $q_1 = 1 - q_0 = P(M_1)$, respectively. Consider deciding between the models M_0 and M_1. We wish to evaluate the posterior probabilities of each model, that is, $P(M_1 \mid y) = 1 - P(M_0 \mid y)$. When applying Bayes' theorem to obtain these probabilities, we will require the marginal predictive densities for the observed data:

$$p_j(y \mid M_j) \equiv \int p_j(y \mid \theta_j) p_j(\theta_j) d\theta_j, \quad j = 0, 1. \tag{10.1}$$

We regard the marginal density in equation (10.1) as the (marginal) "plausibility" of the observed data under model M_j. It also has been termed the (marginal) "likelihood" of the model, M_j, given the observed data. With a flat prior for θ_j, the marginal density $p_j(y)$ is not guaranteed to exist, and often does not, leaving us with no way forward. Consequently, we always assume that priors are proper when obtaining posterior probabilities of different models. We note that while we are using traditional terminology, the marginal predictive density has more recently been called the "prior predictive density"

Applying Bayes' theorem,

$$P(M_1 \mid y) = \frac{q_1 p_1(y)}{q_0 p_0(y) + q_1 p_1(y)}. \tag{10.2}$$

Without any further input, we would tend to choose model M_1 if $P(M_1 \mid y) \geq 0.5$, and model M_0 otherwise. Of course, if we were very concerned about making a mistake of, say, selecting M_1 when in fact the model M_0 is the true model, we might want to make it more difficult to select M_1 by increasing the threshold for model selection from 0.5 to a larger value, perhaps 0.95. In this instance we would be at least 95% certain that M_1 was the true model and we would have $Pr(M_0 \mid y) < 0.05$. A straightforward procedure would select M_1 if $P(M_1 \mid y) \geq k$ for some $k > 0.5$.[1] Making a decision in this way is equivalent to selecting M_1 if the posterior odds satisfy the criterion $P(M_1 \mid y)/\{1 - P(M_1 \mid y)\} > k/(1 - k)$.

As in equation (10.2), Bayes' theorem also leads to

$$P(M_0 \mid y) = \frac{q_0 p_0(y)}{q_0 p_0(y) + q_1 p_1(y)}.$$

---

[1]This kind of thinking can be formalized with a decision-theoretic criterion.

Now we can write posterior odds for M_1 as

$$\underbrace{\frac{P(M_1 \mid y)}{P(M_0 \mid y)}}_{\text{Posterior odds}} = \frac{q_1 p_1(y)/\{q_0 p_0(y) + q_1 p_1(y)\}}{q_0 p_0(y)/\{q_0 p_0(y) + q_1 p_1(y)\}}$$

$$= \frac{q_1 p_1(y)}{q_0 p_0(y)}$$

$$= \underbrace{\frac{P(M_1)}{P(M_0)}}_{\text{Prior odds}} \times \underbrace{\frac{p_1(y \mid M_1)}{p_0(y \mid M_0)}}_{\text{Bayes factor}}. \qquad (10.3)$$

Thus, the BF is the factor by which the prior odds can be multiplied to update to the posterior odds, and this factor is free of q_0 and q_1. Rewriting this, we see that the BF is the odds ratio of posterior to prior odds for M_1 versus M_0. To be specific, we denote this by BF_{10}:

$$BF_{10} = \frac{P(M_1 \mid y)}{P(M_0 \mid y)} \bigg/ \frac{P(M_1)}{P(M_0)}.$$

Similarly, BF_{01} stands for the ratio of posterior to prior odds for M_0 versus M_1 and equals the reciprocal of BF_{10}. Revisiting equation (10.3), from the final expression in it, the BF can also be seen as the ratio of marginal densities of the data under M_1 and M_0, namely, the data densities after integrating out the model-specific parameters with respect to their respective priors: $p_j(y \mid M_j) = \int_{\theta_j} p_j(y \mid \theta_j, M_j) p_j(\theta_j \mid M_j) d\theta_1$, $j = 0, 1$.

Back to choosing a model. If the prior odds are $0.5/0.5 = 1$, and $k = 0.5$, then we would select model M_1 if $BF > 1$. With a different threshold, say with $k = 0.95$, we would select model M_1 if $BF > 0.95/0.05 = 19$, which is considerably more stringent. Now, we would select M_1 if the plausibility of the observed data under M_1 were at least 19 times greater than the plausibility under M_0. Another way to say this is: we would select M_1 if the post-data odds for M_1 versus M_0 were at least 19 times greater than the pre-data odds for it.

Sir Harold Jeffreys was a proponent of the BF and suggested some levels of evidence to aid interpretation of BFs when comparing models. He proposed the admittedly arbitrary grades displayed in Table 10.1 in terms of hypothesis tests. As before, we consider model M_1 to be in the numerator and model M_0 to be in the denominator of the BF. Here is an example of calculation and use of Bayes factor.

Example 10.1. Recall the VetBP data set (in Sections 2.3 and 2.4, for example) regarding blood pressure in veterans; θ is the probability that a random veteran has uncontrolled hypertension. Consider testing $H_0 : \theta \leq 0.5$ versus $H_1 : \theta > 0.5$. Thus set $\Omega_0 = (0.0.5]$ and $\Omega_1 = (0.5, 1)$. The data are binomial with $n = 404$, and the number of veterans with uncontrolled hypertension is 184. With a $U(0, 1)$ prior on θ, $q_0 = q_1 = 0.5$, and $\theta \mid \theta \in \Omega_0 \sim U(0, 0.5)$ and $\theta \mid \theta \in \Omega_1 \sim U(0.5, 1)$. Using

TABLE 10.1: Jeffreys' levels of evidence

$BF_{10}(\mathbf{y}) < 1$	Model M_0 supported
$1 < BF_{10}(\mathbf{y}) < 10^{1/2}$	Evidence against M_0,
	but not worth more than a bare mention
$10^{1/2} < BF_{10}(\mathbf{y}) < 10^1$	Evidence against M_0 *substantial*
$10^1 < BF_{10}(\mathbf{y}) < 10^2$	Evidence against M_0 *strong*
$10^2 < BF_{10}(\mathbf{y})$	Evidence against M_0 *decisive*

(10.1) and R to carry out the computations:

$$
\begin{aligned}
BF_{10} &= \frac{\int_{0.5}^1 Lik(\theta)p_1(\theta)d\theta}{\int_0^{0.5} Lik(\theta)p_0(\theta)d\theta} \\
&= \frac{\int_{0.5}^1 \theta^{1+184-1}(1-\theta)^{1+404-184-1}/q_1 d\theta}{\int_0^{0.5} \theta^{1+184-1}(1-\theta)^{1+404-184-1}/q_0 d\theta} \\
&= \texttt{(1 - pbeta(0.5,185,221))/pbeta(0.5,185,221)} = 0.038,
\end{aligned}
$$

where `pbeta(0.5,185,221) = 0.963` using the R function that gives the area to the left of 0.5 for a $Be(185, 221)$ distribution. As $BF_{10} = 0.038$, the plausibility of the data under M_0 is about 26 (1/0.038) times what it is under M_1. Moreover, since $q_0 = q_1 = 0.5$ means that the prior odds for M_1 are taken to be 1, $P(M_0 \mid y) = 26/(1 + 26) \doteq 0.963$. We would thus likely accept the hypothesis that the proportion of veterans with uncontrolled hypertension is less than 0.5.

Although this example was designed to illustrate explicit calculation of the BF, we note that for most model selection problems it is necessary to use Monte Carlo computational methods to obtain posterior probabilities and/or BFs, a topic considered in Section 10.1.4.

10.1.2 Cautions Regarding Bayes Factors

Bayes factors can be misleading under certain circumstances. In one such case, the situation of testing a point null $H_0 : \theta = 0$ against the alternative hypothesis $H_1 : \theta \neq 0$, it turns out that BF_{10} can depend heavily on the choice of prior, especially when very diffuse priors are used. Of course, an often stated goal of specifying diffuse priors is to minimize the effect of the prior on the posterior. But with BFs, overly diffuse priors can have a huge impact on inferences. This issue has been discussed in the literature extensively for some time (e.g., in [17, 28, 224]).

Diffuse Priors and Bayes Factors. With improper priors, the BF is not a defined finite number, as the marginal densities in its defining ratio are not themselves defined due to the prior not integrating to a finite quantity. It follows that we should not use overly diffuse proper priors either. For example, suppose $Y \sim N(\theta, 1)$, and we want to decide between $H_0 : Y \sim N(\theta, 1)$, $\theta = 0$ and $H_1 : Y \sim N(\theta, 1)$, $\theta \sim$

$N(\mu_0, \sigma_0^2)$. We specify the prior probabilities $P(H_0) = 0.5 = P(H_1)$. It is easy to show that the marginal predictive distribution for $Y \mid H_1$ is $N(\mu_0, 1 + \sigma_0^2)$. Thus

$$BF_{10} = \frac{\frac{1}{\sqrt{1+\sigma_0^2}} e^{-0.5[(y-\mu_0)^2/(1+\sigma_0^2)]}}{e^{-0.5y^2}}.$$

Let us suppose the expert's best guess for θ under the alternative is $\mu_0 = 1$, but that they are incredibly unsure about this guess, so they select $\sigma_0 = 10^7$. Imagine that $y = 5$ is observed. The classical two-sided p-value for testing H_0 is $2(1 - \Phi(5)) \doteq 5.7/10^7$, so virtually any non-Bayesian would be rejecting the null. However, $BF_{10} = 0.027$ and consequently $P(H_0 \mid y = 5) = 0.974$ as the prior probability of H_0 is taken as 0.5. This illustrates the so-called Lindley paradox [224] where a Bayesian, albeit with what we would term a silly prior for any realistic situation, would emphatically accept the null hypothesis while the classical analysis would suggest its strong rejection. The dominant point here is that the result very much depends on the prior specification. If we were to plot the prior for μ, it would be difficult to distinguish it from a constant but improper prior.

Now suppose that our expert was quite unsure about the actual value of θ. When pressed, they gave a best guess of 1.0. After some thought and subject-matter input, they said that θ is between -4 and 6, but they would not attach a probability to the statement that θ is in this interval. With more reflection, they were willing to assert that they were virtually certain that θ is in the substantially wider interval, $(-9.3, 11.3)$. Furthermore, they were ultimately comfortable with the assertion $P(-9.3 < \theta < 11.3) = 0.99$. Assuming that a normal distribution corresponds to their certainty about the value of θ, $\theta \sim N(1, 16)$ matches their belief as expressed by the probability statement. With this prior, $BF_{10} \doteq 40{,}000$ and $P(H_1 \mid y = 5) = 0.9999754$. Repeating the calculation with $\mu_0 = 0$ in place of 1.0 gives virtually the same result. In the previous paragraph, we found that $BF_{10} = 0.027$ with a diffuse prior. So the BF is heavily influenced by the choice of prior. It is essential that careful effort be made to specify a scientifically meaningful prior and not resort to diffuse priors when using BFs.

Testing Hypotheses about Parameters. Consider, in general, a sampling density $p(y \mid \theta)$ and a continuous prior density $p(\theta)$ defined on a parameter set Ω. Testing the null hypothesis $H_0 : \theta \in \Omega_0$ versus the alternative $H_1 : \theta \in \Omega_1$, where Ω_1 is the complement of Ω_0 relative to Ω, covers a large majority of hypothesis testing situations. As before, we treat hypotheses (H_j) and corresponding models (M_j) interchangeably. Assuming $q_j \equiv P(\theta \in \Omega_j) = \int_{\Omega_j} p(\theta) d\theta$ are strictly positive for $j = 0, 1$, the prior under H_j is then

$$p_j(\theta) \equiv p(\theta \mid \theta \in \Omega_j) = p(\theta)/q_j, \quad \theta \in \Omega_j, \; j = 0, 1.$$

A typical instance of this general scenario involves a scalar parameter, θ, with model M_0 corresponding to the hypothesis $H_0 : \theta \leq c_0$, and model M_1 corresponding to the alternative hypothesis, $H_1 : \theta > c_0$. Another instance with two scalar parameters,

θ_1, θ_2, is $H_0 : \theta_1 \leq \theta_2$ versus $H_1 : \theta_1 > \theta_2$. Both of these fit the above framework as long as q_0 and q_1 are both positive.

On the other hand, in the case of a point null hypothesis, like $H_0 : \theta = c_0$, or $\theta_1 = \theta_2$, the above description requires modification as $q_0 = 0$. We must, then, specify a prior probability $q_0 \in (0, 1)$ that reflects our belief that the null hypothesis is true. If H_0 is a simple hypothesis, so that Ω_0 contains a single point, then it completely specifies the sampling distribution for the data. In this case, we can specify the prior under the alternative H_1 as $p_1(\theta) = p(\theta)$ for all $\theta \in \Omega$. This works since $\int_{\Omega_0} p(\theta) d\theta = 0$. If, however, H_0 is not a simple hypothesis, such as $\theta_1 = \theta_2$, further modifications are required. We will not consider such hypotheses in this book but instead recommend the excellent treatment by Berger and co-authors [29, 31, 32, 92] to interested readers.

10.1.3 Choosing among Multiple Models

Let $p_j(y \mid \theta_j)$ and $p_j(\theta_j)$ be the probability density functions for the data and the prior under model M_j, respectively, and let $q_j = P(M_j)$, for $j = 0, 1, \ldots, r$. Define the marginal predictive densities for all $r + 1$ models for the data as in equation (10.1). Then

$$P(M_j \mid y) = \frac{q_j p_j(y)}{\sum_{k=0}^{r} q_k p_k(y)}. \tag{10.4}$$

As before, a straightforward procedure would be to select the model with the largest posterior probability.

If $q_j = 1/(r + 1)$ for all j, we could simply pick the model with the greatest marginal likelihood or plausibility, $p_j(y \mid M_j)$. It is common in this instance to obtain Bayes factors against M_0, namely, $BF_{j0} = p_j(y)/p_0(y)$ for $j = 1, \ldots, r$. We would then select the model, say M_l, that achieves $\max_{j=1,\ldots,r} BF_{j0} = BF_{l0}$, provided $BF_{l0} > 1$, and model M_0 if this is not the case.

10.1.4 Computing Bayes Factors via Sampling

Recall that the Bayes factor, $BF_{i0} = p_i(y)/p_0(y)$, is the ratio of the two marginal predictive densities for the data under models M_i and M_0, respectively. We illustrate with $i = 0, 1$ for simplicity, and we use θ_0 and θ_1 to denote parameters from the two models, even if the two families are distinct, such as gamma and Weibull.

Bayes factors can be difficult to compute analytically but can, in principle, be numerically approximated. Specifically, we sample $\theta_i^{(k)}$, $k = 1, \ldots, m$. from the prior density $p_i(\theta_i)$ and use the approximation

$$p_i(y) \doteq \frac{1}{m} \sum_{k=1}^{m} p_i(y \mid \theta_i^{(k)}). \tag{10.5}$$

Since BFs are actually only evaluated for the data that are observed, the computation is manageable. Also recall that if the priors were improper, the above discussion could be meaningless. Moreover, if the priors are overly diffuse, convergence of the above average to the marginal could be difficult to achieve in practice.

If θ_0 and θ_i *have the same dimension* and a common parameter space, say Ω, a more efficient computational scheme is available by applying Bayes' rule after substituting θ_0 for θ_1 in $p_1(\cdot)$, etc. Write

$$
\begin{aligned}
BF_{10} &= \frac{\int_\Omega p_1(y \mid \theta_1)p_1(\theta_1)d\theta_1}{\int_\Omega p_0(y \mid \theta_0)p_0(\theta_0)d\theta_0} \\
&= \frac{\int_\Omega \frac{p_1(y|\theta_0)p_1(\theta_0)}{p_0(y|\theta_0)p_0(\theta_0)}p_0(y \mid \theta_0)p_0(\theta_0)d\theta_0}{p_0(y)} \\
&= \int_\Omega \frac{p_1(y \mid \theta_0)p_1(\theta_0)}{p_0(y \mid \theta_0)p_0(\theta_0)}p_0(\theta_0 \mid y)d\theta_0 \\
&\equiv \int_\Omega w(\theta_0)p_0(\theta_0 \mid y)d\theta_0.
\end{aligned}
$$

The third line follows from the second line by applying Bayes' theorem: $p_0(\theta_0 \mid y) = p_0(y \mid \theta_0)p_0(\theta_0)/p_0(y)$. The requirement to have the same parameter space is needed at the third and fourth equalities for the integrals to be meaningful. Sampling $\theta_0^{(k)}$, $k = 1, \ldots, m$, from the posterior density $p_0(\theta_0 \mid y)$, we obtain the approximation

$$
BF_{10} \doteq \frac{1}{m} \sum_{k=1}^m \frac{p_1(y \mid \theta_0^{(k)})p_1(\theta_0^{(k)})}{p_0(y \mid \theta_0^{(k)})p_0(\theta_0^{(k)})} \equiv \frac{1}{m} \sum_{k=1}^m w(\theta_0^{(k)}).
$$

Thus, we can obtain the BF by post-processing the posterior output (samples from $p_0(\theta_0 \mid y)$) from the analysis of M_0 and calculating a simple arithmetic average. This is easily done in R. If more convenient for sampling, the roles of M_0 and M_1 can be reversed so posterior samples from M_1 could be post-processed instead. Of course, in this case the definition of $w(\cdot)$ must be modified accordingly.

For good numerical results, the function $w(\cdot)$ must be stable, as was the case in importance sampling (Chapter 4). A successful implementation may require a sensible reparameterization of one or both models. Typically, comparison of regression models of equal dimensions diminish the need for this. An example is link selection in binary regression. For the case of the trauma data discussed in Chapter 8, consider these link functions: logistic (M_1), probit (M_2), and complementary log-log (M_3), as in Section 8.6. Bayes factors can be used to indicate which of the three is most appropriate.

A particularly useful prior specification here is the conditional means priors (CMPs). In prior elicitation, the CMP allows us to focus on interpretable probabilities, keeping away from regression coefficients, which have varying meaning depending on the link function. Moreover, the posterior simulation monitoring can also remain focused on these probabilities, as they can be treated as link-invariant parameters. To implement CMPs in model selection, recall that we begin with a selection of covariate vectors $\tilde{x}_i$ that are convenient for eliciting $\tilde{\theta}_i = P(Y_i \mid \tilde{x}_i, \beta)$. Note that these θ_i equal $\text{expit}(\tilde{x}_i\beta)$ for logistic, $\Phi(\tilde{x}_i\beta)$ for probit, and $\exp\{e^{-(\tilde{x}_i\beta)}\}$ for the complementary log-log. Inverses of these functions define βs in each model.

This single specification of priors for the $\tilde{\theta}$s can be used to induce appropriate but distinct priors on regression coefficients for the three link functions. With a little effort this CMP approach can be extended to many other model selection applications.

Example 10.2. Bayes Factors for the LE Data. We want to compare link functions for modeling the risk of lymphedema (LE). We are considering link functions corresponding to models M_1, M_2, and M_3 given above. The code in `LymphedemaBF.txt` under Chapter 10 on the book's website illustrates how one can calculate the BF to compare model M_3 (complementary log-log link) to M_1 (logistic link). We have used the method described above for computing the BF.

Suppose we have elicited a prior for the risk of LE for the women grouped by high and low node counts, as in Example 8.6. Let $\tilde{\theta}_1$ be the elicited prior risk for the high node count group, with corresponding prior uncertainty characterized by a beta distribution, $\tilde{\theta}_1 \sim Be(a_1, b_1)$. Similarly, $\tilde{\theta}_2$ is the elicited risk for the group of women in the low node count group, with $\tilde{\theta}_2 \sim Be(a_2, b_2)$. The elicited prior on the risk scale induces a prior for the regression coefficients in the logistic model, because of the relationship between the logits and the coefficients. In particular,

$$\begin{bmatrix} 1 & 1 \\ 0 & 1 \end{bmatrix} \begin{pmatrix} \beta_1 \\ \beta_2 \end{pmatrix} = \begin{pmatrix} \mathrm{logit}(\tilde{\theta}_1) \\ \mathrm{logit}(\tilde{\theta}_2) \end{pmatrix} \Longleftrightarrow \begin{pmatrix} \beta_1 \\ \beta_2 \end{pmatrix} = \begin{bmatrix} 0 & 1 \\ 1 & -1 \end{bmatrix} \begin{pmatrix} \mathrm{logit}(\tilde{\theta}_1) \\ \mathrm{logit}(\tilde{\theta}_2) \end{pmatrix}.$$

We then use the above to determine the prior for the regression coefficients. In the BUGS code, we have set $a_1 = a_2 = 2.044$ and $b_1 = b_2 = 13.006$. The matrix $(X')^{-1}$ in the code is the matrix that, on the right-hand side of the equation, premultiplies the vector $[\mathrm{logit}(\tilde{\theta}_1), \mathrm{logit}(\tilde{\theta}_2)]'$. We can use a similar equation for the probit and complementary log-log links by replacing $\mathrm{logit}(\cdot)$ by the appropriate cdf in each case ($\Phi(\cdot)$ and $\log(-\log(\cdot))$, respectively). As a result of running the code, we obtained $BF = 1.004$. From the statistical perspective, there is no difference between the two models. We prefer the logistic for better interpretability of its regression coefficients.

Change of variables from $\tilde{\theta}$ to β gives the induced prior for β. For example, under the complementary log-log transformation we get

$$p(\beta) \propto \prod_{i=1}^{2} \{1 - \exp(-e^{\tilde{x}_i \beta})\}^{a_i - 1} \{\exp(-e^{\tilde{x}_i \beta})\}^{b_i} e^{\tilde{x}_i \beta}.$$

However, this expression is not needed in the BUGS code, as priors can be specified via transformations in BUGS.

Example 10.3. Trauma Data. For the trauma data, we computed the BFs under our informative priors for the same three link functions we discussed above. The results, using code similar to that for Example 10.2, were $BF_{21} = 1.05$, $BF_{13} = 20.7$, and thus

$$BF_{23} = BF_{21}/BF_{31} = BF_{21}BF_{13} = 1.05 \times 20.7 = 21.7.$$

There is a suggestion against the complementary log-log model (M_3), but there is little to choose between the logistic and probit models. Since logistic models are easier to interpret, we prefer the logistic.

10.2 Model Selection Based on Predictive Information Criteria

In this section we discuss methods of model selection that are based on how well a model might predict future observations. We are in agreement with Seymour Geisser [127] that statistical inferences should ultimately focus on observable quantities rather than on unobservable parameters that often do not exist and have been incorporated largely for convenience. He argued that the success of a statistical model should be measured by the quality of the predictions made from it (see Geisser [123, 127] and Christensen and Johnson [78]). In this section we discuss model selection based on such criteria.

There is a range of predictive model selection criteria that can be regarded as approximations to a particular theoretical criterion. These include the Bayesian information criterion (BIC), the Akaike information criterion (AIC), the log pseudo-marginal likelihood (LPML) criterion, the widely applicable information criterion (WAIC), and the deviance information criterion (DIC). We discuss their common motivation and then present the different criteria themselves.

Consider one or more initial parametric models for the data at hand. Of course, the "true" model for the data may or may not be any of these. But the hope and expectation is that there will be one that somehow reasonably reflects the truth. It is possible that more than one, or that none, would. To quote Box [44], "All models are wrong, but some are useful." A simple definition of useful might be "good enough." In what follows we will assume a finite collection of models from which we want to select one. Individual models in the collection could possibly be different parametric families for the sampling distribution of the data.

We begin with $p(y)$ as the probability density function for the "true" probability mechanism that generates the observed data $y = (y_1, \ldots, y_n)$, which could be a member of the collection of models under consideration. Let $\tilde{y} = (\tilde{y}_1, \ldots, \tilde{y}_n)$ be a future data set of the same size, n, that we assume to be generated by this same mechanism. Modeled and "true" distributions for y_i and $\tilde{y}_i$ may depend on a covariate vector x_i. Now consider predicting the new data set, $\tilde{y}$, that is just like the current data y. For example, we may have a standard linear model for the data, $y_i = x_i\beta + \varepsilon_i$, and wish to predict $\tilde{y}_i = x_i\beta + \varepsilon_i^*$, with ε_i and ε_i^* all distributed as independent $N(0, \sigma^2)$ random variables. For simplicity, we use notation that hides the fact that the current data and future data may not be identically distributed, which occurs in regression and other modeling situations. We assume that the y_i are independent, conditional on parameter values for any specified model. From here on, we assume the collection of models under consideration is finite, say $\{M_j : j = 0, 1, \ldots, J\}$. For simplicity of notation, we often refer to model M_j using the subscript j.

One measure of the magnitude of the difference between two distributions is the Kullback–Leibler divergence (KLD). It provides a measure of how different one distribution is from another. For two densities, $p(z)$ and $q(z)$, supported on a common sample space, KLD is the expected logarithm of the ratio $p(z)/q(z)$, with expectation taken under $p(z)$:

$$\text{KLD}(p, q) = \int \log\left(\frac{p(x)}{q(x)}\right) p(x)dx = -\int \log\left(\frac{q(x)}{p(x)}\right) p(x)dx.$$

The KLD is always non-negative, and is strictly positive unless the two density functions are virtually identical. If the two densities are widely discrepant, the value will be large. The KLD, however, is not a distance metric, since it is not symmetric in its arguments and it does not satisfy the triangle inequality.

Recall that the predictive density based on a candidate model, M_j, is $p_j(\tilde{y} \mid y) = \int p_j(\tilde{y} \mid \theta_j)p(\theta_j \mid y)d\theta_j$. If we knew the "true" density $p(\cdot)$, we could use the KLD to assess the discrepancy between the "true" predictive density and one under each candidate model, that is, between $p(\tilde{y})$ and $p_j(\tilde{y} \mid y)$ for all j. We would then select the model, j^*, that has the "closest" predictive density to that from the true model in the Kullback–Leibler sense, that is, the one that has the smallest KLD across models $j = 0, 1, \ldots, J$. Of course, we do not know the true model. Nonetheless, let us define an idealized criterion based on KLD called the Kullback–Leibler criterion (KLC), namely,

$$KLC_j = KLD(p(\cdot), p_j(\cdot \mid y)) = \int p(\tilde{y}) \log\left\{\frac{p(\tilde{y})}{p_i(\tilde{y} \mid y)}\right\} d\tilde{y}. \tag{10.6}$$

Again, since the true model is unknown, it is not possible to calculate KLC_j, much less minimize it to find model j^*. The conceptual goal now is to find a surrogate for the KLC that does not depend on unknown $p(\cdot)$ and that can be used to find the model that is "closest" to the true model in the collection under consideration. We proceed by replacing the KLC with what amounts to an estimate of it and then minimizing that approximating criterion.

Since KLC_j can be written as $\int p(\tilde{y}) \log[p(\tilde{y})]d\tilde{y} - \int p(\tilde{y}) \log[p_i(\tilde{y} \mid y)]d\tilde{y}$, and since the first integral is free of the model specification, it is sufficient to maximize the second term instead of minimizing the KLD. The second term is called the negative cross entropy (NCE):

$$NCE_j = \int p(\tilde{y}) \log[p_j(\tilde{y} \mid y)]d\tilde{y} = E_p\{\log[p_j(\tilde{y} \mid y)]\}.$$

The next step considers a simplified version of this quantity that Gelman et al. [135] term the expected log pointwise predictive density (ELPPD), defined as

$$ELPPD_j = \sum_{i=1}^{n} E_p\{\log[p_j(\tilde{y}_i \mid y)]\}. \tag{10.7}$$

If $p_j(\tilde{y} \mid y) = \prod_i p_j(\tilde{y}_i \mid y)$, then $NCE_j = ELPPD_j$. The $\tilde{y}$s are generally dependent, however, often without and always with conditioning on the data y at hand. The simplification is thus made on purely practical grounds. According to this criterion, we are looking for the model that does the best job of predicting new responses that are modeled to be stochastically like the actual data responses when the new responses are generated by the "true" model. Unfortunately, the problem of not knowing the true model persists as the expectation is with respect to the unknown true model $p(\cdot)$.

To overcome this obstacle, noting the data $y = (y_1, \ldots, y_n)$ are actually drawn from the "true" model, Gelman et al. [135] suggested an alternative to equation (10.7) by defining the *log pointwise predictive density* (LPPD),

$$LPPD_j = \sum_{i=1}^{n} \log[p_j(y_i \mid y)], \tag{10.8}$$

as a computable criterion. It is the sum of the logarithms of the predictive densities for the observed y_i, which can be regarded as an approximation to equation (10.7). It is also an approximation to the log of the M-criterion defined in Laud and Ibrahim [217], again based on ignoring the dependence in the components of $\tilde{y} \mid y$.

If $p_j(y_i \mid y) > p_l(y_i \mid y)$ for all models $l \neq j$ and all observations i, then we prefer M_j to all other models. We would therefore want to select models with large $LPPD_j$. One possible problem with this criterion is that observation $\tilde{y}_i$ is being predicted using all of the data, y, including the corresponding y_i. In regression (and other non-exchangeable) models, using a fit of the model that includes the observation whose future counterpart is being predicted could lead to overly optimistic predictions. It is best to avoid this possibility, as will be the case with the next criterion, after which we also introduce other "information" criteria.

10.2.1 Log Pseudo Marginal Likelihood

A natural way to adjust overly optimistic predictions is to substitute $p_j(y_i \mid y_{(i)})$ for $p_j(y_i \mid y)$ in equation (10.8), where $y_{(i)}$ denotes the data with y_i removed. The method of predicting an observation based on the reduced data set that does not include it is called "leave-one-out cross-validation." The corresponding model selection criterion is termed the log pseudo-marginal likelihood,

$$LPML_j = \sum_{i=1}^{n} \log[p_j(y_i \mid y_{(i)})], \tag{10.9}$$

which was proposed by Geisser and Eddy [128]. The LPML criterion (10.9) has seen increased popularity, in part, because of the relative ease with which it can be computed from MCMC output. It is also intuitive, involving prediction of observed data based on a criterion that leaves out the observations (one at a time) that are being predicted.

For a model, M_j, the term $p_j(y_i \mid y_{(i)})$ is also called the "conditional predictive ordinate" (CPO_i) [124], which also has other uses (see Section 10.3). Gelfand and Dey [129] showed that CPO_i and thus the LPML are easily approximated. They first showed that for model M_j (if the ys are conditionally independent given θ),

$$CPO_i^{-1} = \int \left\{ \frac{1}{p_j(y_i \mid \theta)} \right\} p_j(\theta \mid y) d\theta. \tag{10.10}$$

Then, using a posterior sample $(\theta^{(1)}, \ldots, \theta^{(s)})$, where $\theta^{(l)} \sim p_j(\theta \mid y)$, we have the following Monte Carlo approximation:

$$CPO_i^{-1} \doteq \frac{1}{s} \sum_{l=1}^{s} \frac{1}{p_j(y_i \mid \theta^{(l)})} \, . \tag{10.11}$$

Since

$$LPML_j = \log \prod_{i=1}^{n} p_j(y_i \mid y_{(i)}) = \log \prod_{i=1}^{n} CPO_i,$$

it is easily approximated using equation (10.11).

Geisser and Eddy [128] also discussed the calculation of a pseudo-Bayes factor (PBF) for comparing two models, say M_1 and M_0, namely

$$PBF_{10} = e^{LPML_1 - LPML_0} \, . \tag{10.12}$$

While the PBF does not enjoy the simple interpretation of a Bayes factor as the ratio of posterior to prior odds (as explained in Section 10.1), it approximates the BF in large samples. At the very least it provides a predictive quantification of how well one model fits the data compared to another.

Construction of CPO Statistics. CPO and LPML statistics can be computed using BUGS, JAGS or other Bayesian software in conjunction with R if needed. For a given linear regression model j, the values of CPO_{ij}^{-1} can be computed directly in BUGS by defining nodes for $p_j(y_i|\beta, \tau)^{-1}$. In BUGS, for example, one could include the statements

```
for(i in 1:n){CPOinv[i]<-
    sqrt(2*3.14159/tau)*exp(0.5*tau*pow(y[i]-mu[i],2))}
```

in the model code, where the response is y_i. BUGS will output the posterior mean of each `CPOinv[i]`, which gives a numerical approximation to $(CPO)_{ij}^{-1} = E_{\beta,\tau|y}[p_j(y_i|\beta, \tau)^{-1}]$, for $i = 1, \ldots, n$.

The arithmetic needed to obtain $LPML_j$ can be done in R by taking the sum of the logs of the approximate CPO_{ij} values. Running BUGS from R from the outset makes this process simple. The R commands are:

```
CPO <- 1/y.fit$mean$CPOinv # CPO is a vector of length n
LPML <- sum(log(CPO))
```

For non-normal models, $p_j(y_i|\beta, \tau)^{-1}$ should be replaced by appropriate code for the corresponding predictive density $p_j(y_i|\theta)^{-1}$.

10.2.2 Akaike Information Criterion

The Akaike information criterion [4] is a frequentist criterion that is widely used and has been broadly studied for its properties. From a predictive point of view, one can begin with the frequentist analog of $LPPD_i$ by substituting the plug-in density estimate, $p_j(y_i \mid \hat{\theta}_j)$, for $p_j(y_i \mid y)$ in equation (10.8), where $\hat{\theta}_j$ is the maximum likelihood estimate (MLE) of θ under model M_j. This frequentist "predictive" criterion, $\sum_j \log\{p_i(y_j \mid \hat{\theta}_i)\}$, also results in overly optimistic predictions of the y_i, as in the Bayesian case. A "corrective" adjustment would subtract a penalty for this over-optimism. This penalty is k_j, the number of parameters in model M_j. This adjustment leads to what we call a predictive version of the AIC:

$$\sum_i \log[p_j(y_i \mid \hat{\theta}_j)] - k_j.$$

In the literature, this predictive version is modified by multiplying it by -2. This results in

$$AIC_j = -2\sum_i \log[p_j(y_i \mid \hat{\theta}_j)] + 2k_j = -2\log\{Lik(\hat{\theta}_i)\} + 2k_j,$$

which is minus twice the log of the maximized likelihood under model M_j plus twice the number of model parameters. Instead of making this term as large as possible, we use the original criterion, which is $-2 \times AIC_i$ by convention, and find the model that makes this term as small as possible, to be consistent with the overall approach.

The goal with this criterion is to make it as small as possible, subject to not overfitting. Here adding twice the number of model parameters makes the criterion larger, and increasingly penalizes models that include a larger number of parameters. The term "overfitting" arises since, with a fixed sample size n, letting k_j grow due to expanding models results in decreasing the first term (the goodness-of-fit measure). Too many parameters in a model will fit the current data better but decrease actual predictive ability in future samples. Too few parameters will result in poor goodness of fit. The AIC attempts to strike a balance between these two characteristics of a model fit to a data set.

10.2.3   Bayesian Information Criterion

Historically, one of the most important model selection criteria has been the Bayesian information criterion, also called the "Schwarz information criterion," proposed by Schwarz [283]. A neat feature of the BIC is that it can be used to provide a large-sample approximation to the Bayes factor for comparing two models.

The original derivation of the BIC established that selecting the model with the largest posterior probability was equivalent, with large samples, to selecting the model that maximizes

$$\sum_i \log\{p_j(y_i \mid \hat{\theta}_j)\} - \frac{\log(n)}{2}k_j \ .$$

This looks just like the predictive version of the AIC_j criterion, except that the adjustment term has a penalty multiplier of $\log(n)/2$ instead of 1. The larger n is, the greater the adjustment.

As with the AIC, this criterion is also generally multiplied by -2, so that

$$BIC_j = -2\log\{Lik(\hat{\theta}_j)\} + \log(n)k_j,$$

which is still a prediction-based criterion that we wish to minimize. Larger sample sizes result in larger penalties for overfitting. The particular penalty terms for AIC and BIC arise naturally because of their derivations.

Cavanaugh and Neath [67] have shown that, under general conditions,

$$-2\log\{p_j(y)\} \doteq -2\log\{p_j(y \mid \hat{\theta}_j)\} + k_j \log(n) = BIC_j,$$

for large n, where $p_j(\cdot)$ is the marginal predictive pdf for the observed data under M_j. This implies that, for large n,

$$\begin{aligned}
-2\log(BF_{jj'}) &\doteq BIC_j - BIC_{j'} \\
&= -2\log\{p_j(y \mid \hat{\theta}_j)/p_{j'}(y \mid \hat{\theta}_{j'})] + (k_j - k_{j'})\log(n),
\end{aligned}$$

and thus $BF_{jj'} \doteq e^{-0.5(BIC_j - BIC_{j'})}$. Integration is thus not required for the approximation.

Consider the special case with $j = 0$ and $j' = 1$ where M_0 is a special case of M_1; that is, when M_0 is nested in the model M_1, resulting in $k_0 < k_1$. If we let these models correspond to hypotheses H_0 and H_1, respectively, the alternative hypothesis is that M_1 holds but M_0 does not. In this case, we see that $-2\log(BF_{01})$ is minus twice the log of the frequentist generalized likelihood ratio (LR) test statistic for testing H_0 versus H_1, minus $(k_1 - k_0)\log(n)$. The standard large-sample frequentist LR test rejects H_0 in favor of H_1 if $-2\log(LR)$ is larger than a pre-selected quantile of the $\chi^2_{k_1 - k_0}$ distribution. There is, however, no generally accepted criterion for deciding how small BF_{01} should be before we would conclude that H_1 was true. Note as well that the additional penalty term in the BIC could lead to different inference using BIC than the classical LR test. In fact, the LR test will tend to favor the more complex model. Avoiding this is one of the motivations for the information criteria we are discussing.

A confusing feature of the BIC is that it does not depend on the prior, $p_j(\theta_j)$, leading one potentially to think it is not actually Bayesian. But this is just an interesting aspect of this particular *asymptotic* result. The only assumption about the prior is that it must be bounded above in general, and bounded below in a neighborhood of the "true" value of θ_j; in other words, the prior must not exclude the "truth" as a possibility and cannot attach too much weight to any particular value.

10.2.4 Widely Applicable Information Criterion

Watanabe [346] proposed an alternative model-fitting criterion that adjusts for overfitting. Watanabe's measure is called the widely applicable information criterion. Computation involves subtracting a term from $LPPD_j$ to make it less biased for $ELPPD_j$, which amounts to adjusting equation (10.8) for over-optimism.

Construction of the WAIC requires a numerical approximation to the predictive criterion $LPPD_j = \sum_i \log\{p_j(y_i \mid y)\}$. This is accomplished using an MCMC sample from the posterior, $(\theta^{(1)}, \dots, \theta^{(m)})$, where $\theta^{(l)} \sim p_j(\theta \mid y)$, to obtain

$$p_j(y_i \mid y) \doteq \frac{1}{s}\sum_{l=1}^{s} p_j(y_i \mid \theta^{(l)}) \equiv \hat{p}_j(y_i \mid y).$$

The Watanabe penalty adjustment is

$$p_{W_j} = \sum_{i=1}^{n} \text{Var}_{\theta_j|y} \ \log\{p_j(y_i \mid \theta_j)\}.$$

A nice feature of this adjustment is that it will always be non-negative. Gelman et al. [135] discuss two possible penalty adjustments but argue in favor of this one, since they expect numerical approximation to it to be stable. The predictive version of the WAIC is $\sum_j \log\{p_j(y_i \mid y)\} - p_{W_j}$. We again multiply by -2 to be consistent with the other information criteria, and write the WAIC as

$$WAIC_j = -2\sum_i \log\{p_j(y_i \mid y)\} + 2p_{W_j}. \tag{10.13}$$

Watanabe [346] has shown that, under some conditions, $WAIC_j \doteq LPML_j \doteq AIC_j$, for large n.

10.2.5 Deviance Information Criterion

Another model selection criterion is the deviance information criterion due to Spiegelhalter et al. [304]. They motivated the DIC as follows. In the statistical literature, the deviance function is defined as $D(\theta) = -2\log\{Lik(\theta)\}$, which is usually regarded as a goodness-of-fit measure (i.e., discrepancy from a perfect fit to data). Making $D(\theta)$ small is equivalent to making the predictive criterion $\log\{Lik(\theta)\}$ large. For assessing model M_j, the authors defined

$$DIC_j = E_{\theta_j|y}D(\theta_j) + p_{D_j} \equiv \bar{D}_j + p_{D_j}. \tag{10.14}$$

Here, the penalty is a measure of model complexity (or the effective dimension of the model) given by

$$
\begin{aligned}
p_{D_j} &= -2\left\{ E_{\theta_j|y}\log\{p_j(y \mid \theta_j)\} - \log\{p_j(y \mid \hat{\theta}_j^{\text{Bayes}})\} \right\} \\
&\equiv \bar{D}_j - D(\hat{\theta}_j^{\text{Bayes}}),
\end{aligned}
$$

which is the posterior mean deviance minus the deviance evaluated at the posterior mean.[2] By Jensen's inequality, p_{D_j} is non-negative, provided $p_j(y \mid \theta_j)$ is *log-concave* in θ_j. The motivation for this penalty is that, for the normal fixed effects linear model with k regression coefficients and known variance, the penalty reduces to k. Moreover, for a generalized linear model with k regression coefficients, a second-order Taylor expansion shows that the penalty is approximately k.

We now consider the predictive version of this criterion, which is analogous to that in the AIC where $p_j(y_i \mid \hat{\theta}_j^{\text{ML}})$ was substituted for $p_j(y_i \mid y)$ in equation (10.8). Here, if we substitute $p_j(y_i \mid \hat{\theta}_j^{\text{Bayes}})$ into equation (10.8), where $\hat{\theta}_j^{\text{Bayes}}$ is the approximate posterior mean of θ under model M_j based on an MCMC sample,

---

[2]It is interesting that both $\bar{D}_j$ and $D(\hat{\theta}_j^{\text{Bayes}})$ can be regarded as goodness-of-fit statistics from different points of view.

then the predictive criterion is $\sum_{i=1}^{n} \log\{p_j(y_i \mid \hat{\theta}_j^{\text{Bayes}})\} = \log\{p_j(y \mid \hat{\theta}_j^{\text{Bayes}})\}$. This is simply the log-likelihood function evaluated at the posterior mean instead of at the MLE.

Using the original definition of DIC in equation (10.14) and that of p_D just below it, we rewrite equation (10.14) as

$$DIC_j = D(\hat{\beta}_j^{\text{Bayes}}) + 2p_{D_j}, \tag{10.15}$$

which equals

$$DIC_j = -2\log\{Lik(\hat{\theta}_j^{\text{Bayes}})\} + 2p_{D_j}. \tag{10.16}$$

This is the predictive version of the DIC, since it is -2 times a bias-adjusted approximation to the LPPD, which is a goodness-of-fit measure plus a penalty. One can easily use a random sample from the posterior distribution (e.g., samples via MCMC) to compute the DIC. Since the DIC is already available in packages like BUGS and JAGS, we use it fairly often in this book.

An alternative measure of model complexity is half the posterior variance of the deviance, which can be estimated as

$$p'_{D_j} = \frac{1}{2}\text{Var}\left(D(\theta_j)\right) = \frac{1}{2}\frac{1}{M-1}\sum_{m=1}^{M}\left\{D(\theta^{(m)}) - (1/M)\sum_{m=1}^{M}D(\theta^m)\right\}^2.$$

The formula uses an MCMC sample from $p_j(\theta_j \mid y)$. An advantage of p'_{D_j} over the earlier measure p_{D_j} is that it cannot be negative.

Caveat. The quantity p_{D_j} corresponds to the effective dimensionality in a normal linear hierarchical model. The justification starts to get a bit fuzzy as one deviates from exponential families. There will be models for which p_{D_j} does not represent model dimension. It is not recommended, for example, for hierarchical models, a topic in Chapter 14; or if p_{D_j} is negative in which case the DIC is not a useful criterion. An additional concern is that p_D is not invariant to reparameterization.

10.2.6 Model Selection in Linear Regression

We now illustrate some aspects of model selection in the context of linear regression, demonstrating the use of LPML, PBF, DIC and BIC. Candidate models are all linear regression models, distinguished by different covariate combinations and/or transformations of predictor variables. We note that the response (or dependent or outcome) variable is not transformed. It is not possible to compare two models if the dependent variable is transformed differently in each, such as where one model has the original dependent variable and the other model uses its log transformation.

Recall that we have to obtain LPML by post-processing the output after running the code in BUGS, JAGS or Stan. This is easily accomplished by driving such software from R as discussed in Appendix C. The PBF is obtained by simply using its formula once the LPML has been computed for the two models. The DIC is easily obtained as direct output from BUGS or JAGS.

TABLE 10.2: FEV model selection statistics. S = Smoke, A = Age

Model	Predictors	LPML	DIC	BIC
(1)	S	-394.7	789.2	800.7
(2)	A	-356.5	712.6	724.1
(3)	S, A	-356.3	711.9	727.2
(4)	S, A, SA	-351.5	702.4	721.5
(5)	S, A, A^2, SA, SA^2	-350.7	700.3	727.2
(6)	$S, A, SA, (1-S)A^2$	-349.8	698.4	721.4

Example 10.4. FEV data of Example 7.3. Table 10.2 gives LPML, DIC, and BIC statistics for a variety of models predicting FEV from the dichotomous variable S (Smoke) and the continuous covariate A (Age). Code is available on the book's website with filename FEVmodelselect.txt under Chapter 10. Models (1) and (2) are the simple linear regression models, which in the case of model (1) is a two-group model. Model (3) is the ANCOVA (parallel lines) model. Model (4) includes the interaction, yielding separate straight lines for smokers and non-smokers that have different slopes. Model (5) has separate quadratic trends for smokers and non-smokers, and model (6) includes a straight line trend for smokers and quadratic trend for non-smokers. Diffuse, independent $N(0, 1000)$ priors were used for all regression coefficients independently of a $Ga(0.001, 0.001)$ for the precision.

Although model (6) is supported over the other models by all three selection criteria, the values of DIC and LPML for models (4) and (5) are not very different from those for model (6). One might argue that the more parsimonious model (4) should prevail. Although a consensus was reached on model (6) by DIC, BIC, and LPML in this example, different criteria can give rise to different preferred models. The best approach to model selection combines a selection criterion with guidance from subject-matter experts.

We also computed the PBFs for all 15 pairwise comparisons among the six models. Model (1) without age clearly fits worse than any other model: $PBF_{21} = 4 \times 10^{16}$, $PBF_{31} = 5 \times 10^{16}$, $PBF_{41} = 6 \times 10^{18}$, $PBF_{51} = 1 \times 10^{19}$, $PBF_{61} = 3 \times 10^{19}$. Model (2) with age alone fits only slightly worse than the model with parallel lines for age, $PBF_{32} = 1.31$, but the model with age alone clearly fits worse than any of the more sophisticated models: $PBF_{42} = 150.9$, $PBF_{52} = 336.8$, $PBF_{62} = 820.7$. Since it hardly fits better than the model with age alone, the parallel lines model (3), not surprisingly, also fits much worse than any of the more sophisticated models: $PBF_{43} = 115.3$, $PBF_{53} = 257.3$, $PBF_{63} = 627.0$. The real choice is between models (4), (5), and (6) with $PBF_{54} = 2.2$, $PBF_{64} = 5.4$, $PBF_{65} = 2.4$. Model (6), which is bigger than model (4) yet smaller than model (5), is preferred.

10.2.7 Comments on Information Criteria

We find the LPML criterion to be the most intuitive, and since PBF is a function of it (equation (10.12)), we tend to favor the PBF. It has the advantage over the BF that priors need not be proper, and it is also more stable to compute when diffuse proper priors are used.

The large-sample approximation to the Bayes factor using the BIC criterion is also compelling, since BFs are so directly interpretable. The "adjustment" $k \log(n)$ arises naturally from the approximation to the marginal predictive density for each model.

The other criteria involve mathematical justifications as approximations to the ELPPD. A nice feature of the WAIC is that it only involves Bayesian objects and does not rely on "plug-in" estimates of pdfs, namely estimates of the form $p(y \mid \hat{\theta})$, as in the case of the AIC and DIC. Gelman et al. [135] emphasize that the WAIC is based on the predictive densities that a Bayesian would actually use for predictions, rather than plug-in prediction densities. In this sense, it is more strictly Bayesian than the DIC, for example. The WAIC also has the advantage that it is approximately equal to the LPML in large samples. The DIC has the advantage that it has been programmed in software such as BUGS and JAGS, so one need only ask for it in those environments.

Finally, because the definitions of LPML and WAIC only involve integrals that are well defined and do not involve substituting point estimates, they are appropriate for mixed or hierarchical models. It is not obvious that the DIC or the AIC would be appropriate for assessing the quality of mixed models. Gelman et al. [135] also express doubts; also see Celeux et al. [68]. Mixed and hierarchical models are discussed in Chapter 14.

10.2.8 Statistical versus Practical Import in Model Selection

Suppose, through a careful statistical analysis, we come to be quite certain (say 99% posterior probability) that a treatment is effective, and most model selection criteria also agree that the model should include the treatment. There is still a necessity to ascertain whether the magnitude of the effect is sufficient to warrant a change in current medical practice. We thus conclude this section by discussing the distinction between statistical and practical import.

We have discussed situations where posterior probabilities that regression coefficients were positive (or negative) are quite large, say greater than 0.95. We have asserted that the corresponding regression effect was statistically important in this instance. Statistical importance is to be contrasted with practical importance. For example, the analysis of the trauma data with a diffuse prior was reported in Table 8.4. The posterior median and 95% probability interval for the regression coefficient that corresponds to the revised trauma score (RTS) was -0.59 $(-0.96, -0.26)$. The posterior probability that this coefficient is negative is virtually 1, so there is clear statistical importance of this variable. One would not think of removing this variable from the model. Furthermore, looking at Figure 8.1, we can clearly see the practical importance of this variable. For example, the estimated probability of death for

60-year-olds with injury severity of 40 is about 0.6 with the larger RTS and about 0.8 with the smaller RTS. This is quite a noticeable difference and much more relevant to judging practical importance than the actual estimate of the regression coefficient and its uncertainty interval.

Also in the trauma data analysis table, there are inferences for the interaction term between *Age* and type of injury, *TI*. The posterior probability that this coefficient is negative is 0.59, and the posterior median (-0.007) is very close to zero. There is obviously no statistical import here, and the estimate is useless for assessing practical import. Looking at Figure 8.1 again, however, and comparing the left and right side figures, there is a noticeable difference. That is, there is an observable difference in the estimated effect of *Age* on the curves: there is no apparent effect of *TI* for older patients but there is for younger ones. The question beyond the lukewarm statistical importance of the interaction is whether to retain it regardless.

Consider the following generic situation. Investigators want to compare a novel anti-cancer therapy to the standard treatment. In the study, they randomly assign cancer patients to receive the new treatment or the treatment that is the standard of care. Study personnel follow the enrolled patients over time and record which patients survive and which die. The predictor variable of interest in an analysis of survival is the indicator of assignment to receive the new treatment, since this variable's coefficient provides a measure of the treatment's effect on mortality relative to the standard-of-care treatment. With the likelihood of including additional covariates, an analysis may be based on a logistic regression model in which the parameter β_1 is the coefficient that corresponds to the indicator variable for "new" versus standard treatment. Further, suppose $P(\beta_1 > 0 \mid y) = 0.999$, and that the posterior median difference (new minus standard) in survival probabilities at some clinically relevant time (e.g., 30 days after the start of treatment) for individuals who are otherwise comparable is 0.20, with corresponding 95% probability interval $(0.15, 0.25)$. This is a clear story of statistical and practical import. No one would even think of removing the treatment variable from the model.

Now, suppose we found that $P(\beta_1 > 0 \mid y) = 0.96$, and that the posterior median difference and 95% PI were 0.20 $(0.01, 0.29)$. The estimates are the same but we are no longer very certain about the magnitude of the effect, beyond believing that there is an effect. We would surely leave the indicator variable in the model.

Finally, suppose we obtained $P(\beta_1 > 0 \mid y) = 0.83$, and that the posterior median and 95% PI for the difference in survival probabilities were 0.05 $(-0.03, 0.09)$. Here, it is less clear what conclusions to draw.

As another generic situation representative of a somewhat different type of model choice, consider a situation in which we fit a Weibull regression model and a log-normal regression model for the time to death after diagnosis with leukemia, with gender as a covariate of interest. Suppose a model selection criterion has favored the Weibull over the log-normal. The issue of statistical versus practical import remains regarding the effect of gender based on the selected model.

We mention here the work of Laud and Ibrahim [217] that can be used to assess the practical impact of various models from the predictive perspective. They consider three criteria labeled K, L and M, based on Kullback–Leibler, Euclidean, and probability density scales, respectively. K and M are similar in principle to the LPPD and LPML. The criterion L, however, measures models on the scale of the outcome or response variable in its units. This affords an interpretation more directly meaningful to the scientist to weigh models against one another. On the other hand, this measure does not yield interpretations on the probability scale as do BF and PBF. We recommend the use of L as supplementary to the other methods discussed in this section.

Finally, we remind ourselves that just because we have selected a model based on some criterion, there is no guarantee that the model will fit the data well. In other words, just because one model appears to fit the data better than the other models we have considered, the best-fitting model may still not necessarily fit the data well. It is always important to scrutinize a selected model for its fit to the data. We thus proceed to discuss model checking.

10.3 Model Checking (Model Diagnostics)

Suppose we have selected a model using one or more criteria from the previous sections. We would like to know whether the data are consistent or inconsistent with that model. The fact is that the "best" model according to some criterion may still provide a poor fit to the data. More precisely, in considering a model for the data, $p(y \mid \theta_M, M)$, we now ask whether the data look like they could reasonably have come from that distribution. If not, we will have some concern about this choice of model. Bayesian model checking, however, does not just involve the model for the data, since we must also specify a prior distribution, $p(\theta \mid M)$. Having to consider the prior distribution as well as the sampling model adds a layer of complexity to the issue.

10.3.1 Classical Checking

Classical methods of model checking are much more highly developed than are Bayesian methods. A simple example of model checking is the following basic model for the data that assumes that the residuals are normally distributed. We can take residuals from either a frequentist fit of the selected model or a Bayesian fit, and obtain quantile–quantile (Q-Q) plots to see if they look reasonably normal.

There are various tests and checks for constant variance. For example, if one assumes a Poisson model for data, there are methods to check if there is extra-Poisson variability, meaning that the variances are larger than the means. If the Poisson model holds, the variances should equal the means (see Section 9.2.1). The Pearson χ^2 goodness-of-fit statistic for categorical data models is a classical test that one may use to check a model's fit. We occasionally employ such methods and will discuss them when we do.

10.3.2   Box Check

In order to check a Bayesian model's specification, Box (1980) [45] considered using the marginal predictive density, $p(y \mid M) = \int p(y \mid \theta, M)p(\theta \mid M)d\theta$. In particular, he suggested obtaining the *marginal predictive p-value*,

$$p = P\{\tilde{Y} : p(\tilde{Y} \mid M) < p(y \mid M)\}, \quad \tilde{Y} \sim p(\cdot \mid M), \tag{10.17}$$

which is the probability of seeing a new data set (from the same model, M, that was assumed for the observed data) that is less plausible than the observed data, y. If a very small value is obtained, then it might seem very unlikely that the data were generated under model M. The criterion (10.17) is generalized as

$$p = P\{T(\tilde{Y}) > T(y)\}, \quad \tilde{Y} \sim p(\cdot \mid M). \tag{10.18}$$

In equation (10.18), $T(\cdot)$ is some function of the data that reflects goodness of fit, namely where large values would be incompatible with the model, M. Small values of p indicate poor model fit. An advantage of this method is that p is straightforward to compute using simulation. A disadvantage is that it is meaningful only with proper priors so that the marginal densities will be proper.

For example, if the model specifies that the mean of the data is zero, then $T(y) = |\bar{y}|$, the absolute value of the arithmetic average, would be such a function. Similarly, if $\hat{y}_i$ is the model prediction for the observed y_i, $i = 1, \ldots, n$, and $T(y) = \sum_i |y_i - \hat{y}_i|/n$, a small value of p would indicate a poor model fit. Unlike with criterion (10.17), however, it is possible that a large value of p could be a cause for concern. In the latter case, if $T(y) \doteq 0$, for example, p would typically be close to 1, indicating a near perfect model fit. Large values of p should cause concern that the model fit is too good to be true, as might occur, for example, if the number of parameters was close to the number of observations. The penalties included in the criteria discussed in Section 10.2 attempt to account for such overfitting.

Gelman, Meng, and Stern (1996) [137] have recommended the use of the *posterior* predictive *p*-value. This quantity is defined as in equation(10.18) only with $\tilde{Y} \sim p(\cdot \mid y, M) = \int p(\cdot \mid \theta, M)p(\theta \mid y, M)d\theta$. The measure is thus

$$p^* = P(T(\tilde{Y}) > T(y) \mid y), \quad \tilde{Y} \sim p_M(\cdot \mid y).$$

A tremendous advantage is that these quantities are easy to compute and that prior specifications need not be proper. However, Bayarri and Berger (2000, 2004) [21, 22] argue against the use of this criterion because of "double use of data," which unduly favors the model, as the same data were also used to choose the model.

10.3.3   Johnson Check

Valen Johnson [179] developed a Bayesian method of model checking that uses the data only once, is relatively easy to compute, and is intuitively appealing. Johnson has established some remarkable and simple[3] large-sample results.

---

[3]The proofs are not simple!

The development involves a particular form of the classic Pearson χ^2 goodness-of-fit statistic that requires a partition of the data support into K mutually exclusive and exhaustive categories. We begin with a sample from a presumed parametric model,

$$Y_i \mid \theta \overset{iid}{\sim} p(\cdot \mid \theta, M), \quad \theta \sim p(\cdot \mid M).$$

Let $F(\cdot \mid \theta)$ be the corresponding cumulative distribution function, and let $\tilde{\theta}$ be a single sample taken from the posterior, $p(\cdot \mid y, M)$, where $y = (y_1, \ldots, y_n)$, the observed data. For simplicity of exposition, let $F(\cdot) = F(\cdot \mid \tilde{\theta})$. Then let $0 \le a_{k-1} < a_k \le 1$, $k = 1, \ldots, K$; and, for each such $k > 0$, define $C_k = (F^{-1}(a_{k-1}), F^{-1}(a_k)]$ which is a set in the support of the response variable in the data. Notice that the interval C_k corresponds to the a_{k-1} and a_k quantiles of the distribution $F(\cdot \mid \tilde{\theta})$. With $a_0 = 0$ and $a_K = 1$, we have $F^{-1}(0) = -\infty$ and $F^{-1}(1) = \infty$. The collection $\{C_k : k = 1, \ldots, K\}$ forms a partition of the real line, so that every observation, y_i, must fall into precisely one of these sets.

Under the presumed model, and if $\tilde{\theta}$ were the true value of θ, for $k = 1, \ldots, K$ we must have

$$
\begin{aligned}
p_k &\equiv P(Y_i \in C_k \mid \tilde{\theta}, M) = \int_{C_k} p(y_i \mid \tilde{\theta}, M) dy_i \\
&= F(F^{-1}(a_k)) - F(F^{-1}(a_{k-1})) = a_k - a_{k-1}.
\end{aligned}
\tag{10.19}
$$

With $\theta = \tilde{\theta}$ known, the expected number of observations in the data that would be observed in C_k is np_k. The usual χ^2 goodness-of-fit statistic under these circumstances would be

$$R^B(\tilde{\theta}) = \sum_{k=1}^{K} \frac{(m_k(\tilde{\theta}) - np_k)^2}{np_k}, \tag{10.20}$$

where $m_k(\tilde{\theta}) = \sum_{i=1}^{n} I(y_i \in C_k)$ is the observed number of observations in the interval C_k and has expectation np_k.

If $\theta = \tilde{\theta}$ were truly known, this would be identical to the original frequentist Pearson χ^2 statistic for testing the hypothesis that θ was indeed equal to $\tilde{\theta}$. Of course, there would have been a scientific choice for θ under a null hypothesis of interest, and it would have been typically denoted θ_0 rather than $\tilde{\theta}$. With large n, the approximate sampling distribution for the Pearson statistic under the null hypothesis is χ^2_{K-1}, and the hypothesis would be rejected if the statistic was larger than something like the 95th quantile of this distribution.

In fact, Johnson's statistic is defined exactly as above, with $\tilde{\theta}$ a sample from the posterior. Under some conditions, he has shown that with large n and for $\tilde{\theta} \sim p(\theta \mid y, M)$,

$$R^B(\tilde{\theta}) \overset{\cdot}{\sim} \chi^2_{K-1}.$$

This is a remarkable result. It is the simplicity of Johnson's result that leads us to incorporate it into an introductory book.

So, how do we proceed from here? Johnson recommends computing the fraction of times $R^B(\tilde{\theta})$ exceeds the 95th percentile of the χ^2_{K-1} ($u_{0.95}$, say). This is accomplished by calculating the following quantity:

$$p = \sum_{l=1}^{M} I(R^B(\theta^{(l)}) > u_{0.95})/M, \tag{10.21}$$

where $\theta^{(1)}, \ldots, \theta^{(M)}$ are samples from the posterior. If the model fits, we only expect 5% to exceed this value, so $p \doteq 0.05$. We would be concerned if, say, $p = 0.2$, meaning that $R^B(\cdot)$ exceeded the 95th percentile for 20% of the samples. We might also be concerned if $p = 0.005$.

Johnson also considers the statistic

$$A = \sum_{l=1}^{M} I(R^B(\theta^{(l)}) > X_l)/M, \tag{10.22}$$

where $X_1 \ldots, X_M$ are independent draws from χ^2_{K-1}. This is a cool number to obtain; it says something about how different the actual distribution of the goodness-of-fit statistic is from its large-sample distribution. If the two distributions are about the same, then it can be shown that $A \doteq 0.5$. If A is close to 1, then the density for $R^B(\tilde{\theta})$ is concentrated well above the density for X, and if A is close to 0, the reverse would be true. The bottom line is that values of A close to 0.5 are consistent with a good fit and other values are not.

These quantities are all easily calculated in R after selecting and running the model M. To select the C_k, the simplest choice is C_k such that $p_k = 1/K$. For example, with $K = 5$, take $a_0 = 0, a_1 = 0.2, a_2 = 0.4, a_3 = 0.6, a_4 = 0.8, a_5 = 1$. Then, if we were checking whether a data set was distributed as $N(\mu, \sigma^2)$, we would have $(F^{-1}(a), F^{-1}(b)) = (\mu + \sigma\Phi^{-1}(a), \mu + \sigma\Phi^{-1}(b))$, where Φ is the cdf for a normal $N(0, 1)$ variate and $\Phi^{-1}(a)$ is its a quantile. With $\mu = 0, \sigma = 1$, and $K = 5$, we get $C_1 = (-\infty, -0.84], C_2 = (-0.84, -0.25], C_3 = (-0.25, 0.25], C_4 = (0.25, 0.84], C_5 = (0.84, \infty)$.

For selection of K, Johnson [179] recommends $K = n^{0.4}$, rounded. For example, if $n = 100$, $100^{0.4} = 6.3$, and $K = 6$ categories will suffice.

Now a note regarding cases where F is discrete. For example, if the data are binomial, the cdf, $F(\cdot)$, is not continuous. Obtaining the C_k in this case is not as straightforward as in the continuous case, since it is likely not possible to obtain categories that have exactly $p_k = 1/K$ for all k. This problem is easily addressed by simply selecting categories that have approximately the same probabilities. For example, if $n = 15$ and $\theta = 0.3$, we might set $K = 3$. We find the intervals by noting that for a binomially distributed random variable X with $n = 15$ and $\theta = 0.3$, $P(X \leq 3) = 0.3$ and $P(X \leq 5) = 0.72$. With intervals formed by setting $a_1 = 3$ and $a_2 = 5$, we get $p_1 = 0.3$, $p_2 = 0.42$, and $p_3 = 0.28$. The Johnson asymptotics hold as long as $n=15$ is "large enough." With larger values of n, and provided θ is not too small, the normal approximation to the binomial can be used to find categories.

In addition to its simplicity of procedure, a remarkable feature of this Johnson check is that it can be extended to regression and, more generally, to situations where the model for Y_i is even allowed to depend on i. In the regression case, we would write $Y_i \mid x_i, \theta \overset{\text{ind}}{\sim} p_i(\cdot \mid x_i, \theta)$. More generally, we can write $Y_i \mid \theta \overset{\text{ind}}{\sim} p_i(\cdot \mid \theta)$ where we have suppressed the dependence of Y_i on a family of models for notational simplicity. The only part of the above results that changes for this more general case is the definition of the sets C_k, which now depend on i. So define $C_{ik} = (F_i^{-1}(a_{k-1}), F_i^{-1}(a_k)]$ and $m_k(\tilde{\theta}) = \sum_{i=1}^n I(y_i \in C_{ik})$. Then all the above results remain the same.

10.3.4 *Outlier Checking and Influential Observations

Data are not always well behaved. What does this mean? Often, one can model a set of data reasonably well with a parametric model like the normal or log-normal distribution. Sometimes, however, one or a few of the observations are erroneous. Perhaps someone entered the number 10.67 into the data file as 1.067 or 106.7. Sometimes the stipulated data collection protocol is violated. For example, an experiment on cloud seeding for producing rainfall (Cook and Weisberg [86]) specified randomized seeding, or not, on "suitable" days. Unfortunately, cloud seeding was done on one day that was not suitable, and an extraordinary amount of rainfall was recorded. "Mistakes" like these often result in what are called "outlier" observations. In some instances, outliers can have a major effect on the resulting data analysis, though this will not always be the case. It is important in any data analysis to look carefully to see if there are any gross instances of outliers. Outliers will not always be visible to the eye, however, especially if there is a multivariable aspect to the data. Here we present some methods for outlier detection, along with accommodation where appropriate.

Outlier Detection Using Conditional Predictive Ordinates. A useful and natural procedure for outlier detection is to compute the CPO_i, introduced in Section 10.2.1 and equation (10.10), to obtain the index plot of $-\log(CPO_i)$ versus $i = 1, \ldots, n$ for a given model M. In this way we ascertain which observations, y_i, are predicted least well by the model (excluding y_i from the data for the prediction of y_i). The observation fitting worst to the model has the smallest value of CPO_i and consequently the largest value of $-\log(CPO_i)$.

Outlier Detection Using Predictive p-Values. Geisser [126] also suggested calculating the predictive p-values

$$pp_i = P\left(p(\tilde{Y}_i \mid y_{(i)}, M) \leq CPO_i\right), \quad \tilde{Y}_i \sim p(\cdot \mid y_{(i)}, M), \qquad (10.23)$$

for all data points. Interpreting CPO_i as the predictive plausibility of the observed y_j, the predictive p-value is the predictive probability of seeing a less plausible value for $\tilde{Y}_i$ under the assumed model. Small predictive p-values indicate the possibility of lack of fit and signal that the corresponding data points should receive further scrutiny. One can also find transcription errors like the example of 10.67 above in this way. Only when one ascertains that an error of some sort has been made should one consider discarding a data point. If all or most of these predictive p-values are small, then one may infer that the model itself is not fitting the data very well. In such cases model selection should be revisited to find a more appropriate model.

For the normal model with exchangeable data, Johnson and Geisser [183] obtained an explicit expression for pp_i that results in a simple numerical evaluation. To be specific, let $\{Y_i : i = 1, \ldots, n\}$ be a random sample from the $N(\mu, \sigma^2)$ distribution, with $p(\mu, \sigma^2) \propto 1/\sigma^2$. Let $\bar{y} = \sum_i y_i/n$, $s_y^2 = \sum_i (y_i - \bar{y})^2/n$ and define

$$t_i^2 = \frac{(y_i - \bar{y})^2}{n s_y^2 (1 - 1/n)}, \quad T_i^2 = \frac{t_i^2}{1 - t_i^2}.$$

Johnson and Geisser [183] showed that the predictive p-value in equation (10.23) can be analytically obtained for this model as

$$pp_i = P(F(1, n - 2) > T_i^2),$$

where $F(1, n - 2)$ denotes an F distribution with 1 and $n - 2$ degrees of freedom. In this instance it is actually possible to calibrate the magnitude of "outlyingness" of y_i. As a numeric example, suppose $n = 25$, $\bar{y} = 5$, $y_i = 10$, $n s_y^2 = 35$. Then $t_i^2 = 0.744$, $T_i^2 = 2.91$ and using R, the predictive p-value is 1- pf(2.91,1, 24) = 0.1. If we had instead observed $y_j = 12$ with the rest of the data remaining the same, then we would have $\bar{y} = 5.08$ and $25 s_y^2 = 59$. Then $t_i^2 = 0.845$ and $T_i^2 = 5.47$. Now the predictive p-value is 1 - pf(5.47,1, 24) = 0.028. So, it is quite unlikely that we would have observed a value that was as discrepant as $y_j = 12$ under the assumed model. We would next investigate the circumstances of this case thoroughly and decide whether removing the observation is warranted or if one might possibly consider a new model, one that may be more robust in the presence of possible outliers.

Johnson and Geisser [183] also extended these results for the normal linear model. In general, the criterion in equation (10.23) can be obtained by straightforward numerical approximation (see exercises).

Outlier Accommodation in Normal Linear Regression. If the outlying data points are judged not to be outright errors, there are models available to allow for occasional occurrences of large (or small) observations. For example, Johnson, Pearson, and Utts [185] present a Bayesian robust approach to estimation of the mean when outliers are anticipated.

Having many outliers may be indicative of a skewed or multimodal or heavy-tailed distribution. If so, the model should allow for such possibilities. We consider here the heavy-tailed case. A common choice for this is a t distribution with low degrees of freedom. The t distribution can be written as a scale mixture of normals, where the mixing is over the variance. We model each individual's residual (observed minus expected value) as a random variable that follows a normal distribution with mean zero and a variance that is a subject-specific scale factor times a common variance. Mathematically, we write the model as follows:

$$Y_i = x_i'\beta + \varepsilon_i,$$
$$\beta \sim N(b_0, \Sigma_\beta), \quad \varepsilon_i \mid \sigma^2, \lambda_i \sim N(0, \sigma^2/\lambda_i),$$
$$\lambda_i \sim \chi^2(\nu), \quad 1/\sigma^2 \sim Ga(a, b).$$

With this model, $\varepsilon_i \mid \sigma^2 \sim t(\nu, 0, \sigma^2)$. Aside from the added robustness from having t-distributed residuals, we can examine the posterior means of the λ_i and compare them to their expected values, ν. A small value of ν is recommended to allow for heavier tails for the t distribution, so as to minimize the effect of the prior. Wishing the first two moments of ε to be finite, ν in the range from 3 to 5 is appropriate. We use 4 in the following example.

Example 10.5. Carlin and Louis [63] present data from a study of the effectiveness of aspirin in reducing fevers in children. The data set has temperatures in degrees Fahrenheit for 12 five-year-old children just before and one hour after taking aspirin. We are interested in the change in temperature after taking aspirin, so our dependent variable is pre-aspirin temperature minus post-aspirin temperature. It is likely that the temperature change depends on the pre-treatment temperature, and we use that temperature as a covariate. Our analysis will be based on a linear model of change in temperature (Y) as a function of the pre-treatment temperature (T_0). We want to see if there are any outliers, so we assume a scale mixture of normals model for the residuals written as

$$Y = \beta_0 + \beta_1 (T_0 - \text{mean}(T_0)) + \varepsilon,$$
$$(\beta_0, \beta_1)' \sim N_2(0, \Sigma_0), \ \Sigma_0 = 10 \times I,$$
$$\varepsilon \mid \sigma^2, \lambda_i \sim N(0, \sigma^2/\lambda_i),$$
$$\lambda_i \sim \chi^2(4), \ 1/\sigma^2 \sim Ga(0.001, 0.001).$$

We ran the model in **JAGS** (code and data available on the book's website under Chapter 10 with filename **Aspirin.xxx**). Table 10.3 summarizes the posterior distributions of each parameter in the model, and Figure 10.1 shows boxplots of the MCMC samples of each child's λ. We expect each child's λ_i to be around 4, the mean of a $\chi^2(4)$ distribution. We see that child #1 and child #11 may be outliers, since the posterior means for their λs are 2.97 and 2.88, respectively. All other λ_i are between 3.64 (λ_{10}) and 4.78 (λ_{12}), which are fairly close to the expected value. An analyst would typically look more closely at the potential outliers to try to determine why the model may not fit these individual observations as well as others. If, say, one determines that there was a recording error, the data value could be corrected. The proper inference becomes more difficult if no reasons for the outlying values can be found. Each case is different and has to be handled according to the scientific basis and context of the study.

Influence of Individual Observations. In addition to looking for outliers in data, it is perhaps even more important to see what effect particular observations

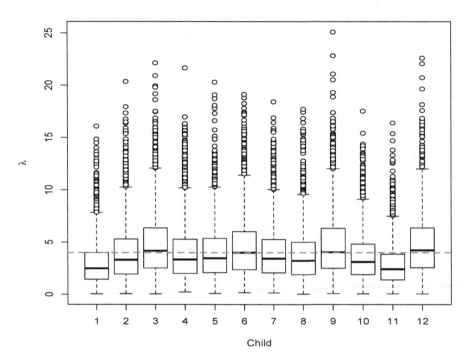

FIGURE 10.1: Boxplots of posterior samples for each child's λ.

have on an analysis. Observations that change inference substantially are termed "influential." Cook [85], Cook and Weisberg [86], and Belseley, Kuh, and Welsch [27] initiated the study of finding influential observations in the classical setting. Johnson and Geisser [183, 184] followed with Bayesian methods for detecting influential observations by considering prediction and estimation. In [183] they defined the predictive influence measure for removing observation i from the data to be

$$KLDP_i = KL(p(\tilde{y} \mid y, M), p(\tilde{y} \mid y_{(i)}), M),$$

where $\tilde{y}$ stands for predictive vector for all observations. This measure is the Kullback–Leibler divergence between the joint predictive density for a future vector that is based on all of the data and the corresponding joint predictive density that is based on all of the data except y_i. If $KLDP_i$ is close to zero, there is little effect on prediction if observation i is held out from the data. The observation corresponding to the largest value may be influential for predictive purposes. Observations with large values of $KLDP$ should thus be subject to scrutiny. If one removes the "most influential" data point and reanalyzes the reduced data set, one looks to see if the inferences are different enough to care about. Again, we may not want to remove such cases just because they are influential but report analyses with and without them, unless permanent removal is scientifically justified.

Johnson and Geisser [184] defined what they term an estimative influence mea-

TABLE 10.3: Posterior summaries from robust regression analysis of pediatric aspirin study data

	Mean	Std dev.	95% predictive interval
β_0	1.76	0.20	(1.36, 2.13)
β_1	0.82	0.24	(0.33, 1.31)
λ_1	2.97	2.10	(0.42, 8.38)
λ_2	3.91	2.65	(0.56, 10.69)
λ_3	4.77	3.05	(0.71, 12.34)
λ_4	3.96	2.69	(0.60, 10.86)
λ_5	4.05	2.67	(0.67, 10.64)
λ_6	4.56	2.90	(0.76, 11.78)
λ_7	3.97	2.60	(0.65, 10.55)
λ_8	3.77	2.55	(0.61, 10.33)
λ_9	4.70	3.04	(0.73, 12.35)
λ_{10}	3.64	2.37	(0.58, 9.68)
λ_{11}	2.88	2.03	(0.42, 8.17)
λ_{12}	4.78	3.00	(0.78, 11.80)
σ	1.11	0.32	(0.65, 1.89)

sure,

$$KLDE_i = KL(p(\gamma \mid y, M), p(\gamma \mid y_{(i)}), M),$$

where $\gamma = g(\theta)$ is a function of the parameters, possibly the identity, that is of particular interest to scientists. For linear and multivariate linear models, the estimative influence measure has explicit formulas [184] for direct computation. In the linear model case, there are good analytic approximations for the predictive influence measure. In general, Monte Carlo techniques are used to approximate these quantities.

While the measures in this subsection are discussed in some generality for a broad class of models, specifics for linear models were developed by Johnson and Geisser [183, 184], some of which are included in the next subsection. For binary response models, a more challenging topic, Johnson [182] discusses the assessment of predictive influence.

10.3.5   Diagnostics for Linear Regression

Standard linear regression models assume independence of observations conditioned on parameters, linearity (in regression coefficients) of the functional relationship, along with normality, and constant variance of the deviations from the regression surface. There are a variety of methods available to check these assumptions based on least squares (LS) estimates, which are the same as the maximum likelihood (ML) estimates in the case of linear regression ([77, Chapter 13]). The methods include looking at an initial scatterplot matrix to determine marginal relationships between the response and each covariate, whether continuous, ordinal, or nominal; residual plots; and tests for non-constant variance. A plot of residuals versus time-order may be appropriate and enlightening too. We recommend these techniques as quite useful in general for assessing whether the normal linear model is appropriate for the data at hand. After reviewing and illustrating these briefly, we discuss Bayesian methods that condition on the observed data and use a more predictive approach as introduced in the preceding subsections of this section.

Residuals are observed deviations of y_i from the fitted values $\hat{y}_i = x_i'\hat{\beta}$, where $\hat{\beta}$ is an estimate of β, typically $(X'X)^{-1}X'y$, the ML (also LS) estimate. Studentized (also called standardized) residuals are residuals that are divided by their *frequentist* estimated standard deviations in repeated data sampling. The *Studentized residual* is

$$S_i \equiv \frac{y_i - x_i'\hat{\beta}}{\sqrt{MSE(1 - h_i)}}, \tag{10.24}$$

where $h_i = x_i'(X'X)^{-1}x_i$ and MSE stands for mean squared error $(y - \hat{y})'(y - \hat{y})/(n-p-1)$, $\hat{y} = X\hat{\beta}$, and $\dim(\beta) = p+1$. The measure h_i is called the "leverage," taking on values between 0 and 1 and increasing with the distance between x_i and $\bar{x}.$, the average of the vectors x_i in the data. If x_i is far removed from the average, leading to $h_i \doteq 1$, the regression surface is pulled or leveraged towards the ith observation, y_i, and the frequentist standard error of $(y_i - x_i'\hat{\beta})$ will be near zero. *Case-deleted residuals* have the same form,

$$T_i \equiv \frac{y_i - x_i'\hat{\beta}_{(i)}}{\sqrt{MSE_{(i)}\{1 + x_i'(X_{(i)}'X_{(i)})^{-1}x_i\}}}, \tag{10.25}$$

except that $MSE_{(i)}$ and the least squares estimate $\hat{\beta}_{(i)}$ are computed with case i removed from the data; similarly, $X_{(i)}$ is X with case (row) i removed. A significance test compares T_i to a $t(n - r - 1)$ distribution.

If we have the correct regression model, residuals when plotted against any variable should look like a band of noise with no discernible pattern. In particular, any fitted trend line should be horizontal at zero. This should be true for variables that are in the model and for variables left out of the model. The most commonly used variable on the x-axis in such plots is made up of the fitted values $\hat{y}_i = x_i'\hat{\beta}$.

Finally, the ε_i should be normal. This can be checked by examining a normal probability (rankit) plot of the residuals. Q-Q plots can also be used. We illustrate with an example.

Example 10.6. FEV Data of Examples 7.3 and 10.4. For the linear regression model with

$$E(FEV \mid Age, Sex) = \beta_1 + \beta_2 Age + \beta_3 Sex + \beta_4 Age \times Sex,$$

the MLEs and the posterior mean of β using proper reference priors (as in Example 10.4) are both approximately $\hat{\beta} = (0.67, 0.21, 1.72, -0.14)'$. Figure 10.2 contains Q-Q and residual plots, separately for smokers and non-smokers. One can fit a

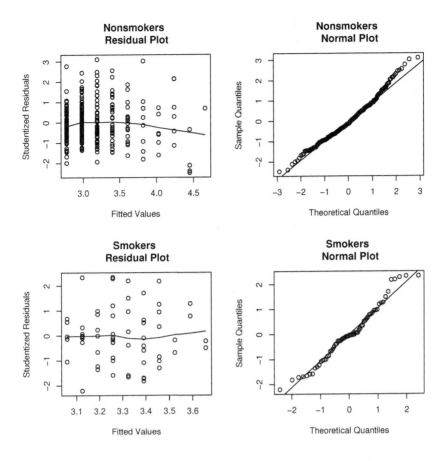

FIGURE 10.2: FEV diagnostic plots for linear trends in age.

nonparametric trend line to the plot of residuals against the fitted values or individual covariates to help visualize deviations from the assumed zero slope (i.e., no association). The trend lines in Figure 10.2 were computed using local weighted scatterplot smoothing (lowess); see Cook and Weisberg [87]. The Q-Q normal plots show that the sample quantiles are larger than the theoretical quantiles, suggesting a slight right skew in these distributions. The skewness appears to be larger for non-smokers. The constant variance condition may also be in question. Among non-smokers, fitted values above 3.75 show larger variance. Since the regression coefficient of age is positive, larger fitted values will tend to relate to older individuals. This suggests a higher variance for older non-smoking children. Data are sparse for this group, however.

Interpreting these plots is obviously subjective. One might conclude that there is no definitive indication of departure from normality or non-constant variance across age, based on these same graphics. A log or other transformation could be applied if normality were in question. In our experience, normal plots frequently deviate from the straight line in the tails.

Johnson and Geisser [183, 184] developed Bayesian methods for detecting the influence that individual cases in the data have on the prediction of future observations and on estimating parameters. While a number of measures were considered there, the simplest one turns out to be proportional to Cook's distance measure [85], namely,

$$D_i = S_i^2 \frac{h_i}{1 - h_i}.$$

This is the square of the Studentized residual in equation (10.24) times a monotone function of the leverage. Cook's motivation was that $D_i = (\hat{\beta} - \hat{\beta}_{(-i)})' X'X (\hat{\beta} - \hat{\beta}_{(-i)})/(p+1)MSE$, which measures the effect of deleting the ith observation on the estimate of β.

Now consider a future case (outcome denoted y_f) that will have predictor information $x_f = x_i$ and that will be predicted using the data $Y_{(i)}$. Then

$$T_{fi} \equiv \frac{y_f - x_i'\hat{\beta}_{(i)}}{\sqrt{MSE_{(i)}[1 + x_i'(X_{(i)}'X_{(i)})^{-1}x_i]}} \bigg| x_i, y_{(i)} \sim t(n - p - 1).$$

T_{fi} is a function of y_f, which is unobserved, but we can use this distribution to evaluate whether the observed value of the case-deleted residual T_i (equation (10.25)) is compatible with the model. We assess this compatibility by calculating the "p-value" $P(|T_{fi}| > |T_i| \mid x_i, y_{(i)})$. Case i is declared an outlier at level α if $|T_i| > t(1 - \alpha/2, n - p - 1)$. It is also shown in [183] that

$$T_i^2 = \frac{(n - r - 1)S_i^2}{n - r - S_i^2},$$

so it is easy to obtain T_i^2 from the Studentized residuals S_i.

10.3.6   Diagnostics for Binary Regression

For deciding among link functions in binary regression, we provided Examples 10.2 and 10.3 as illustrations. However, we did not discuss how to assess model fit with binary data. This is quite challenging.

For grouped data where there are n_i observations corresponding to the same covariate vector, say x_i, it is possible to somewhat mimic the linear regression procedures if the n_i are all moderately large, say greater than 10. It is also possible to produce a plot for model assessment. To see how, let $\bar{y}_i = y_i/n_i$ be the proportion of 1s corresponding to case i. Then $\hat{\theta}_i \equiv \bar{y}_i$ is a natural (nonparametric) estimate of the corresponding success probability θ_i. For logistic regression, the difference between the logit of $\hat{\theta}_i$ (i.e., $\log(\hat{\theta}_i/(1 - \hat{\theta}_i))$) and the model fitted estimate $x_i'\hat{\beta}$ can be treated as a "residual." Here $\hat{\beta}$ is the posterior mean of β under the logistic regression model. (Of course, there are difficulties if $y_i = 0$ or $y_i = n_i$ for any i.) One can also plot $x_i'\hat{\beta}$ versus $\text{logit}(\hat{\theta}_i)$. If the model fits, the plot should look like a straight line with some random scatter around it. Any striking pattern in this scatter would indicate a lack of fit. The process can be repeated for other link functions or for models with different subsets of covariates. The model corresponding to the best-looking straight-line plot could be accepted as the best-fitting model. Of course if none of the plots looks like a straight line, there is evidence against the fit of all models under consideration.

In our experience, the n_i tend to equal 1 more often than not (i.e., data are typically not grouped). We can, of course, proceed with model selection using the BF, LPML, or WAIC, as in Sections 10.1 and 10.2. However, model diagnostics remain challenging. One option is to consider Bayesian nonparametric methods that allow for a broad class of link functions [205], but these are beyond the scope of this book.

10.4   Recap and Readings

We have discussed model selection and assessing model fit in some detail. One can base model selection on posterior probabilities of specific models among a collection of models. An uncomfortable aspect of using posterior probabilities is the necessity to pick prior probabilities for the models under consideration. Imagine trying to assign a prior probability to the hypotheses in a jury trial for murder. What should be the prior probability that the defendant is guilty? This would not be easy, especially as this probability can have a substantive effect on the posterior probability. In a scientific context, one of the authors of this book was apprised that a colleague's prior probability for the hypothesis that the reported phenomenon of extrasensory perception (ESP) actually exists was 10^{-40}. Virtually no amount of data could move this prior probability in the direction of affirming the existence of ESP. Quantifying weight of evidence via Bayes factors avoids the difficulties of specifying prior probabilities for hypotheses in such situations.

Another approach, though not quite as directly interpretable as the BF, is to use one of several predictive information criteria. We gave a summary of advantages and disadvantages of eac.h With large samples, the BIC is a relatively easy criterion to implement and interpret. The DIC has the advantage of being readily available in BUGS and JAGS, but be advised not to use it if the penalty p_D is negative. We find LPML and WAIC quite useful in most situations, including hierarchical models.

In the context of model selection with two models, this is often framed as testing two competing hypotheses. Traditional methods rely on the use of p-values. Although ubiquitous in the medical literature, this emphasis on p-values for scientific purposes has come under severe scrutiny that indicates much caution, perhaps even shunning this approach entirely. In an accessible discussion without excessive mathematics, Goodman argues effectively in favor of the Bayes factor as a proper measure of evidence when testing hypotheses [148, 149]. Other influential articles in this direction are by Berger and Sellke [32], Ioannidis [173], Sellke, Bayarri, and Berger [290], Bayarri and Berger [21], and a statement by the American Statistical Association that includes discussion by several researchers [345].

The final topic was model checking, which is likely the least developed topic in the current Bayesian armamentarium. Looking for outliers using the CPO statistic, model checking using the Box and Johnson methods, and obtaining case influence diagnostics are all straightforward to program and can be recommended for routine use. In some instances we have seen analytic formulas, as is the case for the KLDP and KLDE statistics in linear models.

One final bit of advice. There are one-hundred-dollar analyses of data that have to be done by "tomorrow," there are one-thousand-dollar analyses that have to be done by next week, and there are analyses that really need to be done "right." The caveat *garbage-in, garbage-out* comes to mind. The analysis that must be done by tomorrow has a much higher probability of being *garbage* than if there were sufficient time to get the model "right"; on the other hand it may well be "good enough." Of course there is always a point in a data analysis where it is not worth appreciable effort to obtain "perfection," whatever that might be perceived to be. Data analysis is an art form that takes time and effort. Part of the art is knowing when to keep going and when to stop.

10.5   Exercises

EXERCISE 10.1.   Let the data $\{Y_i : i = 1, \ldots, n\}$ be iid from the model $M_0 : Y_i \sim N(0, 1/\tau)$ or from $M_1 : Y_i \sim N(\mu, 1/\tau)$. Let $p_i(\tau) \propto 1/\tau$ and $p_1(\mu) \propto 1$. Define $\theta_0 = \tau$ and $\theta_1 = (\mu, \tau)'$.

(a) Obtain explicit formulas for $p_i(y)$ and BF_{10}; simplify the formula for the Bayes factor.
(b) Simulate 10 observations from $N(0.1, 1)$ and obtain BF_{10}. Comment.
(c) Repeat (b) with observations from $N(1, 1)$.
(d) Repeat (b) and (c) with $n = 100$.

EXERCISE 10.2.   Suppose we have independent normal observations with unknown mean θ and known precision τ_0:

$$Y_1, \ldots, Y_n \mid \theta \overset{iid}{\sim} N(\theta, 1/\tau_0).$$

Since the likelihood function for θ only depends on $\bar{y} = \sum_i y_i/n$, Bayesian statistical inferences need only depend on $\bar{y}$. We thus simply assume that the observed datum is $\bar{y}$. Then

$$Lik(\theta) \propto \exp\left[-\frac{n\tau_0}{2}(\bar{y} - \theta)^2\right].$$

We wish to test $H_0 : \theta = 0$ versus $H_1 : \theta \neq 0$. The prior under H_0 is $p_0(\theta)$ and must be a point mass assigning probability 1 to $\theta = 0$. Take $p_1(\theta)$ to be a $N(0, 1/\tau_1)$ density. Strictly speaking, $p_1(\theta)$ should not be defined for $\theta = 0$, but any integral over $\theta = 0$ is zero, so it does not matter.

(a) Obtain explicit (analytical) representations for the "marginal" probability density functions for the observed data, $p_i(\bar{y})$, $i = 0, 1$. *Hint*: In performing the second integration, you could first prove that $\bar{y} - \theta$ is independent of θ, given known τ_0 and given $\theta \neq 0$, and then use their independence to ascertain the marginal distribution of their sum (with θ integrated out). Alternatively, you could perform the integration using the complete-the-square formula that we used when deriving the posterior distribution of the mean in the case of a normal-normal model with known variance (see Section 3.2.2).

(b) Obtain BF_{10} and simplify algebraically as best you can.

(c) Then obtain $-2\log(BF_{01})$ and argue that this is larger than a constant k^* if and only if $|z| \equiv \sqrt{n}|\bar{y} - 0|/\sqrt{1/\tau_0} > \tilde{k}$, for a specific value $\tilde{k}$.

(d) Assume the datum $\bar{Y} \mid \theta \sim N(\theta, 10)$, $n = 49$, and the prior $\theta \sim N(0, 1)$. For each of the values $\bar{y}$, $(0, 0.2, 0.4, 0.6, 0.8, 1)$, calculate the corresponding BF, $-2\log(BF)$ and z values. Comment.

(e) Using the same data, write computer code to obtain numerical approximations to the BF values in (d). Comment.

EXERCISE 10.3.   Referring to Exercise 10.2, establish the fact that you will obtain the same marginal Bayes factor formula if you use all of the data or if you restrict the data to be $\bar{y}$, as was done in Exercise 10.2.

*EXERCISE 10.4. *Bayes factors for the LE data.*   Answer the following questions based on the assessment of link functions for the LE data in Example (10.2). Recall that BUGS code is given in the example, and in the files with the name LymphedemaBFdata on the book's website.

(a) Derive the expression for u[i] in the code.

(b) Run the code, or write your own code, and give the BF for comparing the two models.

(c) Revise the code to obtain the BF comparing the complementary log-log model to the probit model. Then give the BFs for comparing complementary log-log to probit, and for comparing probit to logit. Which model do you prefer and why?

EXERCISE 10.5.   Let $Y_1, \ldots, Y_n \mid \theta \overset{iid}{\sim} N(\theta, 1/\tau_0)$ with τ_0 known. Let the hypotheses be $H_0 : \theta = 0$ and $H_1 : \theta \neq 0$, and let M_0 and M_1 be the corresponding model indicators. Let $\theta \mid M_1 \sim N(0, 1)$.

(a) Obtain the analytical BIC formula for each of these models and discuss them in terms of tradeoff between goodness of fit and penalty.

(b) Obtain the approximate BF_{01} formula using the BIC and compare it with the exact analytical form of BF_{01}.

(c) Suppose that $n = 4$, $\tau_0 = 1$, and that the observed data are $(0.158, 0.747, 1.253, 1.841)$. Obtain BIC_i for $i = 0, 1$ and the exact and approximate values for BF_{01}.

EXERCISE 10.6.   Let $Y_1, \ldots, Y_n \mid \theta \overset{iid}{\sim} Exp(\theta)$, with $p(\theta) \propto \theta^2 e^{-5\theta}$. Consider the hypotheses $H_0 : \theta = 1$ versus $H_1 : \theta \neq 1$.

(a) Obtain an analytical formula for BF_{01}.

(b) Using R, obtain the value of the Bayes factor when $n = 50$, $\bar{y} = 2$.

(c) Give a Monte Carlo approximation to the Bayes factor to see how close you can get to the actual value.

(d) Obtain the approximate value of the Bayes factor using the BIC.

(e) Compare results and comment.

EXERCISE 10.7.   Establish that (10.10) is true. *Hint*: First show that

$$CPO_j = p_i(y_j \mid y_{(j)}) = \frac{\int \prod_{l=1}^{n} p_i(y_l \mid \theta)p(\theta)d\theta}{\int \prod_{l \neq j} p_i(y_l \mid \theta)p(\theta)d\theta}.$$

EXERCISE 10.8.   Precisely why is the PBF not a real BF?

EXERCISE 10.9.   Consider the two-sample binomial model with $Y_i \mid \theta_i \overset{\text{ind}}{\sim} Bin(n_i, \theta_i)$, $i = 1, 2$. Suppose $n_1 = n_2 = 25$, and that $y_1 = 3$ and $y_2 = 6$ are observed. Let $\theta_i \sim U(0, 0.5)$, independently, for $i = 1, 2$. For this problem, we consider the models M_1, which allows for distinct θs, and M_0, which equates them.

(a) Write code to obtain point and interval estimates for $\theta_2 - \theta_1$, and also to obtain the posterior probability that $\theta_2 > \theta_1$. Discuss.

(b) Write code to obtain the PBF_{10}. The prior for the common θ is the same $U(0, 0.5)$ distribution. Discuss.

(c) Write code to obtain BF_{10}, and compare with PBF_{10}. They do not have to be the same since they are different criteria.

(d) Repeat all parts above with $n_1 = n_2 = 100$ and with $y_1 = 12$ and $y_2 = 24$.

(e) Now discuss, compare, and contrast all of the above parts together.

EXERCISE 10.10.   For the two-sample binomial problem in Exercise 10.9, obtain the WAIC statistic for both models and both data sets. Discuss. Details for numerical approximation to equation (10.13) are given in Gelman et al. [135], but they are not difficult to figure out on your own. Keep in mind that a population variance can always be approximated by a sample variance, the sample here being an MCMC sample from the posterior.

EXERCISE 10.11.   Show that the three expressions for the DIC given in equation (10.14), (10.15), and (10.16) are the same.

EXERCISE 10.12.   Using the definition of the deviance function, observe that the AIC statistic can be expressed as $\text{AIC} = D(\hat{\theta}^{\text{ML}}) + 2k$, where $\hat{\theta}^{\text{ML}}$ is the maximum likelihood estimate and k is the dimension of the parameter vector. Let $k = 1$ for now.

(a) Assuming the improper prior $p_M(\theta) \propto c$, argue that the posterior mode for θ is the same as the MLE, $\hat{\theta}^{\text{ML}}$.

(b) Obtain a second-order Taylor series expansion for $D(\theta)$ by expanding about $\hat{\theta}^{\mathrm{ML}}$.

(c) Argue that if the DIC is defined using the posterior mode instead of the posterior mean, then DIC $\doteq$ AIC for large n. *Hint*: You can assume that with large n, the posterior mode and the posterior mean are approximately the same.

*EXERCISE 10.13. Repeat Exercise 10.12 with arbitrary k. Let $\hat{\theta} = \hat{\theta}^{\mathrm{ML}}$. *Hint*: Show that

$$\bar{D} \doteq D(\hat{\theta}) + \frac{1}{2} \int (\theta - \hat{\theta})' \ddot{D}(\hat{\theta})(\theta - \hat{\theta}) p_M(\theta \mid y) d\theta,$$

where $\ddot{D}(\theta)$ is the second derivative of $D(\theta)$, the corresponding $k \times k$ matrix of second partial derivatives when k is arbitrary. Note that the integral can be written as $E_{\theta|y}(\theta - \hat{\theta})' \ddot{D}(\hat{\theta})(\theta - \hat{\theta}) = \mathrm{trace}[\ddot{D}(\hat{\theta}) E_{\theta|y}(\theta - \hat{\theta})(\theta - \hat{\theta})'] = \mathrm{trace}[\ddot{D}(\hat{\theta}) \mathrm{cov}_{\theta|y}(\theta)]$. Then use the fact that the large-sample approximation to the posterior is $N_k(\hat{\theta}, 2\ddot{D}(\hat{\theta})^{-1})$.

EXERCISE 10.14. Compute the AIC and DIC statistics for both models and both sample sizes for the two-sample binomial models in Exercise 10.9.

EXERCISE 10.15. Recall that we analyzed the trauma data in Chapter 8 and that the data can be found on the book's website for that chapter. Using the prior of your choice, and with non-standardized covariates, obtain the DIC for each of the three link functions. Comment on which model seems to be preferable.

EXERCISE 10.16. Recall again the LE data with three covariates discussed and analyzed in Chapter 8. Using the prior of your choice, and with non-standardized covariates, obtain the DIC for each of the three link functions. Comment on which model seems to be preferable.

EXERCISE 10.17. For the two-sample binomial problem in Exercise 10.9, obtain the joint marginal predictive densities, $p_i(\tilde{y}_1, \tilde{y}_2)$, $i = 0, 1$, for the $n_1 = n_2 = 25$ case. The joint pdf will factorize as the product of two independent beta-binomial pdfs under model M_1. Simulate from the corresponding marginal predictive distributions and obtain a numerical approximation to (10.17).

EXERCISE 10.18. Suppose a random sample of ten blood donors was taken and that individuals were tested for HIV with a perfect test. A perfect test means that the test's sensitivity, the probability of a positive test outcome given the blood is indeed HIV infected, and specificity, the probability that a negative outcome on the test given that the blood is disease free, are each 100%. (Chapter 15 discusses diagnostic tests.) Suppose that two donors' samples were determined to be positive for HIV and eight were not. Check whether the data are consistent with a model

$$Y_1, \ldots, Y_{10} \mid \theta \overset{\mathrm{iid}}{\sim} Ber(0.01)$$

using the Box p-value criterion (10.17). (You can think of this as having a prior with $P(\theta = 0.01) = 1.0$.) Would the outcome change if it was based on $\sum_{i=1}^{10} y_i \sim Bin(10, 0.01)$? Comment.

EXERCISE 10.19.   Simulate k observations from a $N(\mu, \sigma^2)$ distribution, with $\mu = 10, \sigma = 2$, and with $k = 20, 50, 100$.

(a) Using these data obtain p as defined in equation (10.21), and A as in equation (10.22), for all values of k. Comment.
(b) Now add a spurious observation, $y_{k+1} = 0$, to each of the data sets and repeat (a).

EXERCISE 10.20.   Consider the FEV data with four predictors: *Age*, *Smoke*, *Height*, and *Male*. The data are given on the book's website for Chapter 7 in the file FEVdata-full.xxx.

(a) Obtain p as in equation (10.21) and A as in equation (10.22) for the LE data using the model with two covariates (Age and Smoke) and an informative prior. Comment.
(b) Repeat part (a) using the data with four covariates (Age, Smoke, Height, Male). Use a diffuse proper prior.

EXERCISE 10.21.   Simulate two independent binomial samples with $n_1 = n_2 = 50, \theta_1 = 0.5$, and $\theta_2 = 0.4$. Here, the total sample size is 100, so consider $K = 5$ categories. Select the categories so that a $Bin(100, 0.45)$ random variable has roughly 0.2 probability of being in each category. Using those categories, obtain the Johnson statistics p (equation (10.21)) and A (equation (10.22)) for the model that allows the binomial probabilities to be different. Then repeat under the (incorrect) model assumption that the binomial probabilities are the same. Comment.

EXERCISE 10.22.   Using the fact that $\bar{y} = y_j/n + \{\sum_{l \neq j} y_l\}/n$ and $\sum_l (y_l - \bar{y})^2 = (y_j - \bar{y})^2 + \sum_{l \neq j} (y_l - \bar{y})^2$, fill in the details from the discussion of outlier detection using CPOs about why t_i^2 above is 0.845 when y_j is changed to 12 from 10, with other observations remaining the same.

*EXERCISE 10.23.   For the situation considered in Section 10.2.1 with $\tilde{Y}_j \overset{ind}{\sim}$ $(Y_1, \ldots, Y_n) \mid \theta, M$, $\tilde{Y}_j \overset{ind}{\sim} p(\cdot \mid \theta, M)$, and $Y_i \mid \theta \overset{iid}{\sim} p(\cdot \mid \theta, M)$, do the following.

(a) Show that
$$p(\tilde{y}_j \mid y_{(j)}, M) = CPO_j E_{\theta \mid y} \left[\frac{p(\tilde{y}_j \mid \theta, M)}{p(y_j \mid \theta, M)} \right].$$

(b) Explain why this is a proper density in $\tilde{y}_j$.
(c) Explain how you could numerically approximate the predictive p-values specified in equation (10.23) using this result.

EXERCISE 10.24.   Let $Y_1, \ldots, Y_n$ be iid $N(\mu, 1)$ with $p(\mu) \propto c$, a constant, and let $y = (y_1, \ldots, y_n)$ and $y_{(j)}$ be the vector y with y_j removed.

(a) Obtain the explicit formulas for $p(\mu \mid y)$ and $p(\mu \mid y_{(j)})$.

(b) Then obtain an explicit formula for $KLDE_j$ with $\gamma = \mu$. It may be useful to recognize that $\bar{y} = y_j/n + \sum_{l \neq j} y_l/n = y_j/n + \bar{y}_{(j)}(n-1)/n$.

(c) Explain why it is somehow sensible for detecting influential observations.

(d) Now explain how you would obtain MC samples and how you would use them to approximate the $KLDE_j$ statistic if you did not have formulas.

*EXERCISE 10.25. Continuing with Exercise 10.24, let $\tilde{y} = (\tilde{y}_1, \ldots, \tilde{y}_n)$, with $\tilde{Y}_i \mid \mu \overset{\text{ind}}{\sim} N(\mu, 1)$, independently of Y.

(a) Derive explicit formulas for $p(\tilde{y} \mid y)$ and $p(\tilde{y} \mid y_{(j)})$. They will be multivariate normal with dependence covariance structure. *Hint*: Show that $\tilde{Y} \mid y$ is $N_n(\bar{y}e_n, I_n + e_n e'_n/n)$, where e_n is a vector of n ones.

(b) Obtain an explicit formula for $KLDP_j$. *Hint*: It will be helpful to know that the inverse of the matrix $I_n + e_n e'_n/n$ is $I_n - e_n e'_n/(n+1)$.

(c) Explain why the formula for KLDP is somehow sensible for detecting influential observations.

(d) Explain how you would obtain MC samples and how you would use them to approximate the $KLDP_j$ statistic if you did not have formulas.

EXERCISE 10.26. The FEV data have been analyzed a number of times in this book. The data with two (and four) predictors can be found on the book's website for Chapter 7. Here, we consider model selection with two covariates, *Age* and *Smoke*.

(a) Using proper diffuse priors, run the following linear regression models and obtain the DIC for each: (i) with only the variables *Smoke* and *Age*, (ii) with *Smoke*, *Age*, and a *Smoke*-by-*Age* interaction, (iii) with separate quadratic trends in age for smokers and for non-smokers, and (iv) with a quadratic trend for non-smokers and a separate linear trend for smokers.

(b) Using the model with the smallest DIC statistic, obtain posterior inferences for the regression coefficients and obtain the posterior probability that each regression coefficient is positive. What does this analysis suggest about the associations between FEV and age for smokers and non-smokers? It will help to graph curves of estimated mean response against age for smokers and for non-smokers on the same plot.

EXERCISE 10.27. We continue with model checking for the FEV data, only now using the data set with four predictors, which is on the book's website for Chapter 7. Perform a parallel analysis to what was suggested in Exercise 10.26, only now including the extra two predictor variables, *Height* and *Male*.

EXERCISE 10.28. Consider Exercise 10.26 again. Using model (iv) in part (a), do the following.

(a) Construct the matrices

$$H = X(X'X)^{-1}X', \quad \hat{\varepsilon} = Y - \hat{Y} = Y - X\hat{\beta}, \quad V = \text{diag}(H),$$

$$S = \left(\sqrt{(I-V)MSE} \right)^{-1} \hat{\varepsilon}, \qquad D = V(I-V)^{-1}\text{diag}(S)S,$$

where $\text{diag}(S)$ is a diagonal matrix that is constructed so that the elements of the vector S constitute the diagonals, with zeros off the diagonals, while $\text{diag}(H)$ is a diagonal matrix that has off-diagonal zeros with the diagonal elements of H in its diagonal.

(b) Show that D is just the column vector of Cook's distances with ith element $D_i = S_i^2 \frac{h_i}{1-h_i}$.

(c) Identify the case in the FEV data with the largest Studentized residual and the case with the largest Cook's distance.

(d) Test the hypothesis that the former case belongs to the assumed model.

(e) Remove the case with the largest D_i and rerun the analysis using the same model. Report any substantial differences from the analysis done in Exercise 10.26 using model (iv) of part (a).

EXERCISE 10.29.   Justify that T_{fi} (defined near the end of Section 10.3.5) has the specified t distribution.

EXERCISE 10.30.   Obtain the LPML and DIC statistics for the models in Table 10.2, and for each model, j, construct a plot of $\{(i, CPO_{ij}) : i = 1, \ldots, n\}$. Discuss. The FEV data and BUGS code for analyzing these data can be found on the book's website for Chapter 7.

EXERCISE 10.31.   Consider a proper diffuse prior for the three-sample (log-transformed) DiaSorin data, first assuming equal variances. The DiaSorin data were analyzed in Chapter 7, and the data can be found on the book's website for that chapter.

(a) Give statistical inferences on the untransformed scale for the median values and for predictions. Obtain the DIC and LPML statistics for this model.

(b) Modify your code to handle unequal variances (or precisions) and repeat part (a). Also monitor the ratios of standard deviations, comparing the first and second, first and third, and second and third groups. Is the assumption of equal variances reasonable?

(c) Regardless of your answer to (b), explain how inferences would change if you assumed heterogeneous variances. Are there appreciable differences?

EXERCISE 10.32.   **FEV data analysis project**. Conduct a complete Bayesian linear regression analysis of the *full* FEV data available from the book's website for Chapter 7. These data include the predictor variables *Age*, *Smoke*, *Height* (in inches), and *Male* (yes/no) (1 = Male).

Information for informative prior construction was provided by Dr. David Mannino, M.D. (Division of Pulmonary, Critical Care, and Sleep Medicine and Director of the Pulmonary Epidemiology Research Laboratory at the University of Kentucky). The values are measured in liters. The two numbers are the prior best guess for median FEV followed by the 99th percentile for the median. For 18-year-old female smokers, 70 inches tall: 4.0 and 4.8. For 16-year-old male non-smokers,

70 inches tall: 4.2 and 5.0. For 13-year-old male smokers, 66 inches tall: 3.4 and 4.0. For 12-year-old male non-smokers, 60 inches tall: 2.7 and 3.5.

One issue to be addressed in this study is the determination of normal ranges of FEV for a given type of adolescent. For instance, what range of FEV values is predicted for a 15-year-old male who does not smoke and is 66 inches tall? Do the following in your analysis.

(a) Carry out an exploratory data analysis. This means make yourself familiar with salient features of the data by computing meaningful summaries and plotting the data for descriptions of it that you can communicate easily to Dr. Mannino.

(b) Discuss prior construction, predictor selection (including interactions), and convergence and model diagnostics.

(c) Present posterior inferences for regression parameters and for subpopulation means in appropriately designed tables or figures. Based on your analysis, is smoking related to FEV?

(d) Determine normal FEV ranges for several different types of adolescents, presenting the results in a table.

(e) Perform and discuss a sensitivity analysis.

Chapter 11

Survival Modeling I: Models for Exchangeable Observations

This chapter concerns the analysis of data that arise when studying the time until the occurrence of an event. Such data are often called "time-to-event data," and their analysis is termed "survival analysis." Medical studies often involve such situations. For example, the time until death after diagnosis with leukemia, or the time it takes to develop symptoms of Covid-19 after infection with the SARS-Cov-2 virus. Because one often does not get to record the precise time of the event of interest for each study participant, statisticians have developed methods to handle this mix of complete and incomplete measurements. As one example, a study of the effectiveness of a new anti-cancer drug may focus on time to death of patients as the primary measurement relevant to the drug's potential benefit. While some patients may have died by the time of the analysis (and their time of death known), others may still be alive. In the latter case, we do not know the time of death but we do know a lower bound for it – the time of analysis. This is also informative and relevant to the goal of the study. Another example is when a study outcome is the time the patient experienced some event (e.g., sero-conversion to AIDS), but the records do not allow us to determine an exact time of this event and we only know that the event occurred before a known time. Survival analysis is the collection of methods for analyzing such data in which not all individuals have experienced the event of interest and/or we cannot observe the precise time of the event.

In this chapter, we consider situations without covariates; in other words, the case of exchangeable observations. After delineating some concepts and terminology, we discuss methods based on parametric sampling distributions for the underlying event times. We then introduce Bayesian semiparametric and nonparametric methods.

11.1 Some Concepts and Definitions

We build the discussion of survival-analytic methods by defining key terms and developing some notation. We will generally let T denote a random survival time. Survival times are never negative, so one can use any probability model for positive random variables to characterize survival times. Common distributions that find use in modeling time-to-event data are the log-normal distribution, the exponential distribution, and the Weibull distribution. Some distributions are more convenient mathematically for certain types of models, especially when one is concerned with covariate effects (see Chapter 12).

11.1.1 Survival and Hazard Functions

One key element of survival analysis concerns the so-called hazard function, which we now define. Let the cumulative distribution function for the random survival time T be $F_T(t) = P(T \leq t)$. We call $S_T(t) = 1 - F_T(t) = P(T > t)$ the *survival function*. The density function of T is defined as it is for all continuous random variables (see Appendix A) as the derivative of $F_T(t)$, that is, $f_T(t) = \frac{d}{dt} F_T(t) = \lim_{\Delta t \to 0} \frac{1}{\Delta t} P(T \in [t, t + \Delta t))$. The *hazard function* for T, called the "force of mortality" in demography, is the rate of risk of the event occurring in an instantaneous time interval just beyond t, given that the event has not yet happened (up to and including t). Mathematically, we write

$$h(t) = \lim_{\Delta t \to 0} \frac{1}{\Delta t} P\left(T \in [t, t + \Delta t) \mid T > t\right) = \frac{f(t)}{S(t)}. \qquad (11.1)$$

By definition, $h(t) \geq 0$. The integral of this hazard function, called the *cumulative hazard*, and defined as

$$H(t) = \int_0^t h(s)ds \qquad (11.2)$$

is also non-negative. The relationships among the hazard function, the density function, and the survival function can now be written as

$$h(t) = \frac{f(t)}{S(t)}, \quad f(t) = h(t)S(t), \quad S(t) = \frac{f(t)}{h(t)}, \quad S(t) = e^{-H(t)}. \qquad (11.3)$$

As $\lim_{t \to \infty} S(t) = 0$, we have $\lim_{t \to \infty} H(t) = \infty$. If one knows any of the four functions in expression (11.3), then one knows them all. Specifically, along with equations (11.1) and (11.2), we have

$$h(t) = \frac{d}{dt}\{H(t)\}, \quad H(t) = -\log\{S(t)\}. \qquad (11.4)$$

Also, using the second and last equalities in expression (11.3), we have

$$F(t) = \int_0^t h(s)e^{-\int_0^s h(u)du}ds. \qquad (11.5)$$

Survival analysis consists of models and inference for the sampling distribution of T (discussed in this chapter), often with primary interest in the relationship between explanatory variables and some function of T (the topic of Chapter 12). Inference on the sampling distribution will often focus on estimating $S(t)$ or $h(t)$.

11.1.2 Censoring

We introduce notation that is commonly used in survival analysis. This notation allows us to write mathematical models for situations in which one is not able to observe the actual time that an event occurred, such as in the examples at the beginning of the chapter.

11.1.2.1 Right Censoring

We will consider first the case of right censoring. This is the most common form of censoring in medical studies where we may be prevented from observing the precise time to the event of interest due to another "censoring" event occurring prior to it. The censoring event could be the study team losing contact with the patient (typically called "loss to follow-up") or the time we wish to conduct inference (typically called the "end-of-study time"). Notationally, let C denote the random censoring time. The observed follow-up time Y is the minimum of the time until the event, T, and the censoring time C. With n patients, the observed outcome for patient i is $Y_i = \min(T_i, C_i)$, $i = 1, \ldots, n$. In addition to the observed follow-up time, Y_i, we generally also learn whether the patient experienced the event or the censoring time. Data for survival analysis, therefore, consist of a set of follow-up times and a corresponding set of indicators that let us know if each patient's time is the time until the actual event or if it is a censored time. Let δ_i denote the Bernoulli indicator of whether the event occurred at the time for the ith patient (i.e., the event time is *not* censored). Thus, δ_i equals 1 if we observe the actual event time for individual i, and it equals 0 if we do not observe the actual event at the end of follow-up. The outcome data in survival analysis, therefore, consist of two random quantities, (Y_i, δ_i), for $i = 1, \ldots, n$, where (dropping subscripts)

$$Y = \min(T, C) \quad \text{and} \quad \delta = 1 \text{ if } T \leq C, \ \delta = 0 \text{ if } T > C. \tag{11.6}$$

This also means

$$\delta = 1 \ \Leftrightarrow \ Y = T \quad \text{and} \quad \delta = 0 \ \Leftrightarrow \ Y = C. \tag{11.7}$$

We care about censored data, because we want to include all information in the data set. Even censored observations contain information; a patient still alive 5 years after entering the study tells us something about the treatment, particularly if most patients with this disease tend to die within a year of diagnosis.

11.1.2.2 Left and Interval Censoring

We now turn to two other kinds of censoring we may encounter: left censoring and interval censoring. An example of left censoring is the time of infection for a patient diagnosed with pneumonia. We know the infection preceded the time of diagnosis, but we usually do not get to record the actual time the pathogen caused the infection. Interval censoring occurs when an event time is both left and right censored. Interval censoring would occur, for example, if a woman underwent a series of mammography screening examinations every 2 years, starting at age 50, and has a positive mammogram at age 62. We know the cancer reached a detectable level some time between the most recent cancer-positive mammogram and the previous negative one, but we do not get to record the exact time when the tumor became detectable by mammography.

11.1.2.3   Assumptions for Censoring Mechanism

A common assumption is that censoring is independent of the event of interest, that is, T is independent of C. An example where this assumption makes sense is a clinical study that analyzes the study data 5 years after the first patient enters the study. Patients still alive at the time of analysis will be those early entrants with long lives and the later entrants who have not yet been on-study long enough to have experienced the event. As long as there are no trends in the sorts of patients who enter the study over time and long-lived patients are as likely to enter the study early as late in the course of the enrollment period, it seems reasonable to assume that the time of analysis (i.e., the censoring time) is independent of the failure times. On the other hand, if older patients or sicker patients tend to enter the study in the latter part of enrollment or if the study team tends to censor patients who are about to die prior to their actual death, then it is inappropriate to assume independent censoring.

Another assumption is that the censoring distribution, say $G(c) = P(C \leq c)$, does not depend on any of the same parameters as $S(t)$. This is called *non-informative censoring* or *uninformative censoring*. For example, suppose we observe survival in days for a single patient and see the event (uncensored observation) at $y = 25$. Then 25 would be our estimate of the center of the distribution, say the mean or median time of survival. However, if the observation is censored, $(y, \delta) = (25, 0)$, this would make our estimate of the same central measure something larger than 25. Now suppose we have informative censoring so that the time to event and censoring distributions have a parameter in common. Specifically, let $T \sim Exp(\theta)$ with mean $1/\theta$ and $C \sim Exp(\theta/5)$ with mean $5/\theta$. Seeing a censored observation of 25 now makes us think that the median time to event should be about 4 because of the informative censoring. Non-informative censoring is assumed in most survival analysis studies.

Remark on the need for censoring. Inference would clearly be better if all observations were complete and none censored. This is often not feasible, nor advisable, as if one were to wait until all study participants have died. We may want to publish results sooner rather than wait many years to avoid censoring. Deleting censored observations from the analysis, however, would clearly bias the inference. Thus, the statistical methods for survival analysis incorporate all information, whether complete or partial, for all patients at a pre-chosen time of analysis.

11.1.3   Sampling Distribution (Likelihood) for Exchangeable Data

We need a way to characterize the sampling distribution of the observation times in the presence of censoring. Although any distribution for continuous random variables that do not take negative values would be appropriate, there are a few families of distributions that are useful in survival modeling. These parametric distributions are the exponential, Weibull, log-normal, and gamma. We also discuss nonparametric estimation of survival distributions following the parametric cases in the next two sections, one-sample (Section 11.3) and two-sample (Section 11.4) models. However, the expressions in this subsection are in a general form, suitable for both parametric and nonparametric cases. These expressions are then adapted to the particular situations of the next two sections and their subsections.

11.1.3.1 Right Censored Data

Here, we assume that the only censoring mechanism at work in our data set is right censoring that is independent of the failure times. We consider the observations as pairs, (y_i, δ_i), for each individual in our sample $(i = 1, \ldots, n)$, with y_i and δ_i the ith individual's follow-up time and event indicator, respectively. The sampling distribution for the observations (conditional on any model parameters θ) is a product of the contribution from all observations stemming from the usual exchangeable (conditionally iid) model, although some care is needed in deriving this. We begin by noting that the usual model applies to the pairs (T_i, C_i), $i = 1, \ldots, n$ and can be written as

$$(T_i, C_i) \mid f(\cdot), g(\cdot) \stackrel{\text{iid}}{\sim} f(\cdot)g(\cdot),$$

with $T_i \sim f(\cdot)$ independent of $C_i \sim g(\cdot)$. Thus, as usual, we can write the joint distribution as

$$p\left[\{(t_i, c_i), i = 1, \ldots, n\} \mid f(\cdot), g(\cdot)\right] = \prod_{i=1}^{n} f(t_i)g(c_i).$$

However, unlike previously (see various subsections of Section 3.2), our observed data are $data = \{(y_i, \delta_i), i = 1, \ldots, n\}$, *not* $\{(t_i, c_i), i = 1, \ldots, n\}$. We now appeal to expressions (11.6) and (11.7) to see (Y_i, δ_i) as the one-to-one transformation

$$Y_i = \{T_i\}^{\delta_i}\{C_i\}^{1-\delta_i}, \quad \delta_i = I(T_i \leq C_i),$$

of (T_i, C_i), so that $\{(Y_i, \delta_i), i = 1, \ldots, n \mid f(\cdot), g(\cdot)\}$ are iid since $(T_i, C_i) \mid f(\cdot), g(\cdot)$ are. So, the sampling distribution of the data can be written as $p(data \mid \theta = \{f(\cdot), g(\cdot)\}) = \prod_{i=1}^{n} p(y_i, \delta_i \mid \theta)$. Now, we can write $p(y_i, \delta_i \mid \theta)$ by recalling from expressions (11.6) and (11.7) that $\delta_i = 1 \Leftrightarrow \{(y_i = t_i) \text{ and } (c_i > y_i)\}$ and $\delta_i = 0 \Leftrightarrow \{(y_i = c_i) \text{ and } (t_i > y_i)\}$. This event equivalence and independence of T and C lead to the joint distribution

$$p(y_i, \delta_i, \mid \theta) = \begin{cases} f(y_i)\{1 - G(y_i)\}, & \text{if } \delta_i = 1, \\ P(T_i > y_i \mid \theta) = g(y_i)S(y_i), & \text{if } \delta_i = 0. \end{cases}$$

An alternate way to write the last display is

$$\begin{aligned} p(y_i \mid \delta_i, \theta_i) &= \{f(y_i)\{1 - G(y_i)\}\}^{\delta_i} \{g(y_i)S(y_i)\}^{1-\delta_i} \\ &= \{h(y_i)\{1 - G(y_i)\}\}^{\delta_i} \{g(y_i)\}^{1-\delta_i}S(y_i) \\ &= \{h(y_i)\}^{\delta_i} S(y_i)\{1 - G(y_i)\}^{\delta_i}\{g(y_i)\}^{1-\delta_i}, \end{aligned}$$

where $S(\cdot)$ is the survival function; $h(\cdot)$ is the hazard function corresponding to density $f(\cdot)$, with $f(\cdot) = h(\cdot)S(\cdot)$ from expression (11.3); and $g(\cdot)$ and $G(\cdot)$ are the pdf and cdf of the censoring random variable C, respectively. We can thus write the sampling distribution (likelihood) as

$$p(\{y_i, \delta_i, i = 1, \ldots, n\} \mid \theta) \propto \prod_{i=1}^{n} \{h_i(y_i)\}^{\delta_i} S_i(y_i). \tag{11.8}$$

Notice here the proportionality (rather than equality) for this sampling distribution, caused by omitting the multiplicative terms in $g(\cdot)$ and $G(\cdot)$. This omission would not be possible if there are shared parameters between $f(\cdot)$ and $g(\cdot)$, which are the distributional families of the survival time and the censoring variables. This would be the exceptional case of informative censoring mentioned in the previous subsection.

11.1.3.2   More General Case: Interval Censored Data

Suppose we have event times

$$T_1, \ldots, T_n | \theta \overset{\text{iid}}{\sim} f(t|\theta)$$

but each T_i is possibly censored in such a way that we would only observe that it falls between two numbers $L_i < U_i$. As before, let δ_i denote the indicator random variable of non-censoring. Thus, the observed data are

$$\delta_i = \begin{cases} 1, & \text{if uncensored,} \\ 0, & \text{if censored,} \end{cases}$$

and $T_i = t_i$ if $\delta_i = 1$ or $T_i \in (L_i, U_i)$ if $\delta_i = 0$. The case of right censored data above has $L_i \equiv C_i$ and $U_i \equiv \infty$. Similarly, in the left censored case we would define $L_i = 0$ and $U_i = C_i$ where C_i is the left censoring time.

The sampling distribution for the data (likelihood function) is

$$p(data \mid \theta) = \prod_{i=1}^{n} \{f(t_i|\theta)\}^{\delta_i} \left\{ \int_{L_i}^{U_i} f(t|\theta) dt \right\}^{1-\delta_i}. \tag{11.9}$$

Note that if $\delta_i = 0$, all that is known is $L_i < T_i < U_i$.

11.1.4   Inference and Its Targets

With event times that are conditionally iid from $f(\cdot \mid \theta)$ and subject to right censoring, we work with the sampling distribution in equation (11.8) that uses the hazard and survival functions. Sometimes the following form, a precursor in our development of equation (11.8) using the density instead of the hazard function, is useful:

$$p(\{y_i, \delta_i, i = 1, \ldots, n\} \mid \theta) \propto \prod_{i=1}^{n} \{f_i(y_i \mid \theta)\}^{\delta_i} \{S_i(y_i \mid \theta)\}^{1-\delta_i}. \tag{11.10}$$

In the parametric cases, the functions h, f, and S are more appropriately written as $h(\cdot \mid \theta)$, $f(\cdot \mid \theta)$, and $S(\cdot \mid \theta)$ to make the parameter explicit. Indeed, that is how we have written equation (11.10). With prior $p(\theta)$, the posterior is obtained as usual. Occasionally, the posterior is recognizable, as we shall see with the exponential distribution. More often it is not recognizable, so we rely on MCMC sampling. As we have seen in previous chapters, even when an analytical solution exists, it is often easier to use posterior sampling as our inference targets are typically complicated functions of θ.

Given posterior samples $\{\theta^{(m)} : m = 1, \ldots, M\}$ as MCMC iterates, for any function of θ, say $\gamma = g(\theta)$, we approximate the posterior $p(\gamma \mid data)$ numerically by using the transformed samples $\{\gamma^{(m)} \equiv g(\theta^{(m)}) : m = 1, \ldots, M\}$. We have seen this, of course, in many previous chapters. What is new here are the functions of θ that are the targets of inference and of particular interest in survival analysis. We list a few.

1. **Mean survival time.** While the meaning and importance of this target are obvious, for inference implementation as above, we need to express this mean as a function of θ for the particular parametric model at hand. This requires a usually straightforward derivation or the use of Appendix B.

2. **Median survival time.** Again, the same comments apply here as for the mean, except for the direct use of Appendix B, which does not contain any expressions for the median. The quantile functions in R can be very useful here. Examples are `qexp(0.5,...)`, `qweib(0.5,...)`, `log(qnorm(0.5,...))` and `qlnorm(0.5,...)`, depending on the scale of measurement. Inference for quantiles other than the median is accomplished in a same manner.

3. **Survival probability at a fixed time point.** This is a very common target (e.g., five-year survival after definitive treatment for breast cancer). For some parametric families, $S(\cdot \mid \theta)$ is analytically available as a function of t and θ. We can again use R functions here: `1-pexp(t0,...)`, `1-pweib(t0,...)`, `1-pnorm(log(t0),...)` or the regular cdf functions with `lower.tail=FALSE` indicated in the function call.

4. **Survival function.** The entire estimated survival function can be displayed by plotting $S(t_j \mid \theta)$, $j = 1, \ldots, J$ on a grid of points $\{t_1, \ldots, t_J\}$. At each point, the survival probability is computed as above and averaged over the MCMC samples. If one uses the quantiles of these samples at each time point to make posterior probability intervals (or credible intervals), these should be declared as pointwise intervals with the specified probability. A simultaneous probability *band* can also be computed, but it takes more care and an iterative process to accomplish.

5. **Hazard function.** Parallel to the case of the survival function, one must compute $h(t_j \mid \theta^{(m)})$ for each j, m. One may employ analytic functions when available, or R functions using $h(\cdot) = f(\cdot)/S(\cdot)$. Density functions are available as, for example, `dweib()` in R. For the log-normal distribution, one can use

the `dlnorm()` function; care must be taken to allow for the Jacobian when working with the log-normal if using the R function `dnorm()`.

11.1.5 Prediction

Prediction can be important in survival modeling, especially in the regression setting of Chapter 12. As for most other models, point prediction and point estimation (here, of the population survival function) tend to agree with each other. The *variabilities* or *uncertainties* associated with these, however, are almost always very different in size. Prediction for an individual is much less certain than estimation of a quantity averaged over the population. With T_f denoting a future survival time (conditionally independent of the current data, conditioned on knowing the "true" survival function), the predictive density is

$$f(t_f \mid data) = \int f(t_f \mid \theta)p(\theta \mid data)d\theta.$$

The predictive survival function is similarly obtained as

$$S(t_f \mid data) = \int S(t_f \mid \theta)p(\theta \mid data)d\theta.$$

From these, one can find the predictive median or mean and probability intervals if the integrals are analytically tractable. Such tractability being rare, we often accomplish prediction via simulation. As in previous chapters, we simulate a T_f from the distribution identified by each posterior sample of θ, namely, generate $t_f^{(m)}$ from $S(\cdot \mid \theta^{(m)})$, $m = 1, \ldots, M$. This collection of t_fs approximates the predictive distribution. When $f(\cdot \mid \theta)$ and/or $S(\cdot \mid \theta)$ are available analytically or computationally (as in R), it is possible to carry out the above integrals as averages of MCMC samples of them. This avoids simulating T_f, and has better numerical accuracy.

11.1.6 Plotting Survival and Hazard Functions

As discussed in Section 11.1.4, primary objects of inference for time-to-event data are the survival curve and the hazard function. To be displayed effectively, information about these quantities should be plotted. Consider a general parametric model for survival data that depends on a vector of parameters θ and, possibly, on a vector of covariate information x. For a one-sample problem (Section 11.3), x never changes and can be ignored. For a two-sample problem (Section 11.4), x identifies the two groups and θ contains parameters for both groups. More complicated models involving x are discussed in Chapter 12.

To estimate $S(t|x, \theta)$ for all $t > 0$, we use simulated $\theta^{(1)}, \ldots, \theta^{(M)}$ from the posterior distribution of θ. For each $\theta^{(m)}$, we compute $S(t|x, \theta^{(m)})$. Since we cannot evaluate the survival function at all $t > 0$, we do this over a fine grid, perhaps $t = 0, 0.01, 0.02, \ldots, T_J$, where T_J is just bigger than the largest observed time in the data. Figure 11.1 shows the first 10 sampled posterior survival curves for the data in Example 11.3. Details of the data are given there along with modeling and inference in Section 11.3.1.1. The figure shown here is meant to help visualize what posterior samples of the survival function $S(t|x, \theta^{(m)})$ might look like. While the smoothness and shape of the curves are determined by the parametric model one uses, the variability seen is interesting and driven by the data and the prior on model parameters.

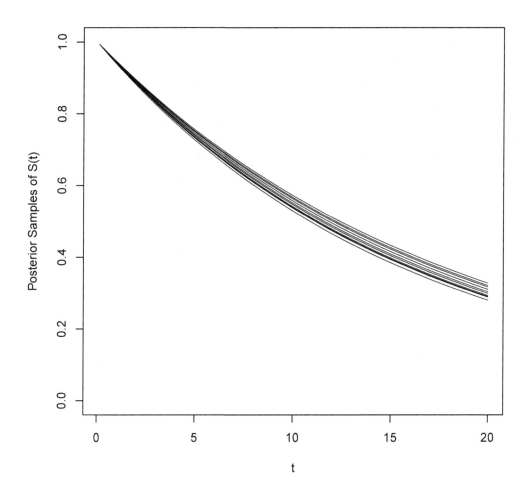

FIGURE 11.1: Ten instances of $S(t)$ from posterior samples of the survival functions with model and data from Example 11.3.

From these samples, the posterior mean of the survival function and, if desired, of the hazard function can be approximated as

$$\hat{S}(t|\theta) \doteq \frac{1}{M} \sum_{m=1}^{M} S(t|\theta^{(m)}) \quad \text{and} \quad \hat{h}(t|\theta) \doteq \frac{1}{M} \sum_{m=1}^{M} h(t|\theta^{(m)}),$$

where $h(t|\theta^{(m)}$ can be computed as $f(t|\theta^{(m)})/S(t|\theta^{(m)})$ if necessary. For simplicity, we have suppressed the possible dependence of these functions on a covariate vector x.

11.2   An Empirical Survival Function: The Kaplan–Meier Estimate

The main target of inference in survival analysis is the survival function $S(t) = P(T > t)$ which equals $1 - F(t)$, where $F(t) = P(T \leq t)$ is the cdf. Without censored data, we have the well-known empirical distribution function $F_n(t) = \frac{1}{n} \sum_{i=1}^{n} I(t_i \leq t)$ as an omnibus estimate of $F(t)$ without specifying a distributional form via a parametric family such as the exponential, Weibull or log-normal. A natural question then is how can this F_n be modified to accommodate censoring, beginning with its most common form of right censoring. Kaplan and Meier discussed such an estimator in 1958 [202]. This has become ubiquitous in describing survival data. Before explaining its construction, we consider data from a clinical trial to focus attention on a specific analysis.

Example 11.1. A Cancer Clinical Trial. The Cancer and Leukemia Group B (CALGB) conducted a randomized clinical trial to compare the benefits of three dose regimen intensities (high, moderate, and low) of a three-drug combination to treat non-metastatic breast cancer. The study, CALGB 8541, randomized over 1,500 women to one of the three treatment regimens. The file `CALGB8541.csv` under Chapter 11 on the book's website contains information collected in this trial, as shown in Berry et al. [37]. We give a brief description of the trial and the data set here, and use it in various examples in this and the next chapter.

Arm 1 (the high-intensity regimen) of the randomized trial consisted of women who received the most dose-intense regimen: four 28-day cycles of cyclophosphamide (600 mg/m^2 on day 1), doxorubicin (60 mg/m^2 on day 1), and 5-fluorouracil (600 mg/m^2 on days 1 and 8). Arm 2 (moderate intensity) patients received lower dose levels of the drugs (400, 40, 400 mg/m^2 on days 1 and 8), but in six 28-day cycles. Arm 3 received the low-intensity regimen made up in the same cycles as those in arm 1 but at the lowest levels of the drugs (300, 30, 300 mg/m^2, respectively).

The data set contains several variables: `seqno`, `study`, `arm`, `er`, `pgr`, `npn`, `tsizecm`, `premeno`, `survyrs`, `survstat`, `dfsyrs`, and `dfsstat`. As needed in the examples that use this data set, we will describe the information contained in each. For now, `seqno` is the sequence number of study participants; `study` always equals 1 for this trial, so we can ignore it; `survyrs` and `survstat`, respectively, contain the survival time in years and its *censoring* status (0 if uncensored time of death, 1 if right censored). Note that in the notation of Sections 11.1.2 and 11.1.3, this variable represents $\delta - 1$ and *not* δ itself. The variables `dfsyrs` and `dfsstat` are similar, except they refer to disease-free survival. This means if `dfsstat=0`, then `dfsyrs` is the time at which either death or disease relapse or recurrence occurred; if `dfsstat=1`, then `dfsyrs` is the time at which the patient was last known to be alive without relapse or recurrence of disease (but the patient's disease or survival status is not available beyond this point). Other variables in the data set contain tumor and patient information that we will describe as needed, mostly in Chapter 12.

There are 519, 517, and 513 subjects in arms 1, 2, and 3, respectively. Of these, right censored observations number 265, 231, and 244 for the survival outcome and 224, 188, and 197 for disease-free survival. The maximum follow-up time is about 20 years in each arm. Focusing on arm 1 for this example, how might one construct an empirical estimate of $S(t)$ for overall survival at some selected values of time t? The smallest right censoring time for overall survival is 3.47 years, and there are 67 deaths before this time ranging from 0.64 to 3.45 years. $S(3.46)$ is easy to estimate since there are no censored observations before 3.46; we simply form the ratio $(519 - 67)/519 = 0.871$, which is the relative frequency of survival times known to be greater than 3.46 without ambiguity. Now consider $t = 4.00$. While there are 17 more deaths after 3.45 and by 4.00 years, for a total of 84 deaths by 4.00 years, there are no more censoring events in this period. Here, it is not clear how to compute the relative frequency of deaths after 4.00 years. We know there are at least $519 - 85 = 434$ patients alive beyond 4 years, but what about the patient who was right censored at 3.47 years? This patient may or may not have died by 4 years; we simply do not know.

In general, with no censored observations, the empirical estimate is simply the relative frequency of observations greater than t_0, that is, $S_n(t_0) = \frac{1}{n} \sum_{i=1}^{n} I(t_i > t_0) = 1 - F_n(t_0)$. Notice that even in the presence of right censored observations, $S_n(t_0)$ is computable if all of the right censored cases occur *after* t_0. However, if one or more are less than or equal to t_0, it is not clear how to compute $S_n(t_0)$, that is, how many of those censored observations with times less than t_0 might have contributed uncensored event times had we followed them longer.

To address this problem, an empirical estimate is formed based on a previously existing product estimate that was used with life-table data. For continuous time data it is called the Kaplan–Meier product-limit estimate or, simply, the Kaplan–Meier (or K-M) estimate. Here is how it works. Consider right censored data $\{(y_i, \delta_i), i = 1, \ldots, n\}$ as defined in equations (11.6) and (11.7). Let $t_1^* < \cdots < t_k^*$ denote the $k > 1$ ordered times at which events occur, with $k \leq n$. Collectively, these times come from the observations with $\delta = 1$. However, k may not equal the count of uncensored observations if there are multiple observations with events at the same time point(s), that is, if not all the y_i with $\delta_i = 1$ are distinct; in yet other words, multiple events at any t_j^* are allowed.

Now let e_j denote the number of events at t_j^*, and n_j denote the number of patients known to be at risk of the event just prior to time t_j^*. So, n_j is the number of observations with $y \geq t_j^*$. In words, it is the number of patients who have neither experienced the event nor been censored before t_j^*. This leads to the fraction $(n_j - e_j)/n_j$ as a natural relative frequency estimate of the conditional probability $P(T > t_j^* \mid T \geq t_j^*)$. Note that this works for any t, not just an observed event time, because no events at t means $e_j = 0$ and the conditional probability estimate equals 1. We

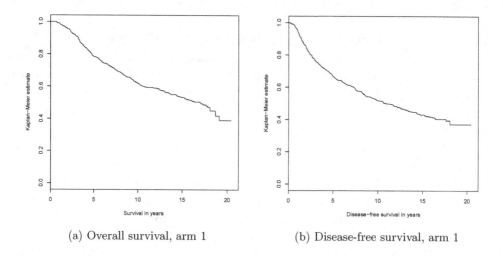

(a) Overall survival, arm 1   (b) Disease-free survival, arm 1

FIGURE 11.2: Empirical (Kaplan–Meier product limit) estimates of overall and disease-free survival.

now write the K-M estimate as

$$S_n(t) = \prod_{j:t_j^* \le t} \frac{n_j - e_j}{n_j}. \tag{11.11}$$

Notice that this is a non-increasing step function in t, constant between successive event times. It equals 1 at $t = 0$ if there are no events at time 0, and equals $(n - e_1)/n$ if there are. Taking $0/0$ to be 1, $S_n(t) = 0$, $t \ge t_k^*$ if there are no censored observations at or beyond t_k^*, that is, the largest event time exceeds the largest right censoring time in the data. However, if the largest event time does not exceed the largest right censoring time, $S_n(t) = S_n(t_k^*)$, $t \ge t_k^*$. In other words, there is no strict decrease in $S_n(t)$ beyond the largest event time.

Example 11.2. K-M Estimate for CALGB8541 Data: Example 11.1, Continued. Figure 11.2 shows the K-M estimates for survival and disease-free survival for arm 1 of the trial. The estimates were obtained by using the R package survival.

11.3   Models for Samples from a Single Population

One-sample models involve sampling from a homogeneous population in which individual observations are seen, as in Chapter 3, as exchangeable or conditionally iid. For survival data with exact and right censored observations, we developed a general form of the sampling distribution (likelihood function), equation (11.8), in the previous section. Here we consider specific cases with analytical details, first with three commonly used parametric families, and then with a flexible nonparametric model similar to that in Section 3.3.

11.3.1   Parametric Models

When we take $f(\cdot)$, and consequently $S(\cdot)$ and $h(\cdot)$, to be in a family of distributions indexed by a parameter θ (possibly a vector), we consider the model to be parametric. We introduce three parametric models that are often used in survival analyses, along with priors and posterior analyses.

11.3.1.1   Exponential Model

The simplest survival model uses the exponential distribution, $Exp(\theta)$. While it arises as the waiting time between events in a Poisson process (see Section 3.2.4), its usefulness is mainly as an introductory model. It is a bit too restrictive to fit most data in practice.

Let $T|\theta \sim Exp(\theta)$. Without right censored observations, the analysis would be identical to that in Section 3.2.4. As there, we use the $Ga(a_0, b_0)$ prior here. It is easy to see that

$$f(t \mid \theta) = \theta e^{-\theta t}, \quad S(t \mid \theta) = e^{-\theta t}, \quad h(t \mid \theta) = \theta, \quad t > 0.$$

The median, $t_{0.5}$, satisfies $0.5 = \exp(-\theta t_{0.5})$, so that $t_{0.5} = \log(2)/\theta = 0.69/\theta$. The hazard function is obtained as $h(t \mid \theta) = f(t \mid \theta)/S(t \mid \theta) = \theta e^{-\theta t}/e^{-\theta t} = \theta$, which is constant in t. Thus, if the time to event has an exponential distribution, the hazard of an event occurring is the same no matter what the time. This constant hazard reflects the *memoryless property* of the exponential: the probability of surviving an additional time y given survival up to t, $P(T > t + y \mid T > t)$, does not depend on t; it equals $e^{-\theta y}$. The hazard (which is a conditional instantaneous rate) of an event after, say, 100 years is the same as the hazard of the event at any other time, 0 included. Interpreted this way, the memoryless property is also called the "no-aging property."

Now consider data $y_i = \min\{T_i, C_i\}$, $\delta_i = I(y_i = T_i)$, and $T_i \overset{iid}{\sim} Exp(\theta)$. With the prior $\theta \sim Ga(a, b)$, using equation (11.8), we have

$$
\begin{aligned}
p(\theta \mid data) \quad &\propto \quad p(data \mid \theta)p(\theta) \\
&\propto \quad \left\{ \prod_{i=1}^{n} \theta^{\delta_i} e^{-\theta y_i} \right\} \theta^{a_0 - 1} e^{-\theta b_0} \\
&\propto \quad \theta^{a_0 + n_u - 1} e^{-\theta \left(b_0 + \sum_{i=1}^{n} y_i \right)},
\end{aligned}
$$

where $n_u = \sum_{i=1}^{n} \delta_i$ is the number of uncensored observations. Recognizing the last expression above as the kernel of a gamma, we write

$$\theta \mid data \sim Ga(a_1, b_1), \tag{11.12}$$

where $a_1 = a_0 + n_u$ and $b_1 = b_0 + n\bar{y}$. As in Section 3.2.4, the gamma prior is conjugate for the exponential, even with right censored data. While sampling approximations to posteriors are typically needed for other models, the analytic results in this simple parametric family are nice to see and can serve as building blocks for more flexible models. With this posterior, it is straightforward to obtain posterior probability (or credibility) intervals for θ. We simply find ℓ and u such that

$$1 - \alpha = P\left(\ell \le \theta \le u \,\middle|\, data\right).$$

Taking ℓ and u as the lower and upper $\alpha/2$ quantiles of the $Ga(a_1, b_1)$ distribution satisfies this equality. These quantiles can be determined computationally by using, for example, the function `qgamma()` in R.

Inference for the survival function $S(t \mid \theta)$ is straightforward too. Any quantile of the posterior distribution of the survival function at any t can be obtained easily by noting that this is a monotonically decreasing function of θ that has a gamma-distributed posterior given the data. To be specific, we have, for example, that the posterior median of $S(t)$ is $\exp\{-\theta_{\text{med}}t\}$, where θ_{med} is the posterior median of θ that one can obtain from the $Ga(a_1, b_1)$ in equation (11.12). For other quantiles, it can be easily shown that the αth quantile of $S(t)$ equals $\exp\{-\theta_{1-\alpha}t\}$, where $\theta_{1-\alpha}$ is the $(1 - \alpha)$th quantile of θ. An alternative to this approach that also works in distributional models that are not so nice analytically as the exponential is posterior sampling of θ followed by plots of $S(\cdot \mid \theta^{(m)})$. This was done and shown in Figure 11.1.

How do we select the prior for θ? The considerations are exactly the same as in Example 3.5 in Section 3.2.4. Essentially, we specify a prior best guess for the median and a large probability (say, 90%) interval for it. These specifications yield a system of two equations for two unknowns. We then use an iterative numerical process to solve for the unknowns a_0 and b_0. Details are given in Example 3.5.

Prediction. Using the $Ga(a_1, b_1)$ posterior, we derive the predictive survival distribution as

$$
\begin{aligned}
S(t_f \mid data) &= \int_0^\infty e^{-\theta t_f} p(\theta \mid data)\, d\theta \\
&= \int_0^\infty e^{-\theta t_f} \frac{b_1^{a_1}}{\Gamma(a_1)} \theta^{a_1 - 1} e^{-b_1 \theta}\, d\theta \\
&= \frac{b_1^{a_1}}{\Gamma(a_1)} \int_0^\infty \theta^{a_1 - 1} e^{-\theta(t_f + b_1)}\, d\theta \\
&= \frac{b_1^{a_1}}{\Gamma(a_1)} \frac{\Gamma(a_1)}{(t_f + b_1)^{a_1}} \\
&= \left(\frac{b_1}{t_f + b_1}\right)^{a_1}.
\end{aligned}
$$

The predictive density is the negative of the derivative of this $S(t_f \mid data)$. Such clean analytical results are rare with censored data.

Example 11.3. Exponential Model Analysis. Let us consider the disease-free survival outcome in arm 1 of the CALGB 8541 trial described in Examples 11.1 and 11.2. Since we have an explicit distributional result for the posterior in expression (11.12), we used R to obtain posterior samples of θ. We employed a diffuse prior with $a_0 = 1.4$ and $b_0 = 5$ that gives $E(1/\theta) = 11.5$ with a 95% interval for $1/\theta$ extending from 1.1 to 57.6 years *a priori*. Using these samples of θ, we constructed a posterior 95% probability interval for $1/\theta$, the mean disease-free survival time. With code available on the book's website in file named `ExpModelAnalysis.R` under Chapter 11, we obtained $E(1/\theta \mid data) = 16.7$ and $P(14.9 < 1/\theta < 18.7 \mid data) = 0.95$. The posterior mean disease-free survival function and a 95% posterior probability band for it are shown in Figure 11.3. As a reference, we also show the Kaplan–Meier curve in the figure.

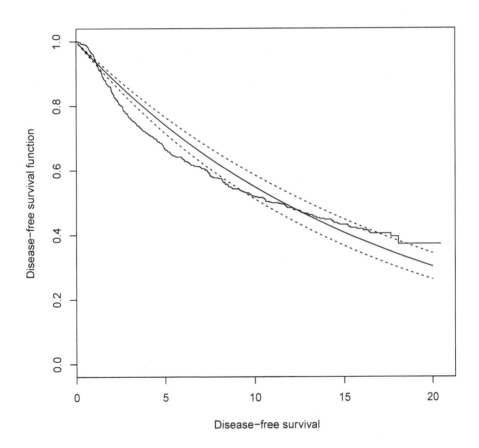

FIGURE 11.3: Posterior mean of $S(t)$ for disease-free survival in arm 1 (Example 11.3). Dashed lines show 95% posterior probability band for $S(t)$. Kaplan–Meier estimate is also shown.

11.3.1.2 Weibull Model

The Weibull distribution is a generalization of the exponential that incorporates a power transformation. If $T \sim Weib\,(\alpha, \lambda)$, then $T^\alpha \sim Exp(\lambda)$; thus α is the power that transforms the Weibull into an exponential. A Weibull with $\alpha = 1$ is an exponential. In our notation from the general presentation at the beginning of Section 11.1.3, $\theta = (\alpha, \lambda)$ for the Weibull sampling distribution.

Define $T \mid \alpha, \lambda \sim Weib\,(\alpha, \lambda)$ if

$$f(t \mid \alpha, \lambda) = \lambda \alpha\, t^{\alpha-1} e^{-\lambda t^\alpha}, \quad S(t \mid \alpha, \lambda) = e^{-\lambda t^\alpha}, \quad t > 0,\ \alpha > 0,\ \lambda > 0.$$

Percentiles of Weibulls are easy to find: the $1 - \beta$ percentile is the value $t_{1-\beta}$ that satisfies $\beta = P(T > t_{1-\beta}) = \exp\{-\lambda t^\alpha_{1-\beta}\}$. Solving, we obtain $t_{1-\beta} = \{-\log(\beta)/\lambda\}^{1/\alpha}$. In particular, the median $t_{0.5}$ is the time at which the survival probability is 0.50, that is, $0.50 = \exp\{-\lambda t^\alpha_{0.5}\}$ so that $t_{0.5} = \{\log(2)/\lambda\}^{1/\alpha}$. The mean is more complicated, but we often focus on medians in survival analysis. The hazard function is

$$h(t \mid \alpha, \lambda) = \frac{f(t \mid \alpha, \lambda)}{S(t \mid \alpha, \lambda)} = \lambda \alpha\, t^{\alpha-1}.$$

The hazard is increasing in t if $\alpha > 1$, and decreasing if $\alpha < 1$.

Now consider data $y_i = \min\{T_i, C_i\}$, $\delta_i = I(y_i = T_i)$, and $T_i \overset{iid}{\sim} Weib\,(\lambda)$, $i = 1, \dots, n$. Using equation (11.8), we have

$$
\begin{aligned}
p(data \mid \alpha, \lambda) &= \prod_{i=1}^{n} \{\lambda \alpha y_i^{\alpha-1}\}^{\delta_i} \exp\left(-\lambda y_i^\alpha\right) \\
&= (\lambda\alpha)^{n_u} \left\{ \prod_{i=1}^{n} y_i^{\delta_i} \right\}^{\alpha-1} \exp\left(-\lambda \sum_{i=1}^{n} y_i^\alpha\right),
\end{aligned}
$$

with $n_u = \sum_{i=1}^{n} \delta_i$. Letting $v = -\sum_{i=1}^{n} \delta_i \log(y_i)$ and $w(\alpha) = \sum_{i=1}^{n} y_i^\alpha$, we have

$$p(data \mid \alpha, \lambda) \propto (\lambda\alpha)^{n_u} e^{-\alpha v} e^{-\lambda w(\alpha)}. \tag{11.13}$$

This is not the functional form of a recognizable joint distribution for (α, λ), unless α is known. If α is known, it is the kernel of a gamma distribution for λ and would lead to the gamma prior as the conjugate family. This, however, is the same result as for the exponential model, essentially stemming from the fact that a Weibull with known α can be turned into an exponential. With α unknown, and $w(\alpha)$ depending on α in a complicated way, we do not have a known prior for (α, λ) that leads to a recognizable, analytically tractable joint posterior distribution. While we must rely on simulations, we can utilize to advantage the conditionally conjugate gamma prior for λ as described in the following.

Recall from Section 4.1.2 that we considered $p(\alpha, \lambda) \propto p(\lambda \mid \alpha)p(\alpha)$ with $\lambda \mid \alpha \propto Ga(a, b)$, and this led to conditional conjugacy for λ as $p(\lambda \mid \alpha, data) = Ga(a + n, b + \sum_{i=1}^{n} y_i^\alpha)$. Now the sampling distribution for the data with possibly some right censored observations in equation (11.13) is of the exact same form as that without right censored observations that we considered in Section 4.1.2. The details are different: $\lambda\alpha$ is raised to power n_u, not n; and in the middle term of products of y_i the product is only over uncensored observations. So, just as in Section 4.1.2, this leads to $\lambda \mid \alpha \propto Ga(a + n_u, b + \sum_{i=1}^{n} y_i^{\alpha})$ and

$$p(\alpha \mid \lambda, \boldsymbol{y}) \propto \alpha^{n_u} \left\{ \prod_{i=1}^{n} y_i^{\delta_i} \right\}^{\alpha-1} e^{-\lambda(\sum_{i=1}^{n} y_i^{\alpha})} p(\alpha).$$

It remains to specify the form of $p(\alpha)$. Again, we turn to the uncensored case in Chapter 4. In particular, in Example 4.4 we used the prior obtained via an auxiliary, Pareto-distributed, ϕ (first introduced in the context of gamma observations in Example 4.3). To be specific here, the prior for α is the marginal distribution stemming from

$$p(\alpha, \phi) \propto p(\alpha \mid \phi) p(\phi) \propto \left\{ \frac{1}{\phi} I_{(0,\phi)}(\alpha) \right\} \frac{I_{(c,\infty)}(\phi)}{\phi^{(d+1)}}, \quad c > 0,\ d > 0\,,$$

that is, $\alpha \mid \phi \propto U(0, \phi)$, $\phi \propto Par(c, d)$. This distribution has some useful properties as a prior for the shape parameter in the Weibull model.[1] We develop these properties in Exercise 11.8.

For posterior Gibbs sampling, we can directly adapt the full conditionals of Example 4.4:

$$p(\phi \mid \alpha, \lambda, data) \propto \phi^{-(d+2)} I_{(\max\{c,\alpha\},\infty)}(\phi),$$

$$p(\alpha \mid \phi, \lambda, data) \propto \alpha^{n_u} \left\{ \prod_{i=1}^{n} y_i^{\delta_i} \right\}^{\alpha} e^{-\lambda \sum_{i=1}^{n} y_i^{\alpha}} I_{(0,\phi)}(\alpha),$$

$$p(\lambda \mid \alpha, \phi, data) = p(\lambda \mid \alpha, data) = Ga\left(a + n_u, b + \sum_{i=1}^{n} y_i^{\alpha}\right).$$

As mentioned in Example 4.4, the full conditional for α is log-concave, so the R code given there is usable here with minor changes as would be indicated by the notational and likelihood changes above.

We now turn to the problem of specifying the parameters in the prior for α and λ. This is a more challenging task here, since there is no nice interpretation, even for λ when $\alpha \neq 1$.[2] Moreover, α is difficult to think about. Our idea is to pick alternative interpretable quantities that are easy to think about, specify distributional aspects of these, and translate this information to solve for the parameters in the distributions for α and λ. We have used this technique many times in preceding chapters; for example, in specifying prior parameters in the examples in Sections 3.2.1–3.2.4 (see Example 3.5, in particular). A natural choice here for one

---

[1] Also for the gamma shape parameter; we used it in Section 4.4.1, Example 4.3. Unlike in the gamma case, however, this prior continues to be useful for the right censored case for the Weibull.

[2] For a fixed α, a scale change of t keeps the transformed variable in the Weibull family as a member with the same α but the new λ depends on α.

alternative quantity is the median survival $t_{0.5} = (\log(2)/\lambda)^{1/\alpha}$; another is a high percentile such as the 90th, denoted $t_{0.9}$, so that $0.1 = P(T > t_{0.9}) = e^{-\lambda t_{0.9}^{\alpha}}$. The technique then proceeds by solving for the model parameters α and λ in terms of $t_{0.5}$ and $t_{0.9}$. We find it convenient here to consider α and λ in sequence.

Although individual values of α are difficult to interpret, the hazard function is $h(t \mid \alpha, \lambda) = \lambda \alpha t^{\alpha-1}$, so that $\alpha = 1$ is the dividing value between decreasing and increasing hazard in time. In many biomedical applications it may be possible to assess a prior probability that the hazard is decreasing, that is, specify $p_{\text{dhr}} = P(\alpha < 1)$. This would occur, for instance, if the risk of an event such as death after a surgery is the highest soon after the surgery and diminishes as recovery proceeds. Increasing hazard might be considered if time 0 corresponds to diagnosis of early stage cancer. It is reasonable to specify an informed choice for p_{dhr}. or take it as $1/2$.

To focus on the prior for α, it turns out (see Exercise 11.8) that its marginal distribution is a mixture of a uniform and a Pareto. In particular,

$$\alpha \sim \pi \, U(0, c) + (1 - \pi) \, Par(c, d).$$

We also have

$$P(\alpha < 1) = \begin{cases} 1 - \dfrac{c^d}{d+1}, & c < 1, \\ -\dfrac{d}{(d+1)c}, & c \geq 1. \end{cases}$$

Now, from the distributions table in Appendix B, the variance of $Par(c, d)$ is finite only if $d > 2$. We suggest $d = 3$ for typical use to keep the variance of α finite yet reasonably large. Also, using the above expression for $P(\alpha < 1) = p_{\text{dhr}}$ and solving for c, we get

$$c = \begin{cases} \dfrac{d}{d+1}/p_{\text{dhr}}, & p_{\text{dhr}} \leq \dfrac{d}{d+1}, \\ \{(d+1)(1 - p_{\text{dhr}})\}^{1/d}, & p_{\text{dhr}} > \dfrac{d}{d+1}. \end{cases}$$

With these choices, $d = 3$ and c as above, we can proceed to specify a and b in the prior for λ. Here, we would like to use the expression for the $1-\beta$ quantile of the Weibull-distributed T, namely, $t_{1-\beta} = \{-\log(\beta)/\lambda\}^{1/\alpha}$. If we fix a reasonable value of α (say, α_*) according to its prior, we can use this quantile expression to advantage in specifying a and b. One such choice for α_* is its prior mean $E(\alpha) = 0.5cd/(d-1)$ if $d > 1$ (see Exercise 11.8). Next, denoting the elicited best value for the prior Weibull median $t_{0.5}$ by $t_{0.5}^*$, we solve $t_{0.5}^* = (\log(2)/\lambda)^{1/\alpha_*}$ to get $\lambda_* = 0.69/(t_{0.5}^*)^{\alpha_*}$. Then, with λ_* as the mode, $(a-1)/b$, of the prior $\lambda \sim Ga(a, b)$, we have $a = 1 + \lambda_* b$. Finally, one more elicitation from the scientist expert allows determination of both a and b. For this, denote by $u_{0.95}$ the expert-specified value for the prior 95th percentile for the median of event time T, $P(t_{0.5} \leq u_{0.95}) = 0.95$. This represents the uncertainty in the expert's point value $t_{0.5}^*$ for the median of T. We can now write

$$0.95 = P\{(\log(2)/\lambda)^{1/\alpha_*} \leq u_{0.95}\} = P\{0.69/u_{0.95}^{\alpha_*} \leq \lambda\}.$$

Thus $0.69/u_{0.95}^{\alpha_*}$ is the 5th percentile of $\lambda \sim Ga(1 + \lambda_* b, b)$. We can determine

b by trial and error using `pgamma()` or `qgamma()` in R. See code in the file `WeibModelAnalysis.R` on the book's website under Chapter 11.

An alternative to the uniform-Pareto hierarchical prior for α (see Example 4.4) is to take $\xi \equiv \log(\alpha) \sim N(c, d)$ where $c = \log(\alpha_*)$. With $P(\alpha \leq u_{0.95}) = 0.95$, we get $P(\xi \leq \log(u_{0.95})) = 0.95$. Standardizing gives $0.95 = P\{(\xi - c)/\sqrt{d} \leq (\log(u_\alpha) - c)/\sqrt{d}\}$. Since 1.645 is the 95th percentile of the standard normal distribution, we have $1.645 = (\log(u_\alpha) - c)/\sqrt{d}$ which gives $d = (log(u_\alpha) - c)^2/1.645^2$. If we take $\alpha_* = 1$ and $u_\alpha = 5$, then $d = 0.957$. With such choices of α_*, c, and d, we can proceed to determine a and b in the prior for λ as explained in the previous paragraph.

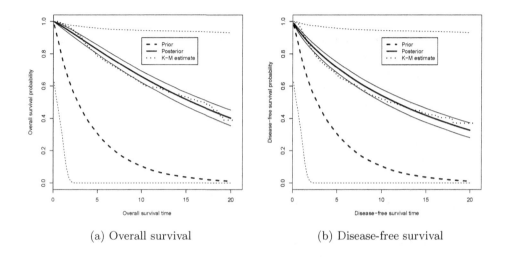

(a) Overall survival   (b) Disease-free survival

FIGURE 11.4: The figures show prior and posterior means of overall and disease-free survival functions, along with pointwise 95% probability intervals, for the Weibull sampling distribution in Example 11.4. The empirical K-M curve is also shown.

Example 11.4. Weibull Model Analysis. To illustrate the analysis for this model, we return to the arm 1 data of Example 11.3. Using the uniform-Pareto hierarchical prior for α, the conditional gamma prior for $\lambda \mid \alpha$, and following the prior elicitation process described above, we made the following choices to represent a relatively low level of information: $d = 3$, $p_{\mathrm{dhr}} = 1/2$, giving $c = 3/2$ and leading to $\alpha_* = 1.125$. Specifying $t^*_{0.5} = 12$, $u_{0.95} = 20$ yielded $\lambda_* = 0.04234$, and computing $0.69/u^{\alpha_*}_{0.95} = 0.02383$ as the 5th percentile of $Ga(1 + \lambda_* b, b)$, we obtained $b = 3.325$ by trial and error. Finally, $a = 1 + \lambda_* b = 1.141$. Relevant code for this entire example is in the file named `WeibModelAnalysis.R` under Chapter 11 on the book's website.

To carry out the analysis, we used an appropriate modification of the R code for inference with the Weibull model first presented in Section 4.1.2. The modification accommodates the sampling distribution in expression (11.13) that allows for right censoring. Results obtained with the above referenced R code are shown in Figure

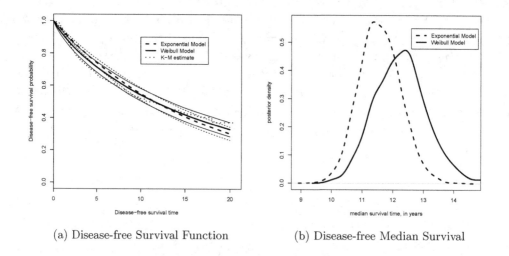

(a) Disease-free Survival Function (b) Disease-free Median Survival

FIGURE 11.5: The figures show posterior comparisons of disease-free survival functions and median survival time along with pointwise 95% probability intervals for the survival function, for the exponential and Weibull models in Examples 11.3 and 11.4. The empirical K-M curve is also shown.

11.4 for both the overall and disease-free survival functions. Also shown are pointwise 95% posterior PIs, and the empirical K-M estimate for reference. We used the same prior parameter settings for both outcomes. The prior mean and 95% PIs are shown too. It is quite clear that this is a low-information prior and the posterior inference is almost entirely determined by the information in the data.

Figure 11.5 shows posterior inference with the exponential and Weibull models. There is some difference in the inference with the two models, especially for the median survival time. The respective posterior medians and 95% posterior PIs for them are: exponential model, 11.55 (10.32, 12.95); Weibull model, 12.27 (10.71, 14.04).

11.3.1.3 Log-Normal Model

Analysis for the log-normal sampling model is similar to treatment of ordinary normal data. If there are no censored cases and we transform the data with logarithms, the likelihood function takes the same form that it did in Section 3.2.2. Adding censored observations alters the likelihood and the posterior but not the prior. Neither reference priors nor prior elicitation changes because of censoring. The "reference" prior is still $p(\mu, \tau) \propto 1/\tau$ (τ is the precision) but the posterior is more complicated with censoring. Our standard prior for this model is a normal distribution for μ and an independent gamma distribution for τ. We sometimes specify a uniform distribution for σ. As illustrated in Section 3.2.2, priors are induced from information on the median and another convenient percentile of the distribution for T. Prior elicitations and posterior inferences about medians and other percentiles transform easily from the original scale to the log scale and back again. The model can be written as

$$\log(T_i)|\mu,\tau \overset{\text{iid}}{\sim} N(\mu, 1/\tau) \quad \text{or} \quad T_i|\mu,\tau \overset{\text{iid}}{\sim} LN(\mu, 1/\tau)$$

with

$$\mu \sim N(m, v) \quad ind \quad \tau \sim Ga(a, b).$$

Here, we have the density and survival functions

$$f(t|\mu,\tau) = \frac{\sqrt{\tau}}{\sqrt{2\pi}\,t} \exp\left\{-\frac{\tau}{2}(\log(t) - \mu)^2\right\},$$

$$S(t|\mu,\tau) = 1 - \Phi\left\{\sqrt{\tau}[\log(t) - \mu]\right\},$$

where $\Phi(\cdot)$ is the cdf for the $N(0,1)$ distribution. The median $t_{0.5}$ satisfies $0.50 = P(T \leq t_{0.5}) = P(\log(T) \leq \log(t_{0.5}))$, so $\log(t_{0.5}) = \mu$, the center of symmetry of the $N(\mu, 1/\tau)$ distribution. Obviously then, $t_{0.5} = e^\mu$. The distribution of T is skewed, so the mean is not as useful as the median and slightly more difficult to obtain. The hazard function does not simplify beyond being the ratio of the two expressions for f and S above. However, the α percentile of the log-normal distribution has an explicit form: $\gamma = e^{\mu + z_\alpha \sigma}$, where $\sigma = 1/\sqrt{\tau}$ and z_α is the α percentile of the $N(0,1)$. This occurs because $P(T \leq e^{\mu + z_\alpha \sigma}) = P(\log(T) \leq \mu + z_\alpha \sigma) = P((\log(T) - \mu)/\sigma \leq z_\alpha) = \alpha$.

For analysis of this model with a data set, we refer to Exercise 11.9. Depending on the software you use (BUGS, JAGS, or Stan), you will need to code the model as described in Appendix C. They each use a different mechanism for specification of censored observations.

11.3.2 Nonparametric Models

An important part of inference with time-to-event data concerns estimating the risk of death over time. The most common way of presenting this inference is by way of the survival curve. That is, we compute an estimate of $S(t)$. The Kaplan–Meier or product-limit estimator is a popular method most often used for estimation of the survival probability curve [202, 204]. This is an empirical method that also has justification as a nonparametric maximum likelihood estimate ([210]).

One approach to Bayesian nonparametric inference is based on the Dirichlet process (Ferguson [108]). We introduced this towards the end of Chapter 3. To recall, the Dirichlet process (DP) is a way to characterize a distribution on the set of distributions. In Section 3.3 we presented the DP via its stick-breaking construction and proceeded to introduce Dirichlet process mixtures (DPMs) of normal distributions as a model for an unknown density. Here we work with the DP itself and write

$$t_1, \ldots, t_n \mid F \overset{\text{iid}}{\sim} F, \quad F \sim DP(M, F_0), \tag{11.14}$$

as a model for uncensored data. It turns out [108] that with such conditionally iid observations, the posterior of F is

$$F \mid t_1, \ldots, t_n \sim DP\left(M + n, \frac{M}{M+n}F_0 + \frac{n}{M+n}\frac{1}{n}\sum_{i=1}^{n}\delta_{t_i}\right), \tag{11.15}$$

where δ_t indicates unit point mass at t. Thus, the DP is a conjugate prior for the distribution function, and lends itself quite naturally to estimating a distribution function or survival function.

The above discussion does not include censored observations. It turns out that the posterior distribution with censored observations is a mixture of DPs. Several authors have described posterior inference with a DP prior in the presence of censoring, including Susarla and van Ryzin [313], Blum and Susarla [43], and Ferguson and Phadia [109]. Kuo and Smith [209] described the use of the Gibbs sampler to generate random samples from the posterior distribution of the survival curve based on a DP prior. They consider left, right, and interval censoring. Rosner [273] illustrated the use of a DP prior for monitoring clinical trials, which typically include right censored observations. Posterior sampling consists of two steps in this approach. In the first step, one computes the posterior, conditional on the uncensored observations. This posterior is just a DP as in expression (11.15) and requires no sampling. The next step predicts the future failure times for the censored observations. This step uses MCMC methods to carry out posterior inference. Within each iteration, the MCMC imputes a possible future failure time based on the current posterior DP. One can either use the posterior, conditional on the observed failure times and the failure times imputed at the previous iterations, or one can update the posterior after each imputation within a chain. Regardless of the approach taken, one ends up with a mixture of DPs, thanks to the imputations for the censored observations. After convergence, one uses the posterior samples for inference, since they are random samples from the correct posterior distribution.

Before we describe another, recently developed, model that is based on a DP mixture, we note that the advantage of these flexible nonparametric models over the Kaplan–Meier empirical estimate stems from the Bayesian inferential framework. While the posterior mean based on the DP prior and the Kaplan–Meier estimate are generally very close to each other under low-information priors, one can carry out predictive inference much more easily within a Bayesian framework. The advantage of posterior prediction is evident if one is monitoring an ongoing study, for example, and one wants to estimate the probability that the study will reach a solid conclusion after accrual of patients ends and planned follow-up is complete (i.e., the end-of-study analysis). One can easily impute the future event times for currently censored observations and for future enrollees into the study. If projecting to end-of-study time, one can simply treat imputed event times as censored at the end of the study if they exceed that date. The general form of the algorithm in R-like statements is shown in Figure 11.6 and is also available on the book's website for this chapter in a file named `GibbsDP.R`.

Example 11.5. DP Prior Model. We illustrate the algorithm by estimating the disease-free survival from the clinical trial described in Example 11.1. We focus again on arm 1 in this example, namely, the group that received the most dose-intense regimen. Figure 11.7 shows prior and posterior mean survival functions and the Kaplan–Meier estimate of the disease-free survival probability for the 519 women randomized to receive this regimen. The prior mean, F_0, is a piecewise

```
for = (iter in 1:(MaxIter-1)) {
    PostDirichletParms[iter,] = TempDirichletParms
    ProjectedFailTime = rep(NA, nCensor)
    for = (j in 1:nCensor) {
#   Grab the remaining time for the censored observation.
        StartIndx = findInterval(CensorTime[j], TimeGrid)
        PotentialFailTimes = TimeGrid[(StartIndx+1):nGrid]
#   Use multinomial sampling over the remaining time grid to
#   generate a future failure time for the censored observation.
#   The multinomial probabilities are proportional to the
#   parameters from vector TempDirichletParms corresponding
#   to the part of the time grid to the right of the censored time.
        ProjectedFailTime[j] =
            sample(PotentialFailTimes, 1,
                prob=Probs[iter, (StartIndx+1):nGrid])
    }
#   Add the imputed failure times to the current Dirichlet
#   distribution parameter vector.
    MatchIndx = match(ProjectedFailTime, TimeGrid)
    oMatchIndx = order(MatchIndx)
    TempTable = table(MatchIndx)
    for (i in 1:length(TempTable)) {
        loc = as.integer(names(TempTable)[i])
        PostDirichletParms[iter, loc] = TempDirichletParms[loc] + TempTable[i]
    }
#   Generate a sample from the posterior Dirichlet distribution
#   (with the imputed failure times at this iteration)
#   via random gammas.
    Probs[iter+1,] = rdirichlet(1, PostDirichletParms[iter,])
}
```

FIGURE 11.6: General form of the algorithm in R-like statements. This code is available on the book's website for this chapter in a file named `GibbsDP.R`.

exponential function consisting of the following two hazard rates: during the first year of follow-up, the hazard was 0.1, switching to a constant of 0.2 thereafter. Figure 11.7a shows what happens when the prior mass parameter is $M = 2$ in the DP prior. By contrast, the prior mass parameter was $M = 100$ in Figure 11.7b. In both cases, we ran the Gibbs sampler for 500 iterations and discarded the first 100 as burn-in.

In Figure 11.7a, the Kaplan–Meier estimate and the posterior mean are almost indistinguishable. The prior mean is far from the data and does not appear to have influenced inference in this example. When the prior mass is 100, as in Figure 11.7b, which is roughly one-third as large as the number of events in the data (295), the prior has more influence on posterior inference.

One can also illustrate the precision in particular estimates. For example, the posterior distributions of the disease-free survival at 1, 5, and 10 years are shown in Figure 11.8.

We now describe a method originally proposed by Kottas [207], especially as developed by Shi [293] and in Shi et al. [295, 296]. The accompanying R package DPWeibull [294] implementing these methods makes computations quite accessible for analyses encountered in this and the next chapter. The model used is one we described in Section 3.3.2, the Dirichlet process mixture, here made up of Weibull

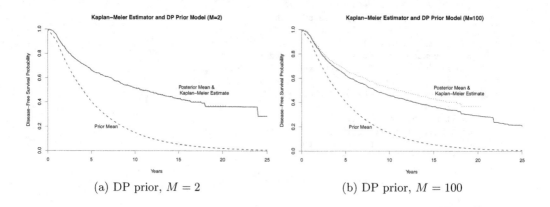

(a) DP prior, $M = 2$ (b) DP prior, $M = 100$

FIGURE 11.7: The figures show the prior and posterior means of disease-free survival, and the Kaplan–Meier estimate.

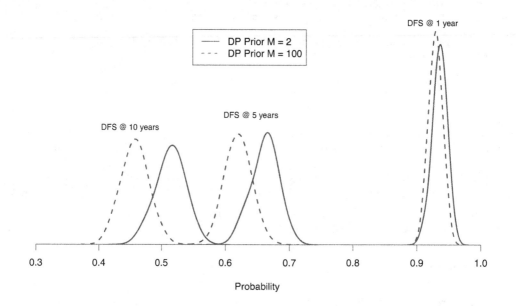

FIGURE 11.8: The posterior estimates of disease-free survival at 1, 5, and 10 years with prior $F \sim DP(M, F_0)$, where F_0 is the piecewise exponential function described in the text. When $M = 100$, the prior has greater influence on posterior estimates, especially at later times when there is less information.

distribution components. In particular, we can write a simpler version of the model as

$$T_i \mid \alpha_i, \lambda_i \overset{\text{ind}}{\sim} Weib(\alpha_i, \lambda_i), \quad (\alpha_i, \lambda_i) \mid G \overset{\text{iid}}{\sim} G, \quad G \sim DP(\nu, G_0). \tag{11.16}$$

To specify the prior for this model, we must make choices for ν and G_0. The Bayesian nonparametric models literature strongly recommends a gamma distribution for ν, and a hierarchical prior for G_0. Shi et al. [296] follow these recommendations to specify priors for a particular standardization of the data with the intention of constructing a rich set of Weibull components for the DPM that have good probability content in the relevant range of the data, while also allowing for possibly long-tailed distributions. We skip the details here as our intention is to use this methodology for applications and to illustrate the type of inferences it allows. We note, however, that the method in Shi et al. [296] is designed to include situations in which very little information is available for determining substantive priors, that is, to include low-information omnibus (LIO) priors (see Section 8.4.3). If substantive prior information is available, currently there is a need for appropriate prior elicitation methods for this model. We expect that such methods will be developed in the near future following similar developments for other Bayesian nonparametric models.

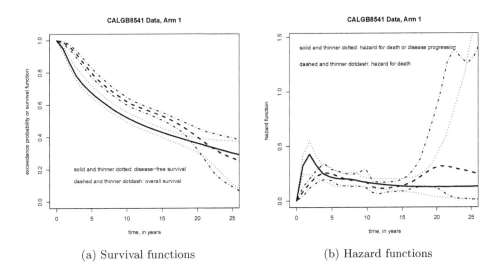

(a) Survival functions   (b) Hazard functions

FIGURE 11.9: The figures show posterior means of overall and disease-free survival, and corresponding hazard functions for a Dirichlet process mixture of Weibulls analysis of the clinical trial data in Example 11.6. Also included are pointwise 95% posterior probability intervals.

Example 11.6. DPM of Weibulls Model. We return again to data from arm 1 of the CALGB8541 trial introduced in Example 11.1 and continued in Example 11.5. Here we illustrate the use of the DPM of Weibulls model in expression (11.16). With the DPWeibull package in R, the code (in file DPMWeibullmodelCALGB.R) is fairly simple. Figure 11.9 shows posterior mean survival and hazard functions for both overall and disease-free survival, along with their corresponding 95% posterior probability intervals. The output object generated by the function dpweib contains posterior samples which can be post-processed to obtain full posterior inference for many other quantities, such as mean and median survival times or survival probabilities at chosen time points as in Figure 11.8. We illustrate this further in Example 12.4.

In the survival analysis literature, there are many alternatives to the DP method described above. An early method specifying a prior on the space of increasing hazard functions is developed in Dykstra and Laud [100] and Laud [215]. Some extensions and computations can be found in [216, 342]. In the past two decades these priors have been generalized and adapted to various survival analysis situations. Another method is based on piecewise exponentials, considered in Ibrahim et al. [171]. We describe this method in some detail and show its use in the next chapter on regression methods in survival analysis.

11.4   Two-Sample Models

As in Chapter 5, comparison of two populations is a very commonly encountered situation in medical studies. Classic examples include a comparison of patient outcomes with a treatment versus placebo, studying sex differences in outcomes, or examining adult versus pediatric populations. In Chapter 5 we considered responses that were normally distributed or binary or in the form of counts. Here the focus is on time-to-event outcomes with possibly censored data. The generic two-population-comparison design begins with independent sampling from the two populations.

With independent, possibly censored, samples from two populations $i = 1, 2$, the observations are written as $y = \{y_{ij} = \min(T_{ij}, \delta_{ij}) : i = 1, 2; j = 1, \ldots, n_i\}$ where the non-censoring indicators are defined as $\delta_{ij} = I(T_{ij} \leq C_{ij})$ for right censoring and as $\delta_{ij} = I(L_{ij} < T_{ij} \leq U_{ij})$ for interval censoring. The task is to compare the populations' survival prospects. This involves comparing their survival curves, say, $S_1(t)$ and $S_2(t)$, or comparing the densities for the groups, $f_1(t)$ and $f_2(t)$. The top row of Figure 11.10 illustrates this idea. Alternatively, one could compare the hazard functions $h_1(t)$ and $h_2(t)$, perhaps by examining the hazard ratio $h_1(t)/h_2(t)$, as illustrated in the bottom row of Figure 11.10. The relative median $t_{0.5}^{(1)}/t_{0.5}^{(2)}$ is another common target of inference. In the context of randomized intervention and control groups, such group differentiating quantities are often called effect measures.

In Bayesian analysis, the two-sample model is very similar to the corresponding one-sample case, especially when the two samples are independent. Posterior sampling can be done separately for each sample, repeating the one-sample version for each. Then, any effect measures quantifying group differences can be calculated from these samples to obtain the posterior samples of the effect measures of interest. Typically, from a programming standpoint, we accomplish this by writing code in a single program. We provide one example below, and encourage the reader to recognize this "repeat twice" aspect of the problem addressing comparison of two populations in the independent samples and priors case.

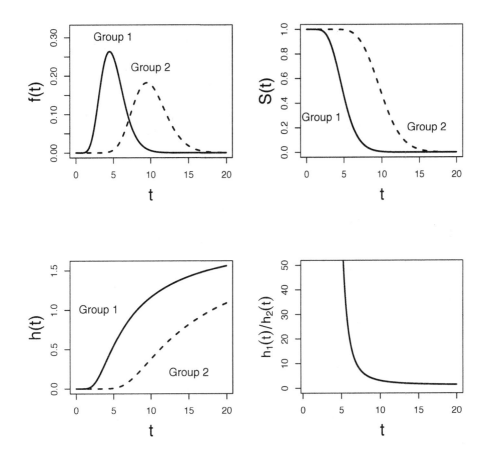

FIGURE 11.10: Illustration of effect measures for comparing two groups in survival analysis.

It is important also to point out that there are exceptions to this. In some cases, the priors in the two models may not be independent. In others, the samples may not be independent. An example of the latter situation is if the study forms pairs of subjects by matching on age and disease stage and randomizing one member of the pair to the treatment and the other to the control regimen. Appropriate care must be exercised in obtaining posterior samples in such paired-data situations.

Before turning to the example, we mention that the two-sample problem can be cast in the framework of regression, using a binary covariate to indicate group or population identity. We pointed this out also in the context of continuous, binary, and count data outcomes, as in Chapters 7, 8 and 9 on regression. These regression models contained the corresponding two-sample cases of Chapter 5. For time-to-event data, we typically use semiparametric formulations that involve an assumption of proportional hazards or accelerated event times as explained in Chap-

TABLE 11.1: WinBUGS output for leukemia data

node	mean	sd	2.5%	median	97.5%
median1	43.030	10.560	27.040	41.490	68.060
median2	13.030	3.234	8.124	12.550	20.650
relmedian	3.495	1.202	1.718	3.303	6.380
S[1]	0.668	0.062	0.541	0.670	0.783
S[2]	0.272	0.082	0.129	0.266	0.447
Sdiff	0.396	0.103	0.183	0.400	0.585
theta1	0.017	0.004	0.010	0.017	0.026
theta2	0.056	0.013	0.034	0.055	0.085

ter 12. As such, these models may not quite contain the two-independent-samples case, not without an additional assumption.

Example 11.7. Leukemia Data. In Example 3.5, we modeled part of the data presented in Feigl and Zelen [107], namely the survival times of 17 $AG+$ (POS $=1$) patients. Here we also include the 16 patients in the $AG-$ (POS $=0$) group and compare the survival times of the two groups. With $i = 1$ for the $AG+$ group, we use the exponential model with a gamma prior described in Section 11.3.1.1, and write

$$T_{ij} \mid \lambda_i \overset{\text{ind}}{\sim} Exp(\theta_i), \; i = 1, 2; \; j = 1, \ldots, n_i, \quad \theta_i \overset{\text{ind}}{\sim} Ga(a_i, b_i), \; i = 1, 2.$$

We construct a prior with the following information. Suppose the best available pre-data value for $t_{0.5}^{(2)}$, the median survival time of $AG-$ patients, is 20 weeks, and we believe that the median is greater than 5 weeks with 95% certainty. With such information, albeit with different numbers, we described in Example 3.5 how a_1 and b_1 can be determined using relatively simple R code. Following this method, we get $\theta_2 \sim Ga(2.31, 37.95)$. For θ_1 we use a $Ga(1.53, 26.4)$, which has mode 0.02 and 95th percentile 0.15. These correspond to a prior guess of $t_{0.5}^{(1)} = 34.5$ weeks and a 5th percentile of 4.6 weeks. As a reference prior, we approximate Jeffreys' prior $p(\theta_1, \theta_2) \propto 1/(\theta_1 \theta_2)$ by independent $Ga(0.001, 0.001)$ priors.

Code for the analysis is on the book's website under Chapter 11 with file names `Leukemia.xxx`. Table 11.1 provides the output when using the informative priors. The prior and posterior distributions for θ_1 and θ_2 are plotted in Figure 11.11. The median time to death for the $AG+$ group is estimated as 41.5 weeks with 95% probability interval $(27, 68)$, much higher than for the $AG-$ group with estimate 12.6 weeks and 95% probability interval $(8, 21)$. The relative median θ_2/θ_1 is roughly 3.3 and probably between 1.7 and 6.4. About two-thirds of $AG+$ patients will live at least 24 weeks, whereas only about a quarter of $AG-$ patients will live 24 weeks or longer. The probability intervals do not overlap. The difference in the 24-week survival probabilities is about 0.4, with a probability interval that is clearly positive.

A sensitivity analysis was conducted using the informative prior and two sets of diffuse priors: $\theta_1, \theta_2 \overset{\text{iid}}{\sim} Ga(0.001, 0.001)$ and $\theta_1, \theta_2 \overset{\text{iid}}{\sim} U(0, 1000)$. The gamma priors

AG Positive

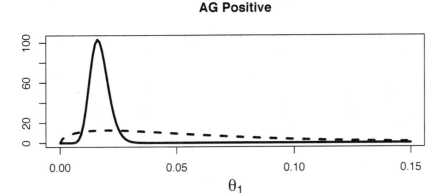

AG Negative

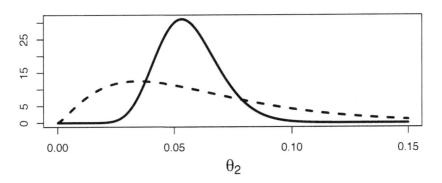

FIGURE 11.11: Prior (dashed lines) and posterior (solid lines) distributions for θ_1 and θ_2.

have mean 1 and variance 1,000. Both priors can be considered diffuse, given what we know about leukemia survival times. Results are given in Table 11.2 along with some from the previous analysis. Even with the relatively small sample sizes, the different priors do not give appreciably different results.

In Section 11.1.6, we described how to generate and plot posterior samples of survival functions on a grid. Following this method, we generated Figure 11.12. Here $S(t \mid \theta)$ has an explicit form so it is easy to evaluate at each grid point. With the MCMC samples, it is also easy to obtain probability intervals from quantiles of these samples. Although not shown, it would be easy to plot hazard functions; but here, for the exponential model, it would be a trivial plot as the hazard is constant in t.

TABLE 11.2: Comparison of posterior medians and 95% probability intervals for three sets of priors (informative, diffuse-gamma, diffuse-uniform in respective rows)

θ_1	θ_2	median1	median2	ratio
0.017	0.055	41.5	12.6	3.3
(0.010, 0.026)	(0.034, 0.085)	(27.0, 68.0)	(8.1, 20.7)	(1.7, 6.4)
0.016	0.055	44.2	12.7	3.5
(0.009, 0.025)	(0.032, 0.087)	(28.3, 74.7)	(8.0, 21.7)	(1.7, 7.0)
0.016	0.055	44.2	12.7	3.5
(0.009, 0.025)	(0.032, 0.087)	(28.3, 74.7)	(8.0, 21.7)	(1.7, 7.0)

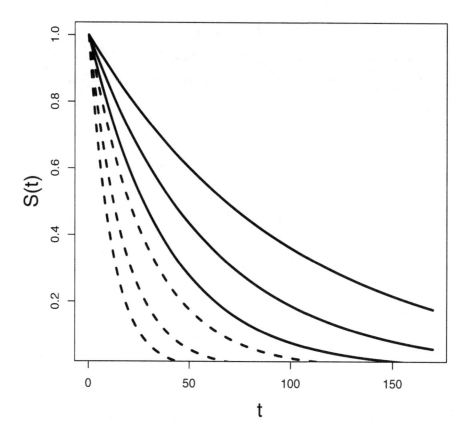

FIGURE 11.12: Posterior survival and 95% pointwise probability bands for $AG+$ (solid lines) and $AG-$ (dashed lines).

11.5   Competing Risks

As mentioned earlier in this chapter, one may be interested in characterizing the risk of failure of a given type (i.e., due to a given cause) when study participants are subject to risks of failing from different causes. If one and only one failure type can be observed, we call the different failure types *competing risks*. For example, a population-based study may follow patients until death but be interested in the cause of death. Some people may die from heart disease, some may have a stroke, others may die from cancer. Deaths can be classified as arising from a single primary cause, despite the presence of other conditions and diseases. Analyzing data in which patients are subject to competing risks is challenging because of a problem of identifiability.

First we will define terms. Let δ index the failure type, that is, $\delta = j$ if the failure is of type j, $j = 1, \ldots, J$.[3] We observe only one failure time, which will be the minimum of the (conceptual) times to failure due to all causes under consideration. That is, we observe $T = \min\{T_1, T_2, \ldots, T_J\}$. We call the instantaneous risk of failure of type j at time t, denoted $h_j(t)$, the *cause-specific hazard*:

$$h_j(t) = \lim_{\Delta t \to 0} \frac{1}{\Delta t} P\Big(T \in [t, t + \Delta t) \cap \delta = j \mid T \geq t\Big).$$

The overall hazard at time t, or the hazard of failure due to any cause, is the sum of the cause-specific hazards, $h(t) = \sum_{j=1}^{J} h_j(t)$. This follows from the J types being mutually exclusive and $(T \in [t, t + \Delta t)) = \cap_{j=1}^{J}(T \in [t, t + \Delta t) \cap \delta = j)$.

Functions of interest in competing risks are: (i) the overall or all-cause mortality represented by the function $F(t) = P(T \leq t)$, that is, the probability of death by time t *regardless of cause*; and (ii) the probability of death by time t *due to each particular cause j*, called the cumulative incidence function (CIF) for cause j and represented by $F_j(t) = P(T \leq t, \delta = j)$. The former is straightforward with all-cause hazard $h(t)$, and follows equation (11.5), so that $F(t) = 1 - \int_0^t h(s) \exp\{-\int_0^s h(u)du\}ds$. The CIF, however, does not follow from the cause-specific hazard for cause j alone. In fact, it is given by

$$F_j(t) = P(T \leq t, \delta = j) = \int_0^t h_j(s) \exp(-H(s))ds,$$

where $H(s) = \sum_{j=1}^{J} \int_0^s h_j(u)du$, is the all-cause cumulative hazard function. While $F(\cdot)$ is a distribution function, the CIF is not because its limit as $t \to \infty$ equals $P(\delta = j)$ which is typically less than 1. Except for this fact, the CIF has other required properties of a distribution function (non-negative, non-decreasing with $F(0) = 0$ for positive random variables), so it is a sub-distribution function.

From a different (i.e., multivariate) point of view, consider the joint survival function for failure times of each type, $S(t_1, t_2, \ldots, t_J) = P(T_1 \geq t_1, T_2 \geq t_2, \ldots, T_J \geq t_J)$. The cause-specific hazard can also be written as

$$h_j(t) = \frac{\frac{-\partial S(t_1, \ldots, t_J)}{\partial t_j}\big|_{t_1 = \ldots = t_J = t}}{S(t, t, \ldots, t)}.$$

---

[3]In this notation, $\delta = 0$ can indicate right censoring for the event if present. For an explanation of basic concepts and functions, censoring is not relevant.

The *net survival function*, $S_j(t)$, is derived from the joint survival function with arguments $t_k = 0$ for all k, except $k = j$: $S_j(t) = S(0, \ldots, t, \ldots, 0)$.

The identifiability problem referred to earlier arises because we only get to observe the failure time for one cause in each individual. The observed failure censors the failure times of all other causes, so we do not get to observe these other causes' potential failure times. Thus, we cannot use the data to verify any hypotheses relating to the dependence structure of the causes' times to failure. In particular, if we assume that each of the J causes acts independently, then the joint survival function is $S(t_1, \ldots, t_J) = \prod_{j=1}^{J} S_j(t)$. This relationship leads to the cause-specific hazard rate being equal to the hazard rate for cause j resulting from the net survival function. We can see this by writing

$$h_j(t) = \frac{\frac{-\partial \prod_{k=1}^{J} S_k(t_k)}{\partial t_j} \big|_{t_1 = \ldots = t_J = t}}{\prod_{k=1}^{J} S_k(t_k)} = \frac{\frac{-\partial S_j(t_j)}{\partial t_j} \big|_{t_j = t}}{S_j(t_j)}.$$

As shown by Tsiatis (1975) [332], one can find an independent risk model that is indistinguishable from a dependent risk model.

Proceeding under the assumption of independent causes, it is possible to estimate the quantities of interest in biomedical applications. These are, typically, the all-cause distribution function, the CIFs for each cause, and the cause-specific hazards. Each of these three quantities has a clearer interpretation in practice, namely, as $P(T \leq t)$, $P(T \leq t, \delta = j)$, and the instantaneous risk of event of type j, respectively. Empirical estimates of the first two follow construction similar to that of the K-M estimate of Section 11.2. Inference is more readily available for these functions from the Bayesian viewpoint. For example, the Dirichlet process mixture of Weibulls model of expression (11.16) is extended to competing risks by Shi, Laud, and Neuner [295]. We refer the reader to this paper for details, but note that the posterior sampling for this model has been implemented in the R package DPWeibull, and provide an example next.

Example 11.8. Paquid Data. The R package riskRegression contains a data set of 2,561 subjects in a prospective study of cerebral aging. The variables in the data set are time, the time to event in years; status, equal to 0 if right censored at time, 1 if event is dementia onset, and 2 if it is death without dementia.

We performed an analysis with these data using the dependent Dirichlet process Weibull model of expression (11.16) and a LIO prior. We used the DPWeibull package in R. The code is available on the book's website under Chapter 11 in the file named Paquid.R. The output object was post-processed in R to generate Figure 11.13. The two CIFs are well separated beyond 2.5 years with the probability of death without dementia exceeding that of dementia prior to death. Even so, 10% of the population is expected to develop dementia (prior to death) by year 9. The posterior distribution of any related inference target, such as the median time to dementia among those that develop it before death, can be obtained by post-processing the posterior samples in the object returned by the function dpweib() in the DPWeibull package.

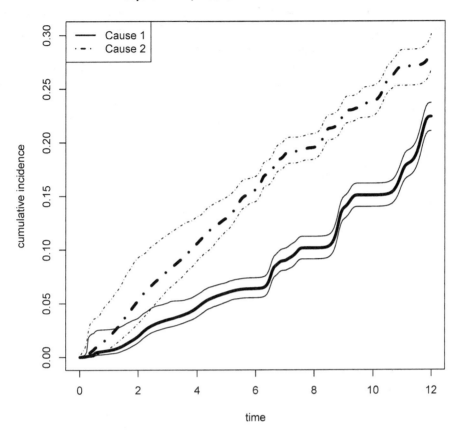

Paquid Data; Cumulative Incidence Functions

FIGURE 11.13: Posterior means of cumulative incidence functions for dementia prior to death (cause 1) and death without dementia (cause 2) in Example 11.8. Thinner lines show pointwise 95% posterior probability limits for the CIFs.

11.6   Recap and Readings

In this chapter we introduced the modeling needs of biomedical studies that primarily focus on the time to a significant medical event from some relevant time zero. One major aspect of such data is that time-to-event is restricted to the positive real line. More importantly, the sampling mechanism and analysis timings often do not allow for observation of the event for each patient. This led to what is termed censored data that required special care in writing the sampling distribution. Inference targets are also somewhat distinct here from those we saw in other chapters. We also considered nonparametric models in this chapter more than in others. This is because of the somewhat common practice of employing such general and flexible models to address time-to-event data. We should point out that parametric models can also be useful if experience in certain scientific areas justifies their use.

As we have encountered in several previous chapters, regression analyses are much more common in biomedical research than are exchangeable (or conditionally iid) sampling studies of a single homogeneous population. Time-to-event studies are no exception to this. The next chapter addresses regression in this context. Much of the current literature routinely includes regression of various types. We chose to separate the exchangeable data case in a separate chapter for pedagogical reasons. The new concepts that relate to censoring and to inference targets such as survival and hazard functions are easier to introduce without having to model how certain covariates might affect these inference targets, particularly in the presence of censoring. As most literature includes regression and treats the exchangeable data situation as a special case, we defer recommending readings until the end of the next chapter.

11.7 Exercises

EXERCISE 11.1.   Show that if $T \sim \text{Weib}(\alpha, \lambda)$, then $T^\alpha \sim \text{Exp}(\lambda)$.

EXERCISE 11.2.   Let $W \equiv \log(T) \sim N(\mu, 1/\tau)$.

(a) Derive the density and survival function for T.

(b) Show that the likelihood, and therefore the Bayesian analysis, does not depend on whether we transform the data before analyzing them in the no-censoring case.

(c) Show that this result remains true when the data are censored.

EXERCISE 11.3.   Plot hazard, density, and survival functions for the Weibull and log-normal distributions that have the following (median, 90th percentile) pairs: $(1, 20)$, $(20, 30)$, and $(50, 70)$. Compare these Weibull and log-normal models by visual inspection.

EXERCISE 11.4.   With right censoring, the data are unambiguously defined by the vectors y and δ. We now define the data for interval censoring as two vectors ξ and η where

$$\xi_i = \begin{cases} t_i, & \text{if uncensored,} \\ L_i, & \text{if censored,} \end{cases} \quad \text{and} \quad \eta_i = \begin{cases} 0, & \text{if uncensored,} \\ U_i, & \text{if censored.} \end{cases}$$

Observing that $\delta_i = 1 - I_{(0,\infty)}(\eta_i)$, write the likelihood in terms of ξ and η.

EXERCISE 11.5.   Turnbull and Weiss (1978) [334] reported data on 191 California high school boys who were asked, "When did you first use marijuana?" The data only noted ages in years, so we regard the ages as interval censored. Thus age 18 is the interval $[18, 18.99)$ in our analysis. Twelve boys indicated use before a given age, so those data are left censored. In addition, 89 boys had never used marijuana before the time of the survey, so were right censored. We regarded left and right censored observations for a given year as being in the middle of the year, thus a (left or right) censored observation for year 18 is taken as censored at 18.5 years. The data are in files with the word `marijuana` in their names on the website.

(a) Carry out a log-normal model analysis using low-information priors. Choose three interesting targets of inference and plot the posterior distributions for these.

(b) Carry out a Weibull model analysis of the same data and inference targets.

(c) Compare inferences based on the two models. Which model would you prefer, or does it matter?

EXERCISE 11.6. *Leukemia data.* Using relatively low-information priors, give plots of survival and hazard functions for the two groups in the leukemia study using:

(a) the log-normal model,

(b) the Weibull model, and

(c) the exponential model.

(d) Make comparative comments on the results of parts (a), (b) and (c).

EXERCISE 11.7. This exercise deals with priors only.

(a) For the Weibull model with a log-normal prior on α, $\log(\alpha) \sim N(c, d)$ or $\alpha \sim LN(c, d)$ and a gamma prior $\lambda \sim Ga(a, b)$ on λ, obtain the prior for (α, λ) that has median $t_{0.5} = 20$, $P(\alpha < 1) = 0.2$, $c = \log(\alpha_*) = 0$, and $P(0.69/\lambda < 50 \,|\, \alpha = 1) = 0.95$.

(b) Plot the implied prior distributions on the median and the 20-year survival probability.

(c) For the Weibull model with the uniform-Pareto prior on α and an independent gamma prior for λ, compute prior parameters with the given information. If insufficient, make reasonable additions to the information.

(d) Repeat (b) with the prior determined in (c).

(e) Compare the induced distributions from (b) and (d).

(f) Now use the exponential model for the data, with a gamma prior on its rate parameter θ. Specify the parameters of the gamma prior for λ. In doing so, you may need to ignore some of the given information if not usable.

(g) Repeat (b) with the model and prior of (f) and compare with results from (b) and (d). Comment on how the induced prior on the median using the exponential model conforms with the specified prior information on the median.

EXERCISE 11.8. Consider the uniform-Pareto hierarchical prior on α for the

Weibull model in Section 11.3.1.2. Note that most of the expressions that you are asked to derive are stated in Section 11.3.1.2.

(a) Derive the marginal distribution of α and express it as a mixture of a uniform and a Pareto, identifying the mixture probabilities.

(b) Derive the mean and variance of α. Use conditions on the parameters as necessary.

(c) Obtain an expression for $P(\alpha \leq 1)$.

(d) Obtain an expression for $F_\alpha(x) = P(\alpha \leq x)$ for $x > 0$.

(e) Find an expression for the median of α.

EXERCISE 11.9. *Log-normal model analysis.* With the arm 1 disease-free survival data from the CALGB 8541 trial (Example 11.4), use WinBUGS, JAGS or Stan to obtain posterior samples of (α, λ) for the log-normal model. For prior specification, use the settings elicited in Section 11.3.1.2. Refer to Appendix C for specifying a model with censored data in the software you use.

(a) Graph prior and posterior densities of α on the same plot.

(b) Graph prior and posterior densities of λ on the same plot.

(c) Plot posterior mean and 95% pointwise PIs for the survival function.

(d) Plot posterior mean and 95% pointwise PIs for the hazard function.

(e) Plot prior and posterior median survival time.

Chapter 12

Survival Modeling II: Time-to-Event Regression Models

In Chapter 11, we introduced the complexities associated with the analysis of censored time-to-event data and discussed some estimation methods. We now turn to regression analysis of censored data. As in other regression methods, we are interested in discovering or determining associations between explanatory variables and time until the occurrence of an event when that time may be censored. We discuss parametric, semiparametric, and nonparametric methods for censored time-to-event data. We continue using the same notation for censored times as in Chapter 11, namely, individual i's outcome is a pair of observations (y_i, δ_i), with δ_i an indicator of whether y_i is an observed failure time or a censored time. In addition, we now include a vector of p explanatory variables for individual i, x_i.

12.1   Accelerated Failure-Time Regression Models

Parametric regression models for failure-time data generally consider a linear model for the logarithm of the failure times. A commonly used class of parametric regression models for these data is the accelerated failure-time (AFT) model,

$$\log(T_i) = x_i'\beta + \sigma\varepsilon_i, \quad \varepsilon_i \overset{iid}{\sim} F_\varepsilon(\cdot). \tag{12.1}$$

In model (12.1), ε_i is a residual term with cdf $F_\varepsilon(\cdot)$, and σ is a scale parameter. The β are, of course, the regression coefficients. The "survival" function is $S_\varepsilon(w) = 1 - F_\varepsilon(w)$ and the "hazard" function is $h_\varepsilon(w) = f_\varepsilon(w)/S_\varepsilon(w)$, where $f_\varepsilon(w)$ is the pdf corresponding to $F_\varepsilon(w)$. If we want to indicate that a random variable T is characterized by any AFT model, we will write $T \overset{ind}{\sim} AFT(F_\varepsilon, \beta, \tau \mid x)$, leaving out the subscript i.

These are called accelerated failure-time models because of the following property. Let $V = e^{\sigma\varepsilon}$, and let $S_0(c) = P(V > c)$. Model (12.1) implies, then, that $T = e^{x'\beta}V$. As a result,

$$P(T > t \mid X = x, \beta) = P(V > te^{-x'\beta} \mid X = x, \beta)$$
$$= S_0\{t \exp(-x'\beta)\}$$
$$= S_0(te^{-\beta_1 - \tilde{x}'\tilde{\beta}}),$$

where $\tilde{\beta}$ and $\tilde{x}$ are just β and x with the first components removed. If $\tilde{x} = 0$, the survival function is just $S_0(te^{-\beta_1})$. We see, then, that the effect of the covariates $\tilde{x}$ on the survival probability is to rescale the time by a factor of $\exp(-\tilde{x}'\tilde{\beta})$.

In the preceding, the observed failure times T follow different distributions, according to the assumed form of the distribution of the random variable ε (F_ε), conditioning on the coefficients. When $\varepsilon \sim N(0, 1)$, we have a log-normal AFT. If instead the density function of ε is $f(w) = \exp(w - e^w)$, $-\infty < w < \infty$, which corresponds to the extreme value distribution, we get a Weibull AFT. Now, the survival function for T is

$$S(t \mid x, \beta, \sigma) = \exp\left\{-\exp\left(\frac{\ln(t) - x'\beta}{\sigma}\right)\right\}.$$

Letting $S_0(t) = \exp(-t^{1/\sigma})$ be the survival function of a Weibull distribution, we get

$$S(t \mid x, \beta) = \exp\left\{-t^{1/\sigma} \exp\left(\frac{-x'\beta}{\sigma}\right)\right\}$$
$$= \exp\left\{-[t\exp(-x'\beta)]^{1/\sigma}\right\} = S_0\{t\exp(-x'\beta)\}.$$

If $\sigma = 1$, the sampling distribution of the failure times is the exponential distribution.

When fitting model (12.1) to data, we need the survival function. Individual i's covariate vector is x_i, and their failure time is T_i, possibly censored. The survival function is

$$\begin{aligned}
S(t \mid x, \beta, \sigma^2) &= P(T > t \mid x, \beta, \sigma^2) \\
&= P\left\{\log(T) > \log(t) \mid x, \beta, \sigma^2\right\} \\
&= P\left[\{\log(T) - x'\beta\}/\sigma > \{\log(t) - x'\beta\}/\sigma \mid x, \beta, \sigma^2\right] \\
&= P\left[\varepsilon > \{\log(t) - x'\beta\}/\sigma \mid x, \beta, \sigma^2\right] \\
&= S_\varepsilon\left[\{\log(t) - x'\beta\}/\sigma\right] \\
&= 1 - F_\varepsilon\left[\{\log(t) - x'\beta\}/\sigma\right].
\end{aligned} \tag{12.2}$$

The density and hazard functions that correspond to the regression model (12.2) are

$$f(t \mid x, \beta, \sigma^2) = \frac{1}{\sigma t} f_\varepsilon\left[\{\log(t) - x'\beta\}/\sigma\right],$$
$$h(t \mid x, \beta, \sigma^2) = \frac{1}{\sigma t} h_\varepsilon\left[\{\log(t) - x'\beta\}/\sigma\right].$$

If F_ε is the standard normal distribution (i.e., $\varepsilon \sim N(0, 1)$), then

$$f(t_i \mid x_i, \beta, \sigma^2) = \frac{1}{\sqrt{2\pi\sigma^2}} \frac{1}{t_i} \exp\left[-\frac{1}{2\sigma^2} \{\log(t_i) - x_i'\beta\}^2\right],$$

and $T_i \sim LN(x_i'\beta, \sigma^2)$. If ε has the extreme value distribution, then $T_i \sim Weib(1/\sigma, e^{-x_i'\beta/\sigma})$.

In the regression part of model (12.1), the β vector consists of the regression coefficients. We note that e^{μ} is the median of a random variable with a $LN(\mu, \sigma^2)$ distribution. We can then easily show that the median of T is $e^{x'\beta}$ if we consider T to follow a log-normal AFT model. We include an intercept in the regression model, so $x_{i1} = 1$ and x_i has $p+1$ elements, namely, a 1 and individual i's p covariates. We again often standardize the covariates, which makes it easier to elicit priors on observable quantities that are functions of the βs. For example, if $x_i = (1, 0, \dots, 0)'$, which corresponds to someone with average values for continuous covariates and the baseline values for discrete covariates, then β_1 is the regression parameter for a standard reference individual.

Recall that a particular AFT model includes the distributional assumption $\varepsilon \sim F_{\varepsilon}(\cdot)$. Let $\tilde{t}_{\varepsilon}$ be the median of this distribution (i.e., $F_{\varepsilon}(\tilde{t}_{\varepsilon}) = 0.5$). If $T \sim \text{AFT}(F_{\varepsilon}, \beta, \sigma^2 \mid x)$, then the median time until the event (t_m) satisfies $0.5 = S(t_m \mid x, \beta, \sigma^2)$. From the survival function in equation (12.2), we have

$$0.5 = 1 - F_{\varepsilon}\left[\{\log(t_m) - x'\beta\}/\sigma\right]$$

which means that

$$\tilde{t}_{\varepsilon} = \{\log(t_m) - x'\beta\}/\sigma$$

or, equivalently,

$$t_m = \exp(x'\beta + \tilde{t}_{\varepsilon}\sigma).$$

Since t_m is a function of the covariates x, we also write $t_m(x)$.

If F_{ε} has median zero, then $\tilde{t}_{\varepsilon} = 0$ and $t_m(x) = \exp(x'\beta)$. This will be the case if ε has a standard normal distribution or a logistic distribution, for example. We can also rewrite the extreme value distribution so $\tilde{t}_{\varepsilon} = 0$, namely,

$$F_{\varepsilon}(u) = 1 - \exp\{-\log(2)e^u\}. \tag{12.3}$$

For eliciting priors, we will often be interested in the relative median. Comparing someone whose covariate is x_1, possibly a vector, to someone with covariate equal to x_2, we find the relative median is $\exp\{(x_1 - x_2)\beta\}$.

Biomedical researchers are also generally interested in hazard ratios in much the same way they characterize covariate effects via relative risks when considering binary outcomes. When considering covariates x_1 and x_2, the hazard ratio with an AFT model is

$$HR = \frac{h(t \mid x_1, \beta, \sigma^2)}{h(t \mid x_2, \beta, \sigma^2)} = \frac{h_{\varepsilon}\left(\{\log(t) - x_1'\beta\}/\sigma\right)}{h_{\varepsilon}\left(\{\log(t) - x_2'\beta\}/\sigma\right)}.$$

As we have throughout the book, we often focus on prediction. In survival analysis, one might think of predictive survival probabilities in one of two ways. A predictive probability associated with covariate x may apply to the individual if that individual has that covariate (or set of covariate values) or as a prediction of the fraction of the population with covariate x that survive. Considering the proportion of the population surviving interpretation, we can approximate predictive survival probabilities at time t as $S(t \mid x, \beta, \sigma^2) = 1 - F_\varepsilon \left[\{\log(t) - x'\beta\} / \sigma \right]$. We can then generate pointwise probability intervals for predictive survival probabilities at multiple times, showing uncertainty along with the prediction.

Example 12.1. Cancer of the Larynx. Kardaun [203] published an analysis of 90 men with cancer of the larynx, and Klein and Moeschberger [204] included this data set in their survival analysis textbook. The outcome is months from diagnosis until death or censoring for each of the men, and there are with three covariates: the stage of the disease at diagnosis (*Stage*), the year of diagnosis (*Yr*), and the age at diagnosis (*Age*). In our analysis, we consider stage 1 the baseline or comparator category and create indicator variables for each stage ($S_{ij} = 1$ if the ith man's stage of disease is $j = 2, 3,$ or 4; 0 otherwise). The analysis considers the standardized versions of age (*sAge*) and year of diagnosis (*sYr*). The resulting regression model, leaving out person i's subscripts for ease of reading, is

$$\log(T) = \beta_1 + \beta_2 \, S_2 + \beta_3 \, S_3 + \beta_4 \, S_4 + \beta_5 \, sAge + \beta_6 \, sYr + \sigma\varepsilon,$$

with $\varepsilon \sim N(0, 1)$.

With this model, the median time to death from diagnosis is e^{β_1} for a man whose age and year of diagnosis (from 1900) equal the average age of 64.6 years and 74.2, respectively. The median survival time of a man whose disease is stage 2, relative to a man with stage 1 disease, is e^{β_1} when both are of average age and their year of diagnosis equals the average diagnosis year. An increase in a man's age of one sample standard deviation unit (10.8 years) leads to a change in the median time to death of e^{β_5} when the two men were otherwise diagnosed in the same year with the same stage of disease. Similarly, a one sample standard deviation unit (2.2 years) difference in year of diagnosis (all other covariates the same) will lead to a relative median time to death equal to e^{β_6}.

We fit a log-normal AFT model to the data using BUGS. The book's website has the BUGS program, as well as versions for JAGS and Stan. The files have `LarynxLogNormal` in the name. (Each of these programs handles censoring differently.) Table 12.1 contains summary statistics for the posterior distributions of the model parameters. The 95% posterior (or data-informed) PI for the effect of stage 2 disease on median time to death relative to stage 1 (e^{β_2}) does not show much effect. Stages 3 and 4 do appear to be associated with much shorter median times to death from diagnosis (i.e., e^{β_3} and e^{β_4}). For stage 4 disease, we are 95% certain that stage 1 disease at diagnosis is associated with longer median time to death that is between 3 ($\approx 1/0.36$) times and 20 ($\approx 1/0.05$) times longer. The coefficient for age (β_5) has more probability below zero, suggesting that older patients tend to have shorter survival from diagnosis. Diagnosis in later years (β_6) appears to lead to better survival, but the coefficient is not very far from zero, relative to its uncertainty. Furthermore, we would expect more time since diagnosis to be associated with greater risk of dying.

Since the 95% PIs for the age and the year of diagnosis coefficients contain 0, there is not much statistical import. We can consider posterior probabilities as evidence of an association. For age, $P(\beta_5 < 0 \mid D) = 0.90$, indicating that most of

TABLE 12.1: Log-normal regression fit to the larynx cancer data

Node	mean	sd	2.5%	median	97.5%
β_1	2.33	0.32	1.75	2.32	3.01
β_2	−0.25	0.51	−1.25	−0.25	0.76
β_3	−0.97	0.41	−1.81	−0.96	−0.17
β_4	−2.02	0.53	−3.09	−2.00	−1.01
β_5	−0.22	0.17	−0.56	−0.22	0.10
β_6	0.13	0.19	−0.24	0.12	0.52
e^{β_2} St2/St1	0.89	0.49	0.29	0.78	2.11
e^{β_3} St3/St1	0.41	0.17	0.17	0.38	0.83
e^{β_4} St4/St1	0.15	0.08	0.05	0.14	0.36
$e^{\beta_3-\beta_4}$ St3/St4	3.23	1.83	1.07	2.80	7.89
e^{β_5} $(Age+1\text{sd})/Age$	0.81	0.14	0.57	0.80	1.11
e^{β_6} $(Yr+1\text{sd})/Yr$	1.15	0.22	0.80	1.12	1.63
σ	1.40	0.17	1.12	1.38	1.76

the support is for values below zero. For year of diagnosis, the probability that the coefficient is positive is $P(\beta_6 > 0 \mid D) = 0.74$. The evidence appears stronger for an age effect on survival than for the year of diagnosis affecting survival.

We also evaluate each covariate's effect on survival by comparing median survival times and survival probabilities. Table 12.2 shows estimates of median survival times and 5-month survival probabilities for different stages. Specifically, we can compare median survival times for men who were 50 years old to that of men 70 years old when diagnosed, conditioning on the year of diagnosis being 1971 or 1977. A 50-year-old man diagnosed with stage 2 cancer of the larynx in 1971 has a median time to death of around 9 months. If this same man were diagnosed in 1977 instead, however, the model estimated median time to death is 12 months. Median survival times for 70-year-old men diagnosed in 1971 or 1977 were around 6 or 8 months, respectively, which is a smaller difference. We note that the relative medians are about 1.33 with the later year of diagnosis, which is the same for the 50-year-old men and for the 70-year-old men. A comparable examination of median survival time effects among men with stage 4 disease shows very little effect in terms of months. The differences in medians are roughly one-half to three-quarters of a month. Stage 4 disease has such a poor prognosis in these data that there is relatively little practical difference.

The analysis suggests that there is a substantial difference between stage 3 and stage 4 disease. Table 12.1 contains some summary statistics for the effect of stage 3 relative to stage 4. The posterior median of the relative median survivals is 2.8, and the 95% PI is (1.07, 7.89). In fact, the posterior probability that the stage 3 median survival is longer than it is for stage 4 disease is almost 1 ($P(e^{(\beta_3-\beta_4)} > 1 \mid D) = 0.981$). We are 98% certain that those with stage 3 disease will live longer

TABLE 12.2: Median survival times and 5-month survival probabilities estimated from a log-normal regression analysis of the larynx data

	Node	mean	sd	2.5%	median	97.5%
Stage 2 Medians	$Age = 50, Yr = 71$	10.6	6.9	3.1	8.9	28.2
	$Age = 50, Yr = 77$	14.5	9.9	4.5	12.0	39.3
	$Age = 70, Yr = 71$	6.8	3.8	2.3	5.9	16.3
	$Age = 70, Yr = 77$	9.3	5.1	3.4	8.0	22.5
Stage 4 Medians	$Age = 50, Yr = 71$	1.83	1.18	0.48	1.55	4.93
	$Age = 50, Yr = 77$	2.42	1.40	0.80	2.10	5.99
	$Age = 70, Yr = 71$	1.18	0.66	0.36	1.03	2.83
	$Age = 70, Yr = 77$	1.55	0.72	0.62	1.40	3.35
Stage 1 5-month surv.	$Age = 50, Yr = 71$	0.72	0.10	0.51	0.73	0.88
	$Age = 50, Yr = 77$	0.78	0.10	0.56	0.79	0.94
	$Age = 70, Yr = 71$	0.62	0.09	0.43	0.62	0.79
	$Age = 70, Yr = 77$	0.69	0.10	0.48	0.70	0.87
Stage 3 5-month surv.	$Age = 50, Yr = 71$	0.46	0.12	0.24	0.46	0.70
	$Age = 50, Yr = 77$	0.55	0.12	0.31	0.55	0.78
	$Age = 70, Yr = 71$	0.35	0.10	0.17	0.35	0.56
	$Age = 70, Yr = 77$	0.44	0.11	0.23	0.43	0.66

TABLE 12.3: Weibull regression fit to the larynx cancer data

Node	mean	sd	2.5%	med	97.5%
β_1	2.22	0.29	1.71	2.20	2.86
β_2	−0.14	0.49	−1.07	−0.15	0.86
β_3	−0.66	0.38	−1.45	−0.65	0.05
β_4	−1.69	0.46	−2.64	−1.68	−0.83
β_5	−0.21	0.16	−0.54	−0.21	0.09
β_6	0.09	0.18	−0.24	0.08	0.45
e^{β_2} St2/St1	0.99	0.54	0.35	0.87	2.37
e^{β_3} St3/St1	0.55	0.21	0.24	0.52	1.04
e^{β_4} St4/St1	0.20	0.10	0.07	0.19	0.43
e^{β_5} $(Age +1sd)/Age$	0.82	0.13	0.58	0.81	1.11
e^{β_6} $(Yr +1sd)/Yr$	1.10	0.20	0.78	1.08	1.58
σ	1.007	0.14	0.77	0.99	1.32

TABLE 12.4: Median survival times and 5-month survival probabilities estimated from a Weibull regression analysis of the larynx data

	Node	mean	sd	2.5%	med	97.5%
Stage 2	$Age = 50, Yr = 77$	13.64	8.67	4.86	11.42	35.72
Medians	$Age = 70, Yr = 77$	8.67	5.26	3.43	7.71	22.3
Stage 4	$Age = 50, Yr = 77$	2.75	1.36	1.10	2.45	6.19
Medians	$Age = 70, Yr = 77$	1.77	0.66	0.87	1.7	3.39
Stage 1	$Age = 50, Yr = 77$	0.76	0.09	0.55	0.77	0.90
5-month surv.	$Age = 70, Yr = 77$	0.67	0.10	0.45	0.68	0.84
Stage 3	$Age = 50, Yr = 77$	0.59	0.12	0.33	0.60	0.81
5-month surv.	$Age = 70, Yr = 77$	0.47	0.13	0.22	0.47	0.71

than those with stage 4 disease if the two men are diagnosed in the same year and are the same age at the time.

Table 12.2 contains posterior calculations that allow us to compare 5-month survival probabilities for men with the same ages and diagnosed in the same two years we have been examining. Not unexpectedly, 50-year-old men diagnosed with stage 1 disease in 1977 have substantially better 5-month survival probabilities than do 70-year-old men diagnosed in 1971 with stage 3 disease; the 95% PIs do not overlap, according to the table.

As shown earlier, we get a Weibull AFT model when F_ε is the extreme value distribution. Specifically, we have that $T \sim Weib(1/\sigma, e^{x'\beta/\sigma})$. With the modified version of the pdf that has median 0, $F_\varepsilon(u) = 1 - \exp\{-\log(2)e^u\}$, we get

$$T \sim Weib(1/\sigma, \log(2)e^{-x'\beta/\sigma}).$$

We carried out an analysis of the laryngeal cancer data with this form of the Weibull AFT model. The results are in Table 12.3. Comparing the Weibull results to those in Table 12.1, we see that the overall inferences are quite similar with the two models (Weibull and log-normal AFTs). Consider two men with stage 2 disease when diagnosed in 1977. The log-normal AFT model (Table 12.2) indicates a median survival of 12 months if the man is 50 years old when diagnosed and 8 months if the man is 70 years old at diagnosis. The Weibull AFT analysis (Table 12.4) gave estimated median survival times of 11.4 months and 7.7 months for a man 50 years old and 70 years old, respectively. This quantifies the similarity of age effect on the more direct scale of median survival and is a reflection of the similarity of inferences for the age regression coefficient: -0.22 (95% PI $(-0.56, 0.10)$) with the log-normal AFT and -0.21 $(-0.54, 0.09)$ with the Weibull AFT.

12.1.1   Prior Distributions for AFT Parameters

The parameters in the AFT model are (β, σ^2), the regression coefficients and the variance, much like we saw in Chapter 7. We could consider the standard reference prior $p(\beta, \tau) \propto 1/\tau$ (τ equal to the precision) or some variant of it (see Ibrahim and Laud [172]).

With a log-normal AFT, we could consider the prior from Section 7.3, that is, $p(\beta, \sigma^2) = p(\beta)p(\sigma^2)$, with a normal distribution for the former and an inverse-gamma distribution for the latter. (If one works with the precision, one works with a gamma distribution for $\tau = 1/\sigma^2$.) Without censoring, this prior would be conjugate for log-normal data. With censored data, however, we no longer have a conjugate model. We also do not have conjugacy if the AFT model has a residual distribution (F_ε) that is neither normal nor log-normal. With large samples, however, the posterior distribution β will be approximately normal, so we might consider using this normal-inverse-gamma prior anyway.

As is our preference, we seek to specify prior distributions for observable or more commonplace measurements and not directly on the regression coefficients in complex models. Bedrick, Christensen, and Johnson [25] proposed specifying priors on median survival times and thereby inducing prior distributions on the βs in AFT models. They assumed independence of the βs and σ^2 (or $\tau = 1/\sigma^2$) *a priori*, which allows one to specify priors $p(\beta)$ separately from priors $p(\sigma^2)$.

12.1.1.1   Specifying $p(\beta)$

As stated when we introduced the AFT model, the median survival time t_m equals $e^{x'\beta}$ if the median of F_ε is zero. Therefore, with the right distribution for the residuals (i.e., the εs), we can ask our experts their opinions about median survival times for individuals with various different covariate values. We start by considering a set of $p+1$ linearly independent vectors of covariates. The ith covariate vector is denoted $\tilde{x}_i$ and consists of a specific constellation of covariate values that define an individual whose median survival we elicit from the expert. That is, $\tilde{x}_i = (1, \tilde{x}_{i1}, \ldots, \tilde{x}_{ip})'$, where $\tilde{x}_{ij}$ is the value of the jth covariate of the individual defined by $\tilde{x}_i$.

For someone with covariate vector $\tilde{x}_i$, the median survival time is $t_{m_i} = e^{\tilde{x}_i'\beta}$. Let the matrix $\tilde{X} = (\tilde{x}_{i1}, \ldots, \tilde{x}_{p+1})'$ and define the vector of expert-elicited medians $t_m = (t_{m_1}, \ldots, t_{m_{p+1}})'$. Then $\boldsymbol{t}_m = \exp(\tilde{X}\beta)$ and $\beta = \tilde{X}^{-1} \log(\boldsymbol{t}_m)$ (if $\tilde{X}$ is nonsingular). If the expert can express an opinion about each median independently of the others, we can assume prior independence of the t_{m_i} and consider the joint prior $p(\boldsymbol{t}_m) = \prod_{i=1}^{p+1} p_i(t_{m_i})$, where $p_i(t_{m_i})$ is the prior distribution for this particular median.

We are eliciting priors on the scale of the data, so we have to consider the induced prior on the βs as a transformation of variables if we write out the densities. (See Appendix A for a review of transformation of random variables.) In our setting, one can show that the Jacobian of the transformation is proportional to $\prod_{i=1}^{p+1} e^{\tilde{x}_i'\beta}$. If we use BUGS or JAGS, we are able to specify the prior distribution for the medians and let the MCMC induce the prior on the βs.

It is often convenient to consider a log-normal prior for the medians when inducing a prior for the βs, although any distribution on the positive real line will do. With a log-normal distribution for the median, we treat the elicited median survival times as medians of the respective distributions. That is, if the expert's best guess for t_{m_i} is $\tilde{m}_{0i}$, we set the median of $p(t_{m_i})$ to be $\tilde{m}_{0i}$. We determine the variance of the log-normal prior distribution by eliciting an upper (or lower) percentile for the median survival time for each set of individuals defined by the $\tilde{x}_i$. That is, we ask the expert for an upper (or lower) bound for the median t_{m_i} that they are, say, 95% certain is above (or below) the median. This upper bound leads to a prior standard deviation for the prior distribution of the median survival time for an individual with covariates $\tilde{x}_i$. Call the resulting standard deviation $\tilde{\sigma}_{0i}$. This process is much like what we did in Chapter 7 and elsewhere in the book. With a log-normal prior, we have

$$t_{m_i} \overset{\text{ind}}{\sim} LN(\log(\tilde{m}_{0i}), \tilde{\sigma}_{0i}^2)$$

or

$$\log(t_{m_i}) \overset{\text{ind}}{\sim} N(\log(\tilde{m}_{0i}), \tilde{\sigma}_{0i}^2).$$

If we want to move beyond normal or log-normal priors, we can consider any AFT in which the residual distribution has median 0. We would specify the prior via the following (where the residual $\varepsilon \sim F_\varepsilon$):

$$\frac{\log(t_{mi}) - \log(\tilde{m}_{0i})}{\sigma_{0i}} \overset{\text{ind}}{\sim} F_\varepsilon. \tag{12.4}$$

The Weibull AFT model is considered for prior elicitation by Bedrick, Christensen, and Johnson [25], along with other AFT models. Just as we described for the log-normal case, the prior for the median survival times characterized in expression (12.4) induces the prior density for the βs from the relationship $\beta = \tilde{X}^{-1}\log(t_m)$. Also, as before, we determine σ_{0i}^2 by asking the expert for an upper bound $\tilde{u}_i$ such that $P(t_{mi} < \tilde{u}_i) = \alpha$. Then, with q_α the 100αth percentile of F_ε, we find the standard deviation σ_{0i} by solving the following equation for it:

$$q_\alpha = \frac{\log(\tilde{u}_i) - \log(\tilde{m}_{0i})}{\sigma_{0i}}.$$

For example, consider the Weibull AFT as given in equation (12.3). If $q_{0.95}$ is the 95th percentile of the residual distribution, then $F_\varepsilon(q_{0.95}) = 0.95$. From equation (12.3), we have $F_\varepsilon(q_{0.95}) = 1 - \exp\{-\log(2)e^{q_{0.95}}\}$. Therefore, $0.95 = 1 - \exp\{-\log(2)e^{q_{0.95}}\}$ and $-\log(2)e^{q_{0.95}} = \log(0.05)$, or $q_{0.95} = \log\{\log(0.05)/(-\log(2))\} = 1.46$.

Example 12.2. Effect of Chemotherapy to Treat Breast Cancer. We illustrate using an elicited prior within a parametric AFT regression model using data from a randomized clinical trial carried out by the Cancer and Leukemia Group B [161]. The study randomized more than 3,000 women with breast cancer having nodal involvement to one of six treatment regimens. The study followed a factorial design that evaluated three doses of the anticancer agent doxorubicin with or without paclitaxel (Taxol), another anticancer drug. In this analysis, we will look at the possibility of an interaction between paclitaxel and estrogen-receptor status.

Our elicited priors are for median disease-free survival. Disease-free survival (DFS) is a common outcome measure in oncology and is defined as the time until relapse, recurrence, or death, whichever occurs first. We apply the model in expression (12.1) with a Weibull residual distribution. Based on historical studies at the time this study was designed, the expectation was that the median DFS would be around 7 years for these women, and the covariates would lead to a deviation from this baseline. Table 12.5 shows the prior estimates for the medians, 95th percentiles, and standard deviations in the analysis. In the table, we used the following abbreviations for the covariates. Paclitaxel is coded T, ER status is ER, having four or more positive lymph nodes is $LN4+$, and the interaction of paclitaxel and ER status is $T{:}ER$.

TABLE 12.5: Specification of the prior based on disease-free survival (years) in the breast cancer example

i	Int.	T	ER	$LN4+$	$T{:}ER$	$\tilde{m}_{0i}$	95%	$\tilde{\sigma}_{0i}$
1	1	0	0	0	0	7.0	12.0	0.369
2	1	1	0	0	0	8.5	13.5	0.317
3	1	0	1	0	0	8.0	13.0	0.333
4	1	0	0	1	0	6.0	11.0	0.415
5	1	1	1	0	1	9.0	14.0	0.303

Summary statistics from the posterior distribution are shown in Table 12.6. We notice that the interaction between paclitaxel and ER status appears to be negative, and there appears to be some strength to this deviation from zero. The posterior mean is -0.154 and the 95% PI is $(-0.36, 0.04)$. In fact, the posterior probability that the interaction term is negative is 0.94, based on the MCMC. We also see that one's DFS is expected to be shorter if one has four or more positive lymph nodes on examination. The posterior mean is -0.43 and the 95% PI is $(-0.52, -0.33)$, which is far from zero in terms of the estimate's posterior standard deviation.

A plot of the hazard functions provides some insight into the nature of the interaction. Figure 12.1a contains posterior mean estimates of survival curves for four groups of women in the trial, all of whom had four or more positive lymph nodes. Figure 12.1b shows the posterior mean hazard functions for women in these same four groups. We see that the benefit of paclitaxel in terms of reducing the risk of an event is larger among women who are ER negative than it is for women who are ER positive.

Partial Prior Information for β.   In Sections 7.3.4 and 8.4.2 we saw that one

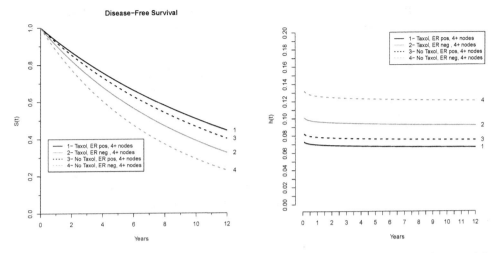

(a) Disease-free survival from Weibull AFT model.

(b) Hazards from Weibull AFT model.

FIGURE 12.1: Posterior estimates of the disease-free survival probabilities and hazard functions from an AFT model with an interaction between Taxol and ER status among women with four or more positive lymph nodes.

can specify fewer than all $p+1$ quantities (medians in the AFT case) to induce priors on the regression coefficients. As in the other regression settings, we first standardize all continuous covariates. Suppose we specify independent prior distributions on $q < p + 1$ median survival times $t_{mi} = e^{\tilde{x}'_i \beta}$, $i = 1, \ldots, q$. With the q covariate vectors, we have a $q \times (p + 1)$ matrix $\tilde{X} = (\tilde{X}_1, 0)$, with $\tilde{X}_1$ a $q \times q$ non-singular matrix and the remaining columns set to 0. Suppose that β_1^* is the set of coefficients most relevant to the specified medians. We can rearrange the vector β into (β_1^*, β_2^*). We then have $t_{mi} = e^{\tilde{x}'_i \beta_1^*}$, $i = 1, \ldots, q$, which will induce a prior distribution for $\beta_1^* = \tilde{X}'_1 \log(t_m)$. For the remaining regression coefficients (β_2^*), we consider independent reference priors. As before, we have specified more informed priors for a subset of the regression coefficients and less informed priors for the remaining ones.

12.1.1.2 Specifying $p(\sigma)$

We specify the prior distribution for σ (or $\tau = 1/\sigma^2$) in much the same way as with models we have already discussed, including when we specified the standard deviation of the prior for β in Section 12.1.1.1. If the residual distribution in our AFT model has median 0, then we can think about another percentile of the survival distribution of T, the time until the event of interest. The steps are similar to those we discuss in reference to expression (12.4). The difference is that we were thinking about uncertainty regarding the median in expression (12.4), but now we

TABLE 12.6: Summary of posterior distribution of Weibull AFT regression parameters from an analysis of women with four or more positive lymph nodes treated in a breast cancer randomized clinical trial

β	Moments		Posterior percentiles				
	Mean	Std dev.	2.5	25	50	75	97.5
Int.	2.520	0.059	2.406	2.481	2.520	2.560	2.637
T	0.276	0.079	0.116	0.222	0.276	0.329	0.431
ER	0.485	0.073	0.346	0.435	0.486	0.537	0.625
$LN4+$	−0.430	0.050	−0.523	−0.464	−0.431	−0.398	−0.331
$T{:}ER$	−0.154	0.103	−0.364	−0.220	−0.153	−0.087	0.042
shape	0.980	0.023	0.937	0.964	0.981	0.995	1.026

are considering uncertainty or variation of the survival times around some central value.

One may be concerned that variation may increase with the central tendency of the failure times. Populations in which times to the event tend to take longer may exhibit larger variation in failure times than populations with shorter failure times. If we specify the same scale term σ for all populations (see expression (12.1)) then we will automatically have more variation in groups that tend to show longer times until the occurrence of the event and less variation among those in the populations that tend to experience the event sooner. Since AFT regression models refer to $\log(T)$, it reasonable to assume that σ may be the same across the covariate-defined subpopulations in our data analysis. (See also Section 7.3.3.2.) As a consequence, we may also just focus on one of the covariate-defined subgroups to determine an informed prior distribution for σ.

Let us reconsider the breast cancer trial we analyzed in Example 12.2 and use the group defined by covariate vector $\tilde{x}_1$ for our purpose. Recall that our best guess of the median DFS for this group is $\tilde{m}_1$. As we stated in the example, our expectation was that the median disease-free survival in that population of women was 7 years. We might think that 90% of women diagnosed with similar breast cancer conditions would relapse, experience a disease recurrence, or die within 15 years. Let $q_{0.9}$ be the proposed 90th percentile of the time to event outcome T for the group defined by covariate vector $\tilde{x}_1$. From the AFT regression model (12.1), $\exp(\tilde{x}_1'\beta + \sigma q_{0.9}) = \tilde{m}_1 \exp(\sigma q_{0.9})$. (Recall that we are assuming that F_ε has $q_{0.5} = 0$.) If the best guess for this percentile is 15 years and we consider this quantity to be the center of the 90th percentile, we can combine this information with the best guess for the median $\tilde{m}_1$ and solve for σ_{01}:

$$0.5 = P\{\tilde{m}_1 \exp(\sigma q_{0.9}) \leq 15 \mid \tilde{m}_1 = 7\}$$

$$= P\left\{\frac{\log\left(\tilde{m}_1 e^{\sigma q_{0.9}}\right) - \log(\tilde{m}_1)}{q_{0.9}} \leq \frac{\log(15) - \log(7)}{q_{0.9}} \middle| \tilde{m}_1 = 7\right\}$$

$$= P\left(\sigma \leq \frac{0.7621}{q_{0.9}}\right).$$

If our AFT has a Weibull distribution, then $q_{0.9} = 1.201$. With a log-normal AFT model, $q_{0.9} = 1.282$. Another distribution that appears in AFT analyses is the log-logistic distribution, for which $q_{0.9} = 2.197$. We remind the reader that these percentiles are on the scale of $\log(T)$, as is the AFT model. For the Weibull distribution in Example 12.2, we find $\sigma_0 = 0.635$. This σ_0 is our "best guess." We can let $p(\sigma) \sim U(0, \sigma_{\max})$, where $\sigma_{\max}$ is a clear upper bound for the standard deviation. We used 4 as the upper bound in Example 12.2, feeling quite certain that the variation in disease-free survival times would not be as large as $\exp(4)$.

Alternatively, we might want to treat σ_0 as the median of the prior distribution of σ in the AFT model. We could then specify another percentile for this parameter or for the precision $\tau = 1/\sigma^2$, as we have done in earlier chapters. In Section 5.3.2, we discussed how to determine an informed gamma prior for a parameter. We can do the same thing in this situation. Considering $\tau_0 = 1/\sigma_0^2$ to be the mode of $p(\tau)$ and $\tau \sim Ga(a_0, b_0)$, we can follow the procedures we followed in Section 5.3.2 to determine a_0 and b_0.

12.1.2 Sensitivity Analysis

As with all data analyses, it is important to examine if the inferences are sensitive to assumptions. When we carry out a Bayesian analysis, we are not only interested in assumptions regarding the sampling distribution posited for the data but may also be curious about the sensitivity of inferences to assumptions about prior distributions. In the survival analysis setting, we can examine posterior survival probabilities at individual time points or the entire posterior mean survival curve under different prior assumptions as a way to evaluate sensitivity to assumptions about priors—particularly priors for the regression coefficients. We want to bring knowledge into our analyses, but we also want to be able to demonstrate to others that we are not just presenting our prior views in the posterior inferences. A simple approach to sensitivity analysis is to reanalyze the data with vaguer (i.e., more diffuse) prior distributions. In the extreme, one can analyze the data with a standard reference prior $p(\beta, \sigma^2) \propto 1/\sigma^2$ (or in terms of $\tau = 1/\sigma^2$, $p(\beta, \tau) \propto 1/\tau$) and compare the results to the analysis with more informed priors. Large discrepancies in posterior means, particularly with respect to important outcomes, may suggest that one take a closer look to see what is going on.

Such a sensitivity analysis may also help elucidate the relative importance of individual covariates on the final inference. Regression coefficients in AFTs relate to the effect of a covariate on the logarithm of time, which may not be a very intuitive scale for many researchers. Showing survival curves or survival probabilities at different times may be more immediately understood and appreciated. For example, fitting a model to learn about the association between duration of treatment and time to relapse may yield a posterior distribution for the treatment duration's regression coefficient that is positive but spans 0. If adding 6 months of treatment does not lead to much separation of the survival curves out to 10 years, then one may have a better sense of the practical import (or lack thereof) of the covariate than one gets from the posterior distribution of the treatment duration's regression coefficient.

An important tool to help sensitivity analyses is the ability to compare a more restrictive model to one that is less restrictive but may include the former model as a special case. The next section relaxes the AFT model's assumption about the distribution of the residual term (i.e., the assumption about the distribution of $\log(T)$) by making no assumptions about the underlying hazard function.

12.2   Proportional Hazards: A Semiparametric Model

While fully parametric regression models, such as the AFT models we have discussed, often offer advantages, especially when they are fairly close to the truth, these models could lead one's inference astray. The distributions we considered for AFT models were all unimodal. Given the relationship between the hazard function and the density function, these unimodal densities may not be able to characterize different but real hazard functions. For example, the risk of another stroke may be high right after experiencing one and undergoing an invasive procedure. Thereafter, the risk may decline sharply only to start to rise again after a fairly long time. Such a U-shaped hazard function will be difficult to capture with the AFT models we discussed in Section 12.1.

Here we consider a ubiquitous approach that is semiparametric. We call this model semiparametric because it combines a parametric regression model involving covariates with a flexible and loosely defined model for the hazard function. The semiparametric model that we discuss here is the proportional hazards regression model of Cox (1972) [88]. The innovation of the so-called Cox model is that it separates inference about the effects of covariates on survival from inference on the underlying hazard. We now discuss the proportional hazards model and Bayesian inference with it.

Recall from Section 11.1.1 that the hazard function at time t provides the instantaneous probability of having the event at that moment, given that the event has not yet occurred. In general, we find it preferable to model the hazard function rather than the survival function. If we let $h_i(t)$ represent the hazard function at time t for the ith individual, then we have several options for relating this hazard function to this individual's covariates. Cox [88] proposed the partial likelihood model. In this model, the hazard function decomposes into a part that is a function of time only and a component that is a function of the covariates but does not depend on time. The part of the hazard function that depends on time but not the covariates is called the *baseline hazard function*, and we denote it by $h_0(t)$. The baseline hazard is common to all observations in the data set. Covariates affect an individual's hazard through the product of the baseline hazard and a function of the covariates but not time, $g(x_i'\beta)$. Thus, $h_i(t) = h_0(t) \times g(x_i'\beta)$. Although most any mathematical function could be used for the function of the covariates, the most commonly used regression function is $g(x_i'\beta) = \exp(x_i'\beta)$. This model for the hazard function is commonly called the Cox model, namely,

$$h_i(t) = h_0(t)\exp(x_i'\beta). \tag{12.5}$$

We note that in this model, the hazard (or instantaneous risk of an event) at time t increases as $x_i'\beta$ gets larger.

The cumulative hazard has a convenient form,

$$H(t \mid x_i, \beta) = \int_0^t h(s \mid x_i, \beta)ds = e^{x_i'\beta}\int_0^t h_0(s)ds = e^{x_i'\beta}H_0(t),$$

where $H_0(t) = \int_0^t h_0(u)du$ is the baseline cumulative hazard function. We write $H_i(t) = H(t \mid x_i, \beta)$ interchangeably. Because of the assumption that the covariate effects are constant over time, the effect on the hazard function is the same as the effect on the cumulative hazard function. We note that one does not need to include an intercept in the βs. The baseline hazard function takes the place of the intercept in this model.

The effect of covariates on the survival function $S_i(t) = S(t \mid x_i, \beta) = \exp\{-H_i(t)\}$ is

$$S(t \mid x, \beta) = \exp\{-e^{x'\beta}H_0(t)\} = \left(\exp\{-H_0(t)\}\right)^{e^{x'\beta}} = \{S_0(t)\}^{e^{x'\beta}}.$$

Unlike the AFT models, where the covariates rescale time, the covariates in the Cox model raise the baseline survival function to a power. If $x_1'\beta > x_2'\beta$, then $S(t \mid x_1, \beta) < S(t \mid x_2, \beta)$ for all time t. This relationship follows from the fact that the survival function is less than 1, so raising it to a positive power results in a smaller number.

As noted, the proportional hazards model assumes that the covariate effects on the hazard function are constant over time. Consider two distinct values for a covariate x_1 and x_2. The ratio of the hazard function with x_2 to the hazard function with x_1 is

$$HR(x_2, x_1) = \frac{h(t \mid x_2, \beta)}{h(t \mid x_1, \beta)} = \exp\{(x_2 - x_1)\beta\}.$$

We wrote the hazard ratio for two values of a single covariate, but the same result holds for a vector of covariate values. Because time is not included in the hazard ratio, it is often used as the target of inference relating to the effect of a covariate.

Another consequence of the proportional hazards model is that the hazard functions for two values of a covariate never cross, regardless of the magnitude of the effect. As a consequence, the survival functions will not cross either. If one wants to model a covariate effect that changes over time, then one must consider an interaction of the covariate with time. There are several ways that one might characterize such a time-dependent covariate.

Suppose you have two treatments and that survival is better under the first treatment early in the study but better under the second treatment later on. This constitutes an interaction between treatment and time. Define a variable Trt with $Trt = 1$ for the first treatment and $Trt = 0$ for the second. An appropriate model allows for an effect of Trt up to a particular point in time, say t_c, and for a different effect after that. Let $z(t)$ take the value 0 for $t < t_c$, and the value 1 for $t \geq t_c$. Then write the model

$$h(t \,|\, Trt, z(t)) = \exp\{\beta_1 Trt + \beta_2 Trt \times z(t)\} h_0(t).$$

Under this model, the hazard ratio comparing an individual with $Trt = 1$ to one with $Trt = 0$ is e^{β_1} for $t < t_c$, and is $e^{\beta_1 + \beta_2}$ for $t \geq t_c$. Perhaps surprisingly, the proportional hazards assumption appears to work reasonably well in a wide variety of biomedical applications, particularly over relatively short follow-up times.

Unlike the AFT models, median survival times are not simple functions of the regression coefficients. We therefore tend to focus on the hazard ratio and sometimes on survival probabilities at particular times when expressing covariate effects. Hazard ratios are particularly straightforward with the proportional hazards model. If x is a covariate that equals 0 or 1, such as a treatment indicator, then e^{β} is the hazard ratio for $x = 1$ relative to $x = 0$. The regression parameter β is the logarithm of the hazard ratio. The hazard ratio is therefore a directly estimated parameter in the proportional hazards regression model.

The sampling distribution with the proportional hazards model for n observed times (y_i, δ_i), $i = 1, \ldots, n$, is given by

$$p[(y, \delta \,|\, \beta, h_0) = \prod_{i=1}^{n} \{e^{x_i' \beta} h_0(y_i)\}^{\delta_i} \{S_0(y_i)\}^{e^{x_i' \beta}}.$$

We note that the sampling distribution is conditional on the baseline hazard function, as well as on the regression coefficients.

Cox [88] defined the partial likelihood for β, PL(β), as

$$\mathrm{PL}(\beta) \propto \prod_{i=1}^{n} \left\{ \frac{\exp(x_i' \beta)}{\sum_{j \in \mathcal{R}(y_i)} \exp(x_j' \beta)} \right\}^{\delta_i}. \tag{12.6}$$

In the definition of the partial likelihood, $\mathcal{R}(y_i)$ represents the individuals still at risk of the event at the time the ith individual experiences the event. Notice how the baseline hazard function is absent from the partial likelihood (12.6), allowing one to ignore the underlying hazard function. If we assumed that the failure times followed a particular distribution that has an analytically tractable hazard function, such as the exponential distribution, we could evaluate the full likelihood. There are very few such distributions, unfortunately. Hence the widespread use of the Cox model. The values of β that maximize the partial likelihood are generally the targets of interest in a non-Bayesian analysis.

12.2.1   Modeling the Baseline Hazard Function

Bayesian inference for the Cox model will require a prior distribution for the regression parameters (β) and the baseline hazard function $h_0(\cdot)$. Cox's approach brought enormous benefit to frequentist inference by allowing the analysis to treat the baseline hazard function as an ignorable nuisance. The advantage of Cox's formulation is less clear for Bayesian inference, however. Unlike frequentist inference that conditions on the parameters, Bayesian inference provides direct inference on the parameters via posterior distributions, which condition on the data. Bayesian analysis addresses all model parameters, and the baseline hazard function is a part of the model. Posterior inference will either have to provide a joint posterior inference for the regression coefficients and the baseline hazard or, if interest focuses solely on the covariate effects, one will have to provide inference based on the marginal posterior distribution of the regression coefficients. A prior distribution for the regression coefficients is fairly straightforward; a normal prior for the βs is often a reasonable choice. An appropriate prior for the baseline hazard function, however, is a bit more problematic. We now discuss several flexible models for the baseline hazard. By "flexible," we mean that we make few assumptions about the shape of the hazard function. Even though we may not force a particular shape, our models for the baseline hazard function are not without parameters. In fact, we gain flexibility with these models by putting together local parametric models. Thus, our statistical model for the baseline hazard function may well consist of a large number of parameters, despite the full model being called "semiparametric."

We start by breaking up the time axis (i.e., the positive real line) into intervals. Let a partition of K intervals spanning 0 to ∞ be given by $[a_0, a_1), [a_1, a_2), \ldots, [a_{K-1}, a_K)$, where $a_0 = 0$ and $a_K = \infty$. There are many ways one can define the partition. The intervals need not all have the same width, and the grid along the time axis can be as fine as one wants. For fitting the Cox model, one generally forms a grid based on the times of the observed failure times (both censored and uncensored times). One may only use the observed (uncensored) failure times and form the intervals so that each one brackets at least one of the observed (uncensored) failure times.

Let T be the random variable representing the time of an event (i.e., the survival time), and $q_i = P\{T \in [a_{i-1}, a_i) \mid T \geq a_{i-1}, H\}$, where H is the cumulative hazard function corresponding to the distribution of T. Bayesian models for making inference via the proportional hazards model will consider different probability distributions to characterize the q_i. We note that if one's model for the baseline hazard function has independent parameters across the intervals, then one will have K parameters for just the baseline hazard. If the number of parameters in the model

(K plus p, the number of covariates) is greater than the number of uncensored observations, then the model will not be identifiable.

Piecewise Exponential Model. We now describe a fairly straightforward statistical model for the baseline hazard function. The exponential distribution is a simple one-parameter model that sometimes is useful when modeling times until an event. The usefulness of this sampling model derives from its relationship to a Poisson process. That is, if one considers that the number of events that occur in an interval follows a Poisson distribution with parameter λ, then the time in between the events will follow an exponential distribution with parameter λ. We have seen that the gamma distribution is conjugate for the exponential distribution, so a gamma prior on λ will lead to a gamma posterior.

The gamma-exponential model is too restrictive for general use, having just one parameter and a mode that is always at 0. The gamma-exponential model is actually quite useful, however, when one models the failure-time distribution via a piecewise exponential model. Consider our K-interval partition $[a_0, a_1), [a_1, a_2), \ldots, [a_{K-1}, a_K)$. We are going to posit possibly different exponential distributions for T within each interval of our partition. Although we defined $a_K = \infty$, all we need for our analysis of a data set is for a_K to be larger than any observed failure time. Let $I_k = [a_{k-1}, a_k)$, and assume that the baseline hazard function within interval I_k is given by $h_0(t) = \lambda_k, t \in I_k$, $k = 1, \ldots, K$. That is, there is a constant hazard that applies to each interval of the partition, which translates to an exponential sampling distribution within the interval. The λ_k are unknown parameters in the statistical model. We will usually want $\lambda_k > 0$ for each interval to ensure that $h_0(t)$ is a true hazard function. (Recall from Chapter 11 that the cumulative hazard $H_0(c) = \int_0^c h_0(u)du \to \infty$ as $c \to \infty$ to ensure that the survival curve goes to 0 over time.)

The observed data for the ith individual consist of a follow-up time (t_i), an indicator of failure or censoring status (δ_i), and the set of covariates (x_i). Let D be the observed data. We define ν_{ik} to be an indicator that equals 1 if individual i's follow-up time lies in interval I_k and is 0 otherwise. That is, $\nu_{ik} = 1$ if $t_i \in I_k$ and 0 otherwise. Finally, let β be the set of regression coefficients.

The sampling distribution or likelihood with the piecewise exponential model is given by

$$f(t, \delta \mid \beta, \lambda, x) = \prod_{i=1}^{n} \prod_{k=1}^{K} (\lambda_k e^{x_i'\beta})^{\delta_i \nu_{ik}}$$

$$\times \exp\left\{ -\nu_{ik}\left(\lambda_k(t_i - a_{k-1}) + \sum_{j=1}^{k-1} \lambda_j(a_j - a_{j-1}) \right) e^{x_i'\beta} \right\}. \tag{12.7}$$

Our interest is in the baseline hazard at the moment, so we will temporarily ignore the covariates. Let TT_k be what is sometimes called the total uptime in interval I_k. TT_k is defined as the sum of the lengths of earlier intervals plus the follow-up times during interval I_k for observation times falling in the interval (i.e.,

$\nu_{ik} = 1$) plus the length of interval I_k for observations times falling later than the upper end of the interval, a_k. We can write this out successively as

$$
TT_1 = \sum_{i=1}^{n} \left\{ \nu_{i1}(t_i - a_0) + I_{\{t_i > a_1\}}(a_1 - a_0) \right\},
$$

$$
TT_2 = TT_1 + \sum_{i=1}^{n} \left\{ \nu_{i2}(t_i - a_1) + I_{\{t_i > a_2\}}(a_2 - a_1) \right\},
$$

$$
\ldots,
$$

$$
TT_j = TT_{k-1} + \sum_{i=1}^{n} \left\{ \nu_{ik}(t_i - a_{k-1}) + I_{\{t_i > a_k\}}(a_k - a_{k-1}) \right\},
$$

$$
\ldots,
$$

$$
TT_K = TT_{K-1} + \sum_{i=1}^{n} \left\{ \nu_{iK}(t_i - a_{K-1}) \right\}.
$$

The last equation follows from the assumption that τ_K exceeds all observed failure times.

We can determine the posterior distribution for the piecewise constant hazards (λ_k, $k = 1, \ldots, K$). Consider independent gamma priors for the exponential rate parameter λ_k in interval I_k, $\lambda_k \sim Ga(\alpha_{0k}, \beta_{0k})$, $k = 1, \ldots, K$. Thanks to the conjugate nature of the statistical model, the posterior distribution in the interval is $\lambda_k \mid D \sim Ga(\alpha_{0k} + n_k, \beta_{0k} + TT_k)$, where n_k is the number of uncensored event times in interval I_k.

The easiest way to add covariates is to assume that the covariates affect the underlying hazard function the same way over time. That is, the hazard effect does not change over time, only the baseline hazard does. This is the proportional hazards assumption. Thus the hazard at time t for patient i with covariates x_i is $h(t) \exp(x' \beta_i)$. While this model allows for a more flexible characterization of the baseline hazard, it, being a proportional hazards model, has the drawback that it assumes that covariate effects are independent of time. Thus, the hazard functions are parallel on the log scale. We illustrate this constant distance on the log scale in Figure 12.2. The figure shows four posterior mean hazard functions from an analysis of the CALGB breast cancer trial. The Y-axis is logarithmic in the figure. One can see in the graph that the distances between group-specific hazard functions remain the same over time.

12.2.2 Counting Process Formulation or Poisson Likelihood Analog.

We now present a formulation of the likelihood that one can use when carrying out posterior inference via MCMC. The same basic approach works in BUGS, JAGS, and Stan, with minor modifications relating to syntax and setting up the data. See Appendix C for more information.

One of the earliest proposals for Bayesian analysis in a proportional hazards model is due to Kalbfleisch (1978) [201]. In this model, we consider a partition, as in the piecewise exponential model, and then posit a gamma process prior for the baseline hazard on the partition. This approach allows one to estimate the

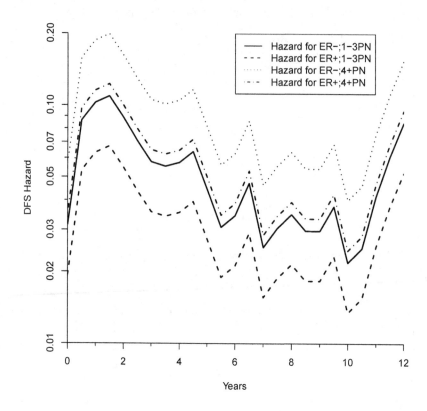

FIGURE 12.2: Posterior mean hazard function from a piecewise exponential model of disease-free survival. The data are from CALGB study 9344. Separate hazard functions are shown for each set of covariate values.

underlying hazard function nonparametrically. The development follows from the counting process formulation first presented by Andersen and Gill (1982) [6] and later by Clayton (1994) [80] within a Bayesian context. It builds on the formulation of the similarity of the likelihood with a multinomial-Poisson likelihood, as pointed out by Holford [168] and Olivier and Laird [211].

Ignoring the partition for the moment, we first consider continuous time. We characterize the observed events as arising from a counting process $N_i(t)$ associated with each individual in the study population. These processes count the number of events of interest that occur to the ith individual until time t. (We assume that only one event can occur in our case.) For this stochastic process, let $I_i(t)dt = E(dN_i(t) \mid F_{t-})$ be the associated intensity process, which is related to a hazard function. In this formulation, $dN_i(t)$ is the increment of the counting process N_i over a short half-open interval $[t, t + dt)$, and F_{t-} denotes the available data up to time t. That is, $dN_i(t)$ equals 0, except at the ith individual's event time, when it takes the value 1. With this definition, $E(dN_i(t) \mid F_{t-})$ is the probability of an event for the ith individual in $[t, t + dt)$. The instantaneous hazard function for individual i corresponds to the limit of this expectation as dt goes to 0. With the proportional hazards formulation, we assume that the instantaneous hazard equals

$$I_i(t) = Y_i(t)h_0(t)\exp(x'\beta_i).$$

In the above formula, $Y_i(t)$ is a process that corresponds to the ith individual being at risk of an event at time t. That is, $Y_i(t) = 1$ at time t if the individual is still in the risk set at time t and 0 otherwise. The rest of the right-hand side of the equation is the Cox model we presented earlier.

The data, therefore, consist of realizations of the processes $N_i(t)$ and $Y_i(t)$, along with the covariates x_i for each individual $i = 1, \ldots, n$. The parameters in the model are the regression coefficients β and the integrated baseline hazard ($H(t) = \int_0^t h_0(u)du$). We estimate the integrated baseline via our nonparametric model.

The joint posterior distribution for the parameters is given by $p(\beta, H_0 \mid D) \propto p(D \mid \beta, H_0) p(\beta)p(H_0)$. Assuming that the censoring is ignorable, we can write the likelihood based on the sampling distribution as $p(D \mid \beta, H_0) \propto \prod_{i=1}^n \left\{ \prod_{t \geq 0} I_i(t)^{dN_i(t)} \right\} \exp\{-I_i(t)dt\}$. If we consider the increments $dN_i(t)$ as independent Poisson random variables with means (rates) $I_i(t)dt$ in the short interval $[t, t + dt)$, then we would get the same likelihood. That is, we can treat $dN_i(t) \sim Po(I_i(t)dt)$. Letting $dH_0(t)$ represent the jump in the integrated baseline hazard in $[t, t + dt)$, we have, as before, $I_i(t) = Y_i(t)\exp(x'\beta_i)dH_0(t)$. The gamma distribution is the conjugate prior for the Poisson distribution, so we consider that the increments ($dH_0(t)$) have independent gamma distributions. As in Kalbfleisch [201], we posit the distributional assumption on the increments $dH_0(t) \sim Ga(c \times h_0^*(t), c)$, where the parameter c represents prior uncertainty associated with the prior guess for the baseline hazard function, $h_0^*(t)$.

12.2.3 Prior Distributions for Parameters in Proportional Hazards Regression Models

The gamma process prior formulation lends itself well to situations in which we have prior information about the baseline hazard. One can also carry out a Bayesian analysis in which one considers less informative priors for the independent increments of the cumulative baseline hazard. Prior specification of the regression effects (β) completes the model. One can use a convenient vague prior, such as $\beta \sim N(0, 10^6)$, for example. We now discuss informed prior distributions for the λ_k followed by a discussion related to the regression coefficients, the βs.

12.2.3.1 Prior Distributions for Hazard Functions in Each Interval

We are assuming that a constant hazard rate applies within each interval. Recall our K-interval partition over $(0, \infty)$ is $[a_0, a_1), [a_1, a_2), \ldots, [a_{K-1}, a_K)$, with $a_0 = 0$ and $a_K = \infty$. We denote the ith interval by $I_i = [a_{k-1}, a_k)$, and assume that the baseline hazard function within interval I_k is $h_0(t) = \lambda_k$, $t \in I_k$, $k = 1, \ldots, K$. If we assumed a single exponential sampling model for all of the failure times (i.e., $h_0(t) = \lambda$ for all times t), then the integrated hazard function in the ith interval would be $H(a_k) - H(a_{k-1}) = \lambda \times (a_k - a_{k-1})$. We would like to relax the assumption that the same rate parameter (λ) applies in each interval, since that assumption seems unlikely to be true in most settings, particularly over long periods of time. Instead, we want a prior model that may consider the exponential model to be the prior mean of the hazard function but will also allow for interval-to-interval variation. We will specify the gamma process approach in a manner that will allow heterogeneity of hazard rates across intervals.

Let λ_k be the constant hazard rate in the kth interval $[a_{k-1}, a_k)$. Our prior model is

$$\lambda_k \overset{\text{ind}}{\sim} Ga(\lambda^* c, c), \quad k = 1, \ldots, K.$$

The prior mean hazard rate is $\lambda^* = E(\lambda_k) = E\{h_0(t)\}$ for all k and at any time point. In case the intervals in our partition are of different widths, we may want to incorporate it into the prior by multiplying c by the width in each interval. The prior model becomes $\lambda_k \sim Ga\{\lambda^* c(a_k - a_{i-1}), c(a_k - a_{k-1})\}$ for interval I_k. For ease of notation, we will simply write $\lambda_k \sim Ga(\lambda^* c_k, c_k)$ for the kth interval.

We need c and λ^* to specify the prior distribution. We focus on c first. The prior mean and variance of $\lambda \sim Ga(\lambda^* c, c)$ are λ^* and λ^*/c, respectively. If c is large, then the prior variance will be small and the prior mean will have relatively more weight in the posterior, leading to the posterior mean being closer to λ^*. If, on the other hand, c is small, then the posterior mean may deviate more from the prior mean and may be relatively farther from λ^*. If c is too small, the posterior means of the λ_k may jump around a lot, leading to overfitting. Many choose $c = 0.001$ to form a reference prior, although this seems arbitrary.

What value shall we use for λ^*? Recall that we are assuming the same prior mean for each interval and, basically, a prior mean that is an exponential distribution. The median for the $Exp(\lambda^*)$ distribution is $\log(2)/\lambda^*$. If we have a fairly good prior guess t_m for the median, then we can set $\lambda^* = \log(2)/t_m$. We could also put a prior distribution (e.g., $Ga(a, b)$) on λ^* with a "best guess" and percentile, as we have done in earlier examples of gamma priors (such as the gamma-Poisson model in Section 5.3.2).

12.2.3.2   Prior Distribution for the Log Hazard Ratios

In the proportional hazards model, the βs are the logarithms of the hazard ratios. Since hazard ratios are a scale that researchers are familiar with, we can elicit prior information directly on the scale of e^{β_j} for the jth covariate. It is quite common to consider a normal prior distribution for each β, with mutual independence for these parameters. The normal distribution is not conjugate in this case but does correspond to the large-sample distribution of these parameters. Therefore, a standard reference prior for a covariate would be a normal distribution with zero mean and a large variance. The zero mean corresponds to a prior assumption that the hazard ratio is 1, that is, the covariate does not affect the hazard or survival probabilities, given the functional relationship.

How large should the prior variance be in this reference prior? Depending on the context, it may be very unlikely that one will see really large hazard ratios. In randomized clinical trials, for example, hazard ratios larger than 3 when comparing treatments are quite rare. The 5th percentile of the standard normal distribution is -1.645, and $e^{-1.645} = 0.19$. Since exponentiation preserves percentiles and it is unlikely that a treatment would reduce the risk failure by as much as one-fifth, a prior variance of 1 is probably sufficient in many cases. In general, it would not matter if the prior variance is set to a much larger value, such as 10 or 100.

It is also possible to elicit a prior from knowledgeable individuals as we have in other contexts. Recall that e^{β_j} is the hazard ratio associated with a one-unit increase in the jth covariate. Suppose $\tilde{R}_j$ is the preliminary estimate of the most likely value of the hazard ratio e^{β_j}. Then, the best preliminary estimate of the log hazard ratio for this covariate is $\beta_{0j} = \log(\tilde{R}_j)$.

We will determine the prior variance for β_j based on a prior estimate of a percentile of the hazard ratio. If we are, say, 95% certain that the hazard ratio is less than $\tilde{R}_j^*$, then we can find the prior standard deviation σ_{0j} from

$$0.95 = P(\beta_j \leq \tilde{R}_j^*) = \Phi\left\{\frac{\log(\tilde{R}_j^*) - \log(\tilde{R}_j)}{\sigma_{0j}}\right\},$$

where $\Phi(\cdot)$ is the standard normal cdf. This equation leads to $\sigma_{0j} = \left\{\log(R_j^*) - \log(\tilde{R}_j)\right\}/1.645$ after plugging in the 95th percentile of the standard normal distribution. If we instead elicited a value that the individual was 100α percent certain was below the hazard ratio, we would work with $\alpha = P(\beta_j \geq \tilde{R}_j^*)$ to determine the prior standard deviation.

With continuous covariates, it may be more convenient to get opinions about hazard ratios associated with larger ranges than one unit. For example, if the jth covariate is years of smoking, one could ask for the best guess associated with the effect of 10 years of smoking on the hazard ratio relative to not smoking. If that preliminary estimate is $\tilde{R}_j$ for this covariate, we have $\tilde{R}_j = e^{10\beta_j}$, yielding $\beta_{0j} = \log(\tilde{R}_j)/10$.

Informed priors for interactions are a bit more challenging. Suppose our proportional hazards regression model includes two binary covariates, x_1 and x_2, and their interaction. That is, our model for the hazard at time t is $h(t) = h_0(t)\exp\{\beta_1 x_1 + \beta_2 x_2 + \beta_3(x_1 \times x_2)\}$. With this model, the hazard ratio for $x_1 = 1, x_2 = 1$ relative to $x_1 = 0, x_2 = 0$ is $\exp(\beta_1 + \beta_2 + \beta_3) = e^{\beta_1}e^{\beta_2}e^{\beta_3}$. The hazard ratio for the interaction depends on e^{β_1}, the hazard ratio for covariate x_1, and e^{β_2}, the hazard ratio for covariate x_2. Suppose we have β_{01} and β_{02} as our prior values for covariates 1 and 2, respectively. Furthermore, let $\tilde{R}_3$ be an elicited prior hazard ratio for the interaction (i.e., the case when both covariates equal 1 relative to when they are both equal to 0). Then we have $\tilde{R}_3 = e^{\beta_{01}}e^{\beta_{02}}e^{\beta_3}$, from which we get our prior best guess for the interaction term $\beta_{03} = \log(\tilde{R}_3)/(\beta_{01}\beta_{02})$. Having assumed that the βs are *a priori* independent, we can use an estimate of a percentile ($\tilde{R}_3^*$) and the normal prior distribution for β_3 to determine the standard deviation in β_3's prior. As we did above for the general regression coefficients, we find (with the condition that $P(\tilde{R}_3 \leq \tilde{R}_3^* \mid \beta_1, \beta_2) = \alpha$)

$$\alpha = P\left(e^{\beta_{01}} e^{\beta_{02}} e^{\beta_3} \leq \tilde{R}_3^* \Big| \beta_1 = \beta_{01}, \beta_2 = \beta_{02}\right)$$

$$= P\left(e^{\beta_3} \leq \frac{\tilde{R}_3^*}{e^{\beta_{01}} e^{\beta_{02}}} \Big| \beta_1 = \beta_{01}, \beta_2 = \beta_{02}\right)$$

$$= P\left(\frac{\beta_3 - \beta_{03}}{\sigma_{03}} \leq \frac{\log(\tilde{R}_3^* e^{-\beta_{01}} e^{-\beta_{02}}) - \log(\tilde{R}_{03} e^{-\beta_{01}} e^{-\beta_{02}})}{\sigma_{03}}\right)$$

$$= \Phi\left\{\frac{\log(\tilde{R}_3^*/\tilde{R}_{03})}{\sigma_{03}}\right\},$$

for some probability α. We can then find $\sigma_{03} = \log(\tilde{R}_3^*/\tilde{R}_{03})/z_\alpha$, where z_α is the 100αth percentile of the standard normal distribution.

As in other regression analyses, it may be easier to determine informed priors for a subset of the βs. In such situations, one may combine the informed priors with reference priors for the remaining βs.

Example 12.3. Proportional Hazards Analysis of Breast Cancer Study.

We revisit the analysis in Example 12.2. We now analyze disease-free survival among these women using a proportional hazards regression model. We again fit a model with four covariates, namely, an indicator for the drug paclitaxel (T), an indicator for the tumor being positive for the estrogen receptor (ER), an indicator for there being four or more positive lymph nodes upon examination during surgery $(LN4+)$, and an interaction between paclitaxel and estrogen receptor positivity $(T{:}ER)$.

We first determined the grid we would use to analyze these data. The study randomized 3,102 women to six treatment regimens, and there were 1,228 events in the data set. The last failure occurred 9.88 years after randomization, and the longest follow-up time was 10.96 years. Given the large number of events, we chose to create a partition over 11 years with each interval spanning roughly 1 month (i.e., each interval was one-twelfth of a year). We therefore had 132 intervals over the 11 years. Had we created a partition based on the unique event times, we would have had 581 intervals of varying width. We used the monthly intervals to avoid the program being too slow.

Having formed the partition for inference on the hazard function, we next determine the prior parameters. Recall that our statistical model assumes a constant hazard rate within each interval with a gamma prior distribution: $\lambda_k \sim Ga(\lambda^* c_k, c_k)$ for the kth interval. Since our intervals all have the same width $w = 0.083$, $c_k = cw = c \times 0.083$ for all k. For λ^*, we used the prior notion that the median disease-free survival in this population of women with breast cancer is 7 years. That assumption led to $\lambda^* = \log(2)/7$. We set $c = 0.01$, which when multiplied by the width w gave us a very diffuse prior for the rate in each interval.

Since the prior median is set by the prior rate parameter across the partition (λ^*), we assumed that each covariate had negligible effect on the hazard function. We posited a $N(0, 9)$ prior distribution for each of the βs. We chose a variance of

9 because this prior led to a prior 95% probability interval for each hazard ratio that is $(\exp(\pm(1.96 \times 3)))$ or $(0.0028, 357.81)$. It would be extremely unlikely that hazard ratios would be nearly that small or that large.

Table 12.7 contains posterior summary statistics for the regression parameters. We see that the posterior distributions are different with this model than they were with the Weibull AFT model. For one thing, the signs of the estimates are reversed. The effects of paclitaxel (T) and of estrogen receptor status (*ERstatus*) are about the same in magnitude, as are their respective posterior standard deviations. Having four or more positive lymph nodes at surgery remains a major risk factor. The interaction between T and *ERstatus* is positive, but the posterior inference suggests less of a predictive effect (i.e., affecting treatment choice). The posterior probability that the interaction is greater than zero is 0.79 with the proportional hazards model, which is substantially smaller than the value we saw with the Weibull regression model (0.94).

Figure 12.3a contains pointwise posterior mean disease-free survival probability curves for each of four groups of women who had four or more positive lymph nodes at surgery. We can compare these curves to the posterior mean survival curves in Figure 12.1a from the Weibull AFT regression. One thing to notice is that the survival probabilities are higher with the proportional hazards analysis than with the AFT analysis. This difference is attributable to the nonparametric estimation of the baseline hazard function, as opposed to the parametric model's determination of the hazard function. We also notice less of an interaction effect, although we should examine the group-specific hazard functions to see that effect more clearly.

Figure 12.3b shows the hazard functions for the four treatment groups we have been discussing. Since we have a relatively fine grid over the 11 years of follow-up, we used a lowess smoother to plot the posterior mean hazard functions [82]. We applied relatively less smoothing to allow some of the local features to show. Looking at Figure 12.3b, we see that the hazard functions from the proportional hazards analysis show variation over time. It often happens in cancer clinical trials that there is an early rise in the hazard of recurrence or death, followed by reduced risk over time, particularly right after treatment. We also see how the shapes of the hazard functions track each other as a result of the constant hazard ratios. If we plot these hazard functions on the log scale, we will see a constant distance between curves. It is also instructive to compare the estimates of the hazard functions with the AFT model and the proportional hazards model. The Weibull AFT analysis yielded posterior mean hazard functions that were almost horizontal lines (see Figure 12.1a).

12.3 Nonparametric Regression for Survival Analysis

In the Bayesian nonparametric survival analysis literature, there are many nonparametric models available that relax the assumptions of the AFT and Cox models,

TABLE 12.7: Summary of the posterior distribution of the proportional hazards regression parameters from an analysis of women with four or more positive lymph nodes treated in a breast cancer randomized clinical trial

β	Moments		Posterior percentiles				
	Mean	Std dev.	2.5	25	50	75	97.5
T	-0.267	0.076	-0.423	-0.318	-0.265	-0.215	-0.119
ER	-0.518	0.075	-0.661	-0.568	-0.517	-0.467	-0.371
$LN4+$	0.594	0.058	0.485	0.556	0.594	0.632	0.709
$T:ER$	0.083	0.104	-0.116	0.012	0.080	0.151	0.289

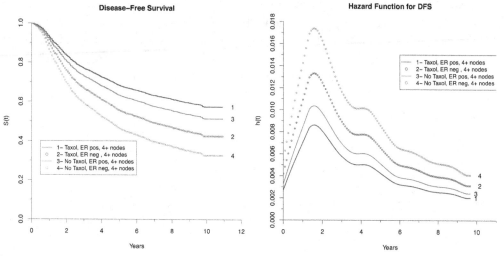

(a) Disease-free survival from a proportional hazards regression model.

(b) Hazards from a proportional hazards regression model.

FIGURE 12.3: Posterior estimates of the disease-free survival probabilities and hazard functions from proportional hazards regression model with an interaction between Taxol and ER status among women with four or more positive lymph nodes.

namely accelerated time and proportional hazards. While this is a large topic in itself, here we introduce one such method recently developed and implemented in an R package. The method is based on a dependent Dirichlet process (DDP), originally defined in MacEachern [234]. An early adoption of the DDP for survival regression is by DeIorio et al. (2009) [90]. The model described here also constructs a DDP by using ideas similar to the Dirichlet process mixture (DPM) of Weibull distributions that we described for exchangeable observations in Example 11.5 in Chapter 11. It also uses, as building blocks, the proportional hazards model described in Section

12.2 with a Weibull baseline hazard. Details and model properties are available in the paper by Shi, Laud, and Neuner [295], and its computational implementation by Shi [294] comprises the R package DPWeibull. Here we provide a very brief description of the model and then show an example of how its analysis can be carried out.

In a simpler form, the model can be written by beginning with

$$T_i \mid \alpha_i, \lambda_i, x_i, \beta \stackrel{\text{ind}}{\sim} Weib(\alpha_i, \lambda_i e^{x_i' \beta_i}), \quad i = 1, \dots, n,$$

where x_i is the covariate vector and β_i is a vector of random covariates associated with observation i. As is usual in regression settings, the entire model is conditional on covariates x_i, $i = 1, \dots, n$. The Weibull parametric proportional hazards model is a baseline or building block for the model. Next, we define a mixture that employs the Dirichlet process, similar to the Weibull DPM model in expression (11.16), jointly for the vector $(\lambda_i, \alpha_i, \beta_i)$. Specifically, dropping the observation identifying subscript i for notational convenience, we have

$$\alpha, \lambda, \beta \sim DP(\nu, G_0), \quad G_0 = p(\alpha, \lambda)p(\beta), \quad \nu \sim Ga(a_\nu, b_\nu).$$

In Shi, Laud, and Neuner [295], convenient choices are also made for $p(\alpha, \lambda)$ and $p(\beta)$. There are choices one may make regarding prior distributions for the parameters (α, λ, β) that can lead to desirable properties for the model and/or allow incorporating a low-information omnibus (LIO) prior. We refer the reader to Shi, Laud, and Neuner for details [295]. We do note, however, that the model results in a stick-breaking representation (Section 3.3.2) for the distribution of event time T.

We now turn to an example to illustrate how this model can be used in analysis, with the help of the R package DPWeibull, when one chooses to use LIO priors.

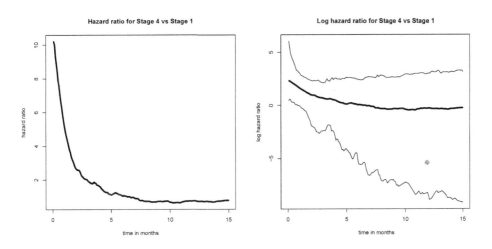

FIGURE 12.4: Posterior estimates of the hazard ratio (stage 4 vs. 1) as a function of time from the dependent Dirichlet process analysis in Example 12.4. The right panel's vertical axis is on the log scale and also shows 95% posterior PIs.

Example 12.4. Dependent Dirichlet Process Model for the Larynx Cancer Data. We return to the data of Example 12.1. The DDP model, being nonparametric, does not directly yield parameter inference. However, its very generality makes it possible to obtain inference for a very wide variety of inferential and predictive targets. For example, while there is not a single hazard ratio for survival after diagnosis of stage 4 vs. stage 1 laryngeal cancer in this model, we can calculate this hazard ratio at each time point from each posterior sample. The R code for accomplishing this uses the DPWeibull package and is available on the book's website under Chapter 12 in a file named `Larynx.R`. The resulting plot is shown in Figure 12.4. The posterior mean hazard ratio is plotted as a function of time in the left half of the figure. This seems to indicate that a constant hazard ratio assumption as in a proportional hazards model may not be appropriate. However, the right half of the figure shows the large uncertainty in this hazard ratio function. A flat line can easily fit within the 95% probability limits. Notice that the variation is so large that we resorted to the logarithm of the hazard ratio for plotting purposes. This large variability is not unexpected with a sample size of 90 patients in a nonparametric survival analysis regression with four stage groups and two other covariates.

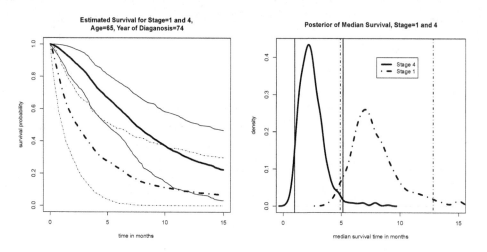

FIGURE 12.5: The left panel shows posterior means and 95% PIs for survival functions for stages 4 and 1. The right panel shows posterior densities of median survival times for patients with disease stages 4 and 1; 95% limits are shown with vertical lines.

Inference for survival functions and median survival times can also be carried out. Figure 12.5 shows the results graphically of an analysis comparing stage 4 disease with stage 1. It is clear that stage 4 disease is associated with much worse survival than stage 1. Other comparisons can also be made by following the code in the `Larynx.R` program mentioned in the previous paragraph. We note that the package provides a `predict()` function that works with an object produced by the `dpweib()` function that contains posterior samples. Estimates can be made at any choice of the covariate values to enable any survival-related inference at these values.

Although we have chosen here to show results graphically, quantitative summaries such as means, medians, percentiles of inferential targets can be easily obtained by standard R functions operating on objects created by the functions `dpweib()` and `predict()` in the package DPWeibull. The package also provides some plot methods for graphical summaries of posterior samples.

12.4 Survival Analysis with Random Effects (Frailty)

We sometimes have to analyze data where we wish to account for the fact that there may be a shared propensity for the event of interest among groups of individuals. We might encounter this issue, for example, when analyzing times until death in an animal study of a supposed carcinogen or treatment for a disease. Animals from the same litter may tend to live longer than animals from another litter in the absence of any intervention. This extra longevity may contribute to longer lifetimes after exposure. Similarly, studies of times to disease onset in familial studies may wish to account for heritable differences across families. If we had measured some observable factors on the individuals when such factors are directly related to the propensity, we could account for the higher or lower risks with covariates. Instead, we will include a random effect. The random effect basically attributes the between-group differences in outcome to some unmeasured quality or characteristic that group members share. This random effect is sometimes called a *frailty*, particularly when we think of it as representing heterogeneity of different groups' tendencies to be more or less sensitive to the outcome. Since adding a random effect simply means that we include a regression parameter that we model with a probability distribution, such models present little challenge in a Bayesian analysis. A common model includes a group-specific parameter added to the linear or log-linear model.

Suppose, for example, there are G groups (e.g., families, litters, clinics) in our data set, with each individual belonging to just one of these groups. We might let b_g be the random effect that we use to characterize the change from the baseline hazard for group g, $g = 1, \ldots, G$. We augment the linear model $(x_i'\beta)$ for the ith individual in our AFT or proportional hazards regression model by adding the appropriate group's $b_{g(i)}$. (In the notation, $g(i)$ represents the group to which the ith individual belongs.) For example, the proportional hazards regression model of the hazard function for individual i in equation (12.5) becomes

$$h_i(t) = h_0(t) \times \exp(x_i'\beta + b_{g(i)}).$$

All individuals in the same group g will share the same baseline hazard $h_0(t)e^{b_g}$. We complete the model by assigning a distribution to the b_g. A common assumption is that $b_g \sim N(0, \sigma_b^2)$, $g = 1, \ldots, G$, with a vague prior distribution on σ_b (or the precision $1/\sigma_b^2$). One might also consider a gamma prior distribution for the hazard ratio e^{b_g}. Regardless of the prior distribution, posterior inference via some MCMC approach proceeds as it does without the additional random effect.

12.5   Recap and Readings

Survival analysis has been a very active area of statistical research for at least 50 years. A good in-depth review of Bayesian methods for survival analysis is the book by Ibrahim, Chen, and Sinha [171].

One of the earliest proposals for Bayesian analysis in a proportional hazards model is due to Kalbfleisch (1978) [201], which we discussed in Section 12.2.2. This approach includes the full likelihood. One might question whether any justification exists for basing Bayesian inference on the partial likelihood proposed by Cox [88]. Sinha, Ibrahim, and Chen [297] address this, and find it reasonable to carry out inference via Cox's partial likelihood in the Bayesian setting. They consider a prior for the hazard function that is degenerate with point mass only at each observed failure time and give an algorithm for generating samples from this partial likelihood-based posterior. Their approach can also be used for frailty models and with time-dependent covariates.

Full likelihood-based approaches, however, are to be preferred as they follow Bayesian principles and generate coherent posterior inferences. There are many such methods available; for example in Laud, Damien, and Walker [216], DeIorio et al. [90], Sparapani et al. [302, 300], and Shi, Laud, and Neuner [295].

Evaluation of influential cases as in Chapter 10 is always an important consideration when carrying out model-based analyses. Johnson [186] introduced case-deletion diagnostics for estimating survival curves in the Bayesian log-normal survival model.

Clayton [81] extended the proportional hazards model for use in studies of familial propensities to experience chronic disease epidemiology. He modeled the data with a random frailty having a gamma distribution. See also Gustafson [156] for a Bayesian presentation of frailty models. Somewhat related are models for multivariate times to events [13, 155]. Also related to this area is the analysis of recurrent events, such as repeat hospitalizations or strokes; see Sparapani et al. [303].

In Section 12.2 we briefly mentioned extending semiparametric regression to allow for time-dependent covariates. We refer readers interested in learning more about time-dependent covariates to Collett [84] or Klein and Moeschberger [204] for results in frequentist survival analysis, and Hanson, Johnson, and Laud [159] for semiparametric Bayesian analyses. Shi, Laud and Neuner [295] include time-dependent covariates for a general nonparametric Bayesian survival model.

Another important area of survival analysis is inference in the presence of competing risks; see Section 11.5. Analyzing data in which patients are subject to competing risks is challenging because of a problem of identifiability. An early Bayesian treatment of semiparametric regression for competing risks is in the dissertation of Fan (2008) [104]; see also Chen et al. (2014) [69]. In a recent paper, Sparapani et al. (2020) bring a tree-ensemble-based Bayesian nonparametric approach to the analysis of times to events that are subject to competing risks [300].

Beyond semiparametric models, Bayesian nonparametric survival models also have been developed in the regression context. DeIorio et al. [90] extend dependent Dirichlet model to allow inference when hazard functions may not be proportional. We presented the DDP Weibull model of Shi, Laud, and Neuner [295] in Section 12.3 that can also address the non-proportional hazards situation. While these and other such models typically use generalizations of the Dirichlet process and mixtures of these, as we have seen, Sparapani et al. [300, 302, 303] take a different approach. They use Bayesian ensembles of binary trees to randomly tessellate the covariate space to model the outcome's dependence on the covariates. This is currently an active area of new developments in regression methods in general, for survival as well as other types of outcomes.

12.6 Exercises

EXERCISE 12.1. Fit an exponential AFT regression model to the larynx cancer data, including the same covariates as in Example 12.1. Since the exponential $Exp(\lambda)$ distribution is a special case of the $Weib(\alpha, \lambda)$ distribution, you can accomplish this by setting $\alpha = 1$. Compare the posterior inference with the exponential AFT model to the log-normal AFT model's results. Compare inferences with those in Tables 12.1 and 12.2.

EXERCISE 12.2. *Larynx cancer data.*

(a) Reanalyze the larynx cancer data using the Weibull AFT regression model. Compare results with the previous analyses in Example 12.1.
(b) Pick either the log-normal or the Weibull AFT regression model and investigate whether adding interaction terms improves the selected model. If it does, modify the model interpretation accordingly.

EXERCISE 12.3. *Log-normal priors.*

(a) Assume a single predictor variable, so each covariate vector is $x_i' = (1, x_{i1})$. Obtain explicit log-normal priors for median survival times t_{m1} and t_{m2} if the best guesses for the two medians are $\tilde{m}_{01} = 10$ and $\tilde{m}_{02} = 20$ and the expert's values of the 95th percentiles are 20 and 30, respectively.
(b) Assume that the single predictor variable is age and that it has been standardized. The average age in the data is 50, and the standard deviation is 5. Write a program to induce the prior on β when you have selected an average age of 50 for the first predictor and an age of 60, two standard deviations above the average, for

the second. Then

$$\tilde{X} = \begin{pmatrix} 1 & 0 \\ 1 & 2 \end{pmatrix}.$$

(c) Rewrite your program for the log-normal so that you solve two equations in two unknowns. Run the program and show the induced priors on the β_i.

EXERCISE 12.4. *Bedrick–Christensen–Johnson priors (see Section 12.1.1).* Repeat parts (a) and (b) of Exercise 12.3 for the Weibull AFT model.

EXERCISE 12.5. *Continuation of Exercise 12.3*

(a) Carry out a Bayesian analysis for Exercise 12.3 that incorporates inducing a partial prior on β, where $p = 1$. We elicit a prior best guess for the median survival in the baseline case, so the first row of $\tilde{X}$ identifies $t_{m1} \equiv \tilde{m}_{01}$. Repeat using the second row of $\tilde{X}$ and let $t_{m1} \equiv \tilde{m}_{02}$.

(b) Now suppose that there is a second covariate, say a dichotomous one relating to the individual's sex (= 1 if male and = 0 if female). Let

$$\tilde{X} = \begin{pmatrix} 1 & 0 & 0 \\ 1 & 2 & 0 \end{pmatrix}$$

and assume that the prior information for the two medians in Exercise 12.3 was actually specified for women. Using this partial prior information, write steps in a program to induce a prior on β.

EXERCISE 12.6. *Case deletion.* Let $D \equiv (y, \delta)$ represent the complete data. Denote the data with the ith case deleted by $D_{(i)}$. Write the ith case data as $d_i = (y_i, \delta_i)$, and let the likelihood based on all the data except d_i be $L(\beta, \sigma \mid D_{(i)}) \equiv L(\beta, \sigma \mid D)/L(\beta, \sigma \mid d_i)$. Prove the following:

$$p(\beta, \sigma \mid D_{(i)}) = \frac{L(\beta, \sigma \mid D_{(i)})p(\beta, \sigma)}{\int L(\beta, \sigma \mid D_{(i)})p(\beta, \sigma)d\beta d\sigma}$$

$$= \frac{p(\beta, \sigma \mid D)/L(\beta, \sigma \mid d_i)}{\int p(\beta, \sigma \mid D)/L(\beta, \sigma \mid d_i)d\beta d\sigma}.$$

EXERCISE 12.7. Show that the Weibull regression model, with an appropriate redefinition of β, satisfies the proportional hazards model (12.5). Give the explicit form for the baseline hazard h_0, the baseline cumulative hazard H_0, and the baseline survivor function S_0.

EXERCISE 12.8. Suppose you have data on time from diagnosis of cancer to death with two dichotomous predictors, sex (S) and race (R). You wish to fit a proportional hazards regression model to the data. Let S be the first variable, taking the value 1 for a female individual and 0 for a male individual. Let R take the value 1 if the person is African-American and 0 for a white person.

(a) With no interaction, construct an informative prior on the two regression coefficients that reflects beliefs that the hazard ratio comparing males to females is 1, with a 5% lower bound of 1/10, and that the hazard ratio for comparing African-American to white individuals is 3/7, with a 95% upper bound of 3/2. Write the necessary steps in an MCMC program (e.g., **BUGS**) to induce the prior on (β_1, β_2).

(b) Now assume an interaction and construct an informative prior for (β_1, β_3) as if you have elicited the following information. Assume a best guess for the hazard ratio comparing a white females to a white males of 5/9 with 95% upper bound 3/2, and a best guess for the hazard ratio comparing African-American females to African-American males is 5 with a lower 95% bound of 4/5. Write the necessary steps in an MCMC program (e.g., **BUGS**) to induce the prior on (β_1, β_3)

(c) Now assume the same elicitation in (b) and add a best guess for the hazard ratio comparing an African-American female to a white female of 1.0 with an upper 95% bound of 3. Find the induced prior on $(\beta_1, \beta_2, \beta_3)$. Write the necessary steps in an MCMC program (e.g., **BUGS**) to induce the full prior. In the same program, induce the prior on the four hazard ratios comparing (i) white females to white males, (ii) African-American females to African-American males, (iii) African-American females to white females, and (iv) African-American males to white males.

(d) Modify the prior in (c) to be only partially informative, using only the first two specifications. Obtain the induced prior on all four hazard ratios.

EXERCISE 12.9. *Full conditional distributions for the proportional hazards model.* Consider the model specified in Sections 12.2 and 12.2.3. Assume the partition with interval $I_k = [a_{k-1}, a_k)$ and a general prior model for each interval's hazard rate $\lambda_k \sim Ga(b_{0k}, d_{0k})$. Further, assume one covariate and the prior $\beta \sim N(\beta_0, \sigma_0^2)$.

(a) Derive the forms of the full conditional distributions for β, the regression coefficients, and for $\lambda_1, \ldots, \lambda_K$ assuming at least one death in every interval.

(b) Explain how to sample each.

(c) Suppose the interval $[a_{k-1}, a_k)$ contains no deaths. Show that with $\lambda_k \sim Ga(b_{0k}, d_{0k})$, the full conditional posterior distribution has the form $\lambda_k \sim Ga\{b_{0k}, g(\lambda_{(k)}, \beta, data)\}$ for some function $g(\cdot)$. If b_{0k} is small and $g(\lambda_{(k)}, \beta, data)$ is large, the distribution focuses on small values. Explain why this might cause computational difficulties. Are computational difficulties more likely to occur when k is large or small?

(d) Consider the prior model $\lambda_k \sim Ga(\lambda^* c, c)$ given in Section 12.2.3, with λ^* the best *a priori* guess for the baseline exponential hazard rate. Obtain the posterior mode for the full conditional of λ_k. Use this value to give a possible explanation of why the selection of the constant c could have a large impact on the posterior.

EXERCISE 12.10. *Larynx cancer data.* Analyze the larynx cancer data from Example 12.1. Compare a PH analysis with the AFT model analyses based on (i) log-normal and (ii) Weibull residual distributions.

EXERCISE 12.11. *Ovarian cancer trial.* Edmonson et al. (1979) described a study that compared the anticancer drug cyclophosphamide to the combination of cyclophosphamide and doxorubicin [101]. The study enrolled 26 women who had ovarian cancer with tumors that were at least 2 centimeters in diameter. After surgery, any residual disease was assessed. The data set includes the following information for each woman; the name of the variable in the data set is in parentheses. The number of days from randomization until the woman died (*futime*), an indicator of whether the woman was still alive at the time of data collection (*fustatus* = 1 if a death and 0 if censored), the woman's age (*age*), an indicator of the extent of residual disease (*resid.ds* = 1 if incomplete, 2 if complete), and indicator of the treatment assignment (*rx* = 1 if single-agent cyclophosphamide, 2 if the combination regimen), and the patient's mobility or performance status (*ecog.ps* = 1 if good and 2 if poor). The data are included with the R package survival and are also available on the book's website with the file name `OvarianCancerTrial.csv`.

(a) Carry out an analysis using log-normal AFT regression.

(b) Carry out an analysis using Weibull AFT regression.

(c) Carry out an analysis using the Weibull proportional hazards model.

(d) Make comparative comments on results from parts (a), (b), and (c).

(e) Carry out an analysis using the DDP Weibull model with LIO priors.

(f) Use results from parts (a)–(e) to make recommendations regarding differences in the treatments with respect to survival.

EXERCISE 12.12.   Modify your program for a Bayesian proportional hazards regression analysis to include a single fixed time-dependent covariate.

EXERCISE 12.13.   Carry out an analysis of the CALGB 8541 trial using the DDP Weibull model and LIO priors.

(a) Determine the posterior distributions for the median disease-free survival in each of the three treatment arms, for the 5-year disease-free survival probabilities for each arm, and for the hazard ratios of arms 2 and 3 relative to arm 1.

(b) What do you conclude about how the three treatment regimens compare with respect to the disease-free survival outcome? Arm 1 is the most dose-intense treatment regimen of the three, although the total dose is the same for arms 1 and 2. What do you think the study tells you about dose versus dose intensity, based on a comparison of arms 1 and 2? Justify your conclusions by quantitative summaries as informed by the data. Also use graphs to communicate your conclusions.

Chapter 13

Clinical Trial Designs

An important goal of biomedical research is to discover the causes of diseases and find effective ways to treat them. Some diseases affect patients acutely, such as pneumonia or other infections. Other diseases may progress to become clinically symptomatic more slowly and last longer, requiring long-term therapy, sometimes for the rest of the person's life. In all cases, however, the research is driven by learning, then developing and testing theories. Sometimes the research is based in a laboratory, either with cell lines, yeast, or mammals. Eventually, though, the research will move to evaluate the therapy in clinical settings, both human and veterinary. Clinical trials are a class of experiments carried out as research in a clinical setting.

There are several very good books that describe key aspects of clinical trials [118, 260]. Aside from the important statistical aspects of clinical trial methodology and practice, these books cover logistics, protocol development, administration, and so on.

This chapter seeks to provide some insight into how Bayesian ideas can be brought to bear on clinical trial design and analysis in order to improve the study. Improvement can relate to the study being more ethical, more efficient, more flexible, more consistent with one's views of inference or science, or some combination of these. We do not intend to be all-inclusive but, rather, seek to provide an overview of the ways some trialists have applied Bayesian thinking to the design of clinical trials and how Bayesian thinking has influenced current views of clinical research. Although we only scratch the surface, we present a fairly broad range of examples to whet the reader's appetite. This topic is a dynamic area of research, and many more applications will appear in the literature. The recent book by Berry et al. provides details of Bayesian adaptive designs [41].

In the following sections, we will first define what we mean by "clinical trial." We will then review the different types of studies often considered as clinical trials and provide some Bayesian approaches to designing these studies.

We do want to point out that there are several flavors of Bayesian designs in the literature. There are two main classifications: fully Bayesian and so-called *stylized* Bayesian designs [231]. The former type of Bayesian design sets the design parameters to maximize the expected value of some utility function that relates to the goals and costs of the study. The other type of design adjusts parameters in the prior distribution or modifies decision rules to achieve desirable frequentist characteristics. We discuss Bayesian designs of both types in this chapter.

13.1   What Are Clinical Trials?

Clinical trials are essentially experiments evaluating different forms of therapy in a setting that is somewhat similar to the setting in which the therapy would be used. Some authors distinguish clinical trials from general clinical studies by reserving the term "trial" for a randomized study. We follow that practice in this chapter, since it allows us to distinguish studies designed to confirm or test hypotheses from studies that are primarily intended for estimation of treatment effects, or even to generate reasonable hypotheses.

One distinguishes clinical studies by their purpose in drug development. The development of pharmaceuticals is traditionally divided into different phases that proceed sequentially. Phase 1 studies seek to learn about toxicity as it relates to dose or schedule. Phase 2 studies generally look for activity, sometimes as a function of dose. Randomized studies that are designed to establish the clinical effectiveness of one therapy over one or several others are phase 3 clinical trials. Phase 3 trials are often the final step in the process of getting regulatory approval for a drug. There are also phase 4 studies that collect data as part of post-marketing surveillance after a drug has received regulatory approval. The goal of such pharmacovigilance is often to collect more information on side effects now that a larger number of people are taking the medication in general clinical settings.

Since we have used the term "effectiveness" already, we want to indicate that the term has a rather technical meaning in the context of clinical research. In general, "efficacy" is related more to the biologic effect of the treatment, whereas "effectiveness" relates more to what one might expect in real-world clinical settings. For example, effectiveness studies will typically have fewer eligibility criteria, in order to allow one to gather information in a broad population of potential patients. Many clinical trialists have proposed simple protocols for large randomized clinical trials to attempt to steer these randomized studies more towards collecting effectiveness data than efficacy data.

Another principle that one finds in effectiveness research is analysis by intention-to-treat. This principle dictates that comparisons of treatments in randomized trials will be based on data from all randomized patients, whether or not the patient took all of the medication and followed the prescribed course of treatment. An analysis of only those patients who took all of their medicine as prescribed would typically be asking questions relating to efficacy. An analysis of patients according to the treatment groups to which they were assigned, ignoring adherence to prescribed treatment, would have a focus on the clinical effectiveness. This analysis considers the treatment effect as one might see it in the real world, where patients choose to adhere or not to prescribed treatment.

A different but related distinction in types of trials is found in Schwartz and Lellouch [282]. They coined the terms "explanatory" and "pragmatic" clinical trials. Explanatory trials focus on the biologic effect of the treatment, while pragmatic trials provide treatment comparisons as they might be realized in actual clinical practice. Schwartz and Lellouch show how the distinction suggests different designs.

13.2 Phase 1 Studies (Dose Finding)

The discussion here will focus mostly on phase 1 study designs in oncology. One reason is that most of the proposals in the statistical literature have been for this application. The other reason is that we have the most experience working with phase 1 studies in oncology.

In a phase 1 study, one picks a starting dose and a set of dose levels to explore. The basis for the starting dose most commonly relates to preliminary animal studies. These animal studies examine toxicity and often include some measure of effect. Toxicity evaluations of many medicines in animals are indeed relevant to learning about toxicity in humans. An early investigation into metabolism showed that if one examines kinetics across species, the logarithms of these measures are linearly related to body surface area on the log scale [117]. Given this cross-species relationship, starting doses are usually some fraction of a dose having a prespecified toxicity risk in a given species, usually whichever species turned out to be the most sensitive. The U.S. Food and Drug Administration issued *Guidance for Industry: Estimating the Maximum Safe Starting Dose in Initial Clinical Trials for Therapeutics in Adult Healthy Volunteers* in 2005 with guidelines for choosing the starting dose [105].

In medical oncology, however, the drugs have often been toxic, and phase 1 studies have enrolled cancer patients rather than healthy volunteers as in drug development for other disease indications. Often, the starting dose for anticancer drugs has been one-tenth of the LD_{10} in mice or one-third of a low-risk but toxic dose in dogs, whichever is smaller [8, 151]. The LD_{10} is the dose that was associated with a 10% mortality (see Section 8.3.1 for more details). The doses above are scaled according to body surface area, since this scale seems to allow cross-species dose–toxicity comparisons [117, 235].

The most commonly used study design for dose escalation in phase 1 oncology studies is the so-called "3+3" design. The algorithm for dose escalation with this design proceeds along the following lines. The first three patients in the study receive the starting dose. If none of these three patients experiences a dose-limiting toxicity (DLT), as defined in the study protocol, the next set of three patients will receive the next higher dose. While often prespecified, the sequence of doses may be more adaptive. For example, some phase I studies specify the dosing increment, often as a function of the degree of toxicity, that the study will follow when escalating the dose, rather than the actual doses.

If one of the three patients treated at a given dose experiences DLT, then the next group of three patients receives this dose of the drug. If two or more patients experience a DLT of the initial three patients or out of all six patients who received the dose under consideration, then the study typically concludes that the maximally tolerated dose (MTD) has been exceeded. If only one of the six has experienced a DLT, then the study will consider the next higher dose level for the next group of three patients. This design stops and declares the MTD to be the highest dose examined for which no more than one patient experienced a DLT.

Often in cancer drug development, treatment of an additional cohort of patients follows the initial 3+3 dose escalation. The purpose is often to gain more information about the toxicity associated with the dose that the dose escalation part of the study suggested is the MTD. Since at most six patients will have generally received the MTD or final schedule of the drug, one will want to monitor toxicity closely in this expansion cohort. One can easily include a Bayesian toxicity monitoring rule based on the posterior distribution of the risk of a DLT. This posterior distribution will include data from the initial dose-escalation part of the study via an informative prior distribution. This prior distribution for the expansion cohort could summarize the information for the MTD as a beta distribution. The two parameters for this prior beta distribution might consider that at most one patient experienced a DLT out of the six patients who received the drug at the MTD. Depending on one's outlook or assessment of the resulting operating characteristics, one might characterize this information about the dose-associated risk of a DLT as $Be(a+1, b+5)$, where the parameters a and b would reflect the *a priori* (i.e., before starting the dose escalation) belief about the risk of a DLT with this dose. For example, if one considered that a Jeffrey's prior distribution characterized that initial uncertainty, then $a = b = 0.5$, and the posterior distribution—after dose escalation but before the expansion cohort—for the risk of DLT at the MTD would follow a $Be(1.5, 5.5)$ distribution.

The following R code implements a toxicity monitoring rule for the expansion cohort. In the code, `ThetaCutOff` is the upper bound of the DLT risk that the investigators do not want to exceed.

```
a.post = a + x
b.post = b + (n-x)
PostDLTRiskTooHigh = 1 - pbeta(ThetaCutOff, a.post, b.post)
if (PostDLTRiskTooHigh <= RiskCutOff) stop
```

The result of applying this code is a set of rules of the form: stop if x out of n patients experience a DLT.

Example 13.1. Toxicity Monitoring in a Clinical Study. Investigators are evaluating a new treatment that has had only limited application clinically. The study will treat up to 15 patients. These investigators wish to set up data-based guidelines to warn them if the treatment is producing more serious adverse events than they deem worth the treatment's potential clinical benefit. Six patients have received the treatment, and one of the patients experienced a DLT. The investigators agree that they want to be warned if the evidence suggests that the risk of a DLT is greater than 30%.

The investigators, including the study statistician, decide to generate a monitoring rule that will trigger a warning if the posterior probability that the DLT risk is greater than 30% is 75% of greater. In other words, the warning will come if the odds are at least 3 : 1 that the DLT risk is 30% or more. Let θ be the DLT risk for the treatment under study. Since one of the first six patients experienced a DLT, the investigators and the statistician decide that a $Be(1.5, 5.5)$ distribution characterizes their current knowledge about θ, the risk of a DLT.

Table 13.1 shows the stopping rules for monitoring toxicity using the $Be(1.5, 5.5)$ prior distribution for the risk of a DLT. The rule calls for stopping if the posterior probability is 75% or more that the risk of DLT is 0.3 or more. The study protocol includes this table that the study statistician generated with the R program above. Including the table in the protocol allows all participating investigators to determine at any time whether or not the current DLT experiences of the patients suggest the treatment may be too toxic.

TABLE 13.1: Toxicity monitoring stopping rules for an expansion cohort of 15 patients

Stopping rule based on the number of DLTs out of n patients	Posterior probability that the toxicity risk > 0.3
Stop if DLT in 3 of 3 patients.	$P(\text{Risk} > 0.3 \mid \text{Data}) = 0.830$
Stop if DLT in 3 of 4 patients.	$P(\text{Risk} > 0.3 \mid \text{Data}) = 0.762$
Stop if DLT in 4 of 5 patients.	$P(\text{Risk} > 0.3 \mid \text{Data}) = 0.867$
Stop if DLT in 4 of 6 patients.	$P(\text{Risk} > 0.3 \mid \text{Data}) = 0.814$
Stop if DLT in 4 of 7 patients.	$P(\text{Risk} > 0.3 \mid \text{Data}) = 0.754$
Stop if DLT in 5 of 8 patients.	$P(\text{Risk} > 0.3 \mid \text{Data}) = 0.853$
Stop if DLT in 5 of 9 patients.	$P(\text{Risk} > 0.3 \mid \text{Data}) = 0.804$
Stop if DLT in 6 of 10 patients.	$P(\text{Risk} > 0.3 \mid \text{Data}) = 0.883$
Stop if DLT in 6 of 11 patients.	$P(\text{Risk} > 0.3 \mid \text{Data}) = 0.843$
Stop if DLT in 6 of 12 patients.	$P(\text{Risk} > 0.3 \mid \text{Data}) = 0.798$
Stop if DLT in 7 of 13 patients.	$P(\text{Risk} > 0.3 \mid \text{Data}) = 0.874$
Stop if DLT in 7 of 14 patients.	$P(\text{Risk} > 0.3 \mid \text{Data}) = 0.836$
Stop if DLT in 7 of 15 patients.	$P(\text{Risk} > 0.3 \mid \text{Data}) = 0.794$

The beta posterior distribution in Example 13.1 follows from the investigators considering that a Jeffreys prior distribution for θ was reasonable before they treated any patients. One might consider the Jeffreys prior (i.e., $Be(0.5, 0.5)$) to be an unusual choice, since this distribution is U-shaped, placing more probability mass away from the center and near 0 and 1. One might, instead, think that a more reasonable choice might put less probability near 1, since there would be little reason to consider applying a treatment that is more likely to have near 100% risk of a DLT than to have a 50% risk.

Many authors have pointed out the inefficiency of the 3+3 design. In particular, there is no underlying model guiding dose selection. Thus, decisions are relatively *ad hoc*, and there is no borrowing information across dose levels. The previous example illustrates the lack of precision in the estimated risk of DLT at the MTD following the initial dose escalation. With only six patients treated at the MTD, the uncertainty of the risk at this dose, as characterized by a 90% predictive interval based on the $Be(1.5, 5.5)$ posterior distribution, is wide: $(0.03, 0.49)$. A model-based approach could allow the information from all patients treated during dose escalation to inform the posterior distribution and might lead to greater precision.

One attempt to improve on the 3+3 design is the continual reassessment method (CRM) of O'Quigley, Pepe, and Fisher [254]. When using the CRM, one first indicates a target risk of DLT (θ) for the dose one will call the MTD. Given the way the 3+3 design decides on the MTD, one would imagine that the target risk is between 16.7% and 33.3% (i.e., between 1 in 6 and 1 in 3). Generally, one chooses 25% or 33%.

Dose escalation with the CRM is built upon a simple (i.e., single-parameter) sigmoidal model to explain the relationship between dose and the risk of toxicity. In their original paper, O'Quigley et al. considered the function in equation (13.1a) with the single parameter a to relate the risk of toxicity at dose d_i.

Other functional forms relating the risk of DLT to the dose of a drug have appeared in the CRM literature. Several authors use equation (13.1b). This prior specification is sometimes called a "skeleton," because it is a simple relationship between each dose level (d_i) and the prior estimate of the risk of toxicity at that dose level ($p_{0,i}$). The parameter in this model is $a \sim p(a)$. In cases where one wants to allow using doses intermediate to the prespecified dose levels, one will prefer to have a function that depends on dose for interpolation. Goodman, Zahurak, and Piantadosi [150] proposed using a logistic regression model as in equation (13.1c). They fixed the intercept parameter b_0 to simplify the model into a one-parameter logistic regression model. Three of the CRM functions that one often sees are the following:

$$f(d_i, a) = \{(\tanh d_i + 1)/2\}^a, \tag{13.1a}$$

$$f(d_i, a) = p_{0,i}^a, \tag{13.1b}$$

$$f(d_i, a) = \exp(b_0 + a \times d_i)/\{1 + \exp(b_0 + a \times d_i)\}. \tag{13.1c}$$

Each of these functions has only one parameter, a. Use of a one-parameter function makes the method efficient but probably not flexible enough to characterize the entire dose–toxicity risk curve. Although this function is unlikely to characterize adequately the dose–toxicity risk curve across all doses, it performs reasonably well over a small part of the curve, much like a straight line might approximate a small part of a curve. As the algorithm assigns doses closer to the target MTD (i.e., the part containing the target toxicity) the model should perform well.

A Bayesian application of the model in dose escalation requires a prior distribution, $p(a)$, to characterize the uncertainty about the parameter and, correspondingly, the uncertainty of the dose–toxicity risk curve. Furthermore, we require the parameter a to be positive in the CRM equation to maintain the relationship of increasing risk with increasing dose. We reparameterize the CRM equations (13.1a)–(13.1c) with $\beta = \exp(a)$. For example, equation (13.1b) becomes $f(d_i, \beta) = p_{0,i}^{\exp(\beta)}$. Now we are sure that the increasing risks across dose levels, namely, $p_{0,1} < \ldots < p_{0,M}$, ensure $d_1 < \ldots < d_M$. A particularly simple and convenient prior for the parameter is $\beta \sim N(0, \sigma_\beta^2)$.

One way to specify a prior distribution is to elicit a prior mean risk of DLT at each of the prespecified dose levels in the study. Consider a study with six dose levels $x_1, \ldots, x_6$. Suppose the clinical experts assign prior estimates of DLT risk at each dose level, $p_{0,1}, \ldots, p_{0,6}$. If we assume the dose–risk function in equation (13.1a), then we can use the inverse function to find the right scale into which to convert the actual doses. The conversion simply finds the rescaled doses $(x_1^*, \ldots, x_6^*)$ such that the dose–risk function fits. That is, $x_i^* = f^{-1}(p_i)$, assuming that $a = 0$, the prior mean.

Rather than use the actual doses, one typically relabels the dose levels when applying the CRM. The prior for the CRM consists of pairs of dose levels and risks $(d_i, p_{0,i}^{\exp(\beta)})$, $i = 1, \ldots, M$ for the M dose levels. Since we assume an increasing risk of toxicity with increasing dose level, we can invert the relationship to find the rescaled dose level. Specifically, we invert the prior relationship, perhaps assuming that the parameter β equals its prior mean. Finally, the rescaled dose levels with $\beta = 0$ are simply $d_i = p_{0,i}$, $i = 1, \ldots, M$. We can also invert the logistic function in equation (13.1c), with $\exp(\beta) = a$, to get rescaled dose levels.

As patients receive the different doses and some patients experience DLTs, Bayesian calculations lead to updated characterizations of the posterior distribution of the parameter and of any function of the parameter. The function of the parameter that is of greatest interest is the point on the dose–toxicity risk curve associated with the target toxicity risk. Using the function in equation (13.1a), we find that the MTD will be dose d^*, the dose that satisfies $f(d^*, \beta) = \theta$.

Posterior inference is fairly straightforward. Suppose there are I dose levels, n_i patients at each dose level, and that y_i of the patients at dose level i experienced a DLT. Then the sampling distribution is binomial and the posterior distribution is proportional to the likelihood times the prior:

$$p(\beta \mid y_1, \ldots, y_I, n_1, \ldots, n_I) \propto \left\{ \prod_{i=1}^{I} f(d_i, \beta)^{y_i} \left[1 - f(d_i, \beta)\right]^{(n_i - y_i)} \right\} p(\beta).$$

One can easily use either model for the risk of a DLT. Based on a grid of possible parameter values, the algorithm generates the posterior distribution by evaluating $p(y \mid \theta) \times p(\theta)$. From the posterior distribution on a grid, one can compute random samples of predicted binary events (toxicity or not) for the next patient and decide on the appropriate dose accordingly.

We include some R code that computes the posterior and the posterior predictive distributions with a one-parameter dose–risk function for the CRM. The sample code includes the one-parameter dose–risk function in equation (13.1a), but one can program any risk function that one considers appropriate. The code easily generalizes to accommodate a two-parameter dose–risk function. For example, if one has a two-parameter logistic regression of the risk on dose, one can apply the grid-based approach given in Gelman et al. [133, Chapter 3].

```
# Define the function that computes the risk as a function of dose.
pYgivenX = function(Dose, a) {
   ((tanh(Dose) + 1) / 2)^a
}
#    Form grid (ParamGrid) for parameter Param.
#    nGrid is the length of the grid. Initialize the vector for evaluating the
#    likelihood for each value of the parameter Param on the grid.
#
ParamGrid = seq(from=0, to=UpperLimitParam, by=0.1)
nGrid = length(ParamGrid)
Likeli = rep(0, nGrid)
#
#    Compute likelihood times prior at each grid value
#    using the function pYgivenX to evaluate the likelihood.
#
for (i in 1:nGrid) {
   LikeliTimesPrior[i] = GetLikeliTimesPrior(ParamGrid[i], Y, Dose)
}
#
#    Normalize posterior: Divide by integral of likelihood times prior.
#
PosteriorParam = LikeliTimesPrior /
   integrate(LikeliTimesPrior, lower=0, upper=3)$integral
#
#    Compute the predictive distribution.
#    First, initialize vector for predictive distribution at grid.
#
PredRisk = rep(0, nGrid)
#
#    Predicted risk is the sampling distribution times the
#    posterior at each grid value. Function pYgivenX
#    evaluates the risk function for a dose at a given value
#    of the parameter Param.
#
for (i in 1:nGrid) {
   PredRisk[i] = pYgivenX(Dose, ParamGrid[i]) * PosteriorParam[i]
}
```

Babb, Rogatko, and Zacks [14] proposed an algorithm for dose escalation with overdose control (EWOC). The goal is to find the highest dose that has posterior probability of exceeding the MTD no greater than some small value α. In EWOC, the MTD is defined as the dose for which the risk of DLT is some prespecified value θ. One can use EWOC in studies with prespecified dose levels and when determining doses between preset minimum and maximum doses.

With EWOC, one first chooses a sigmoidal curve, such as a cumulative distribution function, to characterize the dose–DLT risk curve. Consider the logistic function, with dose d, such that

$$P(\text{DLT} \mid d) = \frac{\exp(\beta_0 + \beta_1 d)}{1 + \exp(\beta_0 + \beta_1 d)}.$$

The assumption is that the risk of DLTs increases with dose (i.e., $\beta_1 > 0$). As with the CRM, one chooses a target DLT risk (θ) to determine the recommended phase 2 dose (RP2D). Knowing β_0 and β_1, one can determine the RP2D from the logistic function. A perhaps more intuitive parameterization is given by ρ_0, the DLT risk at the lowest dose considered in the study, and γ, the MTD or dose associated with the target risk of DLT (θ). After transforming the probability model for (β_0, β_1) to a probability model for (ρ_0, γ), one can find the marginal posterior distribution for the MTD, $p(\gamma \mid data) = \int p(\gamma, \rho_0 \mid data) d\rho_0$ (see Chapter 8). After treating the first patient cohort at the lowest dose ($d_{\min}$), EWOC assigns subsequent cohorts of patients doses such that the posterior probabilities that these doses exceed the MTD (or, equivalently, the MTD is lower than these doses) are some prespecified value α. That is, with γ equal to the MTD, the EWOC dose for the kth cohort is dose $d_k^\star$, such that

$$P(\gamma \leq d^\star \mid data) = \int_{d_{\min}}^{d_k^\star} p(\gamma \mid data) d\gamma = \alpha.$$

Tighiouart, Rogatko, and Babb [330] subsequently defined a prior distribution for (ρ_0, γ) that includes a negative correlation between these two parameters and, thus, has safer operating characteristics without sacrificing efficiency. A program for designing a phase 1 study using EWOC is available from https://biostatistics.csmc.edu/ewocWeb.php.

While many phase 1 studies concern dose finding for a single drug, treatment for several diseases (e.g., cancer, AIDS) involves combinations of drugs. Most phase 1 studies of multiple drugs proceed with an *ad hoc* approach to dose escalation. Thall et al. [317] proposed a Bayesian method for escalating the doses of two drugs within a single phase 1 study. These authors use a six-parameter function to model the toxicity risk associated with the doses of the two drugs. The function has the property that the dose–toxicity risk curve for one of the two agents is a logistic function when the model parameters corresponding to the other agent and the two agents' interaction are zero.

The procedure consists of two stages. In the first stage, successive cohorts of patients receive pairs of doses of the two drugs (d_1, d_2). These dose pairs lie along a line called L_1. This line consists of dose pairs that range from the lowest combination the investigators will consider, doses that are highly likely to be safe, to the pair that consists of the each drug's single-agent MTD, the latter combination likely too toxic. Successive cohorts of patients receive the combinations of doses along L_1 until one has treated n_1 patients. Here, n_1 is a design parameter. The design then moves to the second stage, at which the algorithm assigns to patient cohorts pairs of doses along a contour of predicted equal toxicity risk. This contour is L_2. Stage 2 ends once it has enrolled n_2 patients. That is, the total sample size will be $n_1 + n_2$. The four design parameters are the target toxicity risk, θ, the number of patients in each stage, n_1 and n_2, and the cohort size, c. A program for using this design is available from http://biostatistics.mdanderson.org.

While phase 1 studies typically focus on acute toxicities for dose escalation decisions, some therapies lead to late-occurring adverse events. In such instances, investigators may consider an extended follow-up period over which to collect toxicity information. Aside from the need to consider these late-occurring events when deciding on the recommended phase 2 dose, patients may enter the study before other patients have provided complete follow-up over the extended observation period. Cheung et al. [72] proposed an extension to the CRM approach for phase 1 studies with long periods during which to assess risk of DLTs. This method considers follow-up time when assessing the risk of an adverse event and is called the "time-to-event continual reassessment method" [72]. The basic method weights the modeled risk of an adverse event for each patient's contribution to the likelihood. The weight is a function of the proportion of the total prespecified follow-up time the patient contributes. If a patient has gone 45 days without an adverse event and follow-up will consist of 90 days, then the weight will be 0.5 if the weight function is linear in time. Obviously, nonlinear weight functions are also possible. More information is available in Cheung [71].

13.2.1   Joint Safety and Efficacy Monitoring

As already discussed, some Bayesian designs incorporate monitoring rules based on the posterior probability that a parameter, such as the probability of response, is far from some clinically meaningful target value. Thall and Russell and others [318, 357] have extended this approach to monitor the risk of adverse events and the probability of benefit. In the case of two binary endpoints, such as response and adverse event, the study design considers the multinomial distribution of four possible outcomes. By combining the appropriate categories, one can estimate the marginal posterior probabilities of an adverse event or response. One can then use these marginal posterior probabilities in separate monitoring rules to allow stopping the study if the treatment does not appear to show much efficacy or if it appears to be too toxic.

Consider the following scenario. Several clinicians wish to evaluate the safety and efficacy of a new therapy. Using a list of specific toxicities, coding their symptoms and manifestations as serious or worse, along with criteria for calling the treatment effective, the investigators reduce the outcomes to a pair of binary events: toxicity (yes or no) and efficacy (yes or no). A simple way to combine these events into a single outcome is to consider the four possible combinations, namely, $\{E\bar{T}\}$, $\{\bar{E}\bar{T}\}$, $\{\bar{E}T\}$, and $\{ET\}$, corresponding to "efficacy without toxicity," "no efficacy or toxicity," "no efficacy but toxicity," and "efficacy with toxicity," respectively. For each of these four events, one assigns *a priori* probabilities via a multinomial distribution. These probabilities have, in turn, a Dirichlet distribution prior, and the posterior distribution for these probabilities will then be Dirichlet. Interim stopping rules may relate to the separate marginal probabilities of efficacy and toxicity. For example, one might want the study to stop early if a patient's chance of achieving the efficacy outcome seems to be below a threshold (p_0^{eff}) or if toxicity exceeds a different threshold (p_0^{tox}). With the full posterior distribution for the probabilities of the four combinations, one can easily determine the posterior probability that the risk of serious toxicity exceeds the relevant threshold. That is, one can compute the probability of achieving an efficacy outcome as $p^{\mathrm{eff}} = P(\{E\}) = P\left(\{E\bar{T}\}\right) + P\left(\{ET\}\right)$, where, for ease of explanation, we have left off conditioning on the data to get the posterior probability. With this easily computed posterior probability, one might stop if $P(p^{\text{tox}} > p_0^{\text{tox}} \mid data)$ exceeds a value that corresponds to the level of certainty that one wishes to have before one makes a decision to stop.

Designs for simultaneously finding the right dose while considering efficacy outcomes have also appeared in the literature. Thall and Russell [318] presented an approach that combined safety and efficacy outcomes into ordered categories. Many of the concepts underlying this design find application in many other designs for clinical studies that base study monitoring on Bayesian posterior calculations. In the situation considered by Thall and Russell, one defines three ordered outcomes for each patient in the study. If we assume an underlying risk across patients in the study that depends only on the dose of the drug, then the three ordered outcomes are

$$Y = \begin{cases} 0, & \text{if serious toxicity without any efficacy,} \\ 1, & \text{if efficacy and serious toxicity,} \\ 2, & \text{if efficacy without serious toxicity.} \end{cases} \quad (13.2)$$

They consider a model that is appropriate for ordinal categorical outcomes, such as the proportional odds model, to relate the risk of outcome to dose [238]. We illustrate the model with an example scenario.

Let d be a particular dose in the study, and let $\text{odds}_j(d)$ be the odds that $Y \leq j$ at dose d. With the ordered outcomes shown above, we have

$$\text{odds}_j(d) = \frac{P(Y \leq j \mid \text{dose} = d)}{P(Y > j \mid \text{dose} = d)}, \quad j = 0, 1.$$

Since $P(Y \leq 2 \mid \text{dose} = d) = 1$, $P(Y > 2 \mid \text{dose} = d)$ is undefined, so we do not consider $\text{odds}_2(d)$. The proportional odds model incorporates covariates, such as dose, by assuming that the logarithm of the odds is linear in the covariates. That is,

$$\log\{\text{odds}_j(dose = d)\} = \theta_j + \beta \times d, \quad j = 0, 1.$$

Thus, there are three parameters in the model: $(\theta_0, \theta_1, \beta)$. We note that the slope parameter (β) is assumed the same for all odds, which corresponds to the proportional odds assumption. That is, for any dose, the odds of $Y \leq 1$ divided by the odds of $Y \leq 0$ is $\exp(\theta_1 - \theta_0)$, which does not depend on dose.

Thall and Russell [318] use a slightly different form of the proportional odds model. They characterize the odds of being in the same or higher category, that is, the reciprocal of the usual formulation of the proportional odds model. Furthermore, they set $\theta_1 = \mu + \alpha$ and $\theta_2 = \mu$ Regardless of which form of the model one chooses, there are three model parameters. The next step is to characterize the uncertainty of the model parameters with a prior probability distribution. Rather than work on the scale of the parameters, Thall and Russell describe prior specification based on the associated probability functions $P(Y = j \mid \text{dose} = d)$. As we emphasize in Chapter 6 and throughout the book, it is often easier to elicit priors on the scale that the investigators know than on the scale of the parameters. In many cases, one can go from one scale to the other, as in this case. By showing several different dose–probability curves to the investigators, including examples of extreme cases, one is able to define likely domains for the parameters. That is, one would include cases in which the probability of efficacy without toxicity is below a target threshold across all doses included in the study as one extreme. Another extreme would be a dose–toxicity risk curve that had the risk of toxicity uniformly above an acceptable level at all dose levels. With three parameters in the model, we would need a third scenario—maybe something in the middle. From these sample cases, one can derive a range of possible parameter values. Without any other information, such as which dose–response curves are more likely and which less likely, one can assume that the prior distributions for the parameters are independent and the parameters are uniformly distributed within their respective ranges.

The study's design has to consider the study's goals. In this case, the goal is to find which of several possible doses provides the best chance of efficacy without being too toxic. Operationally, this goal corresponds to finding the dose that has enough probability that $Y = 2$ and low probability that $Y = 0$, referring to equation (13.2). It is up to the study investigators to decide on the respective threshold probabilities or risks. For example, for some diseases a chance greater than 25% that the patient will experience a clinical response without severe toxicity may be an improvement over standard care, while in other settings, the investigators may feel that a threshold of 65% may be a clinically meaningful minimum. Similarly, the study team will decide on toxicity risks that are appropriate for their study population. Call these thresholds p^*_{eff} and p^*_{tox} for efficacy and toxicity, respectively. With these cutoff values, one can formulate the early stopping rules for dose d in terms of futility. That is, one may wish to stop if mounting evidence suggests that $P(Y = 2 \mid \text{dose} = d, \ data) < p^*_{\text{eff}}$. Similarly, one may wish to drop a dose d' from further consideration if it appears too toxic, given the accumulating data; that is, stop dose d' if $P(Y = 0 \mid \text{dose} = d', \ data) > p^*_{\text{tox}}$.

We now have a probability model for the data and threshold probabilities for the chance a patient will achieve a positive outcome (efficacy) and the risk of serious toxicity. As we treat more patients at a given dose, we will learn more about these probabilities. That is, viewing these probabilities as model parameters or functions of model parameter, (e.g., functions of $(\theta_0, \theta_1, \beta)$ in the proportional odds model), we can carry out Bayesian computations that lead to a posterior distribution for these quantities. Thus, even though $P(Y = 2 \mid \text{dose} = d)$ is a probability, it is also a prediction and a function of model parameters. Both of our key outcome monitoring probabilities are functions of the model parameters, namely,

$$P(Y = 2 \mid \text{dose} = d) = g_2(\theta_0, \theta_1, \beta, d) = \frac{1}{1 + e^{(\theta_1 + \beta \times d)}},$$

$$P(Y = 0 \mid \text{dose} = d) = g_0(\theta_0, \theta_1, \beta, d) = \frac{e^{(\theta_0 + \beta \times d)}}{1 + e^{(\theta_0 + \beta \times d)}}. \tag{13.3}$$

Thus, we can talk about uncertainty in these functions, with the uncertainty changing (decreasing, one would hope) with accumulating data as we learn about the parameters. That is, with $g_2(\theta_0, \theta_1, \beta, d) = P(Y = 2 \mid \text{dose} = d)$, we can compute its posterior expected value and also make probability statements about this function.

For example, we can talk about the posterior mean of $P(Y = 2 \mid \text{dose} = d)$ as

$$E\{g_2(\theta_0, \theta_1, \beta, d) \mid data\} = \int \int \int g_2(\theta_0, \theta_1, \beta, d) p(\theta_0, \theta_1, \beta \mid data) d\theta_0 d\theta_1 d\beta.$$

Similarly, we can compute the probability that the chance of efficacy without serious toxicity is below, say, 20% as

$$\int \int \int I\{g_2(\theta_0, \theta_1, \beta, d) < 0.2\} p(\theta_0, \theta_1, \beta \mid data) d\theta_0 d\theta_1 d\beta, \qquad (13.4)$$

where $I\{X < x\}$ is an indicator function that takes the value 1 when the condition $\{X < x\}$ is true and 0 otherwise. Putting this statement into words leads to the cumbersome and, for some, problematic statement about the probability of a probability, namely, the posterior probability that $P(Y = 2 \mid \text{dose} = d) < 0.2$. Despite the awkwardness of such statements, they do allow us to set up monitoring rules for studies based on how certain we become that a patient's chance of a good treatment outcome is too low or that the treatment-associated risk of toxicity is too high. This certainty is the posterior probability calculation in equation (13.4).

The next step in determining the monitoring rule is for the study team to decide how much certainty (in terms of posterior probabilities) they wish before concluding that a particular dose is either not effective enough or too toxic. Let these threshold probabilities be denoted by7 π_1 and π_2 for the thresholds relating to efficacy and toxicity, respectively, borrowing the notation in Thall and Russell. Formally, then, we would want to consider stopping a particular dose ($d^\star$) for lack of sufficient efficacy if $P(\{P(Y = 2 \mid d^\star, data) < p^\star_{\text{eff}}\}) \geq \pi_1$. That is, if we determine that there is high probability (i.e., π_1 or larger) that the treatment-associated chance of efficacy without severe toxicity is below $p^\star_{\text{eff}}$, then we might want to stop for futility. Similarly, we would consider stopping a dose if we find it appears too toxic, as in $P(\{P(Y = 0 \mid d^\star, data) > p^\star_{\text{tox}}\}) \geq \pi_2$. Of course, we can write these statements without the "probability of a probability" by instead using the functions of the parameters in equations (13.3). The equivalent statements would be

$$P\left(\{g_2(\theta_0, \theta_1, \beta) < p^\star_{\text{eff}}\} \mid data\right) \geq \pi_1,$$
$$P\left(\{g_0(\theta_0, \theta_1, \beta) > p^\star_{\text{tox}}\} \mid data\right) \geq \pi_2.$$

As long as we can compute these posterior probabilities, perhaps by resorting to iterative sampling methods outlined in Chapter 4, we can run the study.

One extension of this approach is the following. One might want the study treatment to be a substantial improvement over the standard therapy. If $p^{\text{eff}}_{\text{stnd}} = 0.2$ is the historical chance of efficacy with the standard form of therapy, then one might only be interested in the new therapy if the probability of efficacy with the new therapy is at least 0.4 ($= p^{\text{eff}}_{\text{stnd}} + 0.2$); see also [320].

Quite often, the historical value ($p^{\text{eff}}_{\text{stnd}}$) is an estimate and, therefore, subject to uncertainty. Some have argued that the design should account for this uncertainty by considering its distribution when determining the study design's operating characteristics [319, 320]. Incorporating this uncertainty into the study's design does affect the operating characteristics. If, however, the study does not treat patients with the historical standard therapy, then nothing is learned with respect to the standard. There is no notion of gaining knowledge or certainty as characterized by the transformation from the prior distribution to the posterior distribution. Instead, the stopping criterion based on $p^{\text{eff}} > p^{\text{eff}}_{\text{stnd}}$ now requires greater certainty to stop. In effect, then, placing a distribution on this historical probability of efficacy is really just a sort of trick to achieve better frequentist operating characteristics. One could achieve the same operating characteristics by changing the prior for p^{eff}, making this prior more diffuse. If, as may be the case, the prior for p^{eff} is based on prior data, then one would have to discount those early data to make the prior more diffuse. In this way, the choice is either to discount the early data, making the prior more uncertain, or to add the extra uncertainty to the benchmark criterion $p^{\text{eff}}_{\text{stnd}}$. Logically, if the operating characteristics suggest greater certainty than one feels is warranted, as when the study seems to stop more often with smaller sample sizes than one feels comfortable, then it seems reasonable to associate the investigator's preference with less prior certainty for the current treatment or change the decision rules, rather than place that uncertainty on a parameter about which the study will shed no light.

13.3 Evaluation of a Design's Characteristics

Part of determining whether a given study design is appropriate and will satisfy the needs and desires of the study team requires evaluation of the design's performance under different scenarios. In general, one will have to use computer simulations, since many designs do not lend themselves to closed-form analytic solutions. We now discuss the general strategy for simulating designs that incorporate Bayesian calculations for monitoring or final analysis. The discussion focuses on some general principles, since each study will tend to have its own unique needs.

The study team and reviewers of the protocol generally want to ensure that the study design will allow for safe and efficient achievement of the study's goals. Does the study stop early and often in case of severe toxicity? Can we be confident that, in the end, the right dose will be the one that gets recommended for subsequent study? Answers to these and similar questions will be desired by the team and reviewers of the study. By simulating the trial under various settings, one can provide information to answer these questions. With a statistical model to characterize the study data and the monitoring decision rules, it becomes fairly straightforward to simulate the study multiple times.

The scenarios under which one simulates the study design will represent generally realistic situations, as well as some extreme conditions. The reason why one includes extreme scenarios is not that they represent likely situations. It is to show that the design will act appropriately should these extreme situation arise.

In many cases, the scenarios will represent a single value for the parameter of interest, such as the risk of dose-limiting toxicity at each dose level or the chance of an outcome indicating efficacy or no treatment difference in a randomized clinical trial. One has to distinguish the "true" underlying value of the parameter that one uses in the simulations from the prior distribution that is used for data analysis. The prior distribution for analysis may be vague or diffuse to allow the data to dominate inference. The simulated set of parameters, on the other hand, may be quite precise—in fact, it will often be a single fixed value, as already mentioned. The real difference between the prior distribution and the value or values of the parameters in the simulations, however, is that the prior distribution is used for analysis, while the simulated values are used to evaluate the design. Wang and Gelfand [343] call the distribution characterizing likely parameter values in a given scenario (i.e., the simulation truth) the "sampling priors." They call the prior distribution that is used in the analysis for monitoring and inference the "fitting prior." Whether one considers a single underlying parameter value or not, one needs to keep this distinction in mind. The goal of the simulations is to elucidate and present the characteristics of the study's design under different possible scenarios. Thus, one wants to assume certain parameter values, run the study *in silico*, and summarize the results. Running the study means using the inferential framework that is part of the study's design and planned analyses. This inferential framework includes the analysis or fitting prior distribution that one will use to analyze the trial data. We give an example in Section 13.5.

13.4 Phase 2 Studies (Activity)

The goal of phase 2 studies of pharmaceuticals is generally to provide early evidence of clinical activity. These studies may also evaluate different doses, even though phase 1 studies will have provided information about the dose–toxicity association and established the maximally tolerated dose. In many disease areas, phase 1 studies enroll healthy volunteers, and phase 2 studies are the first studies to treat patients with the new agent. Phase 1 studies of anticancer agents, on the other hand, tend to enroll patients who have relapsed or failed to respond to standard and, perhaps, experimental treatment options. Furthermore, phase 2 studies in oncology will often enlist patients who have received fewer prior therapies than have patients who often enroll in phase 1 studies of new anticancer therapies.

While it is still common to carry out single-arm phase 2 studies, especially in oncology, randomized phase 2 studies are becoming more widespread. Part of the rationale for randomized phase 2 studies concerns the desire to learn about the dose–efficacy relationship. By randomizing patients to different doses, one will collect dose–response data from which one can infer the relationship. Additionally, there may be questions about which of several possible formulations of the drug or dosing schedules might be better for clinical use. It is more efficient to address such questions in smaller phase 2 studies before one goes on to large, randomized phase 3 clinical trials. Yet another impetus for randomization in phase 2 studies is the low frequency of phase 3 studies that demonstrate significant benefit of the new treatment. Without randomization to a control therapy in phase 2, the study may show greater than expected activity because it happened to enroll healthier patients or because of improvements in supportive care or other unmeasured factors.

Phase 2 study designs fall into two broad categories. Some designs seek to estimate treatment activity, while others approach the objective by casting it in terms of testing statistical hypotheses. The ultimate design, particularly the sample size, will depend on the underlying philosophy. If the goal is estimation, the study will often try to achieve a certain precision in the estimate. Phase 2 studies based on hypothesis testing, on the other hand, often base sample size targets on frequentist power considerations, while interim monitoring rules will usually protect the frequentist error probabilities. A third approach to phase 2 study design, one based on decision-theoretic considerations, seeks to maximize some prespecified utility function in expectation. We will now discuss these three approaches in turn after a few preliminaries.

13.4.1   Sample Size

A key question that investigators must address when designing a study concerns the number of individuals to enroll, treat, and follow for the study's endpoint. The standard frequentist approach to sample size determination in the context of hypothesis testing uses the sampling distribution and finds the sample size, n, as the smallest number of observations that achieves a predetermined power for a specific (i.e., fixed) alternative parameter value (θ_a), subject to keeping a specific Type I error probability less than or equal to some upper bound (usually 0.05). The choice of the Type I error probability, α, generally enters into the sample size calculation by defining the part of the sample space that has probability α under the null hypothesis (θ_0), that is, the rejection region. Once the rejection region is defined, one can compute the probability associated with this portion of the sample space under any hypothesis as a function of the sample size. As the sample size increases, the probability of being in the rejection region under θ_a will also increase. The frequentist will typically choose the sample size n for which the probability of being in the rejection region equals the desired power ($1 - \beta$, where β is the Type II error probability).

Frequentist designs incorporate any prior knowledge that relates to the study as one or several constants in the model formulation. For example, the value of the parameter (e.g., treatment effect) for the null and alternative hypotheses may be informed by data from a previous or related clinical study. The prior data may well be an estimate from a small study, in which case there may be considerable uncertainty associated with it. This uncertainty is ignored, however, in the frequentist formulation of the problem. Instead, the estimate is treated as a known constant when designing the study. Similarly, one may need to posit values for other parameters in the sampling model, such as variances. Even in these situations, the general frequentist approach treats the assumed values as constants.

The Bayesian approach, on the other hand, allows one to account for the various levels of uncertainty arising from assumptions. The prior distribution can characterize such uncertainty directly, and the Bayesian formulation includes prior distributions for all model parameters. Similarly, the posterior distribution captures all remaining uncertainty regarding the model parameters after accounting for the information contained in the observations.

There are several approaches that build on the Bayesian framework for determining the sample size for a study. We consider two broad categories. Design approaches in one category consider the primary purpose of the study to be estimation. The investigators want to estimate some quantity with a certain amount of precision. The other category of design consists of fully Bayesian approaches. These include a utility function that constitutes a tradeoff between the inferential or other goal of the study and the cost of each observation [229]. One chooses the sample size that maximizes the expected utility, where expectation is over the outcome's sample space and the parameter space with respect to the sampling distribution and prior distribution, respectively, through the predictive distribution. By including a utility function and taking expectation with respect to all sources of uncertainty, this approach is coherent. Here, "coherent" means that decisions are made with respect to probabilities that, by following the basic axioms of probability theory, are logically consistent.

13.4.2 Precision of Estimates

A Bayesian approach to designing a study that is seeking to provide an estimate with a certain level of precision will have to decide on a particular definition of *precision*. Earlier in the book, we defined precision as the reciprocal of the variance. That definition is a technical one. Here, we mean precision in a generic sense, although any operational definition for a study will be inversely related to the variance, since greater variance indicates less certainty and, hence, less precision.

Bayesian approaches tend to focus on finding a sample size that yields some level of precision in the estimate or some average behavior that satisfies the needs of the study organizers. Cao et al. [60] review and compare several Bayesian criteria for determining a sample size when one wants to achieve a certain precision in the estimate. Precision is based on characteristics of the predictive interval for the quantity one wishes to estimate. The criteria Cao et al. compare are what they call the average coverage criterion (ACC) [1], the average length criterion (ALC) [193], and the worst outcome criterion (WOC) [193]. One applies the ACC by first choosing an interval width l that one desires for a $100(1 - \alpha)\%$ predictive interval. Given l, one then finds the smallest integer that has average coverage at least $1 - \alpha$. The average is with respect to the marginal distribution of the data, $f(y) = \int f(x \mid \theta)p(\theta)d\theta$. That is, one finds the smallest n that satisfies

$$\int \left\{ \int_{a(y,n)}^{a(y,n)+l} f(\theta \mid y, n)d\theta \right\} f(y)dy \geq 1 - \alpha,$$

where $a(y, n)$ is the lower bound of the interval.

The ALC fixes the coverage, $1 - \alpha$, and finds the smallest integer for which the expected width of the interval is no larger than l. Again, one integrates with respect to the marginal density of the data. For this criterion, the interval's width is a function of the data and sample size. Let $w(y, n)$ be a function of the data and sample size that satisfies $\int_{a(y,n)}^{a(y,n)+w(y,n)} f(\theta \mid y, n)d\theta = 1 - \alpha$. The ALC sample size is the smallest integer such that

$$\int w(y, n)f(y)dy \leq l.$$

The WOC seeks to ensure that one achieves the desired coverage and the desired interval width over all possible outcomes. Rather than focus on all possible outcomes, one usually only considers a region of the sample space that has high probability (e.g., 95%). As pointed out by Cao et al. [60], the WOC is the most conservative criterion and leads to the largest sample sizes, compared to the ACC and ALC.

These approaches do not explicitly state a utility function to maximize. As pointed out by Joseph and Wolfson [195] in their discussion of Lindley [229], it is often difficult to specify a utility function in practice. They argue that no utility function may seem appropriate in some cases or satisfy all who design the study. On the other hand, they continue, improving accuracy of an estimate is straightforward, and precise estimates should lead to the right decisions, in general. For example, one might want the study to provide an estimate with a 90% posterior predictive interval width less than or equal to some value, on average. Alternatively, one might seek to achieve some level for the expected or average coverage of the interval.

Example 13.2. Sample Size for Precision: Known Variance. Consider a sample of n observations $y_1, \ldots, y_n$ with $y_i \mid \mu, \sigma^2 \sim N(\mu, \sigma^2)$. Furthermore, assume $\mu \sim N(\mu_0, \sigma^2/n_0)$. From the frequentist standpoint, which assumes fixed μ, the sample size required for a $100(1 - \alpha)\%$ confidence interval to have width l when σ^2 is known is the smallest n that satisfies

$$n \geq \frac{4\sigma^2 z_{1-\alpha/2}^2}{l^2}. \tag{13.5}$$

In equation (13.5), $z_{1-\alpha/2}$ is the $1 - \alpha/2$ quantile of the standard normal distribution.

If we assume that the variance, σ^2, is known, the sample size required for a Bayesian prediction interval with width equal to l to have at least $100(1 - \alpha)\%$ probability of containing the μ is given by

$$n \geq \frac{4\sigma^2 z_{1-\alpha/2}^2}{l^2} - n_0. \tag{13.6}$$

Notice how the *prior sample size*, n_0, adds information in the formula, essentially reducing the required sample size by n_0. In other words, the total sample size requirement is the same as the frequentist's sample size in equation (13.5), but the number of new samples we need to collect is n_0 fewer than we would need without this prior information.

If the variance is known, the sample size required by all three criteria is given by equation (13.6).

It is usually not the case that we know the variance, as we assumed in Example 13.2. We may have one or more previous studies that may provide some information about likely (and unlikely) values of the variance in our study. If we have a strong belief that these earlier studies provide reasonably accurate estimates of the variance we might expect in our study, then we may feel justified treating σ^2 as a known quantity. A Bayesian approach might still treat σ^2 as unknown but with a fairly tight prior distribution.

Example 13.3. Sample Size for Precision: Unknown Variance. If σ^2 is unknown, the Bayesian approach would place a prior distribution on this parameter. As we saw in Chapter 3, a convenient prior distribution for σ^2 is the inverse gamma distribution with parameters (ν, β). With this prior, the sample size required by ACC [60] is the smallest integer n that satisfies

$$n + n_0 \geq \frac{4t^2_{2\nu,1-\alpha/2}}{l^2} \frac{\beta}{\nu} . \tag{13.7}$$

The quantity $t_{\mathrm{df},1-\alpha/2}$ represents the $1 - \alpha/2$ quantile of Student's t distribution with df degrees of freedom.

If one wants to apply the criterion based on average length of the prediction interval (ALC [60]), then the required sample size is the smallest integer n that satisfies

$$2t_{n+2\nu,1-\alpha/2}\sqrt{\frac{2\beta}{(n+2\nu)(n+n_0)} \frac{\Gamma\left(\frac{n+2\nu}{2}\right)\Gamma\left(\frac{2\nu-1}{2}\right)}{\Gamma\left(\frac{n+2\nu-1}{2}\right)\Gamma(\nu)}} \leq l. \tag{13.8}$$

We note that equation (13.8) is undefined if $\nu < 0.5$.

We refer the reader to [60] for the sample size required by WOC.

13.4.3 Decision-Theoretic Sample Size Determination

A strictly Bayesian approach to sample size determination would place the number of patients in the context of a decision problem. That is, one might frame the question of sample size in terms of the cost of recruitment, treatment, and follow-up, balancing these costs against ultimate benefit. Whereas the costs of enrolling and treating patients are easy to imagine, it is often more difficult to find a proper metric on which to place the benefit of the study. From the standpoint of the entity that stands to benefit monetarily, it is more straightforward to allow the utility function to equate benefit to some monetary gain, against which one wants to consider the cost of carrying out the study. From the standpoint of public health or of increasing knowledge—both of which are reasonable benefits to consider as arising from clinical studies—the proper metric is less clear.

The components needed to apply Bayesian decision theory are the following.

First, one needs to specify the space of possible actions one will consider. This action space may consist of nominal discrete points, such as whether or not to stop the study, or the set of actions may be essentially continuous, as when one decides on the number of future patients to enroll. Secondly, there will be a utility function. This utility function can relate each action to a loss function, a gain, or a combination of the two, such as a function that relates cost to benefit. Next, one needs to specify a sampling distribution that characterizes the stochastic nature of the data the study will collect. This distribution often includes model parameters, some of which may relate to the primary study outcome, such as the probability of response or the treatment-specific risk of an event. Finally, one needs a characterization of the uncertainty associated with the model parameters (i.e., prior distributions). One needs to account for all of this uncertainty when deciding which action to take based on the expected utility that would result from each action. Once one has the expected utility for each action, considering a discrete action space to simplify the discussion, one can choose the action that is associated with the maximal expected utility.

Lindley [227, 226] approaches sample size from a Bayesian perspective. He presents a fully Bayesian approach to sample size determination. Lindley argues that the optimal sample size is the number n that maximizes the expected utility over the parameter and sample spaces. The decision may relate to the precision of the estimated treatment effect, with, perhaps, a tradeoff for the cost of collecting each observation.

Consider that the study designers want to make some decision d about the parameter θ at the end of the study. The designers will sample n individuals and collect data $\mathbf{y}$, where the distribution of the data depends in some way on the parameter as characterized by $p(\mathbf{y} \mid \theta)$. The utility function $u(n, \mathbf{y}, d, \theta)$ yields a value for each decision made and value of θ after analyzing the data from the n patients. As mentioned already, the utility may relate to the precision of the estimate, the cost of collecting the data, the benefit of finding a highly effective therapy, or combinations of these. We note that in many situations the decisions, d, may be design characteristics, including the sample size. In this example, though, we separate the sample size decision from the decisions one will make at the end of the study.

Assuming that the observations are conditionally independent and identically distributed, we have that the joint sampling distribution is $p(\mathbf{y} \mid \theta) = \prod_{i=1}^{n} p(y_i \mid \theta)$. We want to find the decision that maximizes the expected utility while accounting for the uncertainty in the parameter value and the variation in the future data for a fixed sample size. That is, we find the expected value of the utility for a given decision and sample size, integrating with respect to $p(\mathbf{y}, \theta \mid d, n)$. We can approach the integration by noting that $p(\mathbf{y}, \theta \mid d, n) = p(\theta \mid d, \mathbf{y}, n)p(\mathbf{y} \mid d, n)$. The two parts on the right-hand side are the posterior distribution times the marginal distribution of the data.

In Lindley's formulation of the problem, $p(\mathbf{y} \mid d, n) = p(\mathbf{y} \mid n)$, because the decision at the end, d, is conditionally independent of θ, given $\mathbf{y}$ and n, so

$$\max_n \left\{ \int \max_d \left(\int u(n, \mathbf{y}, d, \theta) p(\theta \mid d, \mathbf{y}, n) d\theta \right) p(\mathbf{y} \mid n) d\mathbf{y} \right\}. \tag{13.9}$$

Suppose, now, that the utility function is of the form $u(d, \theta) - cn$, where c is the cost per unit sample. In this formulation, the utility is solely a function of the decision d and the parameter θ.

Consider, for example, that we want an interval estimate of θ. The terminal decision may be to chose an interval based on the posterior distribution of θ that has posterior probability $1 - \alpha$ and is of minimum length, as discussed in Section 13.4.2. Lindley contrasts this approach with one in which the terminal decision consists of values a and b that will form the interval estimate (a, b) for θ. The full utility function is $u(a, b, \theta) - cn$, so that the cost of sampling appears in the utility function and the decision problem is coherent in the probabilistic sense. As an aside, a challenge in these sorts of problems is to determine the cost in the same units as the utility function—so-called "utiles." Let the decision, d, be the choice of the endpoints of the interval (i.e., a and b). Ignoring any set-up costs, one would determine the sample size by substituting this utility function into equation (13.9), yielding

$$\max_n \left\{ \int \max_d \left(\int u(d, \theta) p(\theta \mid d, \mathbf{y}, n) d\theta \right) p(\mathbf{y} \mid n) d\mathbf{y} - cn \right\}.$$

This formula is for general utility $u(d, \theta)$. One can make this procedure for interval estimation more aligned with frequentist interval estimation by including coverage (i.e., the probability that $\theta \in (a, b)$). Define the indicator function $\delta(\theta) = 1$ if $\theta \in (a, b)$ and 0 otherwise. Then one can include this in the utility function as $u(d, \theta) = u(a, b) + \delta(\theta)$.

Although we feel that most researchers conduct experiments to lead to a decision, there are studies with the goal of gathering information. There are different information measures in the statistical literature that one may consider to be consistent with the goal of study. One may wish to achieve a certain level of precision of an estimate, as we have already discussed. Alternatively, we may wish to consider a measure of information that is related to knowledge or uncertainty about a state of nature. (Most often, the state of nature corresponds to a parameter or set of parameters in a statistical model.) Inspired by Shannon's theory of information, Lindley [223] proposed entropy of the posterior distribution as the relevant information measure back in 1956. For an experiment that yields n observations $x_1, \ldots, x_n$, where $x \sim p(x)$, the information in the experiment is given by $\sum_i p(x_i) \log\{p(x_i)\}$. Since the experiment seeks to increase our knowledge about the state of nature (i.e., θ in the statistical model), we may characterize the gain in information from an experiment that yields observations $x_1, \ldots, x_n$ in terms of the change in entropy from the prior distribution to the posterior. Averaging over uncertainty, we would consider the average amount of information provided by the observations as

$$\int p(\theta \mid x_1, \ldots, x_n) \log\{p(\theta \mid x_1, \ldots, x_n)\} d\theta - \int p(\theta) \log\{p(\theta)\} d\theta.$$

If we now want to compare experiments (i.e., study designs) during the planning stage, we would also want to account for the uncertainty in the data. That is, we would also integrate over the possible outcomes of the experiment. Let $\mathcal{I}_0 = \int p(\theta) \log\{p(\theta)\} d\theta$, the amount of "knowledge" or information in the prior distribution. After the experiment that yields the observation x, the amount of information provided by the experiment is $\mathcal{I}_1(x) = \int p(\theta \mid x) \log\{p(\theta \mid x)\} d\theta$. The average amount of information an experiment is expected to provide is $E_x[\mathcal{I}_1(x) - \mathcal{I}_0]$, which equals

$$\int \left[\int p(\theta \mid x) \log\{p(\theta \mid x)\} d\theta - \int p(\theta) \log\{p(\theta)\} d\theta \right] p(x) dx. \tag{13.10}$$

This information measure provides a means with which to compare possible experiments. One will choose the design that one expects will provide the most information.

Other researchers have considered entropy in the design of studies. Sebastiani et al. [287] develop other entropy-like information measures. Piantadosi [260] considers the use of entropy when designing translational studies that typically have small sample sizes and seek to learn about biologic effects of a treatment. Recently, Ventz et al. [340] have proposed allocating patients to treatments adaptively based on entropy considerations.

13.5 Interim Analyses and Stopping Rules

An important part of designing a clinical study is knowing when to stop the study. We have discussed planning the size of the study in terms of the target sample size. Investigators, funding agencies, and patients will also want to know the results of a study as soon as one can draw a conclusion from the study's data. Most clinical trials, therefore, include statistical monitoring rules or stopping boundaries. These boundaries may focus only on stopping early if there is sufficient evidence that the new treatment is superior to the control therapy. Many clinical trials also include futility stopping rules that suggest stopping the study earlier than planned when the accruing data indicate that there is little chance the study will conclude in favor of the new therapy's superiority over the control. Any predefined monitoring rules that may lead to stopping the study prior to its planned end (either in terms of accrual or timing) are examples of *adaptive designs*. We discuss several monitoring approaches in this section.

13.5.1 Posterior Probability-Based Stopping Rules

Related to estimation-based designs are monitoring rules based on the posterior distribution of the study's primary measure of treatment effect. Consider a single-arm study for this example. A similar approach is often adopted for safety monitoring based on a high posterior probability that a risk of a serious adverse event exceeds some value. Let θ be the probability of an event, such as a response to therapy or an adverse event, associated with the study treatment. If the outcome is binary, then the sampling distribution is binomial. With a beta prior distribution for $p(\theta)$, the posterior will again be beta, making the calculations easy. Suppose that θ^c is a threshold value of treatment efficacy, such as the minimally clinically relevant chance of a favorable response to therapy. Then one would likely want to consider stopping the study if at any time during the study the probability is low that the current treatment's underlying efficacy is at least θ^c. One might characterize *low* as some value CutOff between 0 and 1 but closer to 0, such as 0.1. Such a rule would be useful for futility monitoring: *stop the study if* $P(\theta \geq \theta^c \mid data) <$ CutOff. Then one would compute the posterior probability of this event $(\theta \geq \theta^c)$ at each interim analysis and decide accordingly whether or not to continue the study. We have included some R statements to show how one might compute this probability in R. In the code, the variable ThetaC is θ^c. Assume that the prior distribution for θ is $Be(a, b)$ with parameters equal to some prespecified values a and b. Further, let x be the current number of individuals achieving the endpoint of interest, such as response to therapy or experiencing an adverse event.

```
a.post = a + x
b.post = b + (n-x)
PostProbEnoughEfficacy = 1 - pbeta(ThetaC, a.post, b.post)
if (PostProbEnoughEfficacy) <= CutOff
    Stop
```

For toxicity monitoring, one might instead want to stop if the posterior probability is high that the risk of a serious adverse event exceeds a threshold value $(\theta^\star)$. In this case, the stopping rule might look like the following: *stop the study if* $P(\theta \geq \theta^\star \mid data) \geq$ CutOff.

Similar monitoring rules based on the posterior probabilities of events relating to some characteristic of the treatment (e.g., response or toxicity) underlie many approaches [357].

13.5.2 Prediction-Based Stopping Rules

Some Bayesian approaches to interim monitoring base the decision to continue a study on the predictive probability of ultimately reaching a conclusion if the study continues to the end. The relationship to estimation is, of course, that the predictive probability calculations incorporate current knowledge about the treatment effect through the posterior probability. Recall that $p(Y_{new} \mid Y_{current}) = \int p(Y_{new} \mid \theta)p(\theta \mid Y_{current})d\theta$, where we have assumed conditional independence of Y_{new} and $Y_{current}$ given θ. Generally, one will predict some function of a test statistic, such as whether the final test will fall in some "rejection" region.

We note that this approach is a sort of inferential hybrid, in that the monitoring rule employs Bayesian inferential calculations of a frequentist test. One reason why we have followed this approach in our own collaborations is the need to satisfy regulators or funding agency officials who tend to require frequentist statistical tests.

Herson [162] proposed using predictive probability calculations when monitoring a phase 2 study in cancer. The motivation was to introduce early termination rules in the desire to reduce the number of patients who may be given ineffective therapy. Since, in general, these studies utilize binary outcomes, such as tumor regression (yes or no), the final outcome of the study will rest on the number of responses among the treated patients. With such a binomial endpoint, there will ultimately be a cutoff number of responses at the end of the study, so that fewer patients will be assigned to the less effective (or ineffective) therapy. Herson, noting that a binomial sampling distribution and a beta prior distribution lead to a beta-binomial predictive distribution, illustrated the calculation of the probability that the final number of responses (R) will be less than the cutoff value (C) at any time during the study. One combines the number of current responses with the predicted number of responses in each of the random samples and computes the proportion of total responses that are less than C. This proportion estimates the predictive probability that the study will ultimately not conclude in favor of the treatment being active enough to warrant further investigation. If this predictive probability of ultimately concluding against the treatment's being active is large enough, one should stop the study for futility. The statistician works with the clinical investigators to set the threshold value corresponding to "large enough" according to the desired operating characteristics for the study.

A simple approach to computing a random sample (NewOutcomes in the code) from a beta-binomial distribution is by simply combining the two functions, as in the following R function.

```
RandomBetaBinomial = function(nRandomSamples, nNewPatients, aPosterior, bPosterior) {
    pVector = rbeta(nRandomSamples, aPosterior, bPosterior)
    NewOutcomes = rbinom(nRandomSamples, nNewPatients, pVector)
}
```

Lee and Liu [218] also present a way to design phase 2 studies with interim monitoring for efficacy and futility based on predictive probabilities. Again, consider the case of a binomial sampling distribution and beta prior. In their approach, they define a test statistic based on data at the end of the study. Let the primary endpoint be response, with θ representing the underlying probability of a response. Consider p_0 to be null response probability, that is, the value such that the treatment is of no further interest if its associated probability of response is p_0 or less. Alternatively, we can say that the treatment is of clinical interest if the event or statement $\{\theta > p_0\}$ is true. The design calls for computing the posterior probability of this event after all planned patients will have entered the study and concluding in favor of the treatment's clinical interest if the posterior probability of this event is above some threshold value, θ^T. Mathematically, we would conclude at the end of the study that the treatment is active enough to warrant further study if $P(\{\theta > p_0\} \mid Y) > \theta^T$. This probability is a new event, namely, the event that the ultimate posterior probability is θ^T or higher that the treatment is active enough to warrant further study. Let $T(Y) = \{P(\{\theta > p_0\} \mid Y) > \theta^T\}$.

$T(Y)$ is an event. But, because it contains a posterior probability, it is a function of the ultimate study data, Y, for fixed p_0, θ^T, and prior for θ. At the end of the study, once all patients have received treatment and their outcomes recorded, $T(Y)$ will equal either 1 or 0, according to whether it is true or not. Before the end of the study, however, $T(Y)$ will be a function of the current data and projected future data. That is, we can speak of the predictive probability or expected value of $T(Y)$ at some intermediate point in the study. Suppose we are partway through the study and have outcome information y_{current} the current cohort of patients. The study will not reach its planned accrual and information goal until collecting information from the remaining patients. Call this future information Y_{new}. With a beta prior for θ and observed binomial data y_{current}, we have a beta posterior distribution, as we have already seen. Additionally, we have a beta-binomial distribution for the future data, Y_{new}. The final test statistic, $T(Y)$, is a function of y_{current} and Y_{new}. We know y_{current} and can project Y_{new} via the predictive distribution, so we can also determine the predictive distribution of $T(Y)$. The design of Lee and Liu calls for stopping the study for futility before enrolling and treating all patients if at an interim analysis the predicted probability that $T(Y) = 1$ is low. Similarly, one would stop the study early and declare the treatment active enough for further study if at an interim analysis the predicted probability that $T(Y) = 1$ is high. As part of designing the study, one quantifies what values would constitute "low" and "high" probabilities for early stopping. Lee and Liu suggest finding these last two threshold values according to the frequentist properties the investigators wish for the study. A program for designing a phase 2 study following the Lee and Liu phase 2 predictive probability design (*Predictive Probability Design (PID-535)*) is available from the software library at the website of the Department of Biostatistics at the University of Texas M. D. Anderson Cancer Center (https://biostatistics.mdanderson.org/SoftwareDownload/).

Sambucini [278] proposes a two-stage design that allows one to choose a different sample size for the second stage, given the results in the first stage. This design applies to studies in which the primary endpoint is a binary outcome. This work extends the two-stage design of Tan et al. [314] by accounting for uncertainty of future data via the predictive distribution. One typically will find the stage 2 sample size on a grid, applying a criterion to the posterior distribution of the probability of clinical benefit. Let y_1 be the number of treatment successes at the end of the first stage that enrolled n_1 patients. Conditional on (y_1, x_1), find the smallest total sample size, $N^\star$, such that

$$p^D \left\{ p^A(\theta > R_U \mid S) \geq \lambda_2 \right\} \geq \gamma_2. \tag{13.11}$$

In the equation, $S = y_1, y_1 + 1, \ldots, y_1 + (N^\star - n_1)$ is the total number of successes at the end of the study. This quantity involves predicting future successes, given that there were y_1 "responses" among the first n_1 patients. The quantities λ_2 and γ_2 are probability thresholds corresponding to the posterior probability of a treatment success (θ) exceeding a clinical threshold value (R_U) with high probability (λ_2) under the scenario characterized by the design prior $p^D(\cdot)$ [343]. The posterior probability in equation (13.11) is with respect to the prior distribution that one will use when analyzing the study's data at the end (i.e., the analysis prior [343]). Once one has determined the final sample size ($N^\star$) and, as a result, the stage 2 sample size ($N^\star - n_1$), one computes the threshold ($r^\star$) for declaring the treatment of clinical interest. Specifically, $r^\star$ is the largest number of successes (out of $N^\star$) such that one would not consider the treatment further. That is, $r^\star$ satisfies $p^A(\theta > R_U \mid S \geq r^\star, N^\star) < \lambda_2$. Again, $p^A(\cdot)$ refers to the analysis prior for θ.

We have found it useful to plan the study with a commonly used test statistic, such as Fisher's exact test for comparing two treatments with respect to a binary endpoint, to satisfy regulators and funding agencies. It is relatively straightforward to implement futility monitoring via predictive probabilities in this setting, as we show in Figure 13.1 and discuss further in Section 13.6. The R code is available on the book's website section for this chapter as a file named `FutilityBinaryRCT.R`.

Example 13.4. *Phase 2 Futility Monitoring.* You are a member of a team planning a randomized controlled study to compare a new form of therapy to the current standard of care for acute myeloid leukemia. The primary endpoint is response. The funding agency requires a frequentist analysis at the end of the study, which will be Fisher's exact test in this example. You want to include an interim analysis for futility halfway through the study. You will apply the code in Figure 13.1 to determine the operating characteristics of your design.

The final analysis will be a one-sided 0.1-level test. Let θ_0 be the probability of response associated with the standard of care and θ_1 be the corresponding probability for the new treatment. Based on many studies with the standard of care, the investigators expect that around 55% of the patients will respond to the standard of care. You propose a $Be(550, 450)$ prior for the probability of response with the standard of care (θ_0), corresponding to the high level of certainty on the part of the investigators. The corresponding 10th and 90th percentiles of this distribution are 53% and 57%, respectively.

The investigators are less certain of the probability of response with the new treatment. Early studies suggest that up to 80% of the patients may respond to the treatment, but it may also not be any better than the current standard. Evaluating several possible beta distributions, you and the rest of the team decide that the prior distribution $\theta_1 \sim Be(7.5, 2.5)$ characterizes the investigators' assessment about the new treatment's clinical efficacy. That is, they expect that around 75% of patients will respond to the new treatment. This prior distribution corresponds to around 80% probability that $0.55 \leq \theta_1 \leq 0.90$ and puts only 8% probability on values of $\theta_1 \leq 0.55$.

You run 1,000 simulations with a $U(0, 1)$ analysis prior for each treatment's probability of response. The design priors in the simulations are the two beta distributions given in the previous paragraph. For each interim analysis, one will compute the predictive power of ultimately rejecting the null hypothesis via Fisher's exact test at the 0.1 level of significance. The study will enroll up 80 patients in each treatment group if it does not stop early. You include an analysis after cohorts of 40 patients enter the study (20 per treatment group). Thus, there are three interim analyses and one final analysis.

```
for (iSim in 1:nSim) {
    for (iGroup in 1:nGroup) {
# Generate data for the new cohort randomized to each of the two treatments
        Control[iGroup, 2] = rbinom(1, n0PerGroup[iGroup], p0)
        Trt[iGroup, 2] = rbinom(1, n1PerGroup[iGroup], p1)
# Parameters for the posterior beta distribution
        TotalControlResponses = sum(Control[1:iGroup, 2])
        TotalControlNoResponse = sum(Control[1:iGroup, 1]) - TotalControlResponses
        aControlPost = aControl + TotalControlRespond
        bControlPost = bControl + TotalControlNoRespond
        TotalTrtResponses = sum(Trt[1:iGroup, 2])
        TotalTrtNoResponse = sum(Trt[1:iGroup, 1]) - TotalTrtResponses
        aTrtPost = aTrt + TotalTrtResponses; bTrtPost = bTrt + TotalTrtNoResponses
# Generate remaining obs from predictive beta-binomial dist'n
        n0Remaining = n0 - n0Entered; n1Remaining = n1 - n1Entered
        Pred.pValue = rep(NA, nPred)
        if (iGroup < nGroup) {
            x0Pred = RandomBetaBinomial(nPred, n0Remaining, aControlPost, bControlPost)
            PredTotalControlResponses = TotalControlResponses + x0Pred
            PredTotalControlNoResponse = TotalControlNoResponse +
                (n0Remaining - x0Pred)
            x1Pred = RandomBetaBinomial(nPred, n1Remaining, aTrtPost, bTrtPost)
            PredTotalTrtResponses = TotalTrtResponses + x1Pred
            PredTotalTrtNoResponse = TotalTrtNoResponse + (n1Remaining - x1Pred)
# Generate future obs'ns and combine with current obs'ns for final test.
            Pred.pValue = rep(NA, nPred)
            for (iPred in 1:nPred) {
                Tab = matrix(c(PredTotalTrtRespond[iPred], PredTotalTrtNoRespond[iPred],
                        PredTotalControlRespond[iPred], PredTotalControlNoRespond[iPred]),
                        ncol=2, byrow=T)
                Pred.pValue[iPred] = fisher.test(Tab, alternative="greater")$p.value
            }
            PredProbReject[iSim, iGroup] =
                sum(Pred.pValue < pValueToReject) / length(Pred.pValue)
            if (PredProbReject[iSim, iGroup] < CutOff) {
                Stop[iSim] = 1.0
                break
            }
        }
    }
    SampleSize[iSim,] = c(n0temp, n1temp)
    if ((iGroup == nGroup) & (Stop[iSim]==0)) {
        TabFinal = matrix(c(TotalTrtRespond, TotalTrtNoRespond,
                        TotalControlRespond, TotalControlNoRespond),
                        ncol=2, byrow=T)
        pValue[iSim] = fisher.test(TabFinal, alternative="g")$p.value
        SampleSize[iSim,] = c(n0temp, n1temp)
    }
}
```

FIGURE 13.1: R code to simulate a randomized clinical trial with futility analyses. The trial's primary endpoint is binary, and the final analysis uses Fisher's exact test. R code available on the book's web site as file **FutilityBinaryRCT.R**.

Table 13.2 shows some of the design's operating characteristics. The table also includes results with design priors that correspond to the underlying treatment-specific probabilities of response being single numbers, as in point null and alternative hypotheses. One sees that the extra uncertainty captured by the design prior increases the fraction of simulated trials that stop for futility and reduces the proportion of trials that ultimately reject the null hypothesis. For reference, a frequentist design without interim analyses would have around 90% power to reject the null hypothesis in favor of the alternative with 80 patients per group, assuming a one-sided 0.1-level Fisher's exact test.

TABLE 13.2: Operating characteristics for a randomized clinical trial that includes futility analyses using predictive probabilities

Control prior	Treatment prior	Stop early for futility	Reject H_0	Average sample size
$\theta_0 = 0.55$	$\theta_1 = 0.55$	69%	8%	52.4 / arm
$\theta_0 = 0.55$	$\theta_1 = 0.75$	5%	88%	77.9 / arm
$\theta_0 \sim Be(550, 450)$	$\theta_1 \sim Be(7.5, 2.5)$	18%	71%	72.7 / arm

13.5.3　Hypothesis Test-Based Stopping Rules

As mentioned earlier, many phase 2 designs are based on frequentist statistical hypothesis tests. If the primary outcome is binary, such as "response," the underlying statistical hypothesis being tested is $H_0 : p \leq p_0$ for some value p_0 representing a probability of success that would not be clinically useful.

Statistical hypothesis tests for phase 2 clinical studies may be evaluated by Bayes factors or posterior probabilities of the hypotheses. Johnson and Cook [180] describe a test-based design approach that uses Bayes factors. Their design is based on using so-called non-local prior densities (Johnson & Rossell [181]) for the prior distribution under the alternative hypotheses. An advantage of non-local priors in this application is a gain in efficiency relative to other Bayesian designs. Many Bayesian designs (or stylized Bayesian designs) characterize prior uncertainty about a treatment-effect parameter under the alternative hypothesis as vague or characterized by a reference prior. These prior distributions place mass across a range of values that includes the null hypothesis. A classic example is testing the point null hypothesis $H_0 : \theta = 0$ against the alternative $H_1 : \theta \neq 0$, with $\theta \sim N(0, \sigma^2)$ under the alternative distribution. By virtue of there being mass around parameter values that are consistent with both the null and the alternative hypotheses, evidence in favor of the null hypothesis over the alternative hypothesis amasses relatively slowly. Non-local densities under the alternative hypothesis, on the other hand, assign no probability to regions of the parameter space that are consistent with the null hypothesis. As a result, evidence in favor of the null against the alternative will increase faster with a non-local alternative prior distribution than it will with a local alternative density that has support in the region of the null hypothesis. Of course, evidence in favor of the alternative will amass quickly when the "true" value of the parameter is far from the null region.

If one is considering two hypotheses and the decision rule is based on the Bayes factor, then one can convert the decision rule to be based on the posterior probability of each hypothesis (see Section 10.1 for more details). Let $P(H_0)$ be the prior probability that hypothesis H_0 is true, and $P(H_1)$ be the prior probability that the alternative hypothesis is true. If $\mathbf{Y}$ represents the data, then the Bayes factor in favor of H_1 over H_0 (BF_{10}) is

$$BF_{10} = [\mathbf{Y} \mid H_1]/[\mathbf{Y} \mid H_0] = \frac{P(H_1 \mid \mathbf{Y})/P(H_0 \mid \mathbf{Y})}{P(H_1)/P(H_0)} \ . \qquad (13.12)$$

Example 13.5. Bayes Factors with Non-Local Prior Distributions. Investigators want to study whether adding a particular drug to a standard regimen of chemotherapy would improve clinical outcomes among patients with non-small cell lung cancer (NSCLC). The clinical outcome of interest is objective response rate (ORR) by the end of 6 months of therapy. A patient experiences an objective response if the patient's tumor decreases in size by at least 30% from baseline, according to commonly used criteria called RECIST [324]. Thus, the clinical endpoint is binary, with objective response defined as success.

The study design calls for interim futility analyses, beginning when 10 patients have enrolled to the study and have either received at least six cycles of therapy or experienced a PFS event.[1] The next interim analysis will occur after 15 patients have either received at least six cycles of therapy or experienced a PFS event. The final analysis will occur after 20 patients have entered and received full therapy (six cycles). The interim analyses are for futility, meaning that there is at most weak evidence that the added drug improves clinical benefit above a predetermined threshold. If the combination therapeutic regimen under study is providing clinical benefit, we want to continue the study and enroll a total of 20 patients. The interim analyses is based on Bayesian hypothesis testing.

We take the expected ORR to be 20% if the second drug does not increase the clinical effectiveness of the standard chemotherapy for NSCLC. This estimate is based on the results of several published studies. We would consider the addition of the experimental drug to yield encouraging clinical improvement if it leads to an ORR that is 35% or higher.

The program BFDesigner[2] allows one to determine a design based on hypothesis testing with Bayes factors in the case of a binomial sampling distribution. Here we use this program to determine interim analysis stopping guidelines.

The study will stop for futility if we see no responses among the first 10 patients or no more than one response in the first 15 patients. We will discard the combination as promising if we see three or fewer responders out of 20 patients. Table 13.3 provides the operating characteristics based on 5,000 simulations.

---

[1]PFS stands for progression-free survival, the time to disease progression or death, whichever comes first.

[2]https://biostatistics.mdanderson.org/SoftwareDownload/

TABLE 13.3: Estimated operating characteristics of the study's design based on 5000 simulations for different possible "true" objective response rates

Scenario	Hypothetical true response rate	Probability stop for futility	Average number of patients treated (percentiles: 10th, 90th)
1	0.10	0.876	15.40 (10, 20)
2	0.15	0.662	17.30 (10, 20)
3	0.20	0.434	18.51 (10, 20)
4	0.25	0.243	19.25 (20, 20)
5	0.30	0.119	19.61 (20, 20)
6	0.35	0.047	19.86 (20, 20)
7	0.40	0.021	19.92 (20, 20)
8	0.45	0.008	19.96 (20, 20)
9	0.50	0.002	19.99 (20, 20)

13.5.4 Decision-Theoretic Stopping Rules

In many instances, the study will lead to a decision—at least, in some generic sense. For example, the decision might relate to rejecting some hypothesis about the activity of the treatment, comparable to a null hypothesis. Another type of decision might relate to the next action to take for the treatment under study, such as whether to test the treatment further in a larger randomized study. The ultimate decision is whether to carry out the study. We outlined the framework for applying Bayesian decision theory in Section 13.4.3. In this section we focus on using decision theory in the context of interim analyses and deciding whether to continue or stop the study (i.e., on sequential decision-making).

A challenging aspect of applying sequential decision-making in study design is the computational part. Computation becomes even more difficult if the clinical trial includes sequential decision-making, in interim analyses as data accrue. The calculations for a Bayesian fully sequential design at time t have to consider all possible outcomes for all possible actions at future times to compute the expected utility. These calculations are usually carried out via dynamic programming [26, 29]. With a finite horizon (call it T), the calculations work backwards sequentially from the last decision time to the first. For illustration, consider a finite and discrete outcome space and a finite and discrete action space. At each time, the algorithm computes the expected utility for each action and each state. Knowing these at the last time point allows one to compute the optimal action for each state at the last time point. Then the algorithm goes to the penultimate decision time $(T - 1)$ and determines the expected utility for each action at each state. That is, if we are at state or outcome Y_j at time $T - 1$ and choose action a_i, we know the probability of reaching each possible outcome at time T from the predictive distribution. Since we have already determined the optimal choice for each outcome at time T and the expected utility for that decision, we know just what to do and what the consequence will be for any possible outcome reached at T. We can then combine the information for each possible outcome at time T with the probability of reaching that outcome from state Y_j at the previous time $T-1$ to determine the expected utility for each decision one might take at $T-1$. These calculations will show which of the possible actions will maximize the expected utility at the end, given one is at Y_j at time $T-1$. The algorithm carries out these calculations for each possible state or outcome at time $T-1$ and yields the optimal action for each outcome one might reach at $T-1$. The algorithm then goes backwards to time $T-2$ and determines the optimal action for each possible state at this time by following the same sort of calculations described for time $T-1$. By working backwards to time 0, we end up with a table of optimal actions for each possible outcome one might observe at each decision time.

The previous example assumed a discrete set of outcomes at each of a finite set of decision times, with a discrete set of actions from which to choose at each time. As the set of possible outcomes or actions increases, the calculations become more difficult, growing exponentially. The problem becomes even more complex if one is dealing with a continuous outcome space, as when one is designing a clinical trial with a continuous primary endpoint, such as change in blood pressure. One can apply numerical methods to find the optimal solution or, at least, a close approximation to the set of optimal decisions. A particularly useful approach is based on generating random trajectories of the clinical study based on the assumed sampling distribution and some prior probability distribution for the parameters in the sampling model. If the outcome space is continuous, the computational burden is still enormous. When there is a sufficient or nearly sufficient summary statistic that one can use, over which one forms a grid, then one can get a reasonably good finite and discrete approximation to the full outcome space [53, 245]. One can then apply backward induction to the finite grid to find an approximate set of optimal decisions.

Carlin et al. [62] illustrate the use of forward sampling when designing a fully sequential Bayesian randomized clinical trial with a normally distributed primary endpoint. Rossell et al. [276] apply gridding and forward simulation to find the optimal phase 2 design and then approximate the boundaries by straight lines, while Ding et al. [97] use these same techniques to determine an optimal design for phase 2 screening trials that have a binary primary outcome. The latter two examples incorporate frequentist concerns in the utility function, providing a fully Bayesian approach that should satisfy frequentist requirements. There are many other examples of study designs based on decision-theoretic considerations [7, 39, 220, 309, 221, 331, 341].

13.6   Phase 3 Study Designs

Large randomized phase 3 studies are generally concerned with clinical questions of pragmatic interest. For example, a study might address the question whether or not a new form of therapy is better than a current standard or accepted way of treating some disease. Other examples include studies by large companies seeking regulatory approval to market a drug or device for some medical condition. Phase 3 studies are often designed and analyzed using frequentist considerations, although the designs of some phase 3 studies have been influenced by Bayesian considerations. Bayesian approaches to study design have been particularly accepted for studies by device manufacturers. The U.S. Food and Drug Administration's Center for Devices and Radiological Health and Center for Biologics Evaluation and Research have issued *Guidance for the Use of Bayesian Statistics in Medical Device Clinical Trials* [106].

A particular impetus for incorporating Bayesian calculation in phase 3 clinical trials is the greater flexibility afforded by this form of inference. Frequentist characteristics are affected by repeated testing of accumulating data, leading to the need to account for the number and timing of the analyses in the design. One approach to account for the inflation of the Type I error (risk of incorrectly rejecting the statistical null hypothesis) is to require more extreme values of the test statistic in order to reject the null hypothesis. Group sequential boundaries generally account for the inflation of the Type I error, and different authors have proposed different ways to compute such boundaries while still leaving the overall Type I error at some desired level.

As a result of the need to account for both the current value of a test statistic and the presence of interim analyses, the frequentist will analyze the data in a way that violates the so-called likelihood principle (cf. Chapter 6). The likelihood principle relates to a fundamental assumption underlying statistical inference. Consider our usual situation, in which we conduct an experiment and collect data (y) where the variation in the samples is characterized by the sampling distribution $[y \mid \theta]$ for some parameter θ. In turn, the likelihood will just be proportional to the joint sampling distribution of the observations. The likelihood principle states that all of the information about θ is contained in the likelihood function, and two different experiments that yield data producing the same value of the same likelihood function should lead to the same inference. Furthermore, two likelihood functions contain the same information about θ if they are proportional to each other. A detailed discussion of the likelihood principle is given by Berger and Wolpert [33].

Since the number and timing of interim analyses can change the p-value and, hence, the inference from an experiment, the frequentist approach violates the likelihood principle. Bayesian inference, on the other hand, conditions on the data and is consistent with the likelihood principle. Heuristically, by looking at the relationship between the posterior distribution and the likelihood, one sees that the same likelihood will lead to the same inference, as long as one considers the same prior distribution (i.e., $p(\theta \mid \mathbf{y}) \propto p(\mathbf{y} \mid \theta) \times p(\theta)$). By conditioning on the observed data through the likelihood, Bayesian posterior inference will not be affected by interim analyses, as long as the interim analyses do not affect the likelihood. By conditioning on the observed data and not what might have occurred, the Bayesian approach leads to study designs that are more flexible than frequentist designs. It should not matter whether the study monitors analyze the accruing data annually, semi-annually, or daily. The observed data are the observed data, and inference should proceed accordingly. Thus, the Bayesian pays no penalty for carrying out interim analyses as long as the likelihood is not affected.

One of the earliest discussions of sequential designs in the medical setting appeared in 1960 with Peter Armitage's book *Sequential Medical Trials* [9]. In his review of this book for the *Journal of the American Statistical Association* that appeared in 1963, F. J. Anscombe argues against the underlying inferential philosophy in Armitage's book, namely, concern for the error probabilities associated with rejecting or failing to reject the statistical null hypothesis [7]. Instead, Anscombe argues in favor of methods that are consistent with the likelihood principle, as well as making many other important points.

Although one would think there would be widespread acceptance of the notion of carrying out clinical studies with interim monitoring, one does not see many sequential designs in clinical studies until the 1980s. Rather than designing studies with monitoring patients one at a time, which would be logistically difficult at the time, group sequential study designs became popular. With these designs, one analyzes the data after cohorts of fixed size enter the study. The original proposals called for particular ways of setting the boundaries for the interim analyses, according to how one wanted the interim analyses to relate to a single analysis at the end of the study [252, 262]. Flexibility was added when Lan and DeMets introduced the notion of a so-called "alpha spending function," allowing a general approach for determining the thresholds for deciding on statistical significance at each interim analysis [213]. This methodology is still very much in use for phase 3 clinical trials.

Freedman and Spiegelhalter wrote many papers advocating Bayesian designs in clinical trials [111, 112, 113, 114, 115, 116, 305, 306, 307, 308]. They and their coworkers offered examples of the benefits of taking a Bayesian approach. In their implementation of a Bayesian inferential model to clinical trial design, particularly for interim analyses, they couched decisions in terms of "convincing" either a skeptic or enthusiast with respect to the benefit of the new treatment. Specifically, if a person, skeptical of the new treatment's clinical effectiveness before the study, has seen the study's data and is now inclined to favor the new treatment, then one might argue that the new treatment is the winner, so to speak. Similarly, if an enthusiastic supporter of the new therapy prior to the study has now, after seeing the study data, become dubious, then the new treatment is a loser. Carrying these notions to interim analyses allows one to consider stopping the study early, once the enthusiast or skeptic has reversed his or her *a priori* thinking about the new treatment.

Implementation of these ideas within the Bayesian framework requires one to mathematically characterize the prior beliefs of the skeptic and the enthusiast via prior distributions. The characterization and associated prior distributions are made easier by the fact that many—if not most—test statistics have an asymptotic normal distribution. The method would proceed by associating the test statistic with a treatment difference and characterizing the treatment difference from the standpoint of the enthusiast and the skeptic.

For example, consider a randomized clinical trial in which the parameter θ characterizes the difference between two treatments, a new therapy and a standard of care (control), with positive θ indicating superiority of the new treatment over the control. Clinicians generally have in mind some minimal level of treatment benefit that they would require of a new treatment before they would consider using it widely. Call this minimal level of benefit θ_{alt}. Clinicians would prefer the new treatment if its benefit over the control therapy is at least θ_{alt}. Similarly, the current standard is clearly preferable if $\theta < 0$. Preference is somewhat ambiguous if θ lies in the so-called range of equivalence (i.e., $0 < \theta < \theta_{alt}$), however.

The skeptic's prior may place only a small amount of probability on values of the treatment difference that favor the new treatment, reserving most of the prior probability for the region that supports the inferiority of the new treatment over its comparator in the trial (i.e., $\theta < 0$). On the other hand, the enthusiast might center the prior distribution at $\theta = \theta_{alt}$. This person's prior would also put relatively little probability in the region of no benefit (i.e., the region $\theta < 0$), corresponding to the notion that it is relatively unlikely that the new treatment is not superior to the comparator; most of the enthusiast's prior distribution has probability over the region in which $\theta > 0$.

A compromise approach for fully characterizing the skeptical and enthusiastic priors might set the enthusiast's prior to place 10% or 20% prior probability in the region that corresponds to the new treatment's clinical improvement being the same as or worse than the expected outcome with the control treatment (i.e., $\theta < 0$). Similarly, the skeptic's prior might place only 5% or 10% probability in the region of treatment benefit (i.e., $\theta > \theta_{alt}$). Assuming a normally distributed test statistic, one would calibrate the prior variances to achieve these probabilities. Figure 13.2 illustrates a skeptical and enthusiastic prior.

Example 13.6. Interim Analysis for Randomized Study with Skeptical and Enthusiastic Priors.
Clinical investigators designed a randomized clinical trial, and it is time for an interim analysis. You will analyze the data and let the study's data safety monitoring committee know if the data suggest that the study should stop now or continue.

The study compares two treatments for breast cancer. One group of patients receives drug A, and the other group receives the combination of drug A and drug B. The study's primary endpoint is progression-free survival (PFS), defined in Example 13.5. The investigators chose a sample size and follow-up time to provide 80% power to detect a hazard ratio of 0.692. (This hazard ratio corresponds to increasing median PFS from 9 months to 13 months, assuming an exponential distribution, since the median equals $\log(2)/\lambda$ for the $Exp(\lambda)$ distribution.) The final analysis will be a two-sided log rank test with significance declared at the 5% level.

It is common to consider the hazard ratio as the primary endpoint in a random-

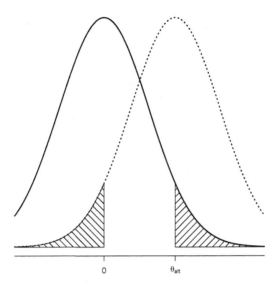

FIGURE 13.2: The difference between the two priors used in the study's design. The skeptic's prior (solid curve) is on the left and centered at 0; the enthusiast's prior (dashed curve) is on the right and centered at θ_{alt}. The shaded region on the left shows the probability that the enthusiast assigns to treatment effects less than or equal to 0. The shaded region on the right indicates the probability the skeptic assigns to large treatment differences greater than or equal to θ_{alt}.

ized clinical trial with a time-to-event endpoint. One reason is that the proportional hazards model (i.e., the Cox model) provides a flexible way to compare groups in the presence of censoring without making any assumptions about the form of the underlying hazard function [88]. Instead, one simply assumes that the ratio of the two group-specific hazard functions is constant over time, no matter the shape of the hazards. While this may seem unrealistic in many settings, it is a surprisingly robust assumption and is nearly ubiquitous in the applied clinical trial literature.

Consider the large-sample approximation to the distribution of the logarithm of the hazard ratio [333]. Under the null hypothesis that the hazard ratio is 1, the log rank test has variance approximately $d/4$, where d is the number of events in the analysis data set. Furthermore, the log rank test statistic is proportional to the log hazard ratio under the null hypothesis and so-call local alternatives [333]. We will use this large-sample approximation for the test statistic to approximate the likelihood.

Let δ be the logarithm of the hazard ratio. We will consider two prior distributions for δ, a skeptical and an enthusiastic prior. In both cases, we will consider $\delta \sim N(\delta_0, \sigma_\delta^2)$. We first consider the skeptical prior. The skeptic will consider that adding drug B to drug A provides no additional benefit. The skeptic's corresponding prior mean will be 0 for the log hazard ratio.

There are currently 263 events. Among patients randomized to receive drug A, there are 135 events; there are 128 events among patients randomized to the combination A + B. At the time of your analysis, the observed hazard ratio is 0.83 (A+B vs. B). The parameter of interest is θ, the logarithm of the hazard ratio (A+B vs. B). Given the specifications of the trial's design, the range of equivalence is $(\ln(0.692), \ln(1))$ or $(-0.368, 0)$.

A skeptical prior distribution for θ might have mean equal to 0, corresponding to no treatment difference. The skeptic's prior variance would characterize this person's prior belief that $P(\theta \geq \theta_{\mathrm{alt}}) = 0.05$. Using the relationship $n_0 = ((\sigma \times 1.645)/\theta_{\mathrm{alt}})^2$, where $\sigma = 2$, the skeptic's variance would have $n_0 = 80$. Therefore, the skeptical prior would be $\theta \sim N(0, 4/80)$.

Using similar logic, an enthusiastic prior distribution for θ might have prior mean equal to $\theta_{\mathrm{alt}} = \ln(0.692) = -0.368$. The enthusiast would base the prior variance on the notion that $P(\theta \leq 0) = 0.05$. As a result, the enthusiast's prior distribution is $\theta \sim N(-0.368, 4/80)$.

Using conjugacy, the skeptic's posterior is $\theta \mid data \sim N(-0.143, 0.0117)$, and the enthusiast's posterior is $\theta \mid data \sim N(-0.229, 0.0117)$. Figure 13.3 shows the posterior skeptical and enthusiastic distributions along with the likelihood. The figure includes vertical lines at $\theta = 0$ and at $\theta = \theta_{\mathrm{alt}}$ to show the range of equivalence, as well as changes from the prior means.

One might calculate key posterior probabilities for the skeptic and enthusiast. Here, smaller hazard ratios indicate improvement by the treatment over the control. The skeptic would now assign probabilities to regions of θ, such as $P(\theta \geq 0 \mid data) = 0.093$, $P(\theta \leq \theta_{\mathrm{alt}} \mid data) = 0.018$, and $P(\theta_{\mathrm{alt}} \geq \theta \leq 0 \mid data) = 0.889$. The enthusiast's corresponding posterior probabilities are $P(\theta \geq 0 \mid data) = 0.098$, $P(\theta \leq \theta_{\mathrm{alt}} \mid data) = 0.098$ and $P(\theta_{\mathrm{alt}} \geq \theta \leq 0 \mid data) = 0.885$.

Figure 13.3 shows the likelihood function and the two posterior densities. The posterior distributions for the enthusiast and the skeptic are fairly close to each other now. Although there is strong evidence that the hazard ratio is less than 1, it seems that the estimated treatment effect is in the range of equivalence $(\theta_{\mathrm{alt}}, 0)$. In fact, the posterior probabilities that θ lies in this range are 0.89 for the skeptic and 0.88 for the enthusiast. Given the large sample size, it seems unlikely that the study will find that the log hazard ratio is less than θ_{alt}. A data safety monitoring committee might want to consider stopping the study rather than continuing it at this point. The study should probably close.

13.7   Response-Adaptive Randomization

A major reason for designing clinical trials with early stopping rules is the ethical concern that the wider patient population—including patients yet to enroll in the study—should benefit from newer and improved therapies as soon as the improvement has been demonstrated in well-designed clinical trials. Likewise, policymakers should withdraw ineffective therapies from clinical practice. One can expand on this viewpoint by arguing that patients entering the study should benefit

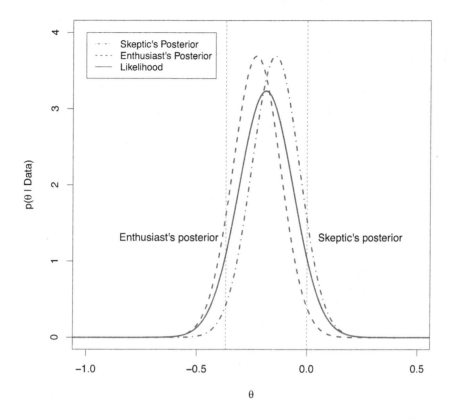

FIGURE 13.3: Posterior densities for the skeptic and enthusiast. Vertical lines show the range of equivalence.

from the knowledge already gained about the relative benefits of the treatments under study. That is, if the accumulating evidence suggests that one treatment may actually be superior to the other or others in the trial, then why not give the better-performing treatment to incoming patients? One way to achieve this preferential treatment assignment is by adapting the randomization probabilities to favor the better-performing treatments. Such considerations have given rise to so-called play-the-winner rules [360], biased-coin or Pólya urn schemes [348, 349], and other implementations of response-based adaptive randomization. A related problem of adapting choices over time to increase one's reward is often called the multi-armed bandit problem [38, 145].

A particularly important randomized trial that used an urn-based adaptive randomization method was the ECMO trial of Bartlett et al. [18] reported in 1985. The basis of the randomization is an imaginary urn that contains balls marked for the different treatments. In this study, some balls would be marked "ECMO" and the others would be marked, say, "control." The randomization scheme called for randomly drawing a ball from the urn, assigning the associated treatment to the patient. The ball would return to the urn. If the patient survived, another ball for the assigned treatment would go into the urn. If the patient died, a ball that corresponds to the other treatment would go into the urn.

When the trial began, the imaginary urn contained just two balls, one ball for "ECMO" and one ball for the standard of care. The first treatment assignment was to ECMO. The neonate lived, so the urn now contained three balls, two for ECMO and one for the control. The second baby received the control treatment and died. After the first two participants, the imaginary urn contained four ECMO balls and only one control ball, since the control patient died but the ECMO baby lived. All subsequent assignments were to ECMO, and each of these babies lived. The trial ended with nine babies assigned to ECMO—all of whom survived—and just one baby assigned to the standard of care who unfortunately died.

The particular implementation of an adaptive randomization method in this ECMO trial of neonates reached a conclusion that failed to convince a large number of pediatricians and led to subsequent trials of this treatment [255, 110]. Some interesting discussion of the statistical and ethical issues relating to this example appeared in the journal *Statistical Science* in papers by Ware in 1989 and Royall in 1991, with associated discussion [277, 344].

Perhaps because of the controversy that surrounded the ECMO trials or for other reasons, response-adaptive designs did not find much application in clinical trials until the end of the twentieth century. The ASTIN study was a particularly interesting study that combined adaptive dose finding within a randomized clinical trial [208]. The statistical details of this study can be found in Berry et al. [40]. Response-based adaptive randomization now enjoys fairly widespread interest.

There are several ways that one may determine randomization probabilities to adapt to accruing information about treatments and their associated clinical outcomes. Generally, one will choose some clinical outcome measure that is relevant for comparing the treatments under evaluation. The randomization probabilities will be functions of this outcome measure.

For example, suppose that there is a binary measure of clinical relevance, such as tumor shrinkage beyond some threshold percentage of baseline or the eradication of symptoms. Furthermore, let us consider a study that is comparing a new treatment to a standard of care. We might want to base randomization probabilities on the probability that the new treatment provides a better outcome than the standard of care. A simple implementation of response-adaptive randomization would assign a patient to the new treatment (A) with probability $P(A > B \mid D_t)$, where D_t represents the data up to time t, the time the patient enters the study. That is, we allocate patients to a treatment according to the posterior probability that the particular treatment is better than the other one.

The literature contains different proposals for relating the function $P(A > B \mid D_t)$ to a measure of clinical benefit. For example, suppose that one is using a binary clinical endpoint. Let p_j be the probability of clinical success with treatment j $(j = 0, 1)$, with the control being denoted by $j = 0$. One may then use $P(p_1 > p_0 \mid D_t)$ for the probability of assigning a patient to the new treatment (and 1 minus this posterior probability as the probability of assignment to the control treatment).

Suppose instead that one wishes to use a time-to-event endpoint, such as survival, for evaluating the benefit of each treatment under study. One might consider using the median survival in the randomization probability in place of the probability of success (p_j). That is, if m_j is the median survival for treatment j $(j = 0, 1)$, then one might assign a patient to the new treatment with probability equal to $P(m_1 > m_0 \mid D_t)$. If one assumes that the failure times follow an exponential distribution with rate parameter λ and that the prior distribution for λ is $Ga(a, b)$, then the posterior distribution for λ is also gamma, as we show in Chapter 3. Furthermore, using the theory for transformations of random variables, if $\lambda \sim Ga(a, b)$, then $m = \ln(2)/\lambda \sim InvGa(a, b')$, where $b' = \ln(2)/b$.

Recalling the issues that arose around the urn sampling-based treatment allocation in the ECMO trial mentioned earlier in this section, we generally prefer postponing modifying randomization probabilities until after the trial has accrued and treated several patients. If the trial adapts the randomization probabilities at the start of the trial, one will run the risk of assigning a larger number of patients to the inferior treatment [315, 347]. This unexpected outcome may occur because the posterior probability estimates are relatively unstable early in the study, especially if one starts with a fairly diffuse prior distribution for the treatment effects. Maintaining equal randomization for a while reduces this risk [347].

Aside from waiting until one has information on some minimum number of patients before changing from equal randomization to an allocation ratio that favors the better-performing treatment, one may consider approaches that smooth the randomization probabilities to make them more stable, especially early in the study. That is, one can modify the probabilities in a way that alters how quickly they react to accruing data. This attenuation can be accomplished by picking a constant $0 \leq \gamma \leq 1$ and randomizing a patient who enters the study at time t to the new treatment with probability

$$R_1(t) = \frac{\{P(Trt_1 > Trt_0 \mid D_t)\}^\gamma}{\{P(Trt_0 > Trt_1 \mid D_t)\}^\gamma + \{P(Trt_1 > Trt_0 \mid D_t)\}^\gamma}. \tag{13.13}$$

The function $R_1(t)$ will lead to equal randomization if $\gamma = 0$. Randomization will adapt completely to the relative clinical benefit if $\gamma = 1$. When there are only two treatments, $R_1(t) = 0.5$ whenever $P(Trt_1 > Trt_0 \mid D_t) = 0.5$.

One may also wish to let the exponent γ change as more patients enter the study. That is, we want greater stability in the randomization probabilities (i.e., less wild variation) early in the trial, when data from relatively few patients are available. As more patients enter the trial and contribute outcome information, we will be willing to allow full adaptive randomization. Thall and Wathen [322] proposed making the exponent a function of the current and final sample sizes. That is, the exponent will increase as the accrual gets closer to the target sample size. The specific suggestion is that if n patients have entered the trial at time t, the exponent in the random allocation function becomes $\gamma(t, n) = n/2N$, where N is the target sample size. Early in the trial, there will be very few patients, and $n/2N$ will be close to zero. As more patients provide outcome data, the exponent approaches $1/2$.

The use of the attenuation factor γ (or some function $\gamma(t,n)$) is not particularly Bayesian. In effect, this approach is discounting the posterior distribution. For a Bayesian, the posterior distribution summarizes the person's knowledge or uncertainty in light of available information and data. Because the attenuation factor's role is to keep the randomization probabilities from changing too quickly in an attempt to mitigate potential concerns by frequentists, particularly by slowing decision-making to improve frequentist operating characteristics, we call the use of γ a stylized Bayesian design.

If the trial is evaluating three or more treatments, then there are two primary ways one may adapt randomization probabilities to favor the better-performing treatments. One approach makes the randomization probabilities a function of the posterior probability that each treatment is the best performer among the treatments under evaluation. The other approach either chooses a fixed threshold value for each treatment to surpass or considers one of the treatments to be the standard that the remaining treatments need to beat.

Suppose that the clinical outcome is binary (e.g., response to treatment) and that the probability of response with any new treatment would have to be at least p^* to be considered worth further investigation. If the trial is evaluating J treatments, we might make the randomization probability for treatment j

$$r_j = \frac{\{P(p_j > p^* \mid D_t)\}^\gamma}{\sum_{k=1}^{J}\{P(p_j > p^* \mid D_t)\}^\gamma}, \quad j = 1, \ldots, J \, .$$

Note that the function r_j may include the exponent γ as an attenuation factor as discussed earlier in this section.

If one of the J treatments is a standard therapy that serves as a control in the study, then one can easily modify the allocation probabilities r_j. Let p_1 be the response probability associated with the control therapy. One might set the probability of randomizing a patient to treatment j to

$$r_j = \frac{\{P(p_j > p_1 \mid D_t)\}^\gamma}{\sum_{k=1}^{J}\{P(p_j > p_1 \mid D_t)\}^\gamma}, \quad j = 1, \ldots, J \, .$$

We might set $P(p_1 > p_1 \mid D_t) = 0.5$.

Yuan et al. [357] pointed out some problems with this randomization function when there is a control treatment among the therapies under evaluation. One problem is that the randomization probability for the control treatment arm will never drop below 0.2 no matter how much better the other treatments are performing. Another problem is that the randomization probabilities may be sensitive to which of the treatments one sets as the control. Consider a trial with three treatments, with the arm labeled 1 the control therapy and the other two treatments the new ones. Suppose that the control and one of the new treatments have the same probability of response and that treatment 3 is inferior to these two treatments (i.e., $p_1 = p_2$ and $p_3 < p_1 = p_2$). In such a situation, the randomization probability for the control treatment will be greater than for arm 2, on average, even though they are equally effective. That is, $r_1 > r_2$, even though $p_1 = p_2$.

A related problem occurs when the control treatment is considerably worse than the other treatments. Again, suppose the trial is evaluating three treatments and that we label the control treatment with the number 1. If the probability of response with the control is much lower than it is for the two new treatments, then the randomization probabilities for treatments 2 and 3 will be the same (or close to the same), even when their respective response probabilities are considerably different. For example, suppose the true response probabilities are $p_1 = 0.20$, $p_2 = 0.70$, $p_3 = 0.85$ for the control and two new treatments. On average, the randomization probabilities will be $r_1 = 0.20$, $r_2 = 0.40$, $r_3 = 0.40$ for the three treatments. Yuan and Yin [358] propose an algorithm that they call "moving-average adaptive randomization" to overcome the sensitivity of the randomization probabilities to the treatment label. Note that basing each treatment's randomization probability on the posterior probability that it is the best avoids the problem of sensitivity to labeling.

Although we have illustrated outcome-adaptive randomization with examples based on trials with binary clinical outcomes, the methods lend themselves to clinical outcomes of any data type. For example, if a trial is evaluating treatments for hypertension, one might consider the mean change in blood pressure from baseline as the clinical outcome on which to base treatment allocation probabilities. With three or more treatments, one uses the function

$$r_j \propto P(\mu_j = \max(\mu_1, \ldots, \mu_J) \mid D_t), \quad j = 1, \ldots, J \ ,$$

where μ_j is the mean change from baseline for treatment j. Similarly, one might consider approximating time-to-event distributions with exponential distributions and use the means or medians as the measure of clinical benefit for comparison and for determining randomization probabilities.

13.8 Recap and Readings

There are many variations of study designs for dose escalation with respect to a single outcome and dose finding based on two outcomes. The books by Cheung [71] and Yuan et al. [357] provide a more thorough discussion of dose finding designs than we could in this chapter. Thall and Cook [316] extend the designs in Section 13.2.1 in recognition that different pairs of risks of toxicity and efficacy may be equally desirable. That is, one may be willing to accept a greater risk of serious toxicity in exchange for a greater chance at clinical benefit.

One can find a discussion of Bayesian sample size considerations in several papers that appeared in the journal *Statistician* in 1995. Adcock (1997) reviews frequentist and Bayesian methods for determining sample sizes [2].

A major part of Bayesian analysis concerns making decisions. We have touched on the basic ideas in this chapter. The books by Lindley (1972), DeGroot (2004), and

Parimigiani and Inoue (2009) give a more thorough presentation of this important topic [225, 91, 256].

One can apply decision theory to address concerns other than sample size. For example, Stroud et al. (2001) discuss the design of a study that sought to learn about the pharmacokinetics and pharmacodynamics of an anticancer drug [311]. Patients received the drug in the clinic as a three-hour infusion. The complexity of the drug's pharmacokinetics led to the need to draw blood samples long after the end of the infusion. As a result, patients would have to stay in the hospital overnight, return to the clinic the following day, or remain in the clinic for 24 hours or longer. While the study wanted to estimate a pharmacokinetic parameter with some precision, the investigators did not want to disrupt patients' lives. The utility function sought to balance the goal of precision against a cost related to drawing a blood sample more than 4 hours after the end of the three-hour infusion.

A good summary of Bayesian adaptive designs as of 2011 is contained in Berry et al. [41]. A full presentation of adaptive randomization would include discussion of the ethical considerations, in addition to the statistical and logistic issues. The ethical considerations touch on the generally accepted need for clinical equipoise for participation in a randomized clinical trial. One may consider the views of Armitage and Bather, expressed in 1985, to get a sense of some of the early differences of opinion [10, 11, 19, 20] on the matter of adaptively modifying randomization probabilities in light of accruing information in the trial. Hey et al. (2015) argue against adaptively changing randomization probabilities on ethical grounds [163]. Many authors provide counterarguments in the discussion that followed that paper.

13.9   Exercises

EXERCISE 13.1.   Suppose that you are designing a phase 1 study. You do not know the risk of a dose-limiting toxicity (DLT) and propose starting with a $U(0,1)$ prior for $\theta(1)$, the risk of a DLT at dose level 1.

(a) What is the predictive probability that the first patient will experience a DLT?
(b) Based on the predictive probability of a DLT, does this prior make sense for the lowest dose level? (That is, should one even consider treating a patient with this dose?)
(c) Suppose that one thinks *a priori* that the risk of DLT at the first dose level is 1/3. What do you think would be a reasonable prior distribution for this dose level?
(d) Find the predictive probability of a DLT using your prior distribution from part (c). What do you think of your prior?

EXERCISE 13.2.   Suppose you are the statistician for a phase 1 study of a new anti-cancer drug called bumblebine. The trial will base dose escalation decisions on the CRM design. Patients will enter the study in cohorts of two. There are five dose levels, shown in Table 13.4. You assume that the prior distribution for the slope parameter (a) is log-normal (i.e., $a = e^\beta$, $\beta \sim N(0, 1.34)$).

TABLE 13.4: Table of dose levels, corresponding doses, and prior estimates of DLT risk

Dose Level	Bumblebine dose (mg/m^2)	Initial estimate of DLT risk
1	15.0	0.1
2	17.5	0.2
3	20.0	0.3
4	22.5	0.5
5	25.0	0.6
6	27.5	0.7

(a) Modify the code for the CRM on page 388 to use a logistic function (see equation (13.1c)) with $b_0 = 3$.

(b) Find the rescaled doses according to which the logistic function gives the risks in the last column of Table 13.4.

(c) Suppose the first five patients do not experience a DLT but the sixth patient does. (In other words, the first DLT occurs to the second patient who receives dose level 3.) Find the posterior distribution of β and the slope parameter $(a = e^\beta)$.

(d) The seventh patient has enrolled in the study. What dose level should this patient receive, based on the CRM algorithm?

EXERCISE 13.3. In this exercise, you will determine the sample size necessary to satisfy the average coverage criterion, namely, find the smallest value of n such that a prediction interval of width l has probability $1 - \alpha$ of containing the mean μ. The study will evaluate the effect of a new anti-hypertension medication by measuring the change in blood pressure after six weeks of therapy. Let $y_1, \ldots, y_n$ be the differences in blood pressure measurements for a sample of n patients. Assume $y_i \sim N(\mu, \sigma^2)$, $i = 1, \ldots, n$, $\mu \mid \sigma^2 \sim N(\mu_0, \sigma^2/n_0)$, and that σ^2 is known.

(a) Find the formula for the smallest value of the sample size n that will ensure that average coverage will be at least $1 - \alpha$.

(b) Find the sample size when $\sigma^2 = 50$ $(\sigma = \sqrt{50})$, the *prior sample size* (n_0) is 2, and the prediction interval width is $l = 10$.

(c) Now, assume that σ^2 is unknown. We characterize uncertainty about the variance via $\sigma^2 \sim InvGa(a, b)$, where $a = 0.5$ and $b = 1$. What is the required sample size now?

EXERCISE 13.4. You are designing a randomized clinical trial that will compare two treatments with respect to a binary endpoint. One treatment is the current standard of care and is expected to lead to clinical improvement for 50% of the patients who receive it. The other treatment is a new form of therapy, and the investigators would like to develop this therapy further if it provides benefit to at least 75% of patients. The study will randomize a total of 100 patients, 50 per treatment arm, and the final analysis will be a one-sided Fisher's exact test with a 10% Type 1 error. The investigators would like to include interim analyses for futility after treatment response information is available for 40, 60, and 80 patients. We assume that the response information is available quickly. The investigators feel fairly certain about the expected response rate with the standard therapy, based on data from 400 patients. They are less certain about the response to treatment for patients who receive the new treatment. Thus far, they have treated 20 patients with the new treatment, and 14 of the 20 patients responded to the treatment.

(a) What prior distribution would you consider for the probability that a patient responds if given the standard of care, based on the historical data?

(b) What prior distribution would you consider for the new treatment's response probability?

(c) Using 1,000 simulations, what do you determine to be the probability that the study would stop for futility if the response probabilities for the two treatments are equal to 50%?

(d) In part (c), what is the average number of patients who enter the study?

(e) Using 1,000 simulations, what do you determine to be the probability that the study would stop for futility if the response probability for the new treatment is 75%, while for the standard it is 50%?

(f) What is the average number of patients enrolled in the study in part (e)?

(g) Do your estimates of the study's operating characteristics (parts (c)–(f)) seem appropriate to you?

EXERCISE 13.5.   You have designed a phase 2 study that will enroll a maximum of 30 patients. Suppose the analysis prior for the probability a patient responds (θ) is $Be(2,3)$, corresponding to a prior mean probability of response equal to 40% and a 95% probability interval of $(0.068, 0.806)$. The criterion for deciding that the treatment demonstrates sufficient clinical activity to warrant further study is that the posterior probability that the response probability is greater than 0.33 is 75% or more. That is, we conclude in favor of the treatment if $P(\theta > 0.33 \mid \text{Data}) > 0.75$. After treating 20 patients, the investigators note that four patients responded.

(a) What is the predictive probability that there will be a total of five patients who respond after the study finishes enrollment and treats 30 patients?

(b) Compute the predictive probability of five responses in 30 patients if the "true" underlying probability of response is 0.2, 0.3, 0.4, and 0.5, conditional on four responders among the first 20 patients.

(c) Calculate the criterion in favor of the new treatment for $n = 30$, 50, and 100. That is, determine $P(\theta > 0.33 \mid \text{Data}) > 0.75$ when the trial will enroll a total of 30, 50, and 100 patients, conditional on four responders among the first 20 patients. You may assume that the "true" underlying probability of response equals 0.4.

(d) Should the trial stop after enrolling 30 patients or continue to enroll more patients? If more patients, 50 or 100? Explain your decision.

EXERCISE 13.6.   You are designing a randomized controlled trial with interim analyses to evaluate a new treatment for cancer. The trial will compare a new therapy to the current standard of care, with the latter being the control. You will use skeptical and enthusiastic priors in the trial design to guide interim decision-making. The primary endpoint is survival. The control therapy is associated with a one-year survival probability of 65%. For clinicians to want to use the new therapy, one-year survival probability will have to increase to 75% or more. We will assume that the distribution of survival times is exponential with hazard rates λ_0 for the control and λ_1 for the treatment. Furthermore, we will assume that the logarithm of the hazard ratio (θ) is normally distributed.

(a) Find the hazard ratio (control divided by new treatment), assuming that the new treatment achieves the minimal hazard rate (75%). Also, find the log of the hazard ratio (θ_{alt}).

(b) We now want to determine an appropriate skeptical prior as in Section 13.6. The skeptic's prior mean is 0. We determine the standard deviation of the prior distribution based on the skeptical prior having just 5% probability that $\theta > \theta_{\text{alt}}$. Assuming that θ has a normal distribution and using the value of θ_{alt} from part (a) of this problem, find the standard deviation for the skeptical prior distribution.

(c) Assume that the enthusiastic prior is centered at θ_{alt} and places 10% probability on the region $\theta < 0$. Find the standard deviation of this enthusiastic prior distribution.

(d) The first interim analysis occurs when there are 100 events out of a planned 250 events. At this time, the estimate of the logarithm of the hazard ratio is $\hat{\theta} = -0.288$. Find the corresponding normal likelihood and plot it.

(e) Find the skeptic's posterior distribution and the enthusiast's posterior distribution. Plot the respective densities on the same graph. Plot the likelihood on the same graph with the posterior distributions.

(f) Compute the posterior probability $P(\theta < \theta_{\text{alt}} \mid data)$ for the skeptic and for the enthusiast. Do you think the study should continue?

EXERCISE 13.7.   Consider a randomized clinical trial that is comparing two treatments with respect to times to failure. Assuming that the failure times follow an exponential distribution, we will set up response-adaptive randomization for this study. Let λ_0 and λ_1 be the hazard rates for the control and experimental therapies, respectively. Randomization probabilities will be equal to $P(\mu_1 > \mu_0 \mid data)$, where the mean $\mu_i = 1/\lambda_i$. We could also use the median, which is the more common measure of a distribution of failure times. Letting m_i be the median time to failure with treatment $i = 0, 1$, we have $m_i = \ln(2)/\lambda_i = \ln(2)\mu_i$. Then the randomization probabilities could be based on the posterior medians of the treatment-specific median time to failure.

(a) If $Y \mid \lambda \sim Exp(\lambda)$ and $\lambda \sim Ga(a, b)$, then $\mu = E[Y] = 1/\lambda$. Show that $\mu \sim InvGa(a, b)$. Furthermore, since the median, $m = \ln(2)/\lambda$, show that $m \sim InvGa(a, \ln(2)b)$.

(b) Suppose that a previous clinical study provided an estimate of the median time to failure for the control treatment $\hat{m}_0 = 26$ weeks. Furthermore, the investigators are 95% certain that the median time to failure is less than 52 weeks. Find an informed prior distribution for m_0 and m_1 based on this information and the assumption that the two priors are the same.

(c) Suppose that the study has enrolled 40 patients in 1 year at a rate of one patient every week. Furthermore, suppose that at 1 year there were 12 failures among patients randomized to the control treatment and nine failures among the experimental treatment patients. The total follow-up times for the two treatments are 182.3 for the control group and 322.97 for the experimental treatment. Find the posterior distribution for each treatment's median time to failure (m_0 and m_1) at this interim analysis. Also, find the posterior distribution of the hazard rate for each treatment group.

(d) Using the posterior means of the treatment-specific median time to failure, determine the randomization probabilities if there is no discounting, that is, $\gamma = 1$ in equation (13.13).

Chapter 14

Hierarchical Models and Longitudinal Data

This chapter considers models that have additional complexity beyond those that we have already considered. In all the chapters that considered regression modeling, there was a presumption that important predictor variables were taken into account. Indeed, when designing a study to assess the importance of various predictor variables on a response variable of interest, scientists will do their best to include those variables that they deem important and they are able to measure. There will be situations, however, where this has been done and where it is also suggested that there may be some other factors that (i) were not taken into account and perhaps should have been, (ii) are difficult to measure and are consequently left out of the model, or (iii) are perhaps even impossible to measure. With a slight abuse of the term, we refer to such variables as *latent*. Strictly, the word "latent" implies that such variables are unobservable. Here we extend this interpretation to mean that they are unobservable or unobserved (perhaps due to some form of scientific oversight). This chapter focuses on extending previous models to allow for latent variables.

Generically, we have data y, latent variables γ, and a collection of parameters, θ. We pose a model for the data given the parameters and latents, $p(y \mid \theta, \gamma)$, a model for the latents, $p(\gamma \mid \theta)$, and a prior distribution, $p(\theta)$. This leads to a joint distribution (probability density function)

$$p(y, \gamma, \theta) = p(y \mid \theta, \gamma)p(\gamma \mid \theta)p(\theta),$$

from which it is possible to obtain the joint pdf for unknown and uncertain (θ, γ),

$$p(\theta, \gamma \mid y) \propto p(y, \gamma, \theta),$$

with y regarded as fixed and equal to the observed data. In theory, we can obtain the marginals $p(\theta \mid y) = \int p(\theta, \gamma \mid y)d\gamma$ and $p(\gamma \mid y) = \int p(\theta, \gamma \mid y)d\theta$. The model as described thus far is a generic version of a two-level hierarchical model for the data, with a third level corresponding to the prior. Such models are also termed *multilevel models*.

If we have a vector of future data, z, with model $p(z \mid \theta, \gamma, y)$, where we do not necessarily assume that Z is independent of Y conditional on (θ, γ), then the predictive density is defined as

$$p(z \mid y) = \int p(z \mid \theta, \gamma, y)p(\theta, \gamma \mid y)d\theta d\gamma.$$

Theoretically, it is quite simple to make a full range of statistical inferences based on this model. It is often simple in practice, as well, provided we are able to iteratively sample from the conditional distributions

$$p(\theta \mid \gamma, y), \quad p(\gamma \mid \theta, y), \quad p(z \mid \theta, \gamma, y).$$

This basic structure underlies the rest of this chapter, wherein we illustrate such inferential models across a number of very important areas of statistical modeling.

In the next section, we motivate and, by example, illustrate the concept of hierarchical modeling. Next, we discuss applications of hierarchical structures to regression modeling. In the literature, such models are termed "mixed models," because of the addition of latent (random) effects to standard regression models. We then discuss the important topic of longitudinal and correlated data modeling. In addition, we use the same hierarchical modeling structure to handle meta-analysis. Meta-analysis infers a common effect across a finite number of studies that were designed separately but with the same purpose in mind. For example, one may posit a general model in which each study assessed the effectiveness of a particular drug for treating a particular disease. The essence of a meta-analysis is to combine information from similar studies to make an overall inference about the effectiveness of the treatment.

14.1   Normal Hierarchical Models

We begin with some simple illustrations of models for normally distributed data that involve latent variables. We then give the basic structure of such models.

14.1.1   Simple Examples

Example 14.1. Conception Data. We consider a data set that was given in the classic applied statistics book by Snedecor and Cochran (1967) [299, Example 10.18.1]. The data are percentages of successful artificial inseminations in cows for six bulls. For bull i, n_i series of semen samples were sent out and the percentage of conceptions was determined for each series. Let y_{ij} be the percentage of conceptions in series j for bull i. The data are given in Table 14.1. Observe that we also give the sample means for each bull as $\bar{y}_i = \sum_{j=1}^{n_i} y_{ij}/n_i$.

Snedecor and Cochran consider the following model for these data:

$$Y_{ij} \mid \sigma^2, \gamma_i \perp\!\!\!\perp N(\gamma_i, \sigma^2) \quad \text{and} \quad \gamma_i \perp\!\!\!\perp N(\mu, \sigma_\gamma^2).$$

Observations for different bulls are assumed independent. Observations within bulls would be conditionally independent if the bulls' means were known. The bull-specific means are modeled with their own normal distributions, so within-bull observations are exchangeable. With this model, we assume that bull-specific mean percentages are a random sample from a population with mean μ and standard deviation σ_γ. In our new terminology, the model assumes that the underlying mean

TABLE 14.1: Conception data

Bull	Percentages of conceptions	n_i	$\bar{y}_i$
1	46, 31, 37, 62, 30	5	41.2
2	70, 59	2	64.5
3	52, 44, 57, 40, 67, 64, 70	7	56.3
4	47, 21, 70, 46, 14	5	39.6
5	42, 64, 50, 69, 77, 81, 87	7	67.1
6	35, 68, 59, 38, 57, 76, 57, 76, 57, 29, 60	9	53.2

responses for different bulls are latent and vary from bull to bull. The model also implicitly presumes that there are other bulls in the population (but not in our sample) that also have means that vary around the unknown value μ. The assumption of a normal distribution for the means is common but somewhat arbitrary. We discuss this issue later.

There are two types of variability in these data that are of interest, the within-bull variability, measured by σ, and the between-bull variability, measured by σ_γ. If $\sigma_\gamma \doteq 0$, then there are no differences among bulls, since in this case the mean percentages for all bulls would be close to the same value μ. On the other hand, if σ is small and σ_γ is large, the implication is that some bulls reliably have percentages above μ and others reliably below μ.

We proceed to analyze these data with proper reference priors. We consider $\mu \sim U(0, 100)$, $\sigma \sim U(0, 100)$, and $\sigma_\gamma \sim U(0, 100)$, all independent. These are extremely diffuse priors. Since percentages are all in $(0, 100)$, there would be no point in allowing for μ to take values outside of this interval. Similarly, it would be impossible for the standard deviations to take values outside this interval. It is important that the prior for σ_γ be a proper prior. We discuss this issue later.

Table 14.2 gives output for the analysis. Inferences relate to the latent mean variables, the overall mean, and the two standard deviations along with their ratio. Statistical literature may refer to inferences for the latent means as predictions, since the γ_i are not regarded as parameters in the traditional sense. It is clear that $\sigma_\gamma \neq 0$, which means that there are differences in the latent means. The estimated standard deviations are of the same order of magnitude, though the 95% probability interval for the ratio has an upper limit of 2.2, implying that σ_γ could be as large as 2σ.

The overall average, μ, is estimated to be about 54% with 95% PI $(40.5, 68.1)$. Since the model for the γ_i centered them on μ, it is not surprising that the predicted γ_i range from 45.1 to 63.1. Notice that the predicted values below 0.54 are all greater than the corresponding sample mean values in Table 14.1, and the predicted values above 0.54 are all less than their corresponding sample means. For example, the sample means are 39.6 and 67.1 for bulls 4 and 5, respectively, and the corresponding predicted means are 45.1 and 63.1. These differences are due to the fact that the predictions from this model are shrunk from the sample means towards

TABLE 14.2: Analysis of conception data with diffuse proper prior

	Post. med.	(95% PI)
μ	54.3	$(40.5, 68.1)$
γ_1	46.1	$(32.0, 58.6)$
γ_2	58.4	$(43.2, 77.4)$
γ_3	55.7	$(45.3, 66.5)$
γ_4	45.1	$(30.8, 58.0)$
γ_5	63.1	$(51.6, 75.2)$
γ_6	57.0	$(47.7, 66.9)$
σ	16.1	$(12.5, 21.4)$
σ_γ	10.9	$(1.5, 34.5)$
σ_γ/σ	0.68	$(0.08, 2.2)$

their overall average. We call this the "shrinkage" effect, which plays a large role in Bayesian statistics. We introduced this concept in Chapter 3 and address this effect theoretically in Exercise 14.4.

As a final note in this example, we observe that the predicted percentage of conceptions for bull 5 is 0.63 and for bull 4 is 0.45. The 95% PI for the ratio γ_5/γ_4 is 1.4 $(0.99, 2.2)$, and the predictive probability that the ratio exceeds 1 is 0.964. This is reasonable evidence in favor of the hypothesis that bull 5 is more productive than bull 4. We considered several other diffuse proper priors and results were practically the same. We also ran several chains and checked for convergence. There were no convergence issues. The code for this analysis is in files named `Ch14-Conception` on the book's website.

Example 14.2. Rat Data. We now consider a data set that was analyzed in Gelfand et al. (1990) [130]. The data consist of weights (in grams) of 30 rats at 1, 2, 3, 4, and 5 weeks after birth. The goal is to model each rat's weight over this time period as a linear function of weeks since birth. Since weight measurements are taken on the same rat over the five-week period, one might expect that there will be individual rat characteristics that might result in higher or lower intercepts and slopes across the rats.

We consider the following model. Let y_{ij} be the weight measurement on the ith rat in the jth week. Let x_j take on the values $(-2, -1, 0, 1, 2)$, where we have subtracted 3 (the midpoint) from the actual numbers of weeks. Thus $x_j = -2$ corresponds to week 1, $x_j = 0$ corresponds to week 3, etc. We have thus centered the actual covariate to have a mean 0, which will help to stabilize inferences. The statistical model is

$$Y_{ij} \mid \gamma_i, \sigma^2 \perp\!\!\!\perp N(\gamma_{1i} + \gamma_{2i}x_j, \sigma^2) \quad \text{and} \quad \gamma_i = \begin{pmatrix} \gamma_{i1} \\ \gamma_{i2} \end{pmatrix} \perp\!\!\!\perp N_2(\beta, \Sigma_\gamma),$$

where $\beta' = (\beta_1, \beta_2)$ and Σ_γ is a diagonal matrix with components $(\sigma_{1\gamma}^2, \sigma_{2\gamma}^2)$ on the diagonals. This model assumes that every rat has its own intercept and slope and

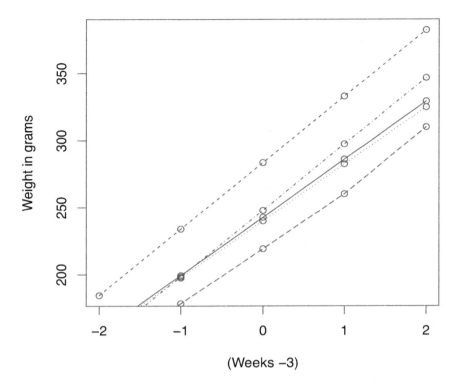

FIGURE 14.1: Plot of predicted growth curves for four rats plus an "average" rat (solid curve).

that these intercepts and slopes vary around an overall intercept β_1 and slope β_2. If $\sigma_{2\gamma} \doteq 0$, the model says that all slopes are approximately β_2; similarly, if $\sigma_{1\gamma} \doteq 0$, all intercepts are approximately the same. If both standard deviations are close to 0, then all rats have approximately the same intercept and slope, or in other words, approximately the same growth curve.

Our main interest in this example is to make inferences about the average growth curve $\beta_1 + \beta_2 x$ for $x \in (-2, -1, 0, 1, 2)$ and to assess how much variability there is in growth curves among rats in terms of slopes and intercepts. We also might be interested in making predictive inferences about a new rat. What would we expect that curve to look like?

In Table 14.3, we have given posterior medians and 95% PIs for the components of β, several γ, and for σ and Σ_γ. It is clear that the intercepts' and slopes' standard deviations are not close to zero and that there is considerably more variability among intercepts than there is among slopes. In Figure 14.1, we have plotted several predicted growth profiles for rats in the data, plus the estimated average growth profile, $\beta_1 + \beta_2 x$, which is plotted with a solid line. This line is identical to the predicted curve for a new rat, say rat 31. Predictions for a new rat are the same as the estimates of the average weights at each time point among all rats. Probability intervals at each of the five points on the curve are wider if predicting an actual set of five future measurements on a new rat, say $\{y_{31,j} : j = 1, \ldots, 5\}$ than they will

TABLE 14.3: Analysis of rat data with diffuse proper prior

	Post. med.	(95 % PI)
β_1	242.6	$(237.0, 248.1)$
β_2	43.3	$(41.8, 44.8)$
γ_{11}	239.9	$(234.6, 245.2)$
γ_{21}	247.8	$(242.5, 253.2)$
γ_{31}	252.5	$(247.1, 257.7)$
γ_{12}	42.5	$(39.0, 45.8)$
γ_{22}	49.5	$(45.9, 53.0)$
γ_{32}	45.4	$(42.1, 48.8)$
σ	6.1	$(5.3, 7.1)$
σ_{1g}	14.6	$(11.4, 19.7)$
σ_{1g}	3.7	$(2.6, 5.2)$

be for predicting $\gamma_{1,31} + \gamma_{2,31}x$ (the predicted weight trajectory), and these intervals will be wider than those corresponding to the average, $\beta_1 + \beta_2 x$. The extra width comes from the variation of a rat's observed weight from its model-predicted weight. The predicted growth curves for rats literally vary around the growth curve that corresponds to the overall average.

In the analysis, we used very diffuse proper priors for all parameters. We used $U(0, 200)$ priors for all three standard deviations and $N(0, 10^5)$ priors for the components of β. All Markov chains converged immediately. The code used and the data are given in files on the book's website that include `Ch14-rat` in the name.

14.1.2 Basics for Two-Level and Three-Level Models for the Data

We now write these models using a generic notation. Let Y_{ij} be a random variable corresponding to an observation. The double subscripts may indicate that this observation is the jth measurement made on the ith experimental unit. For example, there may be repeated observations on a person over time, and Y_{ij} is the measurement made at time t_{ij}, as was the case with the rat data. Alternatively, there may be multiple biopsies of a patient's tumor, and Y_{ij} is the jth biopsy's result. In this instance, the biopsy measurements are said to be clustered within patient.

We can add another level by considering continuous patient outcomes after hospitalization. Consider the structure where there are patients who are treated by physicians who are associated with particular hospitals. We may let Y_{ijk} be the outcome for patient k, who is being treated by physician j who is associated with hospital i. Suppose that there are H hospitals involved, n_i physicians associated with hospital i, and physician j in hospital i has n_{ij} patients. In addition to this structure, there could be vectors of predictor variables associated with hospital i, say v_i $(i = 1, \ldots, H)$, predictor variable vectors that are associated with physician j in hospital i (say w_{ij}), and vectors of patient characteristics, x_{ijk}. Predictors in x_{ijk} could indicate the particular treatment that the patient receives, the patient's overall quality of health, age, blood pressure, etc. At the physician level, years of experience in their specialty is one possible covariate. At the hospital level, there may be quantitative factors available that pertain to the quality of care. Any model that corresponds to this structure would have at least three levels plus a level corresponding to the priors on parameters. At the top level there would be a latent hospital variable (or variables), at the next level there would be a latent physician variable (or variables), and at the third level there would be a model for the data that depends on predictor and latent variables.

We could make this even more interesting by observing perhaps multiple hospitalizations that resulted in observations, Y_{ijkl}. The subscript l corresponds to the lth hospitalization for this patient. In this case, we could have covariates x_{ijkl} for patient k of physician j in hospital i at hospitalization l, covariates v_{ijl} for physician j at hospitalization l, and covariates w_{il} for hospital i at the time of hospitalization l, since all predictor variables could change from one hospitalization to the next. In addition, more latent variables could be added to model specific types of correlation structures for repeated observations on the same patient. For example, if two hospitalizations are a month apart, one might expect greater similarity in responses than if they were 2 years apart. This type of situation suggested adding autoregressive structure to the model. Having said all of this, we refrain for now from specifying a specific model for such a complicated scenario and instead specify a simpler one. A point we wish to make is that the number of levels of the hierarchy, as implied through subscripts, is limited only by what makes sense for the problem at hand. We do need to point out the awkwardness of this notation when programming for data analysis. Different notation is often required.

We begin with two subscripts. For concreteness, let index i refer to hospital i and index k to patient k in hospital i. We allow for hospital-level and patient-level covariates, as well as for latent hospital-level intercepts. The model is

$$Y_{ik} \mid \gamma_i, \theta \perp\!\!\!\perp N(x_{ik}\beta + \gamma_i, \sigma^2),$$
$$\gamma_i \mid \theta \perp\!\!\!\perp N(v_i\delta, \sigma_\gamma^2). \tag{14.1}$$

We have modeled the effect of patient-level covariates as $x_{ik}\beta = \beta_1 + x_{ik2}\beta_2 + \ldots + x_{ikp}\beta_p$, assuming that there are $p-1$ patient-level predictor variables, and hospital covariates as $v_i\delta = v_{i1}\delta_1 + \ldots + v_{iq}\delta_q$ if there are q hospital-level covariates. Note that there is already an intercept in β, so we must not include intercepts for hospital (or physician) regression effects. We specify the prior $p(\theta) = p(\beta, \delta, \sigma_g^2, \sigma^2) = p(\beta, \delta)p(\sigma_\gamma^2)p(\sigma^2)$, where for the moment we imagine proper reference priors for each.

An equivalent model specification for the data is

$$Y_{ik} \mid \gamma_i^*, \theta \perp\!\!\!\perp N(x_{ik}\beta + v_i\delta + \gamma_i^*, \sigma^2),$$
$$\gamma_i^* \mid \theta \perp\!\!\!\perp N(0, \sigma_\gamma^2). \tag{14.2}$$

Both models have a latent effect for hospital, but one (equation (14.1)) is centered on the regression effect involving hospital predictors ($v\delta$), and the other is centered on zero. Therefore, γ_i and γ_i^* have different meanings. Nonetheless, the two models for the data are indeed equivalent. The reason is that the marginal density of the data after integrating out the latent effects from the joint density, namely $p(y \mid \theta) = \int p(y, \gamma \mid \theta) d\gamma$, is precisely the same using either representation.

In the absence of predictor variables, and where, in our notation, hospitals would be regarded as exchangeable, a classic representation of model (14.1) is

$$Y_{ij} \mid \gamma_i, \sigma^2 \stackrel{\text{ind}}{\sim} N(\gamma_i, \sigma^2), \quad i = 1, \ldots, H, \ j = 1, \ldots, n_i,$$
$$\gamma_i \mid \mu, \sigma_\gamma^2 \stackrel{\text{iid}}{\sim} N(\mu, \sigma_\gamma^2). \tag{14.3}$$

The marginal distribution of all the Y_{ij} is identical for all i and j, and the Y_{ij} are pairwise correlated with fixed i. As in the case previously discussed, predictions for the γ_i would be shrunk away from the sample means for each hospital towards the overall mean, μ, because of the shrinkage effect that arises with models like this.

According to the model specification in (14.3) with known (μ, σ_γ^2), if the scientist were told the value of γ_1, the model for $(\gamma_2, \ldots, \gamma_H)$ would not change. Since the full hierarchical model allows for dependence among the γ_i and since it also implies exchangeability, then knowing μ_1 would require the scientist to think that other γ_j might take similar values. Under this model, it makes no sense to consider specifying informative prior information for individual γ_i, beyond what might be specified about (μ, σ_γ^2). If we were to regard the γ_i as unknown but not latent effects, each with its own (independent) prior distribution, it would be difficult to specify those prior distributions for more than a few groups.

We now add a level and consider three indices (i, j, k), with j regarded as physician j, and k as patient k who is treated by physician j in hospital i. The model with covariates and latent effects for hospital and for physician can be represented as

$$Y_{ijk} \mid \gamma_{ij}, \beta, \sigma^2 \perp\!\!\!\perp N(x_{ijk}\beta + \gamma_{ij}, \sigma^2),$$
$$\gamma_{ij} \mid \gamma_i, \delta, \sigma_{1\gamma}^2 \perp\!\!\!\perp N(w_{ij}\lambda + \gamma_i, \sigma_{1\gamma}^2), \tag{14.4}$$
$$\gamma_i \mid \lambda, \sigma_{2\gamma}^2 \perp\!\!\!\perp N(v_i\delta, \sigma_{2\gamma}^2).$$

In equation (14.4), we have modeled hospital covariates as $v_i\delta$, and physician-level covariates as $w_{ij}\lambda = w_{ij1}\lambda_1 + \ldots + w_{ijr}\lambda_r$ if there are r physician-level covariates.

It is possible to write a structurally identical but different version of this model by incorporating all covariates into the vector x_{ijk}. Hospital-level covariates are included, but they do not vary with (j, k). Physician-level covariates are also included, but they do not vary with k. In this instance we can write model (14.4) equivalently as

$$Y_{ijk} \mid \gamma_{ij}^*, \beta, \sigma^2 \perp\!\!\!\perp N(x_{ijk}\beta + \gamma_{ij}^*, \sigma^2),$$
$$\gamma_{ij}^* \mid \gamma_i^*, \sigma_{1\gamma}^2 \perp\!\!\!\perp N(\gamma_i^*, \sigma_{1\gamma}^2), \tag{14.5}$$
$$\gamma_i^* \mid \sigma_{2\gamma}^2 \perp\!\!\!\perp N(0, \sigma_{2\gamma}^2),$$

where hospital covariates (v_i) and physician-level covariates (w_{ij}) have been included in x_{ijk}.

Model (14.4) is called a "centering" model, since latent variables have means that are centered on their corresponding linear covariate effects. Gelfand and Sahu

(1995) [131] have argued that centered hierarchical models may have better convergence properties than uncentered models like (14.5).

We could, of course, keep adding levels. Once the basic two-level and three-level models have been understood, however, one can imagine how to extend to higher levels. In Section 14.3.1, we discuss adding one more level to model (14.4).

Also, as in Example 14.2, any of the above models could include latent effects for slopes in addition to the latent effects for intercepts. We rely on the reader to be able to adapt models in this section to allow for this type of generalization.

14.1.3 Prior Specification

Until now, we have suggested specifying proper reference priors for all parameters. We begin this discussion by specifying proper priors for the parameters $(\mu, \sigma^2, \sigma_\gamma^2)$ in the simpler model (14.3).

In this model, specifying an informative prior for μ should be straightforward, since $\mu = E(\gamma_i \mid \mu, \sigma_\gamma)$ for all i. We ask our expert to think about the average for the population of means. Specifically, we elicit a best guess for μ, and, say, the 95th percentile. The model would specify that $\mu \sim N(\mu_0, b)$, where μ_0 is the best guess and b is selected to obtain the specified value for the percentile. We have done this many times before, so we skip details. The classic diffuse proper prior for μ is something like a $N(0, 10^6)$ distribution. It could also be a sufficiently wide uniform distribution, which we used in the simple examples earlier.

One can specify an informative prior for σ in a similar way as done in Chapter 7. Here, we think about the 90th percentile for an observation for a hospital that would correspond to the average response with mean equal to μ, namely $p_{0.9} = \mu + 1.28\,\sigma$. We would obtain a best guess for this percentile, say p_0. We would be thinking that 90 out of 100 γ_i would be smaller than p_0. With μ_0 our best guess for μ, we obtain a best guess for σ as $\sigma_0 = (p_0 - \mu_0)/1.28$. At this point, we could take a $Ga(c, d)$ prior for σ and set the mode equal to σ_0 ($\sigma_0 = (c-1)/d$), and solve for $c = 1 + d\,\sigma_0$. We could then make the prior diffuse by setting $d = 0.001$, which results in a large variance for the gamma distribution with mode σ_0.

Alternatively, we could select a maximum value for the 90th percentile, say $\tilde{m}$. We would interpret this to mean that $\mu + 1.28\sigma < \tilde{m}$ with probability 1. Conditioning on our best guess for $\mu = \mu_0$, and assuming our prior inferences for μ and σ are independent, we obtain virtual certainty that $\sigma < (\tilde{m} - \mu_0)/1.28$. We could then place a uniform distribution on σ with this upper limit. We leave it as an exercise to obtain a fully informative gamma prior for σ.

Specifying an informative prior for σ_γ is similar to that for σ. Instead of thinking about the 90th percentile of the data outcomes, which is governed by σ, we let $\gamma_{0.9} = \mu + 1.28\sigma_\gamma$ be the 90th percentile of the distribution of the γ_i, which is governed by σ_γ. As before, μ_0 is the expert's best guess for μ, and as always, we assume that knowledge about μ is independent of knowledge about σ_γ. In addition, suppose that, based on scientific input, it is known with virtual certainty that $\gamma_{0.9} < \gamma_{\max}$. Then an appropriate proper diffuse prior for σ_γ is $U(0, \max)$ with $\max = (\gamma_{\max} - \mu_0)/1.28$.

Alternatively, if we let γ_0 be the expert's best guess for $\gamma_{0.9}$, the best guess for σ_γ would be $\sigma_{0g} = (\gamma_0 - \mu_0)/1.28$. Now assume that the expert is 95% sure that $\gamma_{0.9}$ is less than u. Then we have $P(\mu + 1.28\sigma_\gamma < u \mid \mu = \mu_0) = 0.95$, which is equivalent to asserting that $P(\sigma_\gamma < (u - \mu_0)/1.28 \equiv \tilde{\sigma}_\gamma) = 0.95$. We can then select a $Ga(e, f)$ distribution with mode $(e - 1)/f = \sigma_{0\gamma}$ and with 95th percentile $\tilde{\sigma}_\gamma$ as an informative prior for σ_γ.

We note that if H is small, then estimating the variability in the γ_i has to be difficult. Imagine trying to estimate a variance with only two or three observations. In this instance, no one gets to observe the latent γ_i. Yet, we are still attempting to estimate the variance. Of course, this is virtually impossible with only a small number of the latent variables. The point is that if H is small, the posterior for σ_γ will often look just like the prior. There is no harm in this, but the analyst needs to be aware of this possibility when specifying the prior on σ_γ. A sensitivity analysis with respect to the choice of prior for σ_γ—one that considers all inferences—is especially warranted if H is small.

Historically, there has been a tendency to use $Ga(0.001, 0.001)$ priors for the precisions $\tau = 1/\sigma^2$ and $\tau_\gamma = 1/\sigma_\gamma^2$, and an improper flat prior for μ. A nice feature of this specification is that all the full conditionals for model (14.3) are recognizable, so Gibbs sampling is easy. We do not recommend using an improper prior for τ_γ (or σ_γ), however, since this would result in an improper posterior and posterior inferences could be meaningless (Hobert and Casella, 1996, [164]).

The conditionally conjugate prior specification for model (14.3) is

$$\mu \sim N(a, b), \quad \tau \sim Ga(c, d), \quad \tau_\gamma \sim Ga(e, f), \tag{14.6}$$

independently. This means that the full conditionals for each of these are in the same family as the prior and, moreover, the full conditionals for the γ_i are also independent and normal. One can, therefore, easily sample from all posteriors. The reader is asked to establish this result in an exercise.

We conclude this section with a brief discussion about prior specification when regression coefficients and/or additional latent effects are included in the model. Linear regression coefficients can be handled as in Chapter 7, with a flat improper prior, with diffuse proper normal priors, or with partial information conditional means priors. Here, we make these specifications conditional on thinking about experimental units with any latent effects set to their average value. This approach corresponds to setting the latent effects equal to zero in the model representation (14.2), where we modeled latent effects with mean zero.

For a model with two types of latent effect, consider the illustration with hospitals and physicians. There were standard deviations for two latent effects in that example, namely, $\sigma_{1\gamma}$ and $\sigma_{2\gamma}$. We could think about the 90th percentile for each of the corresponding latent effect distributions separately in the same way that we thought about only one of them above. It is probably easiest to place uniform distributions on these standard deviations, with some thought about what the upper value should be. The corresponding latent effects are on the scale of the data, which helps when selecting the upper limit. For example, if all the values in the data are expected to be in the range $(0, 100)$, it would be virtually impossible for any standard deviation to be larger than 100 (see Exercise 14.8).

14.1.4 Meta-Analysis

Meta-analysis often consists of bringing together data from different sources to help produce an overall inference, perhaps to estimate a single effect measure common to all studies. The most common examples include meta-analyses of different clinical trials evaluating some form of therapy. The meta-analysis brings together the data or some summary measures from each of the studies and synthesizes this information in a probabilistically coherent way.

By "probabilistically coherent way" we mean to imply that a non-Bayesian approach to meta-analysis might not be the best way to go. Consider as an example the GUSTO randomized clinical trial [323]. GUSTO randomized more than 41,000 patients to four different thrombolytic treatments. The objective was to determine if one treatment strategy improved survival among patients who suffered a myocardial infarction. The analysis of the trial indicated superior survival among patients randomized to receive accelerated tissue plasminogen activator (t-PA) given with intravenous heparin, compared to the other treatments. Brophy and Joseph (1995) [58] examined the evidence in favor of t-PA in the GUSTO trial in light of other randomized clinical trials that had been carried out and published by the time the GUSTO results appeared in the *New England Journal of Medicine* [323]. In their meta-analysis of the data relating to t-PA, Brophy and Joseph (1995) simply pooled the data without taking a hierarchical approach. Subsequently, they reanalyzed the data with a hierarchical model [57]. They conclude that accounting for the other studies leads to a less optimistic inference regarding the benefit of t-PA.

An important point to remember is that a meta-analysis is an observational study, even though the observations may include only randomized clinical trials. Each randomized clinical trial may epitomize the science of clinical research, but the meta-analysis is, in the end, a random sample of the population of clinical trials of the treatment of interest. Thus, meta-analyses are subject to all of the design and analysis considerations that one would apply when designing and carrying out any observational study.

Why take a hierarchical approach? The advantages for a meta-analysis include relaxing the assumption of exchangeability of patients across studies carried out at different times and with possibly different populations, the ability to make prediction not just for a future patient but also for a future study [281], and the ability to estimate study-specific effects with shrinkage towards the overall mean, to name but a few. The data frequently take the form of a summary statistic obtained from each study, such as a mean, odds ratio, or relative risk, and the associated estimate of uncertainty, such as the standard deviation or standard error.

We give examples of three meta-analyses, one here and two in the binomial regression section of this chapter (Section 14.2).

Example 14.3. Intensive Care Unit Study. This example involves data on 14 clinical trials that study a treatment for decontaminating intensive care unit patients' digestive tracts. We present a similar analysis to that of Christensen et al. (2010) [79]. The thought is that the treatment may help prevent lethal infections. Each of the clinical trials randomized patients to receive either a combination regimen that consisted of systemic antibiotics plus a topical antibiotic or a control therapy. The primary endpoint is mortality, and the main analysis compares the risk of death for the treatment groups via the odds ratio. (We discuss odds ratios in Chapters 5 and 8.) Our meta-analysis of the 14 trials uses the estimated odds ratios from each trial, and our target of inference is the overall or population median odds ratio for mortality for the combination regimen relative to the control treatment.

The data $y = \{y_i : i = 1, \ldots, 14\}$ are in the form of empirical log odds ratios from the various studies. They are available on the book's website for this chapter in file `Ch14-ICU-Metaanalysis.txt`. Our sampling model is

$$Y_i \mid \theta_i, \sigma_i^2 \perp\!\!\!\perp N(\theta_i, \sigma_i^2),$$

and we assume that σ_i^2 is known. In our statistical model, θ_i is the actual underlying log odds ratio for study i. The *known* σ_i^2 is the estimated standard deviation of y_i in study i and is, of course, just an approximation. In our meta-analysis, we use the latent effects model

$$\theta_i \mid \mu, \sigma_i^2, \sigma_g^2 \perp\!\!\!\perp N(\mu, \sigma_g^2).$$

The model characterizes the study-specific log odds ratios as normally distributed quantities that vary about an overall mean log odds ratio μ. We specify proper reference priors for the two parameters,

$$\mu \sim U(-2, 2) \quad \text{and} \quad \sigma_g \sim U(0, 2).$$

This prior specification centers the overall mean log odds ratio at zero and assumes that the between-study variance is not very large. The prior for σ_g^2 seems reasonable, since the scale of the log odds ratios is quite small, as can be seen from the data. As stated above, we wish to infer the median odds ratio, e^μ, across the studies. That is, half of the studies' odds ratios will be less than e^μ, and half will have odds ratios above this central value.

The posterior median odds ratio was $e^{\tilde{\mu}} = 0.82$ with 95% posterior probability interval $(0.66, 1.01)$. In words, our inference is that the midpoint of our estimated odds of death with the combination treatment is around 82% of the odds of dying with the control therapy among studies represented by our sample of 14. Furthermore, we are 95% certain that the median value is as low as 2/3 and as high as 1 (i.e., the same odds). In fact, our analysis indicates a posterior probability of 0.965 that the median is less than 1 (lower mortality risk with the combination treatment). Our meta-analysis provides fairly strong statistical strength to a claim of lower mortality with the combination treatment than with the control.

The estimated odds ratios for the 14 trials are (0.78, 0.77, 0.77, 0.81, 0.82, 0.81, 0.81, 0.82, 0.83, 0.85, 0.86, 0.88, 0.91, 0.92), which are fairly consistent. The estimated value for σ_g is 0.15 $(0.01, 0.44)$. The estimated 20th and 80th percentiles of the induced distribution of odds ratios are $e^{\mu \pm 0.84\,\sigma_g}$ and are estimated to be 0.72 and 0.94, respectively. This means that we would estimate that about 20% of odds ratios would be less than 0.72 and another 20% would be above 0.94. We also considered an extremely diffuse $N(0, 1000)$ prior for μ and a $U(0, 10)$ prior for σ_g. The results were virtually identical.

Unfortunately, since the observed data are already in the form of empirical odds ratios, there is no hope of saying anything about the probabilities of death with the treatments in the studies. So, there is no hope of assessing the practical import of the result.

14.2 Hierarchical Binomial Regression Modeling

We now consider binary response data with latent variables. The concepts are basically the same as with the normal data modeling that we just discussed, but now everything is on a nonlinear scale. The change of scale will have a considerable effect on how we elicit priors involving the variability of the latent variables, since in the logistic model, for example, these variables are on the logit scale rather than on the scale of the data. A different kind of thought process is needed.

As in the normal model case, introducing latent effects introduces correlations among Bernoulli observations when appropriate. The latent variables can adjust for missing or unknown covariates or predictors that are common to a group of observations while not fundamentally changing the nature of the statistical inference.

Example 14.4. Suppose we sample 100 hospitals and then randomly sample a number of patients from each hospital. At the end of each patient's (non-life-threatening) stay, we ask them if they were satisfied with their care in the hospital (yes or no). Patient-reported satisfaction is our binary response. In addition, we track certain hospital characteristics such as the average number of nursing staff per 10 patients and the percentage of physicians who are board certified. We also assume that we could include patient variables, such as age and some kind of assessment of overall health.

Let x_{ij} denote the vector of covariate information for the jth patient in the ith hospital with a 1 in the first slot for the intercept (i.e., $x_{ij1} = 1, j = 1, \ldots, n_i; i = 1, \ldots, 100$). Let y_{ij} be the indicator of the satisfaction for patient j in hospital i, and let $\theta_{ij} = P(y_{ij} = 1 \mid x_{ij})$. Hospital variables are included in the vector x_{ij}, but they do not vary with j. The standard logistic regression model

$$Y_{ij} \mid \theta_{ij} \perp\!\!\!\perp \text{Bernoulli}(\theta_{ij}), \quad \text{logit}(\theta_{ij}) = x_{ij}'\beta$$

allows for the effects of measured hospital and patient characteristics on the probability of satisfaction for any hospital in the data and also to predict patient satisfaction for any new hospital for which we have the appropriate covariates.

We may suspect, however, that important hospital variables have been omitted because they were too expensive to measure or because they were not considered important. To the extent that these are hospital variables and not patient variables, we can accommodate them by incorporating a surrogate, latent hospital effect. While there are always multiple ways to write such a model, we write it as

$$\text{logit}(\theta_{ij}) = \gamma_i + x'_{ij}\beta^*, \quad \gamma_i \perp\!\!\!\perp N(\beta_1, \sigma_\gamma^2). \tag{14.7}$$

We leave the 1 out of x_{ij}, resulting in $x'_{ij}\beta^* = x_{ij1}\beta_2 + \ldots + x_{ij1}\beta_p$, where some of the x_{ijr} values correspond to hospital covariates. We have moved the intercept term so that we could center the latent effects distribution on it. We could have centered the latent effects distribution on the sum of the components of $x'_{ij}\beta$ that correspond to the intercept and hospital covariate effects. Alternatively, we could have left the intercept in $x'_{ij}\beta$ and set the latent effects' means to zero. All three representations correspond to the same model for the data, but the ones not centered on zero may have better Monte Carlo (MC) convergence properties (Gelfand et al. (1995) [131]).

In this model, each hospital is regarded as having been sampled from a population of hospitals. Satisfaction probabilities for patients in each hospital go up or down depending on whether γ_i is greater than or less than β_1. A hospital with $\gamma_i = \beta_1$ is regarded as a "typical" hospital in our subsequent discussion involving prior specification.

Prediction for a new hospital (denoted by subscript f) with hospital and patient covariates x is accomplished by augmenting the existing model. Here, we model

$$Y_f \mid x, \gamma_f, \beta \sim Ber(\theta_f), \quad \text{logit}(\theta_f) = \gamma_f + x\beta,$$
$$\gamma_f \mid \beta_1, \sigma_\gamma^2 \sim N(\beta_1, \sigma_\gamma^2).$$

Monitoring Y_f, however, can only result in a point prediction, since it is a Bernoulli variable. On the other hand, monitoring θ_f will give the same result, since it is a parameter; one can also provide a 95% PI for θ_f. The predicted probability of satisfaction for a new patient in a new hospital will be the same as the point estimate of the proportion of satisfied patients in the new hospital with predictors x, and we will have a 95% PI for this proportion.

The variability in the γ_i, as measured by σ_γ, affects the variability in the probabilities of satisfaction for patients. For example, if $\sigma_\gamma \doteq 0$, then patients who are in hospitals with the same predictor values and who also have the same patient predictor values will all have the same estimated probabilities of satisfaction. If σ_γ is large, then there will be considerable variability among these probabilities.

Finally, this model also correlates responses within each hospital. That is, $\{y_{ij} : j = 1, \ldots, n_i\}$ are all correlated, while responses from different hospitals are independent. The fact that all patients from hospital i share the same latent γ_i effect induces the correlation.

Our next example involves the analysis of toenail fungus data. We apologize for the image this presents, but the problem is real.

Example 14.5. Toenail Fungus. Toenail onychomycosis, known as toenail fungus, is fairly common. It can disfigure and sometimes destroy the nail. It may afflict between 2% and 18% of people worldwide. Onychomycosis can be caused by several types of fungi known as dermatophytes, as well as by non-dermatophytic yeasts or molds. We consider data from a clinical trial on toenail fungus reported by De Backer et al. (1996) [89]. The randomized study compares two oral treatments for dermatophyte onychomycosis infection: terbinafine and intraconazole. These are well-known commercially available treatments.

Specifically, we consider data on an unpleasant side effect: the degree of separation of the nail plate from the nail bed. This is scored in four categories (0, absent; 1, mild; 2, moderate; 3, severe). For the 294 patients in the trial, the response was evaluated at seven visits (approximately in weeks 0, 1, 2, 3, 6, 9, and 12). Times in the data are given with decimal points, so 0.96 would correspond to 0.96 of a week for example. A total of 937 measurements were made on the 146 intraconazole ($Trt_i = 0$) patients, and 971 measurements were made on 148 terbinafine ($Trt_i = 1$) patients. The data were obtained from the pharmaceutical company Novartis at a website that no longer exists, but they are available on the book's website in the files for this chapter. The files have **toenail** in their names.

Following Lesaffre and Spiessens (2001) [219], who also analyzed these data, the responses were dichotomized into categories with toenail separation at the time either (i) absent or mild, or (ii) moderate or severe. Since there were repeated responses on each individual in the sample, they fit a logistic regression model with a latent variable for each individual. Specifically, let $y_{ij} = 1$ if individual i has moderate or severe toenail separation at time j, and let $y_{ij} = 0$ otherwise. Measurements taken at time 0 precede the application of any treatment, and our model needs to reflect this fact. Thus, in the model specification below, we let $z_{ij} = 0$ if $Time_{ij} = 0$ and $z_{ij} = 1$ if $Time_{ij} \neq 0$. The model is

$$
\begin{aligned}
Y_{ij} \mid \theta_{ij} &\perp\!\!\!\perp Ber(\theta_{ij}), \\
\text{logit}\,(\theta_{ij}) &= \beta_2 Trt_i\, z_{ij} + \beta_3 Time_{ij} + \beta_4 Trt_i \times Time_{ij}\, z_{ij} + \gamma_i, \\
\gamma_i \mid \beta_1, \tau, \sigma_\gamma^2 &\perp\!\!\!\perp N(\beta_1, \sigma_\gamma^2),
\end{aligned}
$$

for $i = 1, \ldots, 294$ and $j = 1, \ldots, n_i \leq 7$. The latent effects, γ_i, are centered on the intercept, β_1, and are included to allow for correlation among the repeated observations on the same individual, as well as to account for the possibility that each individual may have a biological tendency to have higher (or lower) probabilities of moderate or severe toenail separation through time. The z_{ij} enforce that treatment effects can only exist after time 0.

Trt is the binary treatment indicator. *Time* is the visit time as measured in four-week periods, which is treated as a continuous covariate although it could also be considered a factor with seven levels. The model also includes an interaction, $Trt \times Time$, that allows for the possibility that the effect of the treatment could be modified by time (effect modification in action).

Let us recall the meaning of the interaction effect using odds ratios. We consider two odds ratios, one comparing the effect of treatment for individual i at time $t_2 \in \{0, 1, 2, 3, 6, 9, 12\}$ and for the same individual at an earlier time t_1. We note that here, $z_i = 1$ is synonymous with $t > 0$. The odds of moderate to severe separation at time t for an individual under $Trt = 1$ are $e^{\beta_2 + (\beta_3 + \beta_4)t + \gamma_i}$ if $t > 0$, and the odds of moderate to severe separation at time t for an individual under $Trt = 0$ are $e^{\beta_3 t + \gamma_i}$, regardless of the value of $t > 0$. Thus if $t > 0$, the odds ratio for assessing the effect of treatment (comparing $Trt = 1$ to $Trt = 0$) at time t is

$$OR(t) = e^{\beta_2 + \beta_4 t}, \quad t > 0.$$

If $OR(t) > 1$, then the probability of moderate to severe separation is greater under $Trt = 1$ than it is under $Trt = 0$, and vice versa if $OR(t) < 1$. If $\beta_4 \doteq 0$, then the treatment effect, as measured by the odds ratio ($OR(t) \doteq e^{\beta_2}$), is the same no matter which t one considers, implying no effect modification due to treatment.

Now we consider the case when $z_i = 0$, which corresponds to time $t = 0$. Random treatment assignments occur at time $t = 0$. We should have no treatment effect at this time, since we can assume that neither treatment has yet been applied. Our model with z_i included reflects this fact and implies that the model is constrained to have $OR(t = 0) = 1$, by definition. We point out, in addition, that since a treatment effect is anticipated at later times, odds ratios for $t > 0$ should subsequently be different from 1.

We obtain the ratio of odds ratios that assess the treatment effect at time $t_2 > t_1$ and the treatment effect at time $t_1 > 0$:

$$OR(t_2)/OR(t_1) = e^{\beta_4(t_2 - t_1)}.$$

If $t_1 = 0$ and $t > 0$,
$$OR(t)/OR(0) = e^{\beta_2 + \beta_4 t} = OR(t).$$

So the ratio of odds ratios, which is used to assess effect modification, takes a different form if $t_1 = 0$ or not. If $t_1 = 0$, it reflects the difference in the treatment effect from time 0, where there is no effect. If $t_1 > 0$, it reflects the change in effect for the two times.

Finally, if both treatments are eventually "effective," one would expect β_4 to be negative and $OR(t_2)/OR(t_1)$ to decrease as t_2 increases for all $t_1 \geq 0$.

We require priors for $\beta = (\beta_1, \beta_2, \beta_3, \beta_4)'$ and σ_γ. We standardized the continuous variable $Time$, by subtracting its mean and dividing by the standard deviation:

$$sTime_i = (Time_i - \text{ave}(Time))/\text{sd}(Time).$$

Since Trt is dichotomous, we consider default proper priors $\beta_i \perp\!\!\!\perp N(0, 1)$, as we did in Chapter 8 in similar situations. We also specified $\sigma_\gamma \sim U(0, 10)$. When analyzing the toenail data, we first tried $U(0, 4)$. It became clear that 4 was too small, since posterior iterates for σ_γ were clearly truncated at the value 4. There was no truncation when we used the value 10. We also considered a reference prior (e.g., dflat() in the BUGS language) and $N(0, 2)$ priors for the βs as a sensitivity analysis. In Chapter 8, we thoroughly discussed informative priors for binomial regression models, and we continue the discussion for handling latent variable parameters in the next section.

Posterior output for the toenail study analysis is given in Table 14.4. Observe that all of the regression coefficients are negative with high probability; specifically, the probabilities are 1, 0.9984, 1, 0.979, respectively. Since $\beta_4 < 0$ with high posterior probability, the interaction effect is clearly statistically important, and the values of $OR(t)$ are expected to decrease as t increases. Posterior medians of $OR(t)$ for $t \in (0.5, 1, 3, 5, 8)$ are $(0.31, 0.24, 0.15, 0.09, 0.007)$, respectively, which indicates clear practical import of the effect modification. The treatment effect is clearly decreasing as a function of time from randomization. After half a week from treatment application, the odds of moderate to severe separation under terbinafine is estimated to be about one-third of the corresponding odds using intraconazole, indicating that terbinafine is the preferred treatment. As time goes on, the estimated $OR(t)$ decreases to 0.007 after 8 weeks, indicating an even greater preference for terbinafine.

Table 14.4 also includes posterior medians for ratios of ORs. These ratios of odds ratios tell us how the $OR(t)$s change relative to $OR(0.5)$; they are decreasing, as we indicated earlier that they would, since the $OR(t)$s are themselves decreasing. This information is already well conveyed by simply looking at the estimated $OR(t)$s. Finally, we note that σ_γ is estimated to be about 4 with 95% probability interval $(3.2, 4.6)$. There is not much to say about this variance parameter, except that it is clearly not close to zero and thus the latent effects clearly belong in the model.

As for the sensitivity analysis, changing to a $N(0, 2)$ prior did result is small changes in inferences. For example, with this prior, the estimate of the interaction effect, β_4, was -0.51 $(-1.11, 0.053)$. Compare this estimate with the result in the table, namely, -0.51 $(-1.06, 0.031)$. Using a reference prior, we obtained -0.51 with 95% PI $(-1.12, 0.10)$. The posterior probability that $\beta_4 < 0$ in the latter case is 0.95. Such differences are hardly worth mentioning. Other changes to the results shown in Table 14.4 were comparable.

Example code using the BUGS language can be found in the files labeled `Ch15-Toenail-sTime` on the book's website. That file contains the program we used to obtain inferences in Table 14.4.

Example 14.6. Dairy Cow Abortion Data. Dr. Mark Thurmond and DR. Sharon Hietala of the Veterinary School at the University of California, Davis collected data on the outcome abortion (yes or no) of individual cows coming from nine herds located in the central valley of California. Prior information was elicited from Dr. Thurmond. Let $y = 1$ correspond to "natural abortion," and $y = 0$ correspond to no abortion. There are two covariate values for each of the 13,145 cows. These are GR (gravidity, the number of previous successful pregnancies) and DO (days open, the number of days between the last successful birth and the current pregnancy). We expect that higher DOs will correlate with higher probabilities of natural abortion, since a longer DO may be a result of a difficult calving for the previous birth. We also expect that higher GR will result in lower probability of natural abortion. We assume a latent herd effect. The goal is to model the probability of abortion as a function of the covariates and a latent effect for herd. We expect that the effect of DO may be modified by GR, so we include an interaction effect.

TABLE 14.4: Posterior summaries for the toenail data. $OR(t)$ compares the odds of moderate to severe separation for $Trt = 1$ (terbinafine) to the corresponding odds for $Trt = 0$ (intraconazole), at time t. Independent $N(0, 1)$ priors for β_i and $U(0, 10)$ prior for σ_γ

Parameter	Posterior median	95% PI
β_1 (Intercept	-3.1	$(-3.8, -2.5)$
β_2 (Trt)	-0.91	$(-1.59, -0.24)$
β_3 ($Time$)	-1.60	$(-1.97, -1.28)$
β_4 ($Trt \times Time$)	-0.51	$(-1.06, 0.031)$
σ_γ	3.9	$(3.2, 4.6)$
$OR(0.5)$	0.31	$(0.14, 0.72)$
$OR(1)$	0.24	$(0.08, 0.69)$
$OR(2)$	0.15	$(0.03, 0.65)$
$OR(3)$	0.09	$(0.01, 0.65)$
$OR(5)$	0.03	$(0.001, 0.68)$
$OR(8)$	0.007	$(0.00006, 0.73)$
$OR(1)/OR(0.5)$	0.78	$(0.59, 1.02)$
$OR(2)/OR(0.5)$	0.47	$(0.20, 1.05)$
$OR(3)/OR(0.5)$	0.02	$(0.0003, 1.26)$

In order to stabilize inferences, we standardized DO and GR as $sDO = (DO - \text{mean}(DO)/\text{sd}(D)$ and $sGR = (GR - \text{mean}(GR))/\text{sd}(GR)$, where $\text{mean}(DO) = 115.8$, $sDO = 59.7$, $\text{mean}(GR) = 3.5$, and $sGR = 1.5$. Now, $sDO = 0$ corresponds to $DO \doteq 116$ days, and $sGR = 0$ corresponds to 3.5 previous successful pregnancies, which, of course, is not a possibility.

The data are outcomes on Bernoulli random variables for dairy cows in nine herds with n_i cows in herd i; we write $y = \{y_{ij} : i = 1, \ldots, k; j = 1, \ldots, n_i\}$. Cow j in herd i has a covariate vector of standardized DO and GR, $x'_{ij} = (sDO_{ij}, sGR_{ij}, sDO_{ij} \times sGR_{ij})$, where we leave the 1 out. The regression coefficient vector is $\beta^* = (\beta_2, \beta_3, \beta_4)'$. The notation reflects the fact that there is no intercept in β^*. The model involves centering the latent effect, γ_i, on the intercept, β_1, which should improve MC convergence properties. The model is

$$Y_{ij} \mid \theta_{ij} \perp\!\!\!\perp Ber(\theta_{ij}), \quad \text{logit}(\theta_{ij}) = \gamma_i + x'_{ij}\beta^*,$$
$$\gamma_i \mid \beta_1, \sigma_\gamma \perp\!\!\!\perp N(\beta_1, \sigma_\gamma^2), \quad i = 1, \ldots, k; j = 1, \ldots, n_i, \tag{14.8}$$

where

$$\theta_{ij} = \text{expit}(\gamma_i + sDO_{ij}\beta_2 + sGR_{ij}\beta_3 + sDO_{ij} \times sGR_{ij}\beta_4).$$

Dr. Thurmond wants to know the effect of the covariates on the probability of abortion for typical herds (e.g., with latent effects set to $\gamma_i = \beta_1$ for all i) over the range of covariate values in the data. The probability of abortion for a "typical" herd and given covariate combination (sDO_f, sGR_f) is

$$P(Y_f = 1 \mid \gamma_f = \beta_1, \beta^*) = \text{expit}(\beta_1 + \beta_2 sDO_f + \beta_3 sGR_f + \beta_4 sDO_f \times sGR_f).$$

He is also interested in knowing the latent effects for herds on these probabilities. This is because certain practices in maintaining herds, not accounted for by GR or DO, may result in either higher (with poor practices) or lower (with good practices) probabilities of abortion. We address this question by setting $sDO_f = sGR_f = 0$ and obtaining posterior medians for

$$P(Y_f = 1 \mid \gamma_i) = \text{expit}(\gamma_i), \quad i = 1, \ldots, 9.$$

We can then look at the differences in estimated probabilities. These estimated probabilities correspond to what might be termed an "average" cow, realizing that $GR = 3.5$ is not a possibility. Other choices can be made for the values of DO_f and GR_f.

Finally, Dr. Thurmond is interested in the practical and statistical import of the interaction effect. This can be addressed by looking at a table of estimated probabilities of abortion, perhaps with the combinations of (sDO, sGR) corresponding to values of DO equal to $(2, 4, 6)$ and values of GR equal to $(60, 116, 172)$ (mean$(GR) \pm 56$ days). We can assess the effect of GR by simply comparing the probabilities of abortion for $GR = 2$ and 4 (or 6) for $DO = 60$, with those probabilities with $DO = 116$, and finally with $DO = 172$. Of course, this assessment can be done with odds ratios as well. Exercise 14.12 addresses these questions in the context of analyzing the cow abortion data.

The data and code are available on the book's website in files with `Ch14-Cowabortion` in the name. We use a partially informative prior for regression coefficients. This prior accounts for our knowledge that the overall average rate of abortions is around 0.12. If we consider the "average cow" in a "typical herd," then the logit of the probability of abortion for such a cow is just β_1. Consequently, the corresponding probability is $\text{expit}(\beta_1)$. Dr. Thurmond has been studying cows in the central valley of California for many years and his best estimate of the probability of abortion for such a cow in such a herd is 0.12. We, therefore, specify $\beta_1 \sim N(-2, b)$, where $-2 \approx \text{logit}(0.12)$. Moreover, since there are over 13,000 observations in the data, we do not require additional specific prior information about the coefficients; the other coefficients are modeled with independent $N(0, b)$ priors. Since all predictors have been standardized, we set $b = 1$ for each. We also set $b = 100$ to check on the sensitivity to that choice.

In addition, we elicited from Dr. Thurmond his best estimate for σ_γ, which was 0.25. (We discuss the elicitation methods in the next section.) In the end, we used a relatively diffuse $U(0, c)$ prior with $c = 2$. We also ran the model with $c = 10$. Results from all analyses were virtually identical, despite the fact that the $N(0, 100)$ and $U(0, 10)$ priors are overly diffuse for reasons discussed in the next section.

14.2.1   Informative Prior Elicitation

There are many possible models with different numbers of levels and parameterizations that correspond to the types of data we have been considering. We have been focusing on the logistic regression model with latent variables, but we could also allow for probit or other regression model structures. Here, we discuss prior elicitation for a common type of situation.

The data are modeled as outcomes on Bernoulli variables for individuals in k groups with n_i individuals in group i, $\{y_{ij} : i = 1, \ldots, k; j = 1, \ldots, n_i\}$. Individual j in group i has covariate vector $\tilde{x}'_{ij} = (x_{ij2}, \ldots, x_{ijp})$, where we leave out the 1 that corresponds to the intercept. The regression coefficient vector is now $\beta^* = (\beta_2, \ldots, \beta_p)'$. The notation reflects the fact that there is no intercept in β^*. The model below involves centering the latent effect, γ_i, on the intercept, β_1. We assume the covariate vector components have been standardized if they are continuous, and that categorical covariates have a reference category taking the value 0. The model is given as

$$\{Y_{ij} : j = 1, \ldots, n_i\} \mid \theta_i \perp\!\!\!\perp Ber(\theta_i), \quad \text{logit}(\theta_i) = \tilde{x}'_{ij}\beta^* + \gamma_i,$$
$$\gamma_i \mid \beta_1, \sigma_\gamma \perp\!\!\!\perp N(\beta_1, \sigma_\gamma^2). \tag{14.9}$$

We continue to define $\beta = (\beta_1, (\beta^*)')'$. The predictor vector is $x = (1, \tilde{x}')'$. Thus, $x'\beta = \beta_1 + \tilde{x}'\beta^*$. The distinctions are necessary because we treat the intercept differently than the regression coefficients in the model; the model centers the latent effects on the intercept β_1.

14.2.1.1   Logit-Normal Prior Specification for β

We illustrate with two predictor variables, say x_1, which is dichotomous, and x_2, which is continuous. Let $sx_2 = [x - \text{mean}(x_2)]/\text{sd}(x_2)$ be the standardized x_2, and $\tilde{x}' = (x_1, sx_2)$. For simplicity, we do not include subscripts in the discussion. Let θ be the generic probability of success, and specify the model as $\text{logit}(\theta) \equiv \gamma + \tilde{x}'\beta^* = \gamma + x_1\beta_2 + sx_2\beta_3$, with $\gamma \sim N(\beta_1, \sigma_\gamma^2)$.

We first consider specification of a prior distribution for β_1. We start by thinking about the probability of "success" for a new individual who is in a *typical* group with $\gamma = \beta_1$ and who also has covariate vector $\tilde{x}'_1 \equiv (x_1 = 0, sx_2 = 0)$. Call this probability $\tilde{\theta}_1$. This individual has an average value of the continuous covariate and falls into the baseline category for x_1, which we regard as reflecting a typical group. Then

$$\text{logit}(\tilde{\theta}_1) = \beta_1.$$

We can specify either a beta prior or a logit-normal prior for $\tilde{\theta}_1$. In Chapter 8, we primarily focused on beta priors. Now, we discuss the logit-normal model, first introduced in Chapter 5. In Example 14.6, we placed a $N(-2, b)$ prior on β_1, which is precisely a logit-normal$(-2, b)$ prior on $\tilde{\theta}_1$.

For our generic problem, let θ_0 be our best guess for $\tilde{\theta}_1$. Then our best guess for β_1 is $\text{logit}(\theta_0)$. Our specification will be

$$\text{logit}(\tilde{\theta}_1) \sim N(a, b),$$

with $a = \text{logit}(\theta_0)$. In order to obtain a fully informative prior on β_1, we need to specify an appropriate value for b. This is accomplished by specifying either an upper 95th percentile (if $\theta_0 > 0.5$) or lower 5th percentile (if $\theta_0 < 0.5$) for our prior on $\tilde{\theta}_1$. Assume that $\theta_0 > 0.5$ and denote the upper percentile as u. Using the logit-normal distribution, we have

$$P(\tilde{\theta}_1 < u) = P\left(\beta_1 < \text{logit}(u)\right)$$
$$= P\{Z < [\text{logit}(u) - \text{logit}(\theta_0)]/\sqrt{b}\} = 0.95.$$

Here, $Z \sim N(0,1)$, since $\beta_1 \sim N(\text{logit}(\theta_0), b)$. We must therefore have $1.645 = [\text{logit}(u) - \text{logit}(\theta_0)]/\sqrt{b}$, so

$$b = \{[\text{logit}(u) - \text{logit}(\theta_0)]/1.645\}^2.$$

This is a conditional means prior.

We next obtain a conditional means prior for $\beta^* = (\beta_2, \beta_3)'$. Define $\tilde{x}_2' = (1, 0)$, which is a predictor vector for a hypothetical subject in the non-baseline category for the first predictor and the average value for the continuous predictor. Define $\tilde{x}_3' = (0, 1)$ for a third hypothetical subject's predictor vector, where this subject is in the baseline category for the first predictor and whose value for the second predictor is one standard deviation above the mean of this variable. Then define $\tilde{\theta}_2 = \text{expit}(\beta_1 + \tilde{x}_2'\beta^*) = \text{expit}(\beta_1 + \beta_2)$ and $\tilde{\theta}_3 = \text{expit}(\beta_1 + \tilde{x}_3'\beta^*) = \text{expit}(\beta_1 + \beta_3)$. We elicit independent logit-normal priors for $\tilde{\theta}_i$ for $i = 1, 2, 3$. Generically, we let $\text{logit}(\tilde{\theta}_i) \perp\!\!\!\perp N(a_i, b_i)$, $i = 1, 2, 3$. In vector and matrix notation, we write

$$\text{logit}(\tilde{\theta}) \sim N_3(\mu_\theta, \Sigma_\theta),$$

where $\mu_\theta' = (a_1, a_2, a_3)$ and $\Sigma_\theta = \text{diag}\{b_1, b_2, b_3\}$.

Since $\beta_1 = \text{logit}(\tilde{\theta}_1)$, $\beta_2 = \text{logit}(\tilde{\theta}_2) - \text{logit}(\tilde{\theta}_1)$, and $\beta_3 = \text{logit}(\tilde{\theta}_3) - \text{logit}(\tilde{\theta}_1)$, we must have

$$\beta = \begin{pmatrix} 1 & 0 & 0 \\ -1 & 1 & 0 \\ -1 & 0 & 1 \end{pmatrix} \text{logit}(\tilde{\theta}) \equiv C \, \text{logit}(\tilde{\theta}),$$

and, using standard properties of the multivariate normal distribution,

$$\beta \sim N(\beta_0, \Sigma_0), \quad \text{with } \beta_0 = C\mu_\theta \text{ and } \Sigma_0 \equiv C\Sigma_\theta C'.$$

Working through the arithmetic, we have $\beta_0' = (a_1, a_2 - a_1, a_3 - a_1)$ and

$$\Sigma_0 = \begin{pmatrix} b_1 & -b_1 & -b_1 \\ -b_1 & b_1 + b_2 & b_1 \\ -b_1 & b_1 & b_1 + b_3 \end{pmatrix}.$$

The induced prior distribution for β is $N(\beta_0, \Sigma_0)$. Observe that the regression coefficients are correlated under this prior.

The demonstration using logit-normal priors to obtain $\beta \sim N_p(\beta_0, \Sigma_0)$ can be extended to the situation with multiple covariates where, of course, additional details are required. The prior probability density function is written as

$$p(\beta) \propto e^{-\frac{1}{2}(\beta - \beta_0)'\Sigma_0^{-1}(\beta - \beta_0)}.$$

14.2.1.2 Conditional Means Prior for β Using Beta Distributions

We could have just as well considered beta distributions rather than logit-normal distributions. The conditional means prior using beta distributions that was discussed in detail in Chapter 8 induces a prior on β that is in the same form as the likelihood function when there are no latent effects. This type of prior is also called a "data augmentation prior." Since we have latent variables centered on β_1, we carry out the elicitation by thinking about probabilities that correspond to p individuals, as we did in Chapter 8. As above in the logit-normal case, we think about such individuals as all being in a *typical* group for whom $\gamma = \beta_1$. As in Chapter 8, we have $\tilde{\theta}_j \perp\!\!\!\perp \text{beta}(a_j, b_j)$. The induced prior on β is

$$p(\beta) \propto \prod_{j=1}^{p} \tilde{\theta}_j^{a_j}(1 - \tilde{\theta}_j)^{b_j}, \qquad \tilde{\theta}_j = \frac{e^{\beta_1 + \tilde{x}_j'\beta^*}}{1 + e^{\beta_1 + \tilde{x}_j'\beta^*}}.$$

In both the logit-normal and beta cases, we could of course specify a partial prior as discussed in Chapter 8. Moreover, we could specify a logit-normal prior on, say, β_1, and then use independent beta priors for the remaining $\tilde{\theta}$s. Alternatively, we could specify $N(0, b)$ priors on the remaining β_i. There are lots of possibilities.

14.2.1.3 Prior for σ_γ

We now elicit information for σ_γ. First, as in Sections 14.2.1.1 and 14.2.1.2, we think about the probability of success for an individual with standardized predictors, say $\tilde{x} = 0$, and who is also in a typical group, so that $\gamma = \beta_1$. This individual has average values for the continuous covariates and reference values for categorical covariates. Next, we obtain a best guess for the corresponding θ, call it θ_0. We now have a best guess for β_1, namely $\text{logit}(\theta_0)$. If $\tilde{x} \neq 0$ (i.e., not a *typical* subject), our best guess for $\beta_1 + \tilde{x}'\beta^*$ is $\text{logit}(\theta_0)$. In this case, our thought process would be different, since we would be considering a success probability for a different type of individual.

We now switch gears and think about success probabilities for individuals across all of the groups. Consider individuals in these groups all having the same covariate vector, say $\tilde{x}$ (possibly 0), but different γs by virtue of being in different groups. We ask our expert for his or her best guess for, say, $\theta_{0.9}$, the 90th percentile of satisfaction probabilities for such groups. What does that mean? Imagine we have 100 groups with individuals having covariates $\tilde{x}$. We expect about 90 of these 100 groups to have success probabilities less than or equal to $\theta_{0.9}$ (i.e., among those individuals in each group with covariates $\tilde{x}$). Let $u_{0.9}$ denote our expert's best guess for $\theta_{0.9}$, and suppose $u_{0.9} = 0.7$. From the normality of γ, we must have $\text{logit}(\theta_{0.9}) = \beta_1 + \tilde{x}'\beta^* + 1.28\sigma_\gamma$. Since our best guess for $\beta_1 + \tilde{x}'\beta^*$ is $\text{logit}(\theta_0)$, our best guess for $\text{logit}(\theta_{0.9})$ must satisfy $\text{logit}(u_{0.9}) = \text{logit}(\theta_0) + 1.28\sigma_\gamma$. Solving the equation, we get a best guess for σ_γ,

$$\sigma_{0\gamma} = [\text{logit}(u_{0.9}) - \text{logit}(\theta_0)]/1.28.$$

Note the similarity with the derivation for σ_γ in a normal model with latent effects. The added complication here was due to the logit scale involving the latent effect, rather than the linear scale under the normal model. Observe that if we were to parameterize the model with $\tau_\gamma = 1/\sigma_\gamma^2$, we would have a best guess for τ_γ of $\tau_{0\gamma} = 1/\sigma_{0\gamma}^2$.

It is often important to select a prior for σ_γ that does not allow for values that are "too large." The reason is that $\operatorname{expit}(\gamma + \tilde{x}'\beta^*)$ will be arbitrarily close to 1 or 0 if $|\gamma|$ (or any $|\beta_i|$) becomes very large.

Our recommended choice for a diffuse yet informed prior for σ_γ uses the above elicitation information in conjunction with a further inquiry about just how large $\theta_{0.9}$ could be. Suppose our expert is virtually certain that $\theta_{0.9} < u_{\max}$. Then we could argue that

$$
\begin{aligned}
1 &\doteq P[\theta_{0.9} < u_{\max} \mid \operatorname{logit}(\theta_0)] \\
&= P[\beta_1 + \tilde{x}'\beta^* + 1.28\sigma_\gamma \leq \operatorname{logit}(u_{\max}) \mid \operatorname{logit}(\theta_0)] \\
&= P[\operatorname{logit}(\theta_0) + 1.28\sigma_\gamma \leq \operatorname{logit}(u_{\max})] \\
&= P[\sigma_\gamma \leq [\operatorname{logit}(u_{\max}) - \operatorname{logit}(\theta_0)]/1.28],
\end{aligned}
$$

where we have assumed that knowledge about β is independent of knowledge about σ_γ. This argument leads to our suggestion of a uniform prior for σ_γ,

$$
\sigma_\gamma \sim U(0, \sigma_{\max}), \quad \sigma_{\max} = [\operatorname{logit}(u_{\max}) - \operatorname{logit}(\theta_0)]/1.28. \tag{14.10}
$$

We note that if our best guess for θ were $\theta_0 = 0.5$ and our best guess for $\theta_{\max}$ were $(0.6, 0.8, 0.9, 0.95, 0.99)$, we would obtain $\sigma_{\max} = (0.32, 1.08, 1.71, 2.30, 3.59)$, respectively. It is difficult to imagine a situation where $\theta_{0.9}$ could be as large as 0.99, so with $\theta_0 = 0.5$ it is hard to imagine selecting a value of $\sigma_{\max}$ as large as even 3. If $\theta_0 = 0.1$ and $u_{\max} = 0.95$, a combination that is also somewhat difficult to imagine, we get a large value for $\sigma_{\max} = 4.01$.

Another way to think about the issue of constraining σ_γ not to be too large is to think about the fact that we have modeled $\gamma_i \sim N(\beta_1, \sigma_\gamma^2)$. Consequently, we expect 95% of the latent values to be in the interval $(\beta_1 \pm 1.96\sigma_\gamma)$. No matter what β_1 is, this interval is bound to be extreme in one way or another if $\sigma_\gamma > 3$.

We briefly discuss how to elicit an informative gamma prior for σ_γ (or for $\tau_\gamma = 1/\sigma_\gamma^2$). Placing a $Ga(a, b)$ prior on σ_γ (or τ_γ), we can set $\sigma_{0\gamma} = (a - 1)/b$ (or $\tau_{0\gamma} = (a - 1)/b$) and solve for a in terms of b, as we have already done a number of times. Setting b to be small corresponds to a large prior variance, which may be undesirable if too much prior mass is attached to large values of σ_γ. If one wishes to take this approach, we recommend selecting b so that simulated values from the gamma prior for σ_γ (or the induced prior on σ_γ with a gamma prior for τ_γ) do not exceed $\sigma_{\max}$ too often. We say a little more about this suggestion at the end of this section.

Alternatively, we can elicit more refined scientific information about $\theta_{0.9}$. Selecting b involves eliciting a value that the expert is, say, 95% sure that $\theta_{0.9}$ could not exceed, say, $\theta_{0.9u}$, namely $P(\theta_{0.9} < \theta_{0.9u}) = 0.95$. Then in exactly the same way that we derived $\sigma_{\max}$ in expression (14.10), we obtain the 95th percentile of a

$Ga(a, b)$ prior for σ_γ,

$$\sigma_{0.95} = (\text{logit}(\theta_{0.9u}) - \text{logit}(\theta_0))/1.28. \tag{14.11}$$

We find b so that the $Ga(1 + \sigma_{0\gamma} b, b)$ distribution has 95th percentile equal to $\sigma_{0.95}$.

We now discuss the now infamous $Ga(c, c)$ prior with small c (e.g., $c = 0.001$) for the precision of the latent effects. Let $\gamma \sim N(0, 1/\tau_\gamma)$, with $\tau_\gamma \sim Ga(c, c)$ for a small value of c. We examine the implication of using such a prior in light of the need to constrain the value of $\sigma_\gamma = 1/\sqrt{\tau_\gamma}$. We considered values of $c = (1, 0.1, 0.01)$ and found that the induced prior on σ_γ with $c = 1$ resulted in $P(\sigma_\gamma > k) = (0.22, 0.06, 0.3)$ for $k = 2, 4, 6$, respectively; with $c = 0.1$ the same probabilities were $(0.73, 0.63, 0.58)$, respectively, and with $c = 0.01$ they were $(0.95, 0.94, 0.93)$. It is clear that we would only consider using $c = 1$ out of these choices.

14.2.2   *Gibbs Sampling

We now obtain the full conditional distributions corresponding to model (14.9) to illustrate the calculation for a common situation. Knowing how to determine the full conditional distributions here will make it easier in other situations. This section is important for anyone who would like to or might need to write their own program instead of one of the software packages available for Bayesian inference, such as BUGS, JAGS, or Stan (see Appendix C). The illustration of Gibbs sampling below corresponds to the type of models we considered for the analysis of the cow abortion data and the toenail data. The most commonly used prior model is a normal prior for β and a gamma prior for the precision τ. Some full conditionals are not recognizable no matter what prior or model one specifies.

We consider two distinct situations for the distribution of the latent effects. The first is identical to model (14.9), in which the distribution of latent effects is centered on the intercept β_1. In the second situation, we let $\tilde{w}_i$ be the $q \times 1$ vector of covariates in $\tilde{x}_{ij}$ that are associated with group i and that do not vary with j. We then replace the vector of individual covariates $\tilde{x}_{ij}$, literally and notionally, with a new $(p - q) \times 1$ vector $\tilde{x}_{ij}$ that has only predictor values that vary with j. Thus, individuals are allowed to have covariates $\tilde{x}_{ij}$, and groups have covariates $\tilde{w}_i$. The only part of the model that changes is that $\gamma_i \perp\!\!\!\perp N(\beta_1 + \tilde{w}_i'\lambda^*, \sigma^2)$, where λ^* is a vector of regression coefficients associated with group-level covariates. Equivalently, we let $w_i = (1, \tilde{w}_i')'$ and $\lambda' = (\beta_1, (\lambda^*)')'$, so that $w_i'\lambda = \beta_1 + \tilde{w}_i'\lambda^*$. We write

$$\gamma_i \perp\!\!\!\perp N(w_i'\lambda, \sigma_\gamma^2), \quad i = 1, \ldots, k. \tag{14.12}$$

14.2.2.1   Centering on β_1

Consider the prior $p(\beta, \tau_\gamma) = p(\beta)p(\tau_\gamma)$. We write $p(\beta) = p(\beta_1)p(\beta^*|\beta_1)$ when we consider β_1 separately from β^*, the regression coefficients for covariates (other than the intercept). Let $\gamma = \{\gamma_i : i = 1, \ldots, k\}$. Then $p(\beta, \tau_\gamma, \gamma) = p(\beta)p(\tau_\gamma)p(\gamma \mid \beta, \tau_\gamma) = p(\beta)p(\tau_\gamma)p(\gamma \mid \beta_1, \tau_\gamma)$. Thus, the joint density for the data, the latent effects, and the parameters is

$$p(y, \gamma, \beta_1, \beta^*, \tau_\gamma) = p(y \mid \gamma, \beta^*)p(\beta)p(\tau_\gamma))p(\gamma|\beta_1, \tau_\gamma)$$

$$\propto \left[\prod_{i=1}^{k} \prod_{j=1}^{n_i} \left(\frac{e^{x'_{ij}\beta^* + \gamma_i}}{1 + e^{x'_{ij}\beta^* + \gamma_i}} \right)^{y_{ij}} \left(\frac{1}{1 + e^{x'_{ij}\beta^* + \gamma_i}} \right)^{1 - y_{ij}} \right] \quad (14.13)$$

$$\times \left[\prod_{i=1}^{k} \tau_\gamma^{1/2} e^{-\frac{\tau_\gamma}{2}(\gamma_i - \beta_1)^2} \right] p(\beta)p(\tau_\gamma).$$

The full conditional posterior distributions are

$$p(\beta \mid y, \gamma, \tau_\gamma), \quad p(\gamma \mid y, \beta, \tau_\gamma), \quad \text{and} \quad p(\tau_\gamma \mid y, \beta, \gamma).$$

We obtain all conditional distributions by simply lifting the part of equation (14.13) that depends on the variable of interest.

Consider the specific situation with

$$\tau_\gamma \sim Ga(a', b') \quad \text{and} \quad \beta \sim N(\beta_0, \Sigma_0),$$

where $a' = a/2, b' = b/2$. (Dividing by 2 makes the formulas a little nicer.) From equation (14.13), after some simplification, we obtain

$$p(y, \gamma, \beta_1, \beta^*, \tau_\gamma)$$

$$\propto \left[\prod_{i=1}^{k} \prod_{j=1}^{n_i} \left(\frac{e^{x'_{ij}\beta^* + \gamma_i}}{1 + e^{x'_{ij}\beta^* + \gamma_i}} \right)^{y_{ij}} \left(\frac{1}{1 + e^{x'_{ij}\beta^* + \gamma_i}} \right)^{1 - y_{ij}} \right]$$

$$\times \left[\tau_\gamma^{k/2} e^{-\frac{\tau_\gamma}{2} \sum_{i=1}^{k}(\gamma_i - \beta_1)^2} \right] \quad (14.14)$$

$$\times \left[e^{\left\{ -\frac{1}{2}(\beta - \beta_0)' \Sigma_0^{-1}(\beta - \beta_0) \right\}} \right] \times \left[\tau_\gamma^{\frac{a}{2} - 1} e^{-\frac{1}{2}b\tau_\gamma} \right].$$

Observe that the first term is free of β_1. It is immediate from equation (14.14) that

$$\tau_\gamma \mid y, \beta_1, \gamma \sim Ga\left((a + k)/2, \left[b + \sum_{i=1}^{k}(\gamma_i - \beta_1)^2 \right] /2 \right).$$

Next we see from equation (14.14) that the γ_i are conditionally independent with

$$p(\gamma_i \mid y, \beta, \tau_\gamma) \propto \prod_{i,j} \left(\frac{e^{x'_{ij}\beta^* + \gamma_i}}{1 + e^{x'_{ij}\beta^* + \gamma_i}} \right)^{y_{ij}} \left(\frac{1}{1 + e^{x'_{ij}\beta^* + \gamma_i}} \right)^{1 - y_{ij}} e^{-\frac{\tau_\gamma}{2}(\gamma_i - \beta_1)^2}.$$

This is not a recognizable distribution. At least it is a scalar distribution, making it easier to sample from via adaptive rejection sampling, since it is log-concave.

We note that

$$\sum_{i}(\gamma_i - \beta_1)^2 = \sum_{i}(\gamma_i - \bar{\gamma})^2 + k(\beta_1 - \bar{\gamma})^2, \quad (14.15)$$

where $\bar{\gamma} = \sum_{i=1}^{k} \gamma_i / k$. Substituting equation (14.15) into equation (14.14), we have

$$p(\beta \mid y, \gamma, \tau_\gamma) \propto \left[\prod_{i=1}^{k} \prod_{j=1}^{n_i} \left(\frac{e^{x'_{ij}\beta^* + \gamma_i}}{1 + e^{x'_{ij}\tilde{\beta} + \gamma_i}} \right)^{y_{ij}} \left(\frac{1}{1 + e^{x'_{ij}\beta^* + \gamma_i}} \right)^{1-y_{ij}} \right]$$

$$\times \left[\exp\left(-\frac{k\tau_\gamma}{2}(\beta_1 - \bar{\gamma})^2 \right) \right] \qquad (14.16)$$

$$\times \left[\exp\left(-\frac{1}{2}(\beta - \beta_0)' \Sigma_0^{-1}(\beta - \beta_0) \right) \right],$$

which is again not recognizable as a distribution. It can be sampled, however, using a Metropolis sampler. Alternatively, we could sample β_j from the distribution $p(\beta_j \mid y, \beta_{(-j)}, \gamma, \tau_\gamma)$ for $j = 1, \ldots, p$. Here, $\beta_{(-j)}$ denotes the $p-1$ vector that is β with β_j removed. This approach is termed "Gibbs within Gibbs" sampling, since we sample from the joint full conditional for β by sampling from the full conditionals for the components of β. Tierney (1994) [327] justified this approach theoretically. We obtain $p(\beta_j \mid y, \beta_{(-j)}, \gamma, \tau_\gamma)$ by factoring out the part of equation (14.16) that involves β_j, and then sample from that unknown univariate distribution using adaptive rejection sampling (since it will be log-concave) or by using some other method, such as slice sampling.

Alternatively, in order to sample from the full conditional for β, we could sample sequentially from $p(\beta_1 \mid y, \gamma, \tau_\gamma)$, followed by sampling from $p(\beta^* \mid y, \gamma, \beta_1, \tau_\gamma)$. In this instance, we will be sampling from a known normal distribution for β_1, followed by an unknown distribution for β^*. To see this, first replace the multivariate normal prior for β with $p(\beta_1)p(\beta^* \mid \beta_1)$ in equation (14.16). We recognize that $\beta_1 \sim N(c, 1/d)$ for appropriate (c, d), and that the conditional prior distribution for $\beta^* \mid \beta_1$ is also normal with a known mean vector and covariance matrix that can be obtained using standard multivariate normal results (Johnson and Wichern, 2002) [178]. Substituting this into equation (14.16), we have

$$p(\beta_1 \mid y, \gamma, \tau_\gamma) \propto \exp\left\{ -0.5 \left[k\tau_\gamma (\beta_1 - \bar{\gamma})^2 + d(\beta_1 - c)^2 \right] \right\}$$

$$\propto \exp\left\{ -0.5(k\tau_\gamma + d)(\beta_1 - \hat{\beta}_1)^2 \right\},$$

where we have used the complete-the-square method. We have

$$\beta_1 \mid y, \gamma, \tau_\gamma \sim N(\hat{\beta}_1, 1/(\tau_\gamma + d)), \quad \hat{\beta}_1 = w\bar{\gamma} + (1 - w)c,$$

where $w = [k\tau_\gamma/(k\tau_\gamma + d)]$. Observe that this full conditional does not depend on the data, y.

Finally, from equation (14.16), we obtain

$$p(\beta^* \mid y, \beta_1, \gamma, \tau_\gamma) \propto \left[\prod_{i=1}^{k} \prod_{j=1}^{n_i} \left(\frac{e^{x'_{ij}\beta^* + \gamma_i}}{1 + e^{x'_{ij}\beta^* + \gamma_i}} \right)^{y_{ij}} \left(\frac{1}{1 + e^{x'_{ij}\beta^* + \gamma_i}} \right)^{1-y_{ij}} \right]$$

$$\times \left[\exp\left(-\frac{1}{2}(\beta - \beta_0)' \Sigma_0^{-1}(\beta - \beta_0) \right) \right].$$

One can obtain a sample from this distribution by sampling β_j from $p(\beta_j \mid y, \gamma, \beta_1, \beta^*_{(-j)}, \tau_\gamma)$ $(j \neq 1)$, $j = 2, \ldots, p$, where $\beta^*_{(-j)}$ includes all β^*s except β_j. This is accomplished by *first* obtaining the part of the prior, $p(\beta)$, that depends on β_j, which one can sometimes find by inspection. The inverse of Σ_0 is involved, which could complicate matters unless it is diagonal. It would be simpler to recognize that this function of β_j is proportional to $p(\beta_j \mid \beta_1, \beta^*_{(-j)})$, which, as mentioned above, can be obtained using standard formulas. Then

$$p(\beta_j \mid y, \gamma, \beta_1, \beta^*_{(-j)}) \propto p(y \mid \gamma, \beta^*) p(\beta_j \mid \beta_1, \beta^*_{(-j)}).$$

14.2.2.2 Centering on Group-Level Covariates

We consider the reparameterization of model (14.9) where the latent effects distributions for group i are centered on $w_i'\lambda$, which is given explicitly in expression (14.12).

Gibbs sampling for this model is very similar to when we centered on the intercept β_1. It looks like we now need to think about a prior for λ, which includes β_1. We have already elicited this prior in different notation. Recall our discussion of the $N(\beta_0, \Sigma_0)$ prior specification for β in the logit-normal model for success probabilities. Suppose we had arranged the predictor variables with the group-level covariates, the $\tilde{w}$s, listed first and the individual-level predictors, the $\tilde{x}$s, last. Then (λ, β^*) would have the same prior distribution. We assume this ordering of predictor variables from here on. The conditional means prior using this ordering of variables and based on beta distributions will induce the same data augmentation prior for β as one with a different ordering of variables, only now in a new notation.

The joint probability model is

$$p(y, \gamma, \lambda, \beta, \tau_\gamma) \propto \left[\prod_{i=1}^{k} \prod_{j=1}^{n_i} \left(\frac{e^{x_{ij}'\beta^* + \gamma_i}}{1 + e^{x_{ij}'\tilde{\beta} + \gamma_i}} \right)^{y_{ij}} \left(\frac{1}{1 + e^{x_{ij}'\beta^* + \gamma_i}} \right)^{1 - y_{ij}} \right]$$
$$\times \left[\tau_\gamma^{k/2} e^{-\frac{\tau_\gamma}{2} \sum_{i=1}^{k} (\gamma_i - w_i'\lambda)^2} \right] \qquad (14.17)$$
$$\times \left[e^{-\frac{1}{2}[(\lambda', \beta')' - \beta_0]' \Sigma_0^{-1} ((\lambda', \beta')' - \beta_0)} \right]$$
$$\times \left[\tau_\gamma^{\frac{a}{2} - 1} e^{-\frac{1}{2} b \tau_\gamma} \right].$$

We immediately obtain, independently,

$$p(\gamma_i \mid y, (\lambda, \beta^*), \tau_\gamma) \propto \prod_{i,j} \left(\frac{e^{x_{ij}'\beta^* + \gamma_i}}{1 + e^{x_{ij}'\beta^* + \gamma_i}} \right)^{y_{ij}} \left(\frac{1}{1 + e^{x_{ij}'\beta^* + \gamma_i}} \right)^{1 - y_{ij}}$$
$$\times \left[e^{-\frac{\tau_\gamma}{2} (\gamma_i - w_i'\lambda)^2} \right].$$

We also obtain

$$\tau_\gamma \mid y, \lambda, \gamma \sim Ga\left((k+a)/2, \left[b + \sum_i (\gamma_i - w_i'\lambda)^2 \right] / 2 \right).$$

These full conditionals hold regardless of the choice of prior for (λ, β).

In the logit-normal case, the full conditional for λ is a recognizable normal distribution. We require the following, analogous to what we obtained in (14.15):

$$\sum_i (\gamma_i - w_i'\lambda)^2 = \sum_i (\gamma_i - \hat{\gamma}_i)^2 + (\lambda - \hat{\gamma})'W'W(\lambda - \hat{\gamma}), \qquad (14.18)$$

with $\hat{\gamma} = (W'W)^{-1}W'\gamma$. W in equation (14.18) is the $k \times q$ matrix constructed by stacking the k row vectors w_i' on top of each other, and $\hat{\gamma}_i = w_i'\hat{\gamma}$. We did things just like this in Chapter 7.

We must have $\lambda \sim N(\lambda_0, \Sigma_{00})$, where Σ_{00} is the $q \times q$ submatrix of Σ_0 that corresponds to λ, and λ_0 is the corresponding $q \times 1$ subvector of β_0. Let $(\Sigma_{00})^{-1} = \tau_{00}$, the precision matrix for the prior on λ. These marginal distributions and relationships hold because the joint distribution for (λ, β^*) is multivariate normal. Substituting equation (14.18) into equation (14.17), we have

$$p(\lambda \mid y, \gamma, \beta^*, \tau_\gamma) \propto e^{-0.5[\tau_\gamma(\lambda - \hat{\gamma})'W'W(\lambda - \hat{\gamma}) + (\lambda - \lambda_0)'\tau_{00}(\lambda - \lambda_0)]}.$$

Using the complete-the-square formula for vectors, we obtain

$$p(\lambda \mid y, \gamma, \beta^*, \tau_\gamma) \propto e^{-0.5(\lambda - \lambda^*)'(\tau_\gamma W'W + \tau_{00})(\lambda - \lambda^*)},$$

where

$$\lambda^* = \tau_\gamma(\tau_\gamma W'W + \tau_{00})^{-1}W'W\hat{\gamma} + (\tau_\gamma W'W + \tau_{00})^{-1}\tau_{00}\lambda_0.$$

Thus

$$\lambda \mid y, \gamma, \beta^*, \tau_\gamma \sim N\left(\lambda^*, (\tau_\gamma W'W + \tau_{00})^{-1}\right).$$

The full conditional for β^* is obtained in the same way as in the previous subsection.

14.2.3 Meta-Analysis: Ganzfeld Studies of ESP

We consider a meta-analysis of 56 studies that were designed to assess whether a particular type of extrasensory perception (ESP) is possible and for which we have available data. Each study's design explores the possibility that two individuals, under experimental conditions, can communicate with each other when they are separated and in the absence of the usual means of communication. If this were possible, it would be a form of psychic, or *psi*, experience called ESP. Ganzfeld is German for "whole field"; the reason for this name will become apparent. In most ganzfeld studies, there is a sender and a receiver. These two individuals are in separate acoustically shielded rooms. The session begins by each person listening to a relaxation tape. For the next 15 to 30 minutes, the sender looks at a target image on a television screen. The target may be a static photograph or a short movie segment that plays repeatedly. The sender attempts to transmit information about the target to the receiver. The receiver is seated in a reclining chair. The receiver is wearing headphones playing white noise while a whole field of red light is shining in the receiver's eyes. The light is diffused with halved ping-pong balls placed over the receiver's eyes. The theory is that the ears and eyes are receiving input, but with no sense or pattern, so the mind, looking for input, hopefully will receive the information being sent by the sender. During this time period, the receiver provides an ongoing verbal report, picked up by a microphone, of his or her thoughts, images, and feelings. This is called the mentation period.

At the end of the mentation period, the receiver is shown four possible choices of targets, all of the same type (i.e., static photograph or movie segment). One is the correct target, and the other three are decoys. The receiver must choose the one that the receiver thinks best matches the description he or she gave during the mentation period. An experimenter, who does not know the correct answer but who has listened during the mentation period, will provide information about what was said if requested by the receiver. If the correct target is chosen by the receiver, the session is a hit; otherwise, it is a miss.

Before a study begins, a target pool is assembled, usually consisting of hundreds of potential targets (photographs and/or video segments). The pool is then organized into sets of four targets that are of the same type (photo or video) but that otherwise are as dissimilar as possible. For each session, one of the sets of four is randomly selected, and then one of the potential targets in the chosen set of four is randomly selected to be the actual target. The remaining three are the decoys used for judging. Therefore, the target is randomly selected from a larger pool in such a way that the probability that it will best match what the receiver said is 0.25 by chance alone, as it is for each decoy.

The 56 studies that we include all met criteria for methodological rigor and adherence to standard ganzfeld procedures. Data from these studies are listed in Table 14.5, with the number of sessions n_i, the number of hits y_i, and the empirical hit rate $\hat{\theta}_i$. The studies we included were conducted by many different investigators and at a variety of laboratories in multiple countries. For more details about the data, see Utts et al. (2010) [339].

We analyze the data using a hierarchical model that assumes a constant probability of a hit within a study but allows for the possibility of different hit probabilities across studies. This is an important assumption, since the studies are generally performed with different subjects and different experimenters in different parts of the world. There are lots of latent factors that can contribute to differing hit probabilities across the studies.

Let θ_i be the probability of a hit for study i, $i = 1, 2, \ldots, 56$. We have n_i sessions with y_i hits in study i. We assume

$$Y_i \mid \theta_i \perp\!\!\!\perp Bin(n_i, \theta_i).$$

We are motivated to estimate the median hit rate in the population of all studies, and we are interested in assessing the variability in hit rate probabilities across the same population of studies. We make posterior inferences for the median(θ) and percentiles $(\theta_{0.1}, \theta_{0.9})$, where median($\theta$) is just $\theta_{0.5}$, and θ_α is the 100αth percentile of the population distribution of hit rate probabilities. Thus, 10% of the hit rate probabilities will be less than $\theta_{0.1}$, half less than $\theta_{0.5}$, and so on.

TABLE 14.5: Number of sessions (n_i), hits (y_i) and hit rates $(\hat{\theta}_i = y_i/n_i)$ for the 56 studies

i	n_i	y_i	$\hat{\theta}_i$	i	n_i	y_i	$\hat{\theta}_i$	i	n_i	y_i	$\hat{\theta}_i$	i	n_i	y_i	$\hat{\theta}_i$
1	32	14	0.44	15	60	27	0.45	29	50	12	0.24	43	30	14	0.47
2	7	6	0.86	16	48	10	0.21	30	50	12	0.24	44	30	11	0.37
3	30	13	0.43	17	22	8	0.36	31	50	9	0.18	45	97	32	0.33
4	30	7	0.23	18	9	3	0.33	32	51	19	0.37	46	22	2	0.09
5	20	2	0.10	19	35	10	0.29	33	29	12	0.41	47	50	13	0.26
6	10	9	0.90	20	50	12	0.24	34	128	60	0.47	48	32	8	0.25
7	10	4	0.40	21	50	18	0.36	35	32	13	0.41	49	58	11	0.19
8	28	8	0.29	22	50	15	0.30	36	50	11	0.22	50	46	12	0.26
9	10	4	0.40	23	36	12	0.33	37	8	3	0.38	51	20	6	0.30
10	20	7	0.35	24	20	10	0.50	38	40	8	0.20	52	30	6	0.20
11	20	12	0.60	25	7	3	0.43	39	65	24	0.37	53	42	5	0.12
12	100	41	0.41	26	50	15	0.30	40	50	18	0.36	54	32	14	0.44
13	40	13	0.33	27	25	16	0.64	41	30	11	0.37	55	40	16	0.40
14	27	11	0.41	28	50	13	0.26	42	30	11	0.37	56	36	13	0.36

For the next layer of the hierarchical model, we assume a logit-normal distribution for the θ_i:

$$\text{logit}(\theta_i) \perp\!\!\!\perp N(\mu, \sigma_t^2).$$

Note that μ is the median (as well as the mean) of the distribution of $\text{logit}(\theta_i)$, so we must have

$$\text{median}(\theta) = \frac{e^\mu}{1 + e^\mu}.$$

More generally, since $\mu + z_\alpha\, \sigma_t$ is the 100αth percentile of the $N(\mu, \sigma_t^2)$ distribution, we have

$$\theta_\alpha = \frac{e^{\mu + z_\alpha\, \sigma_t}}{1 + e^{\mu + z_\alpha\, \sigma_t}}$$

since the logit function is monotone and increasing.

The standard deviation of the distribution of the θ_i is of interest as well. A small value of σ_t indicates that the true probabilities of success are similar across all possible studies, whereas a large value indicates that there is substantial variability.

The final layer of the hierarchical model consists of a prior distribution on the median of the possible values of θ, which is equivalent to putting a prior distribution on (μ, σ_t). If θ_0 is the prior guess for median(θ), then the prior guess for μ would be $\text{logit}(\theta_0) \equiv \mu_0$.

We allowed for different prior beliefs by using four types of prior distributions for median(θ). We expect that most individuals would specify priors for (μ, σ_t) that included the prior guess of 0.25 for the average hit rate. This results in the prior guess for μ, $\mu_0 = \text{logit}(0.25) = -1.1$. This would seem to be a fair choice for anyone who is skeptical or who was simply ignorant of any data involving ESP. For all four types of priors, we specified $\mu \sim N(\mu_0, c^2)$, where we chose c by selecting a 95th percentile for our knowledge about the median of θ, say u. For all priors on μ, we will specify that there is 95% certainty that median$(\theta) < u$. The four types of prior will involve different choices of u. This specification leads to logit$(u) = $ logit$(\theta_0) + 1.645\,c$, or $c = [$logit$(u) - $logit$(\theta_0)]/1.645$.

For all types of prior distributions, we also used a $U(0, \sigma_{max})$ distribution for σ_t. We first select θ_{max} to be the largest possible value that we believe $\theta_{0.9}$ could be. We then have logit$(\theta_0) + 1.28\,\sigma_t < $ logit(θ_{max}), which leads to $\sigma_{max} = [$logit$(\theta_{max}) - $logit$(\theta_0)]/1.28$.

For a *diffuse* prior, we selected $u = 0.8$, which results in $c = 1.5$ and a $N(-1.1, 2.25)$ prior for μ. The induced prior for median(θ) has 95% prior probability interval $(0.02, 0.87)$. We can allow for even more uncertainty by selecting larger values of u. We also selected $\theta_{max} = 0.99$, which results in $\sigma_{max} = 4.5$. This prior is extremely diffuse, relative to the prior knowledge that, if there is no ESP, the overall hit rate should be 0.25. And we should say that if this type of ESP truly existed with hit rates as high at 0.8, that fact should have already been discovered. So, in fact, there is real prior information available to all of us.

We next considered an *open-minded* person. For this person, we selected $u = 0.41$ and $\theta_{max} = 0.8$. This results in $\mu \sim N(-1.1, 0.20)$, and $\sigma_t \sim U(0, 1.94)$.

A *believer* was speculated to have $\theta_0 = 0.33$, $u = 0.36$ and $\theta_{max} = 0.4$. This results in $\mu \sim N(-0.71, 0.0065)$ and $\sigma_t \sim U(0, 0.24)$. The simulated induced prior for median(θ) looks just right.

Finally, we consider a psi *skeptic*. Here, we set $\theta_0 = 0.25$, $u = 0.255$, and $\theta_{max} = 0.26$. This results in $\mu \sim N(-1.1, 0.000259)$ and $\sigma_t \sim U(0, 0.04)$. We provide code that automatically takes the inputs $(\theta_0, u, \theta_{max})$ and builds the appropriate priors into the analysis.

The data were analyzed using the code **Ch15-Ganzfeld-Metaanalysis** available on the book's website. Table 14.6 gives a summary of some of the results. For each prior, the table shows the median of the corresponding posterior distribution and a 95% probability interval. The table also includes the posterior medians for $\theta_{0.1}$ and $\theta_{0.9}$, under each prior. After all of this work, it is clear that the only prior that gives different results for median(θ) is the skeptic's prior. Their very strong prior was, for practical purposes, unmoved by the data, which was to be expected. The analyses based on the open-minded and diffuse priors are virtually identical to each other. We tried a half dozen other very diffuse priors, like $\mu \sim N(0, 0.01)$ with $\sigma_t \sim U(0, 4)$, and got precisely the same results as with these two priors.

The believer's prior obviously did have some impact on inferences for $\theta_{0.1}$ and $\theta_{0.9}$. Under this prior, the estimate of $|\theta_{0.9} - \theta_{0.1}|$ is much smaller than with the other priors. The implied greater certainty or precision arises because the believer's prior was centered at 0.33, which is where the data sit as well, and it was a rather strong prior in terms of specifying $\theta_{max} = 0.4$.

Point inferences for σ_t were $(0.03, 0.22, 0.42, 0.42)$ under the skeptic's, the believer's, the open-minded, and the diffuse priors, respectively. There was a comparable effect on the widths of the corresponding 95% probability intervals for σ_t.

Last, we calculated the posterior probabilities that median$(\theta) > k$, for $k \in (0.25, 0.28, 0.30)$. For the believer, they are $(1.0, 1.0, 0.997)$; for the open-minded prior, they are $(1.0, 0.996, 0.93)$; for the diffuse prior, they are $(1.0, 0.997, 0.94)$;

TABLE 14.6: Prior guess and 95th percentile for median(θ); posterior median and 95% probability intervals for median(θ), $\theta_{0.1}$ and $\theta_{0.9}$

	Prior inference	Posterior inference		
Prior	med(θ) (95%tile)	med(θ) (95% PI)	$\theta_{0.1}$	$\theta_{0.9}$
Diffuse	0.25 (0.8)	0.33 (0.29, 0.36)	0.22	0.45
Open	0.25 (0.41)	0.33 (0.29, 0.36)	0.22	0.45
Believer	0.33 (0.36)	0.33 (0.31, 0.35)	0.27	0.39
Skeptic	0.25 (0.255)	0.258 (0.252, 0.264)	0.251	0.264

and, interestingly, for the skeptic, they are $(0.997, 0, 0)$. The skeptic's posterior was moved to the right ever so slightly by the data; the posterior interval is $(0.252, 0.264)$. The practical import, however, is nil under this prior, while under all of the other priors, we would say that there is statistical and practical import. This is yet another illustration of how the prior can very much matter. In this instance, it is clear that strong beliefs may need extraordinary amounts of data to overcome them.

In the ganzfeld analysis, the estimated odds of a hit in a "typical" study are $(0.33/0.67 \doteq 1/2)$, compared with the odds under chance $(0.25/0.75 = 1/3)$, resulting in an estimated OR of 1.5. So if the "size of the psi effect" were to be measured using this odds ratio, it is comparable to the size of a treatment effect in many clinical studies that led to a change in clinical practice. It remains unclear how one could actually use the psi effect discussed here. The Bayesian analysis that we propose would be interesting, in part, because we would be obtaining estimated probabilities of events rather than the more opaque odds ratios.

14.3 Hierarchical Longitudinal and Spatial Data Modeling

In Chapter 9 we discussed some traditional methods for analyzing longitudinal data, such as growth curve modeling. In this section we employ and extend the hierarchical modeling techniques discussed in this chapter to handle longitudinal data. Sampling individuals who share a common environment or taking multiple observations on a single unit typically generates dependent observations. Correlation structures discussed in the book so far have involved either a general structure, meaning that there are no constraints on the covariance matrix for a collection of dependent data, or they have involved compound symmetry (CS). Here, we extend that structure to accommodate the longitudinal (or spatial) nature of the data.

Longitudinal data arise when repeated measurements are taken on each unit through time. For example, in a sample of hospitals, we could obtain overall measures of patient satisfaction and collect these measurements on several occasions.

Longitudinal studies are often conducted to assess time trends and the effect of covariates on time trends. We saw in Example 14.5 that a trial designed to compare different toenail fungus treatments might involve a baseline (pre-treatment) measurement on each person prior to treatment assignment, followed by several post-assignment measurements. We may examined different trends in fungus eradication over time and whether the trend depended on the treatment. We could also evaluate whether the treatment or time effects were affected by a participant's particular characteristics. Units are assumed to be independent, but the repeated measurements on the same unit are typically dependent.

Spatial data involve taking measurements of a phenomenon such as cancer incidence in different geographic regions. Some pairs of regions may be in close proximity to one another and others not. Cancer incidences corresponding to regions that are close to one another might be expected to be correlated, and those corresponding to distant regions may be thought to be uncorrelated. Moreover, these spatially observed incidences can be monitored over time. These types of data are called "spatial" and "spatiotemporal." A common phenomenon in longitudinal, spatial, and spatiotemporal data is that the correlation between observations decays with increased separation in time or distance. We do not discuss spatial data here but recommend the excellent treatment by Banerjee et al. (2015) [15].

Example 14.7. Reference Values for IL-1β. Understanding the extent of day-to-day variation in key hormones is important background for evaluating effects of interventions. Do the changes one sees after some intervention reflect the effect of the intervention or just natural variation? Thomas et al. (2009) [325] describe a longitudinal study that investigated variability of several physiological compounds that they measured in healthy adults. The investigators thought one or more might be useful as biomarkers associated with predicting abnormalities or disease. Among these potential biomarkers was interleukin-1β (IL-1β). IL-1β is a pro-inflammatory cytokine protein that already has several clinical applications but might also be useful as a measure of periodontal health.

The investigators measured concentrations of IL-1β in samples of saliva they collected from 30 healthy subjects on six consecutive days. The data for subject i are the vector $y_i = (y_{i1}, y_{i2}, y_{i3}, y_{i4}, y_{i5}, y_{i6})$ that consists of the measured concentrations in units of picograms per milliliter each day for the subject. The logarithms of the IL-1β measurements are shown in Figure 14.2 in a trellis plot that includes a lowess curve [82] showing each subject's trend over the six days. No consistent day-to-day trends appear across the subjects in the plots. Some of the measurements increase over the six days, some decline, and some seem to fluctuate around a central value.

Figure 14.3 shows boxplots of the log of the IL-1β measurements across subjects on each day. These plots do not suggest much change in the mean or variance from day to day. Day-to-day within-subject trajectories are shown in Figure 14.4 and confirm the impressions we have already formed.

We computed the sample correlation matrix for the logarithmically transformed

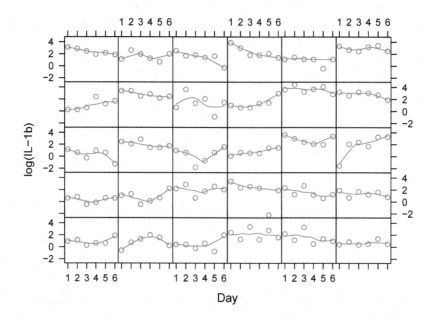

FIGURE 14.2: Trellis plot containing each individual's IL-1β data vector on the log scale.

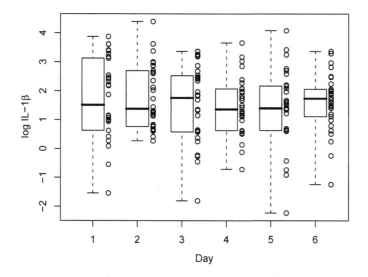

FIGURE 14.3: Boxplots of log(IL-1β).

data as follows:

$$
\begin{pmatrix}
1.00 & 0.62 & 0.57 & 0.51 & 0.26 & 0.18 \\
0.62 & 1.00 & 0.58 & 0.71 & 0.34 & 0.46 \\
0.57 & 0.58 & 1.00 & 0.68 & 0.42 & 0.28 \\
0.51 & 0.71 & 0.68 & 1.00 & 0.44 & 0.37 \\
0.26 & 0.34 & 0.42 & 0.44 & 1.00 & 0.30 \\
0.18 & 0.46 & 0.28 & 0.37 & 0.30 & 1.00
\end{pmatrix} .
$$

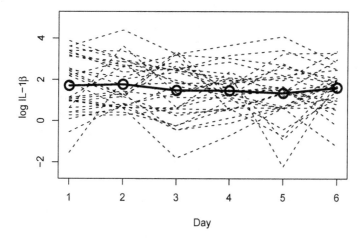

FIGURE 14.4: Spaghetti plot of log(IL-1β) with sample means.

There appears to be substantial correlation across days, which makes us think that we do not want to assume independence of within-subject observations. We also note that the correlations appear to get smaller when we consider days that are farther apart. This phenomenon is not infrequent and might be something we want to consider in our models.

14.3.1 Longitudinal Modeling as Hierarchical Modeling

We consider data in the following form. Let $y = \{y_{ij} : i = 1, \ldots, k; j = 1, \ldots, n_i\}$ be the observed response data, and let $\{(x_{ij}, t_{ij}) : i = 1, \ldots, k; j = 1, \ldots, n_i\}$ be covariate vectors and times of observations for all subjects in the sample. With this notation, y_{ij} is the jth observation on subject i in a sample of k subjects sampled from a population of interest. The time of observation for y_{ij} is t_{ij}, and the p observed covariate values at that time for that subject are in the $(p+1)$-vector x_{ij}, of course with a 1 in the first slot.

Laird and Ware (1982) were possibly the first to recognize the utility of hierarchical models for modeling longitudinal data [212]. The simplest such model is one that we have already seen in this chapter. Let

$$Y_{ij} \mid \gamma, \beta, \sigma^2 \perp\!\!\!\perp N(x'_{ij}\beta + \gamma_i, \sigma^2), \quad j = 1, \ldots, n_i,$$
$$\gamma_i \mid \sigma_g^2 \perp\!\!\!\perp N(0, \sigma_g^2). \tag{14.19}$$

Observe that we are centering the latent effects on 0. Since the predictor variables for each subject are allowed to vary from one time to the next, x_{ij} varies with j, so we cannot center the latent effects on $x'_{ij}\beta$. Covariates that vary in time are called "time-dependent covariates." We could always center on β_1, or if $x_{ij} = x_i$ we could center on $x'_i\beta$. Markov chains may be better behaved in either case. In the text, we choose to center on zero for notational convenience, while in our examples we tend to center on the intercept.

A major drawback to this model for longitudinal data is that $\text{Corr}(Y_{ij}, Y_{ik})$ is the same for all $j \neq k$. This is because $\text{Cov}(Y_{ij}, Y_{ik}) = \text{Cov}(\gamma_i, \gamma_i) = \sigma_g^2$, and $\text{Var}(Y_{ij}) = \sigma^2 + \sigma_g^2$, resulting in $\text{Corr}(Y_{ij}, Y_{ik}) = \sigma_g^2/(\sigma^2 + \sigma_g^2)$, for all $j < k$. This correlation structure is termed "compound symmetry." This structure may be considered to be inadequate, since it is often the case that we expect correlations to be smaller as k increases for any j. Before considering generalizations of this model for longitudinal data that address this issue, we analyze the interleukin-1β data using the CS model (14.19).

Example 14.8. Reference Values for IL-1β. We sometimes have to choose between analyzing data on the raw or original measurement scale or after some transformation, such as a logarithmic transform. Each approach has advantages and disadvantages. Many measurements appear more "normal" (i.e., symmetric) after taking logarithms, which can make modeling assumptions easier to justify, such as a normal sampling distribution. At the same time, interpretation is often easier on the raw scale; logarithms are not the most intuitive scale to consider for most people, unless this scale is in common use among subject-matter experts. We have been analyzing the IL-1β data on the log scale, because the data appear very skewed on their original scale. Despite the analysis being on log-transformed data, we often prefer to present inferences on the original scale, because it is easier to understand.

We used a log-normal sampling model to fit the IL-1β data with the model in expression (14.19). The log-transformed data range from -1.81 to 4.4 log(picograms per milliliter). Since the data are from healthy adults, we assume that the intercept, β_1, is most likely to lie within this range. Of course, we recognize that an analysis of other individuals, particularly unhealthy adults or children, might give rise to a different range. We also make the assumption that the standard deviations σ or σ_g most likely lie between 0 and 2. Our analysis, therefore, starts with $\beta_1 \sim N(0, 4)$ and both σ and σ_g distributed $U(0, 2)$ *a priori*.

Since the goal of the study was to characterize natural changes in IL-1β levels across consecutive days in healthy adults, we make our inferences on the raw or original scale of measurement. We summarize the predictive distribution for a healthy adult's IL-1β level in Table 14.7. The predicted median value for a future IL-1β measurement is 4.7 pg/ml. The corresponding 95% prediction interval is $(0.4, 57.5)$. The fact that the predicted median is not near the center of the interval highlights the skewness of the distribution of values, which appears clearly in the plot of the predictive density, $p(y_f \mid y)$, in Figure 14.5. From the predictive density, we infer that with probability 10%, the future measurement will be larger than 23.7 pg/ml and that there is only a 5% chance that the future IL-1β measurement will be greater than 37.8 pg/ml. Since these measurements reflect a (hopefully representative) group of healthy adults, physicians might want to examine further individuals with measurements above the predictive 90th or 95th percentiles.

Table 14.7 also contains summaries of the posterior distributions of the standard

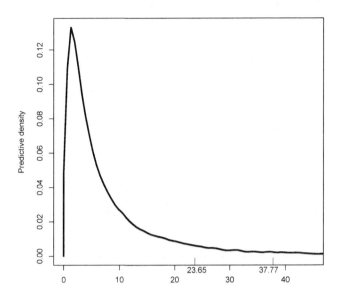

FIGURE 14.5: Predictive density, $p(y_f \mid y)$, for future IL-1β score, Y_f, on untransformed scale.

deviations (σ and σ_g) and the correlation (ρ). The posterior medians of σ and σ_g are about the same size, which we interpret to mean that there is roughly as much variation within individuals as among individuals, based on the sample of healthy adults.

Table 14.7 indicates that we expect 90% of future healthy adults to have IL-1β levels greater than 1.5 pg/ml, the 10th percentile of the predictive distribution. The table also shows the uncertainty associated with our estimate via a 95% prediction interval $(1.0, 2.1)$. Our analysis also suggests that 90% of future healthy adults whom we measure will have IL-1β levels less than 15.3 pg/ml. The corresponding 95% prediction interval is $(10.7, 21.9)$. We generated these predictions for future observations by setting the latent parameter γ equal to the parameter β_1. By doing this, we can get an idea of the variability of the IL-1β levels for typical healthy adults in that we do not take account of variability across individuals, only within individuals.

The book's website contains some code for this example in the section for Chapter 14 in files with `Ch14-IL-1beta` in their name. The example appears again in Exercise 14.18. Note that the untransformed data are modeled with a log-normal distribution in the program. This is equivalent to transforming the data and then modeling them as normal.

The next level of generalization allows for an overall trend in time and latent departures from the overall trend that reflect differences in individuals. This modi-

TABLE 14.7: Posterior results on untransformed scale for IL-1β data. The median outcome for typical patients is e^{β_1}. The α quantile of outcomes is $\exp(\beta_1 + z_\alpha \sigma_g)$ for $\alpha = 0.1$ and 0.9

	median	(95% PI)
y_f	4.7	$(0.4, 57.5)$
$\exp(\beta_1)$	4.7	$(3.4, 6.6)$
$\exp(\beta_1 - 1.28\sigma)$	1.5	$(1.0, 2.1)$
$\exp(\beta_1 + 1.28\sigma)$	15.3	$(10.7, 21.9)$
σ	0.92	$(0.82, 1.03)$
σ_g	0.82	$(0.60, 1.15)$
ρ	0.45	$(0.29, 0.62)$

fication of the model has expectation

$$E(Y_{ij} \mid \beta, \gamma) = x'_{ij}\beta + \beta_{p+1}t_{ij} + \gamma_{1i} + \gamma_{2i}t_{ij}. \tag{14.20}$$

The vector for the latent intercept and slope, $\gamma_i = (\gamma_{1i}, \gamma_{2i})'$, is specified to have a bivariate normal distribution

$$\gamma_i \overset{\perp\!\!\!\perp}{\sim} N_2(0, \Sigma_g), \quad \Sigma_g = \begin{pmatrix} \sigma_{1g}^2 & \sigma_{12g} \\ \sigma_{12g} & \sigma_{2g}^2 \end{pmatrix}.$$

A standard simplification would be to let $\sigma_{12g} = 0$, but a more thorough analysis would explore whether or not this was a reasonable assumption. It is not obvious that knowing the latent intercept would be uninformative for the latent slope.

This model can be written in matrix and vector form. Let $y_i = (y_{i1}, \ldots, y_{in_i})'$, and let $\tilde{X}_i$ be the $n_i \times (p+1)$ matrix that has rows x'_{ij}. The first column is all 1s, the second column contains values for the first predictor for all n_i responses for individual i, and so on. We augment this matrix by appending the column vector $t_i = (t_{i1}, t_{i2}, \ldots, t_{in_i})'$. Thus, we define the matrix $X_i = (\tilde{X}_i, t_i)$ so that X_i is $n_i \times (p+2)$. Let $\beta = (\beta_1, \ldots, \beta_{p+2})'$. Finally, let Z_i be the $n_i \times 2$ matrix that has all 1s in the first column and has the vector t_i in the second column. The conditional mean for Y_i can be expressed as

$$E(Y_i \mid \beta, \gamma) = X_i\beta + Z_i\gamma_i.$$

We write the matrix version of the model for the entire data set $y = (y'_1, \ldots, y'_k)'$. Let X be the $T \times (p+2)$ matrix with all of the X_i stacked on top of each other and where $T = \sum_i n_i$ is the total number of observations in the data. Next define $\gamma = (\gamma'_1, \ldots, \gamma'_k)'$, and the $T \times 2k$ matrix,

$$Z = \begin{pmatrix} Z_1 & 0 & \cdots & 0 \\ 0 & Z_2 & \cdots & 0 \\ & & \ddots & 0 \\ 0 & 0 & \cdots & Z_k \end{pmatrix}.$$

Then we can write

$$Y \mid \gamma, \beta \sim N_T(X\beta + Z\gamma, \sigma^2 I_T), \tag{14.21}$$

where I_T is the $T \times T$ identity matrix. In the statistical literature, this model and its generalizations, some of which are discussed below, are referred to as "linear mixed models." When the expected value is a generalized linear model (see Chapters 8 and 9), such models are sometimes called "generalized linear mixed models." There are entire books dedicated to using these types of models [312].

The next level of generalization could allow for quadratic and higher-level polynomial trends in time, with corresponding latent departures from each. These modifications would simply involve augmenting the matrix X by adding columns that correspond to squared, cubic, etc. functions of the t_{ij}. One would add the same columns to the Z_i and augment the vectors γ_i with corresponding additional latent effects.

In addition, we could add latent effects that reflect individual departures from one or more predictor variables' coefficients. This simply involves adding column vectors to the Z_i that correspond to these variables, and of course adding more latent effect terms to the γ_i.

The γ_i would now be modeled with a higher-dimensional multivariate normal distribution. There would be issues related to modeling the covariance matrix for that distribution. It would generally be the case that the covariance matrix, Σ_g, would be constrained to be a function of a relatively small number of parameters, say $\theta = (\theta_1, \ldots, \theta_q)$. In this case we would write the covariance matrix as $\Sigma_g(\theta)$. Considerable care is needed to guarantee that the resulting matrix is indeed a proper covariance matrix. One must also place a reasonable prior on θ. We refer the reader to Christensen et al. [79, Section 10.3] for illustrations of such covariance structures .

It was the generalized linear mixed model that Laird and Ware (1982) suggested for use in analyzing longitudinal data [212]. The nice feature of their suggestion was the fact that these models do not require having regular data for analysis. Regular data must have equal n_i, times of observation must be the same for all subjects, and they must be equally spaced, which was a requirement for classical methods for repeated measures data. As in the simple latent intercept case, this generalization does not directly address the issue that observations on the same individual that are near in time tend to be more highly correlated than those that are farther apart in time.

We now consider an example that involves modeling trends in time.

Example 14.9.   Dental Data. We will examine the classic example of longitudinal data from the paper by Potthof and Roy (1964) [263]. The data consist of measurements based on X-rays taken every 2 years on 16 young men and 11 young women. Their ages at the time of the X-ray measurements were 8, 10, 12, and 14 years. The data come from a study in which the investigators measured the distance (in millimeters) from the pituitary gland to the pterygomaxillary fissure as an indicator of physiologic growth. In our analysis, we examine the effects of sex and age on the growth rate.

Figure 14.6 shows the data as individual plots for each of the 27 young people in the study. The figure also shows the sample means by age and sex, with separate lines connecting the age-specific means for the young men and young women. Note that we can consider age to be a surrogate for time, since the data collection occurred regularly at equally spaced times (ages 8, 10, 12, and 14). Also, there are no missing observations. Neither regularly spaced data nor no missing data will be the case in practice. The methods we are using here, however, work equally well for non-regularly spaced data.

We first consider a simple model that assumes that the boys and girls have trend lines of growth that are parallel over this age range but may have different intercepts. If we examine Figure 14.6, we can try to imagine two curves based on the sex-specific means. A difference in intercepts would characterize a sex-related difference in size. The effect of time (or aging) manifests itself via the slope of the curves. Since we are assuming parallel curves with possibly different intercepts, our model reflects a belief that males and females between 8 and 14 years of age grow at the same rate but may differ in size during those ages. Looking at the figure suggests that there are different intercepts and that the slopes of the lines are positive.

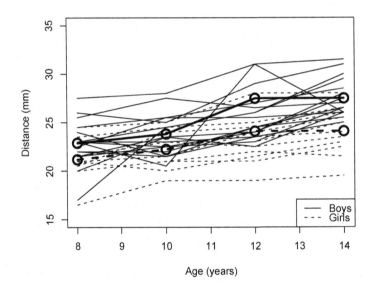

FIGURE 14.6: Plot of the dental data with sample means for boys and girls.

Our model allows for a latent intercept and a latent slope. We model these latent parameters with a bivariate normal distribution that centers the latent intercept ($E[\gamma_{1i}]$) on the overall average intercept β_1. We have standardized the covariate *Age*, creating the variable $sAge_{ij} = (Age_{ij} - 11)/2$. The covariate *Male* is coded as 1 = male and 0 = female. The model is

$$
\begin{aligned}
Y_{ij} \mid \gamma, \beta, \sigma^2 &\perp\!\!\!\perp N(\mu_{ij}, \sigma^2), \quad i = 1, \ldots, 27; j = 1, 2, 3, 4, \\
\mu_{ij} &= \gamma_{1i} + \beta_2 sAge_{ij} + \gamma_{2i} sAge_{ij} + \beta_3 Male_i \\
\gamma_i &\overset{iid}{\sim} N_2(\mu_g, \Sigma_g),
\end{aligned}
\tag{14.22}
$$

where

$$
\gamma_i = \begin{pmatrix} \gamma_{1i} \\ \gamma_{2i} \end{pmatrix}, \quad \mu_g = \begin{pmatrix} \beta_1 \\ 0 \end{pmatrix}, \quad \Sigma_g = \begin{pmatrix} \sigma_{1g}^2 & \sigma_{12g} \\ \sigma_{12g} & \sigma_{2g}^2 \end{pmatrix}.
$$

The average intercept for the females in this model is β_1, and the average intercept for the males is $\beta_1 + \beta_3$. Thus, the model considers the possibility that the two groups will have different average intercepts, according to the value of β_3. We could add an interaction effect to the model, $\beta_4 sAge_{ij} \times Male_i$, to allow for different rates of growth for the two groups. With the interaction effect, the average slopes would be β_2 and $\beta_2 + \beta_4$ for females and males, respectively. We note that these parameters relate to average intercepts and slopes, since we have parameterized the model via $E(\gamma_{1i}) = \beta_1$ and $E(\gamma_{2i}) = 0$. The plots of the data in Figure 14.6 seem to indicate that parallel lines are appropriate, so we leave an interaction term out of the model.

We proceed to specify a diffuse proper prior. We standardized age out of force of habit, just to help with convergence properties. We placed a $N(0, 100)$ prior on all three regression coefficients, and a $U(0,10)$ prior on σ; the range of the data responses is only 12 mm so, in light of this fact, these priors are quite diffuse. We also placed $U(0,10)$ priors on σ_{kg} for $k = 1, 2$. It remains to place a prior on the covariance, σ_{12g}. This cannot be done arbitrarily, since our induced prior on the covariance matrix Σ_g has to be positive definite with probability 1.

Specifying an appropriate prior on σ_{12g} is not difficult. The correlation between γ_{1i} and γ_{2i} is just $\rho_g = \sigma_{12g}/(\sigma_{1g}\sigma_{2g})$; thus, $\sigma_{12j} = \rho_g \sigma_{1g} \sigma_{2g}$. A simple diffuse prior for ρ_g is $U(0,1)$. Having specified proper diffuse priors for $(\sigma_{1g}, \sigma_{2g}, \rho_g)$, we have in effect specified a proper diffuse prior for Σ_g. If we expected a negative relationship between latent intercept and slope, we could allow for negative values for ρ_g.

If we were writing a program to fit the model and only know what we know thus far, we might want to specify the precision matrix in terms of $(\sigma_{1j}, \sigma_{2j}, \rho_g)$. This is, of course, easily accomplished, since we know how to take the inverse of a 2×2 matrix. We leave as an exercise for the reader the case where the γ_i are modeled as bivariate normal and the mean vector and precision matrix are specified appropriately in the code.

Here, instead, we use simple properties of the bivariate normal distribution to write the model for $(\gamma_{1i}, \gamma_{2i})$ as a marginal $N(\beta_1, \sigma_{1g}^2)$ for γ_{1i}, and conditional normal for γ_{2i} given γ_{1i}. The formulas for the mean and variance of our conditional normal are

$$
\begin{aligned}
E(\gamma_{2i} \mid \gamma_{1i}) &= 0 + \rho_g \frac{\sigma_{2g}}{\sigma_{1g}} (\gamma_{1i} - \beta_1), \\
\mathrm{Var}(\gamma_{2i} \mid \gamma_{1i}) &= \sigma_{2g}^2 (1 - \rho_g^2).
\end{aligned}
\tag{14.23}
$$

TABLE 14.8: Posterior inferences for the dental data

	median	(95% PI)
β_1	22.7	$(21.4, 23.9)$
β_2	1.31	$(1.02, 1.61)$
β_3	2.24	$(0.57, 3.92)$
σ	1.35	$(1.13, 1.63)$
σ_{1g}	2.05	$(1.47, 2.92)$
σ_{2g}	0.44	$(0.08, 0.78)$
ρ_g	0.37	$(0.02, 0.85)$

We are finally in a position to analyze the data. Figure 14.7 gives the sample means for males and females across ages, and it gives model-based predicted values, which appear to adhere to the data nicely. The predicted lines are parallel by construction. Again, with these fits it would not really occur to us to try to fit separate slopes, which could be accomplished by adding an interaction term. Parameter estimates are given in Table 14.8. The intercept is not particularly interesting here.

In our model, we created a "standardized" age covariate $sAge = (Age - 11)/2$. This is not a typical standardization but it marks ages in two-year increments. If $sAge = 0$, the age is 11, and if $sAge = 1$, the age is 13, and so on. Thus a difference in standardized ages of 1 corresponds to a difference in actual ages of 2 years. We standardized ages in the model in order to have better Markov chain performance. Consequently, we are able to interpret the estimated coefficient for age as an estimate of the difference between median responses for individuals who are 2 years apart in age, regardless of their actual ages. This (statistically important) age effect is estimated to be 1.31 for males and for females, since there is no interaction in the model. Similarly, the (statistically important) effect of sex is estimated to be 2.24 regardless of age.

Our prior assumed that $\rho_g > 0$. We also ran the model with $\rho_g \sim U(-1, 1)$. The results were virtually identical to those in Table 14.8, with the exception of inferences for ρ_g, which were 0.26 $(-0.47, 0.82)$. The implication is that there does not appear to be very much information in the data for estimating this correlation. In Exercise 14.20 we ask the reader to explore an alternative model for these data that assumes this correlation is zero.

14.3.2   Incorporating Latent Effects with Autoregressive Structure

In this section we expand the basic hierarchical model that we have been using to include latent effects that incorporate an autoregressive correlation structure into the basic model. In simple terms, this means that correlations can be larger between observations that are closer in time than for those that are farther apart. We first generalize the form of model expressed in expression (14.21) to allow for

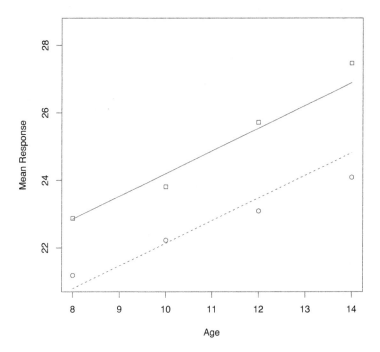

FIGURE 14.7: Plot of model-based predicted outcomes for boys and girls at ages 8, 10, 12, and 14 years. Sample means for boys are squares and for girls are circles.

this structure. For simplicity of exposition, we illustrate by extending the simpler model in expression (14.19). The notation for the data, covariates, and observation times remains the same.

We discuss latent effects with autoregressive structure. For each $i \in \{1, \ldots, k\}$, let $w_i \equiv \{w_i(t) : t \in (t_{i1}, t_{i2}, \ldots, t_{in_i})\}$ be a collection of random variables indexed by time, namely, $w_i = (w_i(t_{i1}), w_i(t_{i2}), \ldots, w_i(t_{in_i}))'$. This is the definition of a discrete time stochastic process that is specific to the given time points. The extended processes $\{w_i(t) : t \in (0, T)\}$ for $T > \max_i(t_{ni})$, $i = 1, \ldots, k$, are regarded as independent continuous time stochastic processes. Practically speaking, it is only discrete time that matters. The vector W_i is modeled as

$$W_i \mid \theta \perp\!\!\!\perp N_{n_i}(0, \Sigma_i(\theta_w)), \quad i = 1, \ldots, k,$$

where $\Sigma_i(\theta_w)$ is, at the moment, a "patterned" covariance matrix that can have many possible forms. We will focus on only one form in this section. Under this assumption, the continuous time process $\{w_i(t) : t \in (0, T)\}$ is called a "Gaussian process." We thus have k independent Gaussian processes for incorporating autoregressive structure into the model for the full data.

Here, we only consider the autoregressive form for $\Sigma_i(\theta_w)$, which simply means that correlations are larger for times that are closer together than for times that are farther apart. We make this precise shortly, but right now, we incorporate w_i

into the model for the data as follows. The generalized version of model (14.21) is

$$Y_i \mid \gamma_i, w_i, \beta, \sigma^2 \perp\!\!\!\perp N_{n_i}(X_i\beta + Z_i\gamma_i + w_i, \sigma^2 I), \quad i = 1, \ldots, k. \tag{14.24}$$

All that remains is to specify a Gaussian process that gives the W_i an autoregressive structure. We accomplish this structure by specifying a covariance "function" for the processes, $\{W_i(s) : s \in (0, T)\}$. We use a covariance function from the literature that specifies

$$\text{Cov}(W_i(t+s), W_i(t)) = \sigma_w^2 \rho_w(s), \quad \text{Var}(W_i(t)) = \sigma_w^2, \quad \rho_w(s) = \rho_w^s, \quad \rho_w > 0.$$

While there are other possible choices for $\rho_w(s)$, this particular one is termed the "exponential covariance function." It follows that

$$\text{Corr}(W_i(t), W_i(t+s)) = \rho_w^s < \text{Corr}(W_i(t), W_i(t+r))) = \rho_w^r, \quad s > r.$$

This immediately gives

$$\Sigma_w(\theta_w) = \sigma_w^2 \begin{pmatrix} 1 & \rho_w^{t_{i2}-t_{i1}} & \rho_w^{t_{i3}-t_{i1}} & \cdots & \rho_w^{t_{in_i}-t_{i1}} \\ \rho_w^{t_{i2}-t_{i1}} & 1 & \rho_w^{t_{i2}-t_{i1}} & \cdots & \rho_w^{t_{i(n_i-1)}-t_{i2}} \\ \ddots & \ddots & \ddots & \ddots \\ \rho_w^{t_{in_i}-t_{i1}} & \rho_w^{t_{in_i}-t_{i2}} & \cdots & \cdots & 1 \end{pmatrix}, \tag{14.25}$$

where $\theta_w = (\sigma_w^2, \rho_w)$. This is the (autoregressive) correlation structure that we have been seeking. We note that the correlation between pairs of observations in the *data* will depend on this structure when w_i is included in the model, and it will depend on the latent structure induced by including γ_i in the model as well.

We now consider the actual correlation structure for the Y_{ij} when there are only random intercepts and Gaussian process terms in the model, namely, $Y_{ij} \mid \gamma_i, w_{ij}, \beta, \sigma^2 \perp\!\!\!\perp N(x_{ij}\beta + \gamma_i + w_{ij}, \sigma^2)$, with γs and ws independent. Then it is easy to obtain

$$\text{Corr}(Y_{ij}, Y_{ik}) = \frac{\sigma_g^2 + \sigma_w^2 \rho_w^{|k-j|}}{\sigma_g^2 + \sigma_w^2 + \sigma^2}. \tag{14.26}$$

We can see that this correlation decreases to $\sigma_g^2/(\sigma_g^2 + \sigma_w^2 + \sigma^2)$ as the difference in time, $|k - j|$, increases. This limit is the same correlation that we had with the compound symmetry model with only latent intercepts in the model.

We also note that the autocorrelations between observations that are $|k-j| = m$ units apart for $m = 1, 2, \ldots, n-1$ are interesting to monitor. This way it is possible to see if compound symmetry is plausible for a given data set. If it is plausible, then these correlations should be approximately equal. On the other hand, if the autocorrelations decrease and then flatten, we have some idea about how much time is needed before the autocorrelation fades.

A major advantage of the autoregressive structure is that the matrices $\Sigma_i(\theta_w)$ can be analytically inverted, which results in precision matrices that are tridiagonal. Details are given in Quintana et al. (2016) [265] who developed a more

TABLE 14.9: Posterior results on untransformed scale for IL-1β data using model with autoregressive structure

	median	(95% PI)
$\exp(\beta_1)$	4.8	$(3.5, 6.7)$
$\exp(\beta_1 - 1.28\sigma)$	1.8	$(1.2, 2.8)$
$\exp(\beta_1 + 1.28\sigma)$	12.7	$(8.4, 19.4)$
σ	0.92	$(0.52, 0.94)$
σ_g	1.0	$(0.05, 1.9)$
σ_w	0.64	$(0.18, 1.03)$
ρ_w	0.53	$(0.08, 0.99)$

general and more flexible model than our model (14.24). Using this result leads to a simple expression for a multivariate normal model for W_i as the product of univariate conditional normals:

$$p(w_i \mid \theta_w) = p(w_{i1} \mid \theta_w)p(w_{i2} \mid w_{i1}, \theta_w)p(w_{i3} \mid w_{i2}, \theta_w) \dots p(w_{in_i} \mid w_{i(n_i-1)}, \theta_w).$$

We have used the fact that

$$p(w_{ij} \mid w_{i1}, w_{i2}...w_{i(j-1)}, \theta_w) = p(w_{ij} \mid w_{i(j-1)}, \theta_w), \quad j = 2, \dots, k,$$

which follows from the tri-diagonal form of the precision matrix, $[\Sigma_i(\theta_w)]^{-1}$. Then, for $j = 1, \dots, n_i - 1$, define $r_{ij} = \rho_w^{|t_{i(j+1)} - t_{ij}|}$. Quintana et al. (2016) [265] have shown that

$$W_{i1} \sim N(0, \sigma_w^2),$$
$$W_{i2} \mid W_{i1} = w_{i1} \sim N\left(w_{i1}r_{i1}, \sigma_w^2(1 - r_{i1}^2)\right),$$
$$\dots,$$
$$W_{ik} \mid W_{i(k-1)} = w_{i(k-1)} \sim N\left(w_{i(k-1)}r_{ik-1}, \sigma_w^2(1 - r_{ik-1}^2)\right),$$
(14.27)

for $k = 2, \dots, n_i$. This makes it straightforward to obtain the full conditional distribution of w_i in the Gibbs sampling algorithm.

Example 14.10. IL-1β Data Revisited. Recall Example 14.8 where we analyzed the IL-1β data that involved six repeated observations on 30 individuals using a model with latent intercepts. The data are plotted in Figure 14.2. Observe that most of the profile plots there either trend continuously upward or downward. This is an indication of high autocorrelation in the data, so we might expect a model that included autoregressive latent effects to improve on the model we fit in this example. This turns out to be the case.

We modified the code from our analysis in Example 14.8 to include the autoregressive terms specified in expression (14.27). Inferences based on model (14.24) with autoregressive correlation structure (14.25) are given in Table 14.9. We used proper diffuse priors for all parameters.

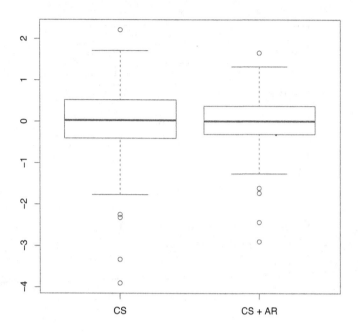

FIGURE 14.8: Boxplot of residuals for the IL-1β data, $y_i - \hat{y}_i, i = 1, \ldots, k$, under model (14.19) on the left ($\hat{y}_i = E(E(Y_i \mid \gamma_i) \mid y) = E(\gamma_i \mid y)$), and under model (14.24) on the right ($\hat{y}_i = E(E(Y_i \mid \gamma_i, w_i) \mid y) = E(\gamma_i + w_i \mid y)$). CS refers to model (14.19) that only allows for compound symmetry, while CS +AR allows for compound symmetry and autoregressive structure.

Results for the overall average median e^{β_1} are virtually identical under the two models. Remaining results show some minor differences in inferences for σ and for the 10th and 90th percentiles for "typical" individuals. (Recall that typical individuals have γ values set to β_1 and w values set to 0.) Inferences for σ_g show a much wider PI than we saw with the non-autoregressive model.

The most interesting aspect of the new model is that it fits the data noticeably better than the model without autoregressive structure. Figure 14.8 shows box-plots of residuals. These plots suggest that the model with autoregressive structure (model (14.24)) has appreciably smaller residuals than the model with only a compound symmetry structure (model (14.19)). Another interesting feature of fitting this model is that predicted values for a future individual at the six specified ages are (10.03, 10.33, 10.58, 10.61, 10.74, 10.94), respectively, indicating a slightly increasing trend over time. Since we saw (Figure 14.2) individual profiles that went down, up, and somewhat flat, the implication is that overall, there was more of a tendency to go up than down. Under the model without autoregressive structure, the predicted values were (10.56, 10.54, 10.51, 10.63, 10.48, 10.58), respectively, and we see no discernible pattern. The book's website for Chapter 14 includes data and code for this analysis. The files include `Ch-14-Interleukin-CSAR` in their names.

14.4   Recap and Readings

We have presented many of examples of the use of hierarchical models, both for normal and binomial models. We have shown how hierarchical models can be used to perform meta-analyses. We have used them to illustrate a general method of performing longitudinal and clustered data analyses. Our most general model illustrated the use of latent effects to incorporate both compound symmetry and autoregressive components in an overall model for longitudinal data. These approaches all involved parametric modeling.

We did not discuss the extension of parametric longitudinal modeling in the case of binomial or other non-normal types of data. Models similar to (14.24) are easy to specify on the logit scale, for example. An additional section in this chapter would just parallel the development in Section 14.3.1 and would use materials from Section 14.2.

The assumption of normality for latent effects can certainly be questioned. Early papers that allowed for nonparametric mixtures of normal distributions as models for latent effects distributions were presented in Kleinman and Ibrahim (1998) [205, 206]. In this chapter we referred to an extension of the parametric model to a semiparametric model for the latent effects; Quintana et al. (2016) [265] extended the model (14.24) to a situation where the processes, W_i, are modeled as Dirichlet process mixtures of the Gaussian processes with autoregressive structure, with the mixing on θ. This extension allows for the possibility of having individuals in the data whose latent effects are clustered, meaning that their latent (w) effects might coincide with those for a subgroup of individuals in the data set. The model also allows for a more general autoregression structure in which correlations of repeated observations on the same individual can have diminishing correlations over time, but where these correlations can diminish at a faster or slower rate than with parametric autoregression structure. Moreover, the correlations can diminish to a value and then remain flat afterwards. Quintana et al. give multiple additional references for this kind of generalization of latent effects models.

Here, we strongly re-emphasize the importance of specifying proper prior distributions for the latent effects' covariance parameters. We illustrated how to do this in the two-dimensional case. We also emphasized the simplicity of placing uniform priors on the latent effects' standard deviation parameters, like σ_g, that were not unnecessarily diffuse in the case of binomial and normal models.

We finally remark that the Thurmond–Hietela cow data were analyzed in Hanson et al. (2003) [158]. They jointly modeled the probability of abortion and time to abortion, using an expanded version of the data we discussed here that included additional covariates not discussed here. A major goal of the survival part of the model was to assess whether early abortions were a result of certain factors. One of the highlights of the analysis involved the joint modeling of latent effects for the survival and binomial regression parts, and another highlight was that the survival distributions were semiparametric rather than parametric. This allowed flexibility in modeling that was similar to that discussed above for generalizing latent effect distributions to nonparametric mixtures of parametric distributions. Survival modeling is discussed in Chapters 11 and 12. This paper may serve as an introduction to joint modeling, which is a topic that is large enough for a book [270, 102].

14.5   Exercises

EXERCISE 14.1.   Reanalyze the conception data in Example 14.1 using several alternative choices of diffuse proper priors for the model parameters. Code and data are on the book's website for Chapter 14 in files with Ch14-Conception in their names. Discuss the effect of changing the prior on posterior inferences. For three priors, including the one used in the example, obtain the predictive probability $P(\gamma_5 > \gamma_6 > \gamma_4)$. Compare the results.

EXERCISE 14.2.   We will reanalyze the rat growth data (Example 14.2). Code and data are on the book's website for Chapter 14 in files with Ch14-rat in their names.

(a) Reanalyze the data using independent $Ga(0.001, 0.001)$ priors for the precisions but leaving the prior on β as is. Discuss the effect changing the prior has on posterior inferences.

(b) Obtain the induced prior on σ_{1g}. Does this prior seem reasonable from a scientific point of view? Why or why not?

(c) Using both priors, obtain inferences for $\gamma_{9,1}/\gamma_{29,1}$ and $\gamma_{2,2}/\gamma_{4,2}$. Discuss.

EXERCISE 14.3.   For the model in expression (14.3) and using the conditionally conjugate prior in expression (14.6), show that the full conditional for μ is normal, for τ is gamma, for τ_γ is gamma, and for γ_i is normal, with the γ_i being *a posteriori* independent. Completely specify these distributions. *Hint*: You will need to apply the complete-the-square formula. Also show and use the fact that $\sum_{ij}(y_{ij} - \gamma_i)^2 = \sum_{ij}(y_{ij} - \bar{y}_i)^2 + \sum_i n_i(\gamma_i - \bar{y}_i)^2$, where $\bar{y}_i = \sum_j y_{ij}/n_i$.

EXERCISE 14.4.   For this exercise, refer to expression (14.3) where an exchangeable model is assumed for analysis-of-variance type data. Argue that $\bar{Y}_i = \sum_j Y_{ij}/n_i \mid \gamma_i, \sigma^2 \sim N(\gamma_i, \sigma^2/n_i)$. Also assume that $\gamma_i \mid \mu, \sigma_g^2 \sim N(\mu, \sigma_g^2)$, and that $(\sigma^2, \mu, \sigma_g^2)$ are known. Show that the conditional distribution $\gamma_i \mid \bar{y}_i \sim N(w\mu + (1-w)\bar{y}_i, \sigma_g^2/(\sigma^2/n_i + \sigma_g^2))$, where $w = (\sigma^2/n_i)/(\sigma^2/n_i) + \sigma_g^2)$. Thus, argue that the Bayesian prediction for γ_i involves shrinkage away from the sample mean to the overall mean.

EXERCISE 14.5.   Show that with $Y = \{Y_{ij} : i = 1, \ldots, H; j = 1, \ldots, n_i\}$, $Y \mid \theta \sim N(\mu(\theta), \Sigma(\theta))$ with precisely the same mean vector and covariance matrix for the models in expressions (14.1) and (14.2).

EXERCISE 14.6. *DiaSorin data.*   Analyze the log-transformed DiaSorin data with three groups using model (14.3) with the diffuse but *proper* prior $\mu \sim N(0, 0.00001)$, $\tau \sim Ga(0.001, 0.001)$, and $\sigma_g \sim U(0, k)$, for several choices of k. Be sure to give some thought to your choices of k and how you would explain your choices. What can be said about any differences or similarities in the three groups? What can be said about the sensitivity of inferences to the choice of k?

EXERCISE 14.7. *Fully informative prior for σ.*   Assume the model in expression (14.3). Let $p_{0.9} = \mu + 1.28\,\sigma$, with p_0 as a best guess for $p_{0.9}$. Recall that our best guess for σ was $\sigma_0 = (p_0 - \mu_0)/1.28$, where μ_0 was our best guess for μ. Assume that the expert is 95% sure that $p_{0.9}$ is less than $\tilde{p}$, conditional on all of the other information. Derive a suitable $Ga(c, d)$ prior for σ_g based on this information. Actually obtain (c, d) if $p_0 = 10$, $\mu_0 = 5$, and $\tilde{p} = 15$.

EXERCISE 14.8.   Show that if a random variable X with pdf $p(x)$ has a finite range, say (r, s), then $\text{sd}(X) < (s - r)$. *Note*: We realize that many distributions have infinite range, in theory. In the real world, however, everything is finite, including the values that data can actually take. In this sense, the range of the data is a reasonable start for determining how much variability there might be in them.

EXERCISE 14.9. *Anesthesia data.*   Perry et al. (1974) studied concentrations of plasma epinephrine in 10 dogs that received three different types of anesthesia [259]. Epinephrine is essentially adrenaline, and one does not want high levels of adrenaline or epinephrine when giving a patient anesthesia. The anesthetic agents were isofluorane (I), halothane (H), and cyclopropane (C). The data from the study are given in Table 14.10, as given in Rice (1995) [269]. The variable *Dogs* constitutes

TABLE 14.10: Anesthesia data

	Dog 1	Dog 2	Dog 3	Dog 4	Dog 5	Dog 6	Dog 7	Dog 8	Dog 9	Dog 10
I	0.28	0.51	1.00	0.39	0.29	0.36	0.32	0.69	0.17	0.33
H	0.30	0.39	0.63	0.68	0.38	0.21	0.88	0.39	0.51	0.32
C	1.07	1.35*	0.69	0.28	1.24	1.53*	0.49	0.56	1.02	0.30

what we call a "blocking factor" in the statistical literature. We wish to compare the three anesthetics in terms of concentration of plasma epinephrine. Repeated observations on the same dog are likely to be correlated, since each dog has its own physiological and biological characteristics. Thus, epinephrine levels within a dog should tend to be higher or lower across all three anesthetics, depending on the particular dog's innate physiology or metabolism for these agents. As we have discussed in this chapter, we characterize such unmeasured sources of between-dog variability using latent effects. We thus include latent effects for the 10 dogs in our model.

Consider the following model for the data:

$$Y_{ij} \mid \gamma, \beta, \sigma^2 \perp\!\!\!\perp \mathrm{N}(\mu_{ij}, \sigma^2), \quad \mu_{ij} = \mu_I I_j + \mu_H H_j + \mu_C C_j + \gamma_i,$$
$$\gamma_i \mid \sigma_g^2 \perp\!\!\!\perp \mathrm{N}(0, \sigma_g^2), \quad i = 1, \ldots, 10; j = 1, 2, 3.$$

Each predictor (i.e., I_j, H_j, and C_j) is an indicator variable for the corresponding anesthetic. The unconditional mean for each anesthetic is the overall mean response for dogs that are being administered that particular anesthetic. This is a simple analysis of variance model with latent effects for dogs. The main goal is to assess which anesthetic has the best performance, and possibly which is worst in terms of mean responses. It is also possible that they are all equally effective or that one is better or worse than the other two, while the other two are equally effective.

(a) Calculate the analytical correlation between any two repeated measurements on any dog; that is, find $\rho \equiv \mathrm{Corr}(Y_{ij}, Y_{ik})$, $k \neq j$, under this model.

(b) Using a proper diffuse prior with $p(\mu_I, \mu_H, \mu_c, \sigma, \sigma_g) = p(\mu_I)p(\mu_H)p(\mu_c)p(\sigma)p(\sigma_g)$, where the μs are all $N(0, 4)$ and the σs are both $U(0, 4)$, analyze the anesthesia data. Obtain posterior inferences for all possible differences in mean responses. Also, obtain the posterior probabilities that $\mu_C > \mu_H$, that $\mu_C > \mu_I$, etc. Finally, look at joint probabilities of the form $\mu_C > \mu_h > \mu_I$. Draw conclusions about which anesthetics are better. Also make inferences about the relative magnitudes of σ and σ_g, and the correlation, ρ.

(c) Perform a sensitivity analysis using some alternate priors and discuss the effects of perturbing the prior on posterior inferences.

(d) Using the prior in (b), fit a model without the latent effects. Compare inferences with those in (b).

(e) Now suppose that the observations in Table 14.10 with asterisks (*) were missing. Redo the analysis by replacing these numbers with NA. If you are using a program that generates posterior samples via MCMC, the program can (and normally will) impute missing values at each iteration of the MCMC sampler, possibly using the full conditional distribution for that missing observation if one is using Gibbs sampling. The entries with asterisks are the largest ones in the data. Compare inferences to those in part (b) and discuss.

(f) Suppose y_{11} were missing. Obtain and precisely identify the name of the full conditional distribution of Y_{11}. *Hint*: It will be a normal distribution.

EXERCISE 14.10.   On the book's website for Chapter 14, we include the data and various programming statements to analyze the intensive care unit study data in Example 14.3. The files have icu in their names. Reanalyze the data and verify the results given in Example 14.3. Obtain a plot of the predictive density for a future odds ratio. This will be a point estimate for the pdf for the "true" distribution of odds ratios. Obtain a posterior estimate of the proportion of odds ratios in the population of odds ratios from which our 14 samples were taken that will be below 0.9, 0.8, and 0.6, respectively, and above 1, 1.1, and 1.5, respectively.

EXERCISE 14.11. The data and program statements to analyze the data from the toenail study (Example 14.5) are on the book's website for this chapter. The files have `toenail` in their names.

(a) Modify the code so that you can create a table of inferences that provides predicted probabilities of moderate or severe separation at times 1, 2, 3, 5, 8, and 10 for a new individual who receives $Trt = 1$ with $\gamma_{384} \mid \sigma_g^2 \sim N(\beta_1, \sigma_g^2)$. Repeat the process for the same individual, assuming now that this person receives $Trt = 0$. The table should be 6×2. Compare the probabilities across times and treatments.
(b) Now perform your own sensitivity analysis and comment.

EXERCISE 14.12.

(a) Fit the model for the cow abortion data analysis in Example 14.6. (The data and some example code are in files with `cowabortion` in their names on the book's website for Chapter 14.) Before making inferences, monitor the chains to check on convergence. Comment. Now rerun the analysis with a $U(0, 10)$ prior for σ_g and normal priors for the βs, with precision 0.01 and the same means. Note that we believe these would be poor choices for reasons given in the prior specification section. What do you notice about the new analysis? (Be warned that the code takes about 2 minutes per thousand iterations.) Finally, make basic inferences using the output.
(b) Now modify the code to obtain estimates of abortion probabilities for "typical" herds, by which we mean herds that correspond to all combinations of (GR, DO), with GR taking values $(2, 4, 6)$ and DO taking values $(60, 116, 120)$. (Keep in mind that these values will need to be standardized if modifying code on the book's website; you would use the means `meangr = 3.485024` and `meando = 115.842` and standard deviations `stdgr = 1.517102` and `stddo = 59.72637`.) Make an appropriate table and make appropriate additional inferences to those made in part (a). The additional inferences should include inferences for effect modification, still for "typical" cows.
(c) Revise your program to make inferences for odds ratios to assess whether the effect of DO is modified by GR. Create an appropriate table.
(d) Using results in parts (a)–(c), address the question of whether the interaction effect is statistically important and practically important.
(e) Modify your program yet again, now to obtain predictive probabilities for cows with specified values for $sGR = 0$ and $sDO = 0$, where these future cows will be from herds $1, 2, \ldots, 9$. That is, make inferences from the predictive probabilities $P(Y_f = 1 \mid sDO = sGR = 0, \gamma_i)$, $i = 1, \ldots, 9$. Comment on how these probabilities vary across herds. Which herds have the best and worst "management policies"?
(f) Modify your program to use the standard parameterization in which the latent effects are centered at zero. Include the intercept in the regression part of the model. Run this program with two chains for around 1,000 iterations and look at

convergence properties of the two chains. What do you notice? The Markov chains for all variables except the random effects will have the same stationary distribution as in part (a). Centering as in part (a) often results in better-behaved chains.

EXERCISE 14.13.   The development surrounding equation (14.11) led to the choice of the informative $Ga(a, b)$ prior for σ_γ.

(a) Using this same development, what would you specify as a prior guess for τ_g, say $\tau_{0\gamma}$?

(b) Now obtain an informative $Ga(a, b)$ prior for τ_γ, where here we specify $P(\theta_{0.9} > \theta_{0.9l}) = 0.95$ instead of $P(\theta_{0.9} < \theta_{0.9u}) = 0.95$. Given the elicited value $\theta_{0.9l}$, our expert is 95% certain that $\theta_{0.9}$ will exceed $\theta_{0.9l}$, giving us a probabilistic lower limit on what the 90th percentile of probabilities could be. In this same context, recall that our best guess for $\beta_1 + \tilde{x}'\beta^*$ is $\text{logit}(\theta_0)$, where we often set $\tilde{x} = 0$ to correspond to a "typical" predictor combination, provided continuous variates are standardized. Find the value for $\tau_{0.95}$, the 95th percentile of the $Ga(a, b)$ distribution, using this information. Then, with the mode $\tau_{0\gamma} = (a - 1)/b$, explain how to find the value of b so that the $Ga(a, b)$ distribution has mode $\tau_{0\gamma}$ and 95th percentile $\tau_{0.95}$.

(c) Consider the cow abortion data scenario. Suppose that $\tilde{x} = 0$ and $\gamma = \beta_0$, so that the corresponding θ is the probability of abortion corresponding to a typical cow in a typical herd. Your best guess for θ is $\theta_0 = 0.15$, and you are 80% certain that $\theta_{0.9}$ is in the interval $(0.05, 0, 25)$. Obtain informative gamma priors for τ_γ and σ_γ using this information.

EXERCISE 14.14.   Consider the cow abortion data in Example 14.6.

(a) Find an informative gamma prior for σ_γ that takes account of the elicited information that $\theta_0 = 0.12$ (best guess for the probability of abortion with $sGR = 0 = sDO$), $u_{0.9} = 0.20$ (best guess for 90th percentile of probabilities of abortion across herds for cows with $sGR = 0 = sDO$), and $\theta_{0.9u} = 0.24$ (95% certainty that 90th percentile of such probabilities is less than 0.24).

(b) Find a uniform prior for σ_γ that corresponds to $\theta_{\max} = 0.3$.

EXERCISE 14.15.   Consider the prior and centering specified for the cow abortion data (Example 14.6). Write the explicit form of the full conditional distributions for β_1, β^*, and γ. (You may wish to look at the code on the book's website for that example to see the precise prior distributions.)

*EXERCISE 14.16.   Consider the cow abortion data (Example 14.6). Assume that the prior guess for the probability of abortion for an average cow in a typical herd is 0.12, as it was there. Also assume that Dr. Thurmond is 95% certain that this probability is less than 0.15.

(a) Obtain a prior on β_1 based on specifying a $Be(a_1, b_1)$ prior for the probability of abortion for a typical herd with standardized DO and GR both equal to zero.

(b) Assume the prior specification for β_1 in (a) and an independent $Be(a_2, b_2)$ prior distribution for the probability of abortion for a typical herd with $DO = \text{mean}(DO)$

and $GR = 4$, so that $sDO = 0$ and $sGR = (4 - \text{mean}(GR))/\text{sd}(GR)$. Further, assume that the best guess for this probability is 0.16 and that Dr. Thurmond is 95% certain that this probability is less than 0.20. Simulate the induced joint prior for (β_1, β_2) and plot smoothed histograms for the two marginals.

(c) Obtain the analytical expression for the induced joint prior for (β_1, β_2).

(d) Repeat (a)–(c) using logit-normal distributions instead of beta distributions.

*EXERCISE 14.17. Suppose that you have specified a $Ga(a, b)$ prior for $\sigma_\gamma = 1/\sqrt{\tau_\gamma}$ but that your program for performing your own Gibbs sampler has been written for a gamma prior for τ_γ.

(a) How might you use the prior information that you elicited and still use your code?

(b) Suppose your original prior was $\sigma_\gamma \sim Ga(3, 2)$. How well do you think your method in (a) would work with this prior?

EXERCISE 14.18. Recall the analysis of the IL-1β data using model (14.19). (The data and example programs can be found on the book's website for this chapter. The files include **IL-1beta** in their names.)

(a) Reproduce the results of Example 14.8. You may wish to modify one of the programs on the book's website or write your own program.

(b) Perform a sensitivity analysis. What do you notice? (You may wish to look at the prior specifications for **beta[1]**, **sig**, and **sigg** in the available programs.)

(c) The variable **ID[ ]** identifies the 30 distinct individuals in the data. Each individual gets his or her own latent effect. Modify your program to infer the predictive distribution for a new individual. That is, model y_f using γ_{31}, or **gam[31]** in your program. (As we pointed out at the end of Example 14.8, the data are untransformed and we model them as log-normal in our programs. The analysis is equivalent to transforming the data and then modeling the log-transformed data as normal.)

EXERCISE 14.19. *Dental data.* Write a program or use one of the programs available on the book's website to analyze the dental data (Example 14.9). (See the book's website for the data and sample program files. The files' names include **dental** in them.) Use the prior specified for the dental data in Example 14.9 and do this in the two ways discussed in that example. In one of the ways, you must find the precision matrix in terms of $(\sigma_{1g}, \sigma_{2g}, \rho_g)$. In the other way, you will program the model described in expression (14.23) and the paragraph preceding these equations.

EXERCISE 14.20.

(a) Either use code from the previous exercise or write a program to analyze the dental data using the priors that were given in Example 14.9. Then perform a sensitivity analysis.

(b) Now expand the model to include an interaction term between *Male* and *Age*. Analyze the data and make inferences for the interaction term. Decide whether the interaction term belongs in the model.

(c) Reanalyze the dental data assuming independence between the intercept and slope latent effects. Compare the analysis with that of part (a). Comment on whether or not an interaction term would be needed in this model.

EXERCISE 14.21. Derive formulas for the variance of Y_{ij} and the covariance between Y_{ij} and Y_{ik} under the random intercepts and slopes model (14.22). Assume that $sAge_{ij} = 0$ and $sAge_{ik} = x$. What can you say about the correlation as x increases?

EXERCISE 14.22. The IL-1β data using model (14.24) with autoregressive correlation structure (14.25) were analyzed using code on the book's website with the name `Interleukin-CSAR`. Results were presented in Table 14.9. Revise the code so that you can estimate autocorrelations between observations that are $1, 2, \ldots, 5$ years apart using equation (14.26).

(a) Run the modified code and monitor convergence using multiple chains. Discuss.
(b) Perform a sensitivity analysis. Discuss.
(c) Modify the same code to analyze the data without the Gaussian process part of the model, which leads to model (14.19). Reproduce the boxplots in Figure 14.8 using R.

EXERCISE 14.23. Establish the formula in equation (14.26) and give formulas for the first three autocorrelations.

Chapter 15

Diagnostic Tests

Diagnosis is an extremely important part of medical practice. Proper diagnosis will help determine the best course of treatment. Physicians are often faced with a patient who presents with a collection of symptoms and who has responded to questions related to them. It is routine for a physician to attempt to make a diagnosis as to what disease or disorder might be associated with these symptoms. In many instances, the physician will not have enough input to make a diagnosis with a high degree of certainty without obtaining additional diagnostic information. Blood and urine are often analyzed to provide such information.

For example, a patient may present with the symptoms "thick, cloudy or bloody discharge from the penis or vagina" and "pain or burning sensation when urinating." There are other symptoms that could be present as well, but it is likely with these symptoms that either a blood or urine test or both would be made to see if the etiologic or infective agent, *Neisseria gonorrhoeae*, could be detected. This agent is the cause of the disease known as gonorrhea. On the other hand, if a patient has detected a lump in her breast, she would likely make an appointment to determine if the lump is suspicious and possibly malignant. If it seems suspicious on physical exam, the patient may undergo a mammogram, and if still uncertain about the nature of the lump, there may be a biopsy of the lump.

If the outcome of analyses of blood, urine, a mammogram, or a biopsy is a "yes," or "no," or a "maybe," then the procedure used to produce the result is called a *diagnostic test*. It is often the case that such tests are designed to result in simply yes or no binary outcomes. A key feature of binary diagnostic tests is that they are seldom 100% accurate. Even in the absence of the condition, a test might say "yes." Similarly, a test may incorrectly declare "no" when the condition is present. When a diagnostic test is perfect, it is often termed a "gold standard" test.

A procedure that ultimately results in a yes or no outcome for some infection or disease may be based on a single assay. For example, a physician may rely on a blood test in the absence of other testing. Alternatively, the diagnostic process may proceed in steps that involve a sequence of yes, no or maybe outcomes before one reaches a final definitive outcome, as would be the case with breast cancer. We call the diagnostic process a *protocol*, whether the process consists of a single assay or a sequence of steps. True gold standard tests often do not really exist. For example, a routine mammogram may not detect a cancerous growth at an early stage, in which case a more definitive biopsy would not be performed. Moreover, a blood test for something like human immunodeficiency virus (HIV) may not detect the virus if it has only been present for a short period of time. Early stages of any infection or disease are often very difficult to detect. In addition, protocols designed to detect an infection may react to some benign biological agent as if it were the infective agent under scrutiny, even though it is not. This is called "cross-reactivity" and results in positive ("yes") outcomes when the infective agent is not present.

A biomarker is a numerical outcome that is based on a measurement of a biological substance that is associated with a particular disease or infection. Most biomarkers may reasonably be regarded as continuous, with higher values indicating a greater chance of the condition being present.

We often use a threshold value of a continuous biomarker, forming a dichotomy. If a patient's biomarker exceeds a cutoff, c, the patient is presumed to have the condition, and if the value is less than c, they are deemed not to have it. The cutoff is selected to optimize the relative costs of a false positive declaration, as when the biomarker exceeds c but patient is healthy, versus a false negative determination. The larger the value of c is, the lower the chance of a false positive and the higher the risk of a false negative declaration. The relationships are reversed for smaller values of c.

Many diagnostic outcomes are indeed yes or no from the outset. For example, a microscopic examination involves looking for an infectious organism with a microscope. The examiner either sees the organism in the material being inspected (possibly stool, urine, or blood) or they do not. Another example is a colonoscopy. If the gastroenterologist fails to see anything suspicious, the result is negative. If the examination identifies something suspicious, the result is "maybe," in which case there is a follow-up procedure and submission of suspicious materials (often polyps) for analysis and a determination of whether or not the disease is present.

The first part of this chapter will deal with binary diagnostic tests under a variety of circumstances. For example, the diagnostic protocol may only involve a single dichotomous outcome (perhaps based on a sequence of single tests). There may instead be more than one protocol, resulting in two or more single-outcome tests. For example, one test may involve a microscopic examination and the other a blood biomarker that has been dichotomized. From a scientific point of view, interest may focus on which test is preferable. If one of the tests has smaller false positive and false negative rates, then it would surely be preferable, unless it was much more costly, in which case that aspect would need to be taken into consideration.

For the sake of brevity in an already long book, we have decided to omit discussion of having multiple biomarkers and situations where a gold standard test does not exist or is too expensive to use for routine diagnosis. We give references to these materials in the recap and readings section at the end of this chapter.

The second part of the chapter deals with biomarkers that are regarded as continuous. In this part of the chapter, we discuss what are called receiver operating characteristic (ROC) curves. Investigators use ROC curves to determine where to place the threshold for declaring the presence or absence of a condition. These curves provide a way to trade off false positive and false negative rates. We also show how diagnosis can be accomplished using the biomarkers without the use of arbitrary cutoff values as in the traditional way. Instead, one obtains a predictive probability of disease and uses this probability as a criterion. We also discuss ROC regression in which covariate information can be used to help with diagnosis in various ways.

15.1 Basics of Diagnosis with One Imperfect Binary Test and with Available Gold Standard Information

Let T refer to the outcome of a diagnostic test that yields a binary outcome, possibly after comparing a continuous marker to some accepted diagnostic threshold. The two outcomes are defined to be $T+$ and $T-$, with $T+$ indicating that the characteristic is present, and $T-$ that it is absent. Notation for the characteristic actually being present is $D+$. We indicate the absence of the condition as $D-$. Just because the test indicates $T+$ or $T-$ does not necessarily prove the presence or absence of the characteristic. As part of developing a diagnostic test for use, research studies determine the test's characteristics relating to its accuracy.

Test accuracies are defined as the proportions of time the test correctly declares $D+$ and $D-$. These proportions are defined to be

$$Se = P(T+ \mid D+) \quad \text{and} \quad Sp = P(T- \mid D-),$$

which are called the *sensitivity* and *specificity* of test T, respectively. The false positive and false negative error rates are

$$P(FP) = P(T+ \mid D-) = 1 - Sp \quad \text{and} \quad P(FN) = P(T- \mid D+) = 1 - Se.$$

If $Se = Sp = 1$, there is no chance of error. In this instance, the test is deemed to be perfect and is often called a gold standard (GS) test or a perfect reference standard test. The term "reference standard" refers to a primary use of such a test to assess the quality of another test that is likely imperfect. This chapter focuses to a large extent on assessing the quality of various tests, both when a GS test is available and when one is not.

Gold standard tests are not necessarily easy to develop and are often quite expensive. It is easily the case that a sequential protocol of the type described for breast cancer screening can result in a final definitive correct outcome. Such protocols are often invasive and/or expensive, as in the case of performing a breast biopsy after a mammogram. When testing for HIV infection, one initially performs a relatively inexpensive but imperfect enzyme-linked immunosorbent assay (ELISA) test. If the outcome is positive, one carries out an expensive western blot test (possibly several of them) until the diagnosis is definitive. Even so, this protocol cannot result in a GS test, because if the ELISA test is negative, the sample unit being tested could still be $D+$, resulting in a false negative outcome.

For now, we assume that a GS test is available, or that by some other means it is possible to know if certain individuals are $D+$ or $D-$. Suppose we have a random sample of n_1 individuals known to be $D+$ and an independent random sample of n_2 individuals known to be $D-$. This is often termed a "training sample." In addition, we apply a suitable test (T) to all individuals for diagnosing $D+$ or $D-$. The outcome for each sample is the number of $T+$ and $T-$ individuals. Let Y_1 be the number of positive outcomes $(T+)$ in the sample of individuals known to be $D+$, and let Y_2 be the number of negative outcomes $(T-)$ in the $D-$ sample. With $Se = P(T+ \mid D+)$ and $Sp = P(T- \mid D-)$,

$$Y_1 \mid Se \sim Bin(n_1, Se), \quad Y_2 \mid Sp \sim Bin(n_2, Sp).$$

We place independent beta priors on Se and Sp, which results in independent beta posteriors for the test accuracies. Statistical inferences are easily obtained using the methods we have already developed in the book.

Alternatively, we could take a random sample of size n from a population that includes both $D+$ and $D-$ individuals. This design is termed "cross-sectional sampling." If a GS test is available in addition to a presumably imperfect test T that has sensitivity Se and specificity Sp, we could apply both tests to all n individuals. Table 15.1 depicts the outcomes from such as study. We can summarize the data with a 2×2 multinomial table of counts, $y = \{y_{ij} : i, j = 0, 1\}$. In Table 15.1, y_{11} is the number of true positive individuals in the sample, y_{10} is the number of false positive outcomes, y_{01} is the number of false negatives, and y_{00} is the number of true negatives. These counts must add to n, the total sample size.

TABLE 15.1: Cross-classification of test outcomes

	$D+$	$D-$	Row sum
$T+$	y_{11}	y_{10}	y_{1+}
$T-$	y_{01}	y_{00}	y_{0+}
Col. Sum	y_{+1}	y_{+0}	n

The column totals give the number of $D+$ and $D-$ individuals, and the row totals give the number of $T+$ and $T-$ individuals. The natural or empirical estimates of the sensitivity and specificity are $\widehat{Se} = y_{11}/y_{+1}$ and $\widehat{Sp} = y_{00}/y_{+0}$, respectively. $\widehat{Se}$ is just the sample proportion of known $D+$ individuals that test positive $(T+)$, and $\widehat{Sp}$ is just the sample proportion of known $D-$ individuals that the test says are negative $(T-)$.

In order to make Bayesian inferences, we need prior distributions. For the sensitivity and specificity, we assume independent beta priors as before. Now the probability model for the data will also depend on the prevalence, $\pi = P(D+)$. We place yet another independent beta prior on π.

We need to specify the likelihood function to proceed further. We define the matrix of probabilities $p = \{p_{ij} : i, j = 0, 1\}$, where

$$p_{11} = P(T+, D+) = P(D+)P(T+ \mid D+) = \pi Se,$$
$$p_{01} = P(T-, D+) = P(D+)P(T- \mid D+) = \pi(1 - Se),$$
$$p_{10} = P(T+, D-) = P(D-)P(T+ \mid D-) = (1 - \pi)(1 - Sp),$$
$$p_{00} = P(T-, D-) = P(D-)P(T- \mid D-) = (1 - \pi)Sp.$$

We write p in tabular form in Table 15.2. The distribution of the data is $Y \mid p \sim Mult_4(n, p)$.

TABLE 15.2: Joint outcome probabilities

	$D+$	$D-$	Row sum
$T+$	$p_{11} = \pi Se$	$p_{10} = (1 - \pi)(1 - Sp)$	$p_{1+} = P(T+)$
$T-$	$p_{01} = \pi(1 - Se)$	$p_{00} = (1 - \pi)Sp$	$p_{0+} = P(T-)$
Col. sum	$p_{+1} = \pi$	$p_{+0} = 1 - \pi$	1

Under multinomial sampling, every entry in the table and every marginal total has a binomial distribution. For example, $Y_{+1} \mid \pi \sim Bin(n, \pi)$ and $Y_{11} \mid \pi, Se \sim Bin(n, \pi Se)$. Also, the multinomial likelihood after simplification is

$$Lik(\pi, Se, Sp) \propto [\pi Se]^{y_{11}} [\pi(1 - Se)]^{y_{01}} [(1 - \pi)(1 - Sp)]^{y_{10}} [(1 - \pi)Sp]^{y_{00}}$$
$$= \pi^{y_{+1}} (1 - \pi)^{y_{+0}} Se^{y_{11}} (1 - Se)^{y_{01}} Sp^{y_{00}} (1 - Sp)^{y_{10}}. \tag{15.1}$$

Observe that the maximum likelihood estimate of the prevalence is just the sample proportion of $D+$ individuals, for the sensitivity it is the proportion of $D+$ samples that are $T+$, and for specificity it is the proportion of $D-$ samples that are $T-$. Clearly, with independent beta priors for the three model parameters, the joint posterior consists of independent beta distributions. We leave it as an exercise to show this fact.

Before we consider an example, we briefly discuss some additional parameters of interest. We actually discussed this same problem from a more elementary point of view in Chapter 3. If an individual has just tested $T+$ for some affliction, they will likely be interested to know whether the they actually have the condition. That is, they want to know their positive predictive value (PPV), namely

$$PPV = P(D+ \mid T+) = \frac{\pi Se}{\pi Se + (1 - \pi)(1 - Sp)}.$$

Similarly, if they have just tested negative, they may be interested to know if they might, in fact, be $D+$, that is,

$$P(D+ \mid T-) = \frac{\pi(1 - Se)}{\pi(1 - Se) + (1 - \pi)Sp} = 1 - NPV,$$

where NPV, the negative predictive value, is the probability of being $D-$ given that you tested $T-$. Although it is more common to report NPV, it may be of greater interest to know the chance that one is $D+$ given that one tested $T-$. We model our uncertainty about the estimates of prevalence and the test accuracies (Sp and Se) with independent beta priors, which leaves us in a position to make realistic inferences that reflect all uncertainty about unknown inputs.

Example 15.1. The cross-classified multinomial data presented in Table 15.3, taken from Weiner (1979) and Pepe (2004) [350, 258], are based on a sample of 1,465 men who were suspected to be suffering from coronary artery disease (CAD). Each man was subjected to an imperfect exercise-based stress test, EST, and to arteriography, which is a method of perfectly determining whether or not coronary heart disease is present. Maximum likelihood estimates are

$$\widehat{Se} = 815/1023 = 0.80, \quad \widehat{Sp} = 327/442 = 0.74, \quad \hat{\pi} = 1023/1465 = 0.70,$$
$$\widehat{PPV} = 815/930 = 0.88, \quad \widehat{NPV} = 327/535 = 0.61.$$

Since the study involved a sample of men "at risk," the estimate of prevalence may not be of much interest for use in the general population. We leave it as an exercise to give a Bayesian analysis of these data.

TABLE 15.3: Cross-classification of EST by disease status

	$CAD+$	$CAD-$	Row sum
$EST+$	815	115	930
$EST-$	208	327	535
Col. sum	1,023	442	1,465

The next situation we consider is one in which there is partial verification of an initial but imperfect test's outcome results. Suppose that one applies test T for a particular infection in a sample of "units." If the outcome of the initial test on a unit is $T+$, the unit will undergo further testing with a perfect test; if the outcome is $T-$, no retesting is done. This is actually the standard protocol for HIV testing of blood donated for transfusion. Of course, if your blood test outcome were positive, you would want to know whether or not you were actually infected. Generally, a relatively inexpensive and highly accurate but imperfect ELISA test is applied to blood donors as an initial screening test. Units that test positive with ELISA ($ELISA+$) are retested with a western blot (WB) test. Regardless of the outcome of the retest, the blood is discarded. If the outcome is $ELISA-$, the blood is then available for transfusion. We do not know the actual status of the units that are $ELISA-$, only that they are negative by the test. It would be incredibly expensive to apply the WB test to all donated units. Moreover, it would be anticipated that the NPV would be close to 1, indicating that most of the ELISA negatives would indeed be disease free. Thus it is generally the case that $ELISA-$ units are not retested. Table 15.4 is a representation of data of this type.

TABLE 15.4: Cross-classification of test outcomes when $T-$ outcomes are not verified with a gold-standard test

	$D+$	$D-$	Row sum
$T+$	y_{11}	y_{10}	y_{1+}
$T-$	NA	NA	y_{0+}
Col. sum	y_{+1}	y_{+0}	n

Suppose we wish to estimate Se and Sp for the ELISA test that is used for testing for HIV infection. Our discussion here applies to generic tests, T, under similar circumstances. In such situations, a random sample of size n units from the population of interest is taken, and all units undergo testing with test T. Let y be the number out of n that are $T+$ and $n - y$ the number that are $T-$. We have $Y \mid \pi, Se, Sp \sim Bin\,(n, P(T+))$, where $P(T+) = P(T+, D+) + P(T+, D-) = \pi Se + (1 - \pi)(1 - Sp)$. Suppose that incorrectly classifying a $D+$ unit as $D-$ might be dangerous or costly. This is certainly the case when testing for HIV since, if an $HIV+$ sample is not detected, the individual involved may not get appropriate treatment and they may infect other individuals unknowingly.

Under the above circumstances, we would surely also be interested in estimating $PPV = P(D+ \mid T+) = \pi Se / [\pi Se + (1 - \pi)(1 - Sp)]$. It is easy to show that PPV is monotone and increasing in Se and in Sp, and that PPV increases to 1 as Sp increases to 1. The false negative rate is $P(D+ \mid T-) = 1 - NPV = \pi(1 - Se) / [\pi(1 - Se) + (1 - \pi)Sp]$. We see that $1 - NPV$ decreases to 0 as Se increases to 1. Therefore, in order to protect the blood supply, it is clearly important to have a very high sensitivity for the ELISA test. Also, for the sake of a person who tests positive by ELISA, it is most important to have a high-quality follow-up test.

Looking at Table 15.4, we see that the counts y_{01} and y_{00} are missing but their sum is available. The data are still multinomial but now there are only three cell probabilities in the multinomial sampling distribution instead of four as in Table 15.1. Now, $Y \mid p_{11}, p_{10}, p_{0+} \sim Mult_3(n, \{p_{11}, p_{10}, p_{0+}\})$. The corresponding likelihood is

$$Lik(\pi, Se, Sp) \propto \pi^{y_{11}}(1 - \pi)^{y_{10}} Se^{y_{11}}(1 - Sp)^{y_{10}} [\pi(1 - Se) + (1 - \pi)Sp]^{y_{0+}}. \quad (15.2)$$

It is clear that the joint posterior will not be recognizable with this likelihood, but we can still carry out Bayesian inference, especially with an iterative computational approach like MCMC.

Example 15.2. UK HIV Data. We consider HIV test data for blood donors from the UK that were previously analyzed by Johnson and Gastwirth (1991) [187]. The data were collected in 1986 with $n = 3{,}122{,}556$ samples that were tested using a Welcome ELISA. Among these samples were $y_{+1} = 373$ positive outcomes that were retested with a western blot test (WB); 64 of those were positive. This results in $y_{11} = 64$ true positives, $y_{10} = 373 - 64 = 312$ false positives, and $y_{+0} = 3{,}122{,}183$ negative outcomes. We encourage the reader to see Gastwirth and Johnson (1990) [122] and Johnson and Gastwirth (1991) [187] for considerable discussion about prior specification.

We selected the main prior used in [187] for our illustration here. We specified $\pi \sim Beta(15, 94092)$, $Se \sim Beta(142, 2)$, and $Sp \sim Beta(1363, 3)$. The prior on π has median 0.00016, and 99th percentile 0.00027, reflecting the belief that the prevalence of HIV in blood donors in the UK in 1986 was quite small, but that we are still relatively uncertain about how small. The median and first percentile for the prior on Se are 0.988 and 0.954, respectively. Thus, we are 99% sure that the ELISA Se is greater than 0.95. The median and first percentile for Sp are 0.998 and 0.995, respectively.

Output from our data analysis is presented in Table 15.5 using our specified prior, prior 1 in the table, and a much less informative prior, prior 2. (The data and programs for these analyses are available in the Chapter 15 section of the book's website. The file names include HIV.) Note that with both priors, the precision for the ELISA Sp is incredible and the same. The results for Sp suggest that we would only expect to see between 8 and 12 false positives per 100,000 HIV tests, with 99.8% certainty. In addition, the prevalence of HIV in the sampled population is expected to be between about 2 and 3 individuals per 100,000 tested, with 95% certainty. Perhaps most importantly, if we consider blood units that have tested $ELISA-$, then we expect between 4 or 5 and 110 out of every 100 million blood units that have passed through the system to carry HIV positive blood. All of these results are virtually the same under both priors.

TABLE 15.5: Posterior inferences for UK HIV data. PM=posterior median. (PI) = probability interval. Prior 1: $\pi \sim Be(15, 94092)$, $Se \sim Be(142, 2)$, $Sp \sim Be(1363, 3)$. Prior 2: $\pi \sim Be(0.5, 99.5)$, $Se \sim Be(142, 2)$, $Sp \sim Be(13.6, 0.03)$.

	Prior 1		Prior 2	
	PM	(PI)	PM	(PI)
Se	0.987	$(0.958, 0.998)$	0.988	$(0.962, 0.998)$
Sp^*	0.99990	$(0.99988, 0.99992)$	0.99990	$(0.99988, 0.99992)$
π $(\times 10^{-5})$	2.48	$(1.97, 3.08)$	2.49	$(1.97, 3.11)$
PPV	0.20	$(0.16, 0.24)$	0.20	$(0.16, 0.24)$
$(1 - NPV)^*$	0.0316	$(0.0045, 0.1098)$	0.0310	$(0.0043, 0.1079)$

*PIs are 99.8%, all other intervals are 95%.

Before finishing the data analysis, we need to discuss results that were developed in [122] and [187]. They investigated the HIV testing problem discussed here from a theoretical standpoint. They assumed the generic situation with a large sample size n, with a low prevalence disease, and where available tests would have high accuracy, which is clearly the case in the current illustration. They also assumed that with a Beta(a, b) prior for π, the parameter a would be considerably smaller than b, with a Beta(a_1, b_1) prior for Se, a_1 would be considerably larger than b_1, and that with a Beta(a_2, b_2) prior for Sp, a_2 would be considerably larger than b_2. Under these assumptions, they showed that the approximate posterior for Se would be the prior for Se. Their approximation to the posterior for Se is $Se \mid y \overset{.}{\sim} Be(142, 2)$ in the case of both priors discussed here. The results for Se in Table 15.5 show very close similarity under both priors 1 and 2 since the marginal priors for Se are the same. When we analyzed these data with a $U(0.9, 1.0)$ prior for Se, we noted in a plot of the posterior for Se that it was precisely the same as the prior.

Recall that we essentially have a missing-data problem here, since we only observe the marginal total of the number that test negative. Instead of a multinomial of dimension 4, we only have dimension 3. Since the sum of the multinomial counts must be n, we went from having three bits of information for estimating three parameters to having only two bits of information for estimating three parameters. Something had to give, and here, while it was not obvious until now, we find that we have no information in the data for estimating Se.

In addition, [187] showed that, under the low prevalence, high accuracy, large sample assumptions, we have

$$\begin{aligned}
\pi \mid y &\overset{.}{\sim} Be(a + y_{11}, b + y_{0+}), \quad Sp \mid y \overset{.}{\sim} Be(a2 + y_{0+}, b2 + y_{10}), \\
PPV \mid y &\overset{.}{\sim} \pi(1 - Se)\mid y, \quad (1 - NPV) \mid y \overset{.}{\sim} \pi/(\pi + 1 - Sp)\mid y,
\end{aligned} \tag{15.3}$$

where the notation $\overset{.}{\sim}$ means "is distributed approximately as." We carried out an analysis in which we calculated these approximations. We found them to be highly accurate, meaning that results using them were virtually identical to the results using no approximation. In addition, we can infer that there is information in the data and the prior for Sp and π, which implies there is also information in the data for NPV under our assumptions. Since there is no information in the data for Se, it is clear that the PPV will be highly affected by the choice of prior for Se.

As a final note on this example, our Bayesian analysis gave 0.9999 for the posterior mean of Sp and all three quantiles $(0.025, 0.5, 0.975)$. We used the beta approximation given in expression (15.3) in R to obtain the 99.8% PIs given in Table 15.5.

15.2   Continuous Biomarkers

We now focus on biomarkers that are continuous. In previous sections we considered continuous biomarkers that had been dichotomized (think ELISA) and others that were actually dichotomous, as in the case of microscopy where one either sees the "organism" or not. For those biomarkers that were continuous, someone decided on a cutoff that turned the outcome into a binary biomarker. Let y be the outcome of a continuous biomarker and suppose that large values of y are associated with an individual having the infection of interest. One might select a value, say k, and give the diagnosis $T+$ if $y \geq k$ and $T-$ if $y < k$. For any particular choice of k, we have $Se(k) = P(Y \geq k \mid D+)$ and $Sp(k) = P(Y < k \mid D-)$.

Figure 15.1 displays density functions for a biomarker's distribution in the $D-$ and $D+$ populations. We see that the area to the right of k under the density function for individuals in the diseased or infected group is $Se(k)$, and the area to the left of k under the density function for healthy individuals is $Sp(k)$. Observe that as $Sp(k)$ increases, $Se(k)$ decreases, and vice versa. Thus, a value of k that results in a good sensitivity may also result in a poor specificity.

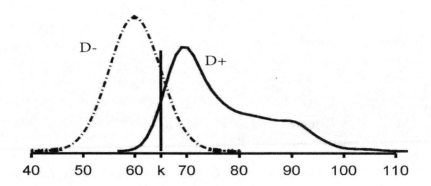

FIGURE 15.1: Possible distributions for a continuous biomarker applied to $D-$ and $D+$ individuals with hypothetical cutoff value k.

How should we select the value of k if we are dichotomizing a continuous biomarker? If we assessed the costs or losses associated with misclassifications, we could develop a decision rule that would choose the value of k that minimizes the expected loss. A simple approach would assign a loss of zero to a correct classification (e.g., $T+$ if $D+$ is the true state) and a non-zero loss for each misclassification (e.g., $T+$ when $D-$ is the true state). The expected loss would be a weighted average of the false negative and false positive losses, where the weights are the probabilities of making the respective misclassifications. We compute these misclassification probabilities based on the underlying probability model, which provides the sensitivity and specificity for any cutoff k. The goal is to find a decision rule that makes this loss small. In general, we will simply take the posterior mean of this quantity for as many rules we wish to consider (e.g., on a grid of possible biomarker cutoffs k) and then select the rule k^*, say, with the smallest value.

Less formally, we will consider the tradeoffs involved in considering estimates of the pairs $(1 - Sp(k), Se(k)) \equiv (FP(k), TP(k))$ for all possible choices of k. The ideal cutoff would yield the value $(0, 1)$, but this would imply that there was a GS test, which is rarely going to be the case. In general, we want $FP(k)$ to be small, and $TP(k)$ to be large. Cutoffs are generally selected by scientists who weigh the benefits and risks associated with having larger Se versus smaller Sp and vice versa.

15.2.1   Receiver Operating Characteristic Curves

A plot of $FP(k)$ versus $Se(k)$ across all possible values of k is called a receiver operating characteristic (ROC) curve. An example of such a plot is given in Figure 15.2. We now discuss how to model continuous biomarker data and how to estimate ROC curves.

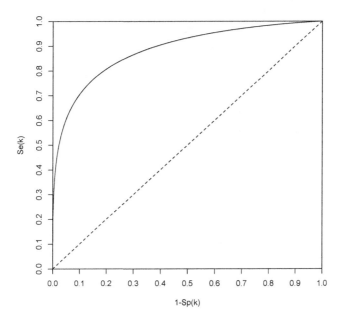

FIGURE 15.2: Plot of ROC curve (solid) with 45-degree line (dashed).

For any cutoff k, a major criterion for a useful biomarker is that $TP(k) = Se(k) = P(Y > k \mid D+) > P(Y > k \mid D-) = FP(k)$. We only consider biomarkers for which ROC curves are above the 45-degree line from $(0,0)$ to $(1,1)$ in the plot given in Figure 15.2. Since ideal ROC curves tend to increase rapidly from $(0,0)$ up to the upper left-hand corner, $(0,1)$, of this plot, the area under the curve (AUC) can be used to determine how useful the biomarker y might be for accurately classifying an individual or diagnosing a condition. If the curve is the 45-degree line, AUC $= 0.5$. If we were to simply toss a coin to decide $T+$ or $T-$ for each value of k, we would have $P(T+ \mid D+, k) = P(T- \mid D-, k) = 0.5$. The ROC curve for this classifier would simply be the 45-degree line and would of course be useless. On the other hand, a perfect classifier would have AUC $= 1$. A perfect classifier can only occur if the support of the biomarker for healthy individuals is (virtually) completely separate from the support for the infected or diseased individuals. AUCs that are close to 1 are indicative of good classifiers, and AUCs near 0.5 indicate poor accuracy for any k.

We need models for $Y \mid D+$ and for $Y \mid D-$. We begin with generic parametric models. Let $Y \mid D+, \theta_1 \sim G_1$, where $G_1(\cdot)$ is a cdf with pdf $g_1(\cdot \mid \theta_1)$, and $Y \mid$

$D-, \theta_0 \sim G_0(\cdot)$ where $G_0(\cdot)$ is a cdf with pdf $g_0(\cdot \mid \theta_0)$. We drop the dependence of the cdfs on parameters for convenience. Survival curves, which are defined as 1 minus the cdf of the associated random variable, are discussed in Chapter 11. Here we define the corresponding survival curves for the cdfs G_0 and G_1 as $S_0(t) = 1 - G_0(t) = P(Y > t \mid D-)$ and $S_1(t) = 1 - G_1(t) = P(Y > t \mid D+)$. Our goal is to obtain an equivalent way of expressing $(TP(k), FP(k))$ by a change of variables, so that the new expression gives the same ROC curve. Almost immediately, we will have a simple expression for the AUC as well.

Consider the change of variables $FP(k) = S_0(k) = t$. Then $k = S_0^{-1}(t)$ and $Se(k) = S_1(k) = S_1[S_0^{-1}(t)]$. Define

$$ROC(t) = S_1[S_0^{-1}(t)]. \tag{15.4}$$

Then the plot of $(S_0(k), S_1(k))$ for all k is our definition of the ROC curve, and this is precisely the same plot as for $(t, ROC(t))$ over all $t \in (0,1)$. Since, in general, $k \in (-\infty, \infty)$, the latter plot is much simpler.

By definition,

$$AUC = \int_0^1 ROC(t)dt = \int_0^1 S_1[S_0^{-1}(t)]dt = \int_{-\infty}^{\infty} S_1(v)g_0(v)dv$$

after changing variables to $v = S_0^{-1}(t)$, which implies that $t = S_0(v)$ and $dt = -g_0(v)dv$. This is just the probability that a biomarker response for a $D+$ individual exceeds an independent biomarker response for a $D-$ individual. To see this, let $Y_1 \sim G_1$ be independent of $Y_0 \sim G_0$. Then

$$
\begin{aligned}
P(Y_1 > Y_0) &= \int_{-\infty}^{\infty} P(Y_1 > Y_0 \mid Y_0 = v)g_0(v)dv \\
&= \int_{-\infty}^{\infty} P(Y_1 > v)g_0(v)dv = \int_{-\infty}^{\infty} S_1(v)g_0(v)dv,
\end{aligned}
$$

where we have used the law of total probability and the independence of Y_1 and Y_0.

Example 15.3. Binormal Model. In this example, we assume that the pdfs g_0 and g_1 are normal. Thus we have that

$$Y_0 \mid D-, \mu_0, \sigma_0^2 \sim N(\mu_0, \sigma_0^2), \quad Y_1 \mid D+, \mu_1, \sigma_1^2 \sim N(\mu_1, \sigma_1^2)$$

independently. We are thus assuming that the continuous (biomarker) outcomes Y_0 and Y_1 are independent and normally distributed, conditional on disease status. This is often called the "binormal" distribution since the specification involves two normal distributions, one for each of two types of individual being sampled. The binormal distribution is illustrated in Figure 15.3.

Eventually, we will have either independent samples from these distributions if GS information is available, or a mixture of these distributions, where $\pi = P(D+)$ will be the mixing proportion. Moreover, it will often be the case that the actual biomarker outcomes are not normally distributed, but a transformation of them

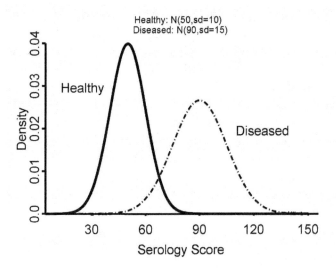

FIGURE 15.3: Binormal distribution.

might be reasonably approximated by a normal distribution. For now, we are simply interested in obtaining the ROC curve and AUC assuming binormality of the biomarker distribution.

Let $\Phi(\cdot)$ and $\phi(\cdot)$ denote the standard normal cdf and pdf, respectively. Then $g_0(y) \propto e^{-0.5(y-\mu_0)^2/\sigma_0^2} \propto \phi([y-\mu_0]/\sigma_0)$, and $g_1(y) \propto e^{-0.5(y-\mu_1)^2/\sigma_1^2} \propto \phi([y-\mu_1]/\sigma_1)$. Then

$$
\begin{aligned}
ROC(t) &= P(Y_1 > S_0^{-1}(t)) = P(Y_1 > G_0^{-1}(1-t)) \\
&= P(Y_1 > \mu_0 + \sigma_0 \Phi^{-1}(1-t)) \\
&= P([Y_1 - \mu_1]/\sigma_1 > [\mu_0 - \mu_1 + \sigma_0 \Phi^{-1}(1-t)]/\sigma_1) \\
&= 1 - \Phi(-a + b\Phi^{-1}(1-t)) \\
&= \Phi(a + b\Phi^{-1}(t)) \quad\quad\quad (15.5)
\end{aligned}
$$

where $a = (\mu_1 - \mu_0)/\sigma_1$ and $b = \sigma_0/\sigma_1$. Exercise 15.15 asks the reader to establish the details that have been skipped in this demonstration.

We move on to the AUC. We have $AUC = P(Y_1 > Y_0) = P(Y_1 - Y_0 > 0)$. But $Y_1 - Y_0 \sim N(\mu_1 - \mu_0, \sigma_1^2 + \sigma_0^2)$, so

$$
AUC = 1 - \Phi\left(\frac{-(\mu_1 - \mu_0)}{\sqrt{\sigma_1^2 + \sigma_0^2}}\right) = \Phi\left(\frac{\mu_1 - \mu_0}{\sqrt{\sigma_1^2 + \sigma_0^2}}\right) = \Phi\left(\frac{a}{\sqrt{1 + b^2}}\right). \quad (15.6)
$$

Thus the more separated the two distributions are, the larger the AUC and the better will be the accuracy of diagnosis using the given biomarker.

15.2.2 Diagnosis Based on Continuous Biomarkers

Dichotomizing continuous biomarkers involves a loss of information. Here we discuss an alternative method of diagnosis that uses the actual value of y that is observed.

Consider Figure 15.4, for example. We see four observed values of a biomarker y and a cutoff $k = 65$. We continue to think of larger values of y being associated with the disease state and smaller values being associated with the non-disease state. With the given cutoff 65, the individual with the value 64 is classified $T-$, while the much smaller value, 40, is also classified $T-$. The value 66 is classified $T+$, while the much larger value 110 is also classified $T+$. There is barely a distinction between 64 and 66, but there is a huge distinction between 40 and 110. Despite the relative nearness of 64 to 66, the use of a cutoff forces classification of individuals with marker values 64 and 66 to be classified the same way they would be if their markers were 40 and 110, respectively. One would expect that $P(D+ \mid y = 110) \gg P(D+ \mid y = 66) \doteq P(D+ \mid y = 64) \gg P(D+ \mid y = 40)$. Using the cutoff 65 to decide is quite blunt by comparison with what could be much more nuanced if the actual values were used for diagnosis.

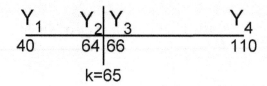

FIGURE 15.4: Dichotomizing a continuous biomarker.

The observed data for the classical problem of diagnosis with only two categories involves sampling two distinct populations of interest. The goal is to use the information in the samples to form a diagnostic rule for allocating each new individual with unknown population origin to one of the two. This is precisely what we have been talking about with the two categories (with or without the condition). R. A. Fisher tackled this problem decades ago with his development of discriminant analysis. Fisher considered the problem of sampling multivariate observations on individuals from two or more distinct populations. He cleverly devised statistical methodology for using the data to allocate individuals with unknown status to one of the populations. From this point of view, the collected data are called "training data." In light of our previous discussion, a training sample involves the ability to ascertain which individuals are infected and which are not through the use of some form of GS information. We assume the GS case. We briefly discuss the no-gold-standard (NGS) case in the recap and readings for this chapter.

Observed continuous biomarker data are represented as $y = \{y_{ij} : i = 0, 1; j = 1, \ldots, n_i\}$, where the index $i = 0$ corresponds to the sample of healthy individuals and $i = 1$ corresponds to infected or diseased individuals. While the y_{ij} can be multivariate, we only consider the univariate case. In the next section we assume binormality for the Y_{ij} when it is time to make statistical inferences.

Consider the generic parametric model for the biomarker data,

$$Y_{ij} \mid D+, \theta_i \perp\!\!\!\perp p_i(\cdot \mid \theta_i), \quad i = 0, 1; j = 1, \ldots, n_i.$$

Let $\theta = (\theta_0, \theta_1)$ be the collection of unknown model parameters. The goal is to use this model and these data to diagnose the unknown disease status of a new individual with observed biomarker value, say y_f, but whose group status Z_f (which takes the values $1 = D+$ or $0 = D-$) is unknown.

Let the unknown prevalence of disease be $\pi = P(D+)$. We assume the same model for the future observation Y_f conditional on disease status. The disease status of the new individual, z_f equals 1 if they are $D+$ and 0 if they are $D-$. *A priori*, $Z_f \sim Ber(\pi)$. The marginal model is the mixture

$$p(y_f \mid \theta, \pi) = P(Z_f = 0)p_0(y_f \mid z_f = 0, \theta_0) + P(Z_f = 1)p_1(v \mid z_f = 1, \theta_1),$$

or equivalently,

$$Y_f \mid \pi, \theta \sim (1 - \pi)\, p_0(\cdot, \theta_0) + \pi\, p_1(\cdot \mid \theta_1).$$

We assume that the current collection of biomarkers, Y, and the new individual's pair (Z_f, Y_f) are independent conditional on (θ, π).

We require a prior distribution for the above parameters. From now on we assume knowledge about these parameters can be specified independently as

$$p(\pi, \theta_0, \theta_1) = p(\pi)p(\theta_0)p(\theta_1).$$

In the case of the binormal distribution $\theta_i = (\mu_i, \sigma_i)$, and we will assume these two parameters can be regarded independently, as well.

Let $\gamma = (\theta, \pi)$. The Bayesian method of diagnosis is to simply obtain the posterior probability of disease,

$$
\begin{aligned}
P(Z = 1 \mid y, y_f) &= P(D+ \mid y, y_f) \\
&= \int P(Z = 1 \mid \gamma, y, y_f)p(\gamma \mid y, y_f)d\gamma \\
&= \int P(Z = 1 \mid \gamma, y_f)p(\gamma \mid y, y_f)d\gamma \qquad (15.7) \\
&= \int \frac{\pi p_1(y_f \mid z = 1, \gamma)}{\pi p_1(y_f \mid z = 1, \gamma) + (1 - \pi)p_0(y_f \mid z = 0, \gamma)}p(\gamma \mid y, y_f)d\gamma \\
&= \int \frac{\pi p_1(y_f \mid z = 1, \theta_1)}{\pi p_1(y_f \mid z = 1, \theta_1) + (1 - \pi)p_0(y_f \mid z = 0, \theta_0)}p(\theta, \pi \mid y, y_f)d\theta d\pi,
\end{aligned}
$$

where we have used Bayes' theorem and the conditional independence of (Z, Y_f) and Y.

Diagnosis without dichotomizing the biomarker by thinking about the Se/Sp tradeoff would follow by calculating $P(Z_f \mid y, y_f)$ and deciding that $Z_f = 1$ if this quantity is sufficiently large (see Thurmond et al., 2002 [326]; Choi et al., 2006 [75]; Norris et al., 2009 [251]). For example, if the ratio is 0.9999, most people would be comfortable saying that the individual was indeed $D+$. For mass screening, one could decide to say $D+$ if this probability exceeds 0.95, say, and $D-$ if it is below 0.05, and remain undecided otherwise. There are obviously many possibilities. If one can quantify the costs or losses associated with making classification errors, one can obtain the posterior risk and decide on a rule on that basis.

15.2.3   Statistical Inference for Binormal Diagnostic Outcome Data: GS Case

While there are many possible forms of data that could be observed, we only consider the univariate binormal case. We have

$$Y_{ij} \mid \mu_0, \mu_1, \sigma_0, \sigma_1 \stackrel{\perp\!\!\!\perp}{\sim} N(\mu_i, \sigma_i^2), \quad i = 0, 1; \ j = 1, \ldots, n_i.$$

These are obviously just two-sample normal data with unequal variances, which were discussed in detail in Chapter 5 and other chapters. The data may well have been transformed to better approximate binormality, using the same transformation for both samples.

Statistical inferences are quite straightforward and were previously discussed for this type of data. We are mainly interested in functions of the model parameters, such as the AUC and the ROC curve. If one uses conjugate priors, the posteriors for the model parameters are available in closed form. Since the parameters of interest are complicated functions of the model parameters, however, we use numerical approaches such as Monte Carlo methods to make our inferences. We have found it more efficient to obtain an MCMC sample from the joint posterior for $(\mu_0, \mu_1, \sigma_0, \sigma_1)$ and then carry out post-processing of the posterior samples to make inferences about the ROC curve, the AUC, and predictive probabilities of disease.

Example 15.4. Diabetes Data: GS Case. Diabetes is a metabolic disease mainly characterized by high blood sugar concentration and insulin deficiency or resistance. Normally, the pancreas releases insulin to help the body store and use sugar from food. Diabetes can occur when the pancreas produces very little or no insulin or when the body does not respond appropriately to insulin. Diabetes is endemic in the U.S. and is a leading cause of blindness, kidney failure, amputations, heart failure, and stroke.

The data considered here were taken from a pilot survey of diabetes in Cairo, Egypt. The data consist of blood glucose measurements (milligrams per deciliter) from 286 subjects. High blood glucose is associated with acquiring diabetes. Based on World Health Organization criteria, 88 subjects were classified as diseased and 198 as healthy (Smith and Thompson, 1996) [298]. Our method of assessing the quality of blood glucose measurements as a biomarker for diagnosing diabetes will be based on gold standard data.

Histograms for subjects classified as diseased and for subjects classified as healthy were obtained and scrutinized. We also plotted a histogram of the data after Box–Cox transformation (Box and Cox, 1964) [46] and decided that the normality assumption was reasonable enough to consider for the untransformed data. We leave it to exercises for the reader to make these considerations on their own. We analyze the data as binormal.

Predictive densities using this model are given in Figure 15.5. The densities overlap considerably, and the center of the distribution for the diabetic subjects is shifted considerably to the right. We also note that the two distributions' standard deviations appear to be quite different, the one for diabetics being considerably larger than that of the healthy subjects. Because of the considerable overlap, there is no hope of having anything near a perfect diagnostic rule for any cutoff, nor is there any hope of having an AUC that is close to 1.

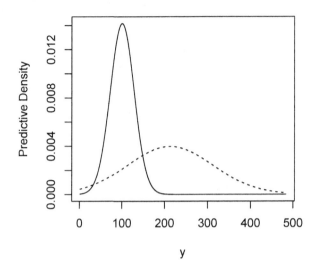

FIGURE 15.5: Predictive densities for healthy (dash) and diabetic (solid) patients.

We treat the problem as if we have virtually no knowledge about the science of this particular study and employ diffuse priors for the model parameters, which are the means and the standard deviations of the two populations. The range of the observed data for the healthy group was $(57, 275)$ mg/dl, and the corresponding range for the diabetic group was $(80, 484)$ mg/dL. The means of the corresponding populations are virtually certain to be within these rather wide ranges. For the two populations' means, our priors are $\mu_0 \sim N(100, 1000)$ and $\mu_1 \sim N(250, 10000)$, which correspond to normal distributions with rather diffuse 95% prior probability intervals for mean glucose levels, $(38, 163)$ and $(50, 450)$, respectively. These intervals are so wide that we hardly admit to having cheated by looking at the data to set the prior distribution.

We selected $\tau_i \perp\!\!\!\perp Ga(0.1, 0.1)$ priors for the precisions. For normal data, these priors are diffuse and generally allow the data to speak for themselves. Induced priors on the standard deviations have 95% prior probability intervals of $(0.32, 40,000,000)$, which is silly but will have little impact on the posterior.

Table 15.6 summarizes the results. The posterior densities of μ_0 and μ_1 are in Figure 15.6. There are clear statistically important differences in these means. Because of the large overlap in the data (see Figure 15.5), however, this is not of much interest to us for diagnosis. The AUC is estimated to be 0.86 with 95% PI $(0.80, 0.91)$; the corresponding posterior density is shown in Figure 15.7. The estimate (0.86) is not a large value, meaning that we do not expect to be able

TABLE 15.6: Posterior medians and 95% PIs for population means, standard deviations, and the AUC for the diabetes data

	Med	(95% PI)
AUC	0.86	$(0.80, 0.91)$
μ_0	100.6	$(96.8, 104.5)$
μ_1	212.8	$(191.8, 233.8)$
σ_0	28.1	$(25.6, 31.2)$
σ_1	100.0	$(86.8, 117.1)$

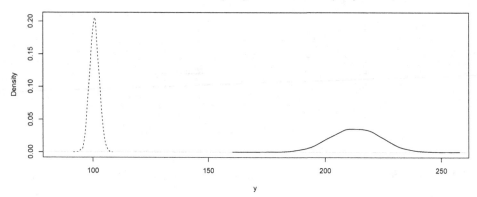

FIGURE 15.6: Posteriors for μ_0 and μ_1 for blood sugar glucose measurements.

to find a cutoff that would give both particularly large Se and Sp values. The estimated ROC curve with pointwise 95% probability limits is given in Figure 15.8.

We can glean from Figure 15.8 that it is possible to have 95% specificity with 75% sensitivity, or 84% specificity with 80% sensitivity. In practice, it will be important to find the corresponding cutoffs. In the former case, it is 146.8 mg/dl, and in the latter case, it is 128.7 mg/dl. We obtain these values using the fact that, with cutoff k, we have $S_0(k) = t$ (see equation (15.4)). Thus, we set $S_0(k) = 0.05$ in the former case (i.e., 95% specificity), and 0.16 in the latter. In the former case, we have $0.05 = 1 - \Phi((k - \mu_0)/\sigma_0) = 1 - \Phi(1.645)$. Solving the equation gives $k = \mu_0 + 1.645\,\sigma_0$. Thus, the estimate of k in this instance is $100.6 + 1.645 \times 28.1 = 146.8$.

15.2.4   ROC Regression: GS Case

It is often the case that there are additional biomarkers and/or covariates that are related to the biomarkers and/or disease status. When multiple biomarkers are available, it is necessary to model them jointly, conditional on disease status. The issue becomes even more interesting and complicated when multiple biomarkers are

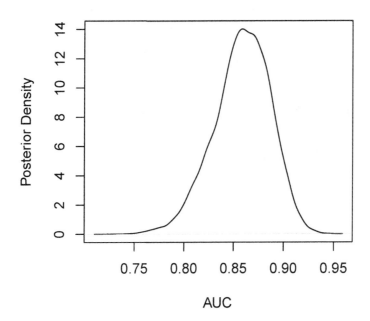

FIGURE 15.7: Posterior density for the AUC.

observed longitudinally, with the goal of diagnosing an infection or illness over time. This effort is beyond the scope of our book. For an illustration with two biomarkers see Norris et al. (2009) [251].

Here we discuss how to use covariate information to improve biomarker-based diagnosis while at the same time possibly making the model identifiable (Branscum et al. (2008, 2015), [50, 49]). The modeling is straightforward as it simply involves specifying a linear model for the biomarker in the disease group, for the healthy group, or both.

We represent the data as $\{(y_{ij}, x_{ij}) : i = 0, 1; j = 1, \ldots, n_i\}$, where the x_{ij} are covariates that are associated with the biomarker of interest. Consequently, these covariates may be indirectly related to disease status. For ease of presentation, we assume x_{ij} is a scalar covariate, such as age, for the jth individual in disease status group i. We set $i = 0$ for the healthy group and $i = 1$ for the "diseased" group. In our next example, we will assess whether it is easier to diagnose diabetes in younger people based on blood glucose than it is in older people.

First, we write the model as a form of binormal linear model.

$$Y_{ij} \mid x_{ij}, \beta, \sigma \perp\!\!\!\perp N(\beta_{i1} + \beta_{i2}\, x_{ij}, \sigma_i^2), \quad i = 0, 1; j = 1, \ldots, n_i, \tag{15.8}$$

where $\beta = [\beta_0, \beta_1] = [(\beta_{01}, \beta_{02}), (\beta_{11}, \beta_{12})]$ and $\sigma = (\sigma_0, \sigma_1)$. This is another situation where a conjugate prior for each regression would make the posterior analyt-

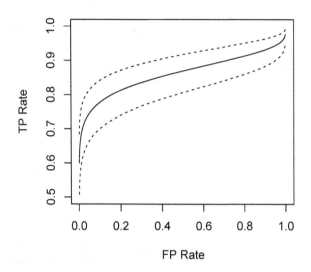

FIGURE 15.8: Posterior median for the ROC curve with pointwise 95% posterior probability intervals.

ically tractable. With conditionally conjugate priors, the Gibbs sampler would be quite easy as well. However, none of this is necessary when using a general MCMC program (e.g., BUGS, JAGS, or Stan), since sampling from the corresponding un-recognizable full conditionals has been automated in those packages.

Here, we could specify normal priors for β_0 and β_1 and independent gamma priors for the precisions $\tau_0 = 1/\sigma_0^2$ and $\tau_1 = 1/\sigma_1^2$, with the τ_i independent of the β_i. This specification results in conditional conjugacy for the pairs (β_i, τ_i), $i = 0, 1$, as was discussed for a single normal regression sample in Chapter 7. We, of course, recommend induced priors via conditional means priors, which we discussed in Chapter 7. Such prior specification was particularly straightforward to do with only one or two predictor variables. We also advocate for the use of uniform priors for the σ_i over appropriately specified ranges, as we have done in previous examples. Conditional conjugacy remains for β_i but not for τ_i, though.

On the other hand, the proper reference prior here specifies $\beta_{i0} \perp\!\!\!\perp \beta_{i1} \sim N(0, 10^6)$ and $\tau_i \perp\!\!\!\perp Ga(0.001, 0.001)$, which is simply an approximation to $p(\beta, \tau) \propto \tau$. In this case, as discussed in Chapter 7, we expect posterior inferences to be quite reasonable. Of course, we always advocate for using informative priors when suitable information is available.

With this model, we can perform ROC regression. In the previous section we assumed $Y_{ij} \mid \mu, \sigma \perp\!\!\!\perp N(\mu_i, \sigma_i^2)$, and we obtained the formulas in equations (15.5) and (15.6) for the ROC and AUC, respectively. These formulas were written as explicit functions of μ and σ. All we need to do now is replace μ_i with $\beta_{i1} + \beta_{i2}\, x$, where x is a particular covariate value of interest. We would generally select several values of x to study. Define

$$a_x = \frac{\beta_{11} - \beta_{01} + (\beta_{12} - \beta_{02})x}{\sigma_1} \quad \text{and} \quad b = \frac{\sigma_0}{\sigma_1}.$$

We see immediately that

$$ROC_x(t) = \Phi(a_x + b\Phi^{-1}(t)) \quad \text{and} \quad AUC_x = \Phi\left(\frac{a_x}{\sqrt{1+b^2}}\right). \tag{15.9}$$

What does this mean? The ROC_x curve plots the false positive rate, $1 - Sp_x(k) = P(Y_0 > k \mid x)$, against the true positive rate, $Se_x(k) = P(Y_1 > k \mid x)$, where these quantities have been modeled to depend on the covariate x. Implicitly, these quantities also depend on (β, σ). As x grows, the difference in the two means, which equals $\beta_{11} - \beta_{01} + (\beta_{12} - \beta_{02})x$, will grow if the slope for the affected population is larger than the slope for the healthy population. In this case, AUC_x increases as x increases, resulting in the possibility of having better diagnostic performance for larger values of x. Of course, if the difference in slopes is negative, diagnostic performance will be better for smaller values of x.

We note that it can easily be the case that β_{02} or β_{12} or both could be negligible. In the case of ROC regression, it will be important to perform an initial analysis to determine if modeling the covariate in healthy and/or non-healthy samples will potentially be worthwhile.

Example 15.5. Diabetes Data with Age as Covariate. We augment the blood glucose data for 286 individuals with their ages. Our analysis uses what we have termed the binormal regression model with the reference prior just discussed. In exercises, we ask the reader to obtain ROC curves that depend on age. Results of our analysis are summarized in Table 15.7, where we include inferences for $AUC_{x=40}$ and $AUC_{x=70}$, the areas under the ROC curves for 40-year-olds and 70-year-olds. In the analysis, we standardized the covariate age by subtracting its sample mean and dividing by its sample standard deviation.

We first fit model 2, which is the model that includes both slopes. Model 1 *excludes* the slope for the diabetes group (β_{12}), since its 95% PI was very wide, $(-36.5, 25.7)$, with zero in the middle. Additional reasons in support of model 1 are that $P(\beta_{12} > 0 \mid y) = 0.37$ and $DIC = 2{,}927$ for model 2, while it was 2,925 for model 1. We also note that all the inferences *not* shown for model 2 were virtually identical to those for model 1, while intervals for the AUCs are appreciably wider than they are in model 1. For better or worse, the implication of choosing model 1 over model 2 is that we are accepting the hypothesis that age is not related to blood glucose measurements in diabetics, but it is in healthy individuals. At the very least, there is no evidence in the data that there is a relationship in the diabetes group, while there is appreciable statistical evidence that there is a relationship in the healthy group where blood glucose appears to increase with age.

Observe that inferences for the intercept and standard deviation for the diabetes group are virtually identical to those obtained in Table 15.6, which is not

TABLE 15.7: Posterior medians and 95% PIs for population means, standard deviations, and AUCs for the diabetes data with covariate *Age*. Model 1 excludes the slope β_{12}, while model 2 includes it

Model 1	$DIC = 2{,}925$	
	Med.	(95% PI)
$AUC_{x=70}$	0.83	$(0.76, 0.88)$
$AUC_{x=40}$	0.87	$(0.81, 0.92)$
β_{01}	101.8	$(98.1, 105.5)$
β_{02}	8.9	$(5.5, 12.4)$
β_{11}	212.5	$(191.2, 233.5)$
$\beta_{12} = 0$	NA	NA
σ_0	26.5	$(24.0, 29.3)$
σ_1	100	$(86.8, 116.9)$
Model 2	$DIC = 2{,}927.0$ $P(\beta_{12} > 0) = 0.37$	
$AUC_{x=70}$	0.81	$(0.68, 0.9)$
$AUC_{x=40}$	0.88	$(0.78, 0.94)$
β_{12}	-5.2	$(-36.5, 25.7)$

surprising, since the model for this group is the same in both analyses. The very small differences in results are simply due to Monte Carlo error. The estimate of the intercept in the healthy group corresponds to average blood glucose for an individual of average age. It is not surprising that inferences for the intercept are similar to (but still different from) the previous analysis that did not take age into account.

The most interesting aspect of the analysis is that the estimated AUCs for 40-year-olds are noticeably different than those for 70-year-olds. Since we clearly have $\beta_{12} - \beta_{02} = -\beta_{02} < 0$, we are in the situation where the AUC decreases as age increases. The estimated value of $AUC_{40} - AUC_{70}$ is 0.04 with 95%PI $(0.025, 0.063)$, and up to four decimal places, the posterior probability that the true difference is positive is 1.0. Thus, it appears that it will be easier to diagnose 40-year-olds than 70-year-olds when using only blood glucose as a biomarker.

15.3   Recap and Readings

We have covered many topics in this chapter, including the assessment of the quality of dichotomous tests and prior specifications for model parameters. We also discussed how to model continuous biomarkers and how to use those models to estimate receiver operating characteristic curves that one can use to ascertain how to select cutoffs for future dichotomous tests. We discussed how to calculate predictive probabilities of disease for individuals who might benefit from a more personal diagnosis based on appropriate biomarkers. We extended the gold standard results to depend on covariates, and we discussed the advantages of taking account of the extra information that comes from this extension.

One of the key goals in diagnostic testing is to ascertain if one test is better than another. Clearly if one test has higher test accuracies than another, it is preferable on those grounds. On the other hand, if it costs 100 times as much to apply the better test and many units will be tested, more thought may be required to make a decision. Making such inferences based on binary tests in the GS case was relatively straightforward, since many useful and relevant tools had already been developed in previous chapters.

Extension to the NGS case is actually much more challenging, since this involves the application of two or more tests to each unit to be tested, the subsequent modeling of often dependent multiple binary test outcomes, and the need to deal with the lack of identifiability that usually ensues in this case. The development of such models starts with Hui and Walter (1980) [169], who discussed the NGS model for two diagnostic test outcome data under the assumption of conditional independence for the two tests and assuming samples from distinct populations of individuals. Using their model, and under their assumptions, it is possible to assess the test accuracies for the two tests and consequently to ascertain whether, say, a new test is preferable to a standard reference test. This work has been the starting point for considerable subsequent work, including Bayesian methods by Joseph et al. (1995) [194], Enøe, Georgiadis, and Johnson (2000) [103], Dendukuri and Joseph (2001) [94], Johnson, Gastwirth, and Pearson (2001) [188], Georgiadis et al. (2003) [141], Branscum, Gardner, and Johnson (2004) [47], Hanson and Johnson's comments relating to Gustafson (2005) [157], Jones et al. (2010) [192], Johnson, Jones, and Gardner (2019) [189], and Johnson, Ward, and Gillen (2017) [190]. For brevity, we do not consider this topic here.

Another topic that we have left out of the presentation involves the relaxation of the assumption of binormality. There are many possible shapes of distributions that nature could be following in any given situation. Branscum, Johnson, and Hanson (2008, 2015) [50, 49] developed semiparametric methods for estimating ROC cures with normal distributions replaced by flexible (nonparametric) classes of distributions. The linear regression form stays the same, so the mean biomarker responses for each group are still linear functions of one or more covariates. In the NGS case, a logistic regression model is used for the latent disease status. The flexibility of the semiparametric approach allows the shape of the distribution around the linear means to be multimodal, skewed, and so on.

15.4   Exercises

EXERCISE 15.1.   Using the multinomial likelihood specified in equation (15.1) in conjunction with independent beta priors for the model parameters, show that the joint posterior is the product of independent beta distributions. Give the specific beta distributions.

EXERCISE 15.2. *CAD data.*   Using your results from Exercise 15.1 with independent $U(0,1)$ priors, analyze the CAD data in Table 15.3. Plot the exact beta posterior densities for (π, Se, Sp) using R or some other computing platform. Also, with the known beta posteriors for the model parameters, obtain plots of the posterior densities for the PPV and NPV using simulation.

EXERCISE 15.3.

(a) Recall the CAD data from Example 15.1. Write your own or use sample code available on the book's website for this chapter to analyze these data. The file names include CAD. Assume that prior information for model parameters is specified in the form of a best estimate and a 0.05 quantile of the prior (the latter in parentheses). For π, we have 0.5 (0.2), for Se we have 0.7 (0.4), and for Sp, 0.7 (0.4), which are all relatively diffuse. Using these priors, reanalyze the CAD data. Compare point estimates with those in Exercise 15.2 and with the maximum likelihood estimates given in the example.

(b) Now modify the prior and the code so that the prevalence is specified to be precisely $\pi = 0.05$ (point mass at 0.05). Reanalyze the data and make comparisons of inferences with those in part (a).

(c) Now suppose that 100 new patients from the same population will be tested. Using the prior in (a), obtain predictive inferences for the number out of the 100 that will (i) test positive and (ii) will be $D+$.

EXERCISE 15.4. *CAD data.*   For the data analysis parts of this exercise, use priors from part (a) of Exercise 15.3. It is a fact that if we condition on column totals in a multinomial table, as in Table 15.3, then individual cell counts in those columns are binomial with success probability equal to the conditional probability of being in the particular cell. Specifically,

$$Y_{11} \mid y_{+1}, \pi, Se, Sp \sim Bin(y_{+1}, Se) \quad \text{and} \quad Y_{00} \mid y_{+0}, \pi, Se, Sp \sim Bin(y_{+0}, Sp),$$

independently.

(a) Show that the conditional distributions above are correct.

(b) Analyze the CAD data assuming that the column totals are fixed. What parameters are estimable under these circumstances?

(c) It is also true that if we condition on row totals, individual cell counts are binomial. Obtain the precise binomial distributions by analogy with the results when conditioning on column totals.

(d) Analyze the data when conditioning on row totals. What parameters are estimable under these circumstances?

EXERCISE 15.5. *HIV Data.*

(a) Analyze the HIV data from Example 15.2 using the large-sample results specified in expression (15.3). Use prior 1 specified in Example 15.2. Compare results with those obtained in Table 15.5.

(b) Use prior 1 in Example 15.2 to analyze the new data set $y = (3, 5, 148675)$, $n = 148{,}693$. These are the data analyzed there only divided by 21 and rounded so that they are actual counts. Compare with inferences in Table 15.5.

(c) Repeat part (a) using the new data in part (b). Comment on the quality of the approximation.

(d) Using the results in expression (15.3), obtain plots of the approximate densities for $(\pi, Sp, PPV, 1 - NPV)$ for the full data and the reduced data (from part (b)).

EXERCISE 15.6. *Canadian HIV data.* A 1986 study of blood donated for transfusion in Canada was performed. There were $n = 94{,}496$ blood units that were tested with an Abbot ELISA with 405 $ELISA+$ outcomes, and with all of these retested with western blot (WB), resulting in 14 $WB+$ outcomes and 391 $WB-$ outcomes. In addition, there was a sample of 627 blood units that were set aside by screeners based on the donors' responses to a questionnaire about risky behavior. These were all tested with the ELISA and WB assays. Counts for $(ELISA+, WB+)$, $(ELISA+, WB-)$, $(ELISA-, WB+)$, $(ELISA-, WB-)$ were $(11, 3, 1, 612)$, respectively. An additional control sample was taken that resulted in counts $(1, 2, 0, 619)$. Individuals in this sample were matched to those in the "risky behavior" sample based on age, sex, and other factors unrelated to the risky behavior. Assume that the WB test is perfect and that all three samples are independent and follow a multinomial distribution with appropriate probabilities for each cell in each multinomial.

(a) Write and simplify the likelihood function for the combined data.

(b) Using the prior $Se \sim Beta(57, 4)$, $Sp \sim Beta(10, 1)$, $\pi \sim Beta(1, 10)$, analyze the combined data. Perform a sensitivity analysis. Keep in mind that the posterior for Se will be very similar to the prior.

EXERCISE 15.7. Consider the derivation of the functional form for the ROC curve in Example 15.3.

(a) Show that $S_0^{-1}(t) = G_0^{-1}(1 - t) = \mu_0 + \sigma_0 \Phi^{-1}(1 - t)$.

(b) Use this result to argue that $ROC(t) = 1 - \Phi(-a - b\Phi^{-1}(1 - t))$, where $a = (\mu_1 - \mu_0)/\sigma_0$ and $b = \sigma_0/\sigma_1$.

(c) Show that $\Phi(x) = 1 - \Phi(-x)$ for any x, and that $-\Phi^{-1}(t) = \Phi^{-1}(1 - t)$.

(d) Thus argue that $ROC(t)$ as defined in equation (15.4) is equal to $\Phi\left[a + b\Phi^{-1}(t)\right]$.

EXERCISE 15.8. Using equation (15.5), do the following:

(a) Give a single plot of the ROC curves for which (i) ($a = 0.5, b = 1$), (ii) ($a = 1.5, b = 1$), and (iii) ($a = 2.5, b = 1$).
(b) Obtain the AUC for each of these three models (see equation (15.6)).

EXERCISE 15.9.   Establish the result in equation (15.7) that justifies going from line 2 to line 3. You need to explicitly use the conditional independence assumption given there. It does take an appropriate but brief technical argument.

EXERCISE 15.10.   Suppose $n_0 = n_1 = 1$, $Y_{01} \mid \mu_0 \sim N(\mu_0, 1)$, $Y_{11} \mid \mu_1 \sim N(\mu_1, 1)$, and $Z_f \sim Ber(\pi^*)$ with π^* a constant. Let $Y_f \mid \mu_0, z_f = 0 \sim N(\mu_0, 1)$ and $Y_f \mid \mu_1, z_f = 1 \sim N(\mu_1, 1)$. Assume that (Z_f, Y_f) is independent of Y conditional on the model parameters. Also let $p(\mu_0, \mu_1) \propto k$ with k a constant.

(a) Determine an analytical formula for $P(Z_f = 1 \mid y, y_f)$ using equation (15.7).
(b) From here on, suppose $\{y_{01} = 0, \ y_{11} = 2\}$ and $\pi^* = 0.5$. Plot $P(Z = 1 \mid y, y_f)$ as a function of y_f and find the value of y_f for which $P(Z_f = 1 \mid y, y_f) = 0.95$ and the value for which it is 0.05.
(c) Simulate predictions from $P(Z_f = 1 \mid y, y_f)$ for several values of y_f. Compare with analytical values from part (b).

EXERCISE 15.11.   In the context of Example 15.4, show that the cutoff corresponding to $Sp = 0.84$ and $Se = 0.80$ is approximately 146.8. Include details that were left out of the derivation of the cutoff 146.8.

EXERCISE 15.12.   In this exercise we will reanalyze the glucose data in Example 15.4. The data and sample code are available on the book's website for Chapter 15. The file names contain `glucose`.

(a) Analyze the glucose data and try to reproduce all of the inferences presented in Example 15.4.
(b) Repeat (a) with $N(0, 10^6)$ priors on the means and $Ga(0.001, 0.001)$ priors on the precisions. Do results change appreciably?
(c) Using untransformed data, and log-transformed data, obtain Q-Q plots for each sample and discuss whether either version appears to be approximately normal and which one appears to be closer to normality.
(d) Formulate appropriate priors for the bi-log-normal case and revise your program to obtain results for the ROC and the AUC. Comment.

EXERCISE 15.13.   Modify your program from Exercise 15.12 to obtain $P(Z_f = 1 \mid y, y_f)$, where (Z_f, Y_f) is the disease status and observed blood glucose outcome for a new patient. Plot these probabilities over a suitable range of values of y_f. What do you see?

EXERCISE 15.14.   Consider the binormal regression model for GS data (y, x) discussed in Section 15.2.4; outcomes in y are biomarkers from diseased and healthy individuals, and values in x are the corresponding covariate values. Let (y_f, x_f, z_f)

be the biomarker outcome, covariate value, and unknown disease status for a future individual whose values are independent of the data conditional on model parameters. We have

$$Y_f \mid x_f = x, z_f = i, \theta_{z_f} \perp\!\!\!\perp N(\beta_{i1} + x\,\beta_{i2}, \sigma_i^2), \quad i = 0, 1.$$

Derive the formula for the predictive probability

$$P(Z_f = 1 \mid x_f = x, y_f, y).$$

Hint: Recall the result in equation (15.7).

EXERCISE 15.15.   In this exercise we reanalyze the data in Example 15.5. We have the data and sample code available on the book's website for Chapter 15 in files with `glucose-regression` in their names. The code is currently set to fit model 2, the model that does not include a slope coefficient for the effect of age on glucose in the diabetes group.

(a) Run the code, and then revise it, to reproduce the results in Table 15.7 for models 1 and 2.

(b) Obtain posterior inferences for ROC_x for $x \in \{30, 40, 60, 70\}$. Plot all four ROC curves on the same plot. Make inferences for the differences $ROC_{30} - ROC_{70}$ and $ROC_{40} - ROC_{60}$. Comment.

(c) Modify your program for part (b) to obtain and plot the predictive probabilities, $P(Z_f = 1 \mid x_f = x, y_f, y)$, as functions of y_f over an appropriate range. Generate four plots, one for each of the values of x specified in part (b). This was defined and discussed in Exercise 15.14 and for the simpler non-regression problem in equation (15.7).

Appendix A

Probability and Random Variables

This appendix simply lists the definitions and rules for probability and random variables that are used throughout this book. It is not intended to serve as an introduction to these topics, but as a reference for precisely what is meant when terms appearing here are used in the text. Our intention is to review material the reader may have already studied or inspire the reader to study the material in greater depth in a suitable textbook.

A.1 Probability Axioms and Rules

Probability is a number attached to an event. For mathematical precision, we begin with any set Ω, looking upon its elements as elementary or atomic events.

Event Space. A collection $\mathcal{A}$ of subsets of Ω is called an event space if it satisfies the following:
  (i) $A \in \mathcal{A}$ implies $A^c \in \mathcal{A}$.
  (ii) $A_1, A_2, \ldots \in \mathcal{A}$ implies $\bigcup_{i=1}^{\infty} A_i \in \mathcal{A}$ and $\bigcap_{i=1}^{\infty} A_i \in \mathcal{A}$.

Elements of an event space are events. When we call something an event, it is taken to be an element of some event space.

Probability Space. A probability space is a triple $(\Omega, \mathcal{A}, \mathcal{P})$, where $\mathcal{A}$ is an event space of Ω. and P is a real-valued function with domain $\mathcal{A}$ satisfying the following:

  (i) $P(\Omega) = 1$.
  (ii) $P(A) \geq 0$ for all $A \in \mathcal{A}$.
  (iii) If $A_1, A_2, \cdots \in \mathcal{A}$ are mutually exclusive events (i.e., as subsets of Ω, $A_i \cap A_j = \emptyset$ (the empty set) for all $i \neq j$) then

$$P\left(\bigcup_{i=1}^{\infty} A_i\right) = \sum_{i=1}^{\infty} P(A_i).$$

From here onward, we take all events to be elements in the event space of some probability space.

Additive Law of Probability. If A and B are two events, then

$$P(A \cup B) = P(A) + P(B) - P(A \cap B).$$

Independence of Two Events. Two events A and B are independent if and only if

$$P(A \cap B) = P(A)P(B).$$

Independence of Multiple Events. Events $A_1, \ldots, A_k$, $k \geq 3$, are mutually independent if and only if

$$P(A_1 \cap A_2 \cap \cdots \cap A_k) = \prod_{i=1}^{k} P(A_i).$$

A similar equality holds for any sub-collection containing at least two but fewer than k events.

Conditional Probability. For two events A and B such that $P(A) > 0$, the conditional probability of B given A is defined as

$$P(B|A) = \frac{P(B \cap A)}{P(A)}.$$

This also results in $P(B \cap A) = P(A)P(B|A)$ if $P(A) > 0$, and $P(B \cap A) = P(B)P(A|B)$ if $P(B) > 0$. Note also that if $P(A) = 0$ or $P(B) = 0$, then $P(B \cap A) = 0$ since $B \cap A$ is contained in A as well as in B.

Law of Total Probability. Let $B_1, \ldots, B_k$ be a finite partition of an event space Ω.[1] Then

$$P(A) = P(A|B_1)\, P(B_1) + \cdots + P(A|B_k)\, P(B_k).$$

Bayes' Theorem. Let $B_1, \ldots, B_k$ be a finite partition of an event space Ω. Let A be an event in Ω with $P(A) > 0$. Then

$$P(B_i|A) = \frac{P(A|B_i)P(B_i)}{P(A|B_1)\, P(B_1) + \cdots + P(A|B_k)P(B_k)}, \quad i = 1, \ldots, k.$$

Note that for two events A and B, Bayes' theorem tells us that $P(B \mid A) = P(A \mid B)P(B)/P(A)$.

---

[1] A finite partition of the event space Ω consists of $B_1 \cup \cdots \cup B_k = \Omega$ and $B_i \cap B_j = \emptyset$, $1 \leq i < j \leq k$ In other words, the partition consists of a finite set of subsets of Ω such that their union is all of Ω and none of the subsets intersect.

A.2   Random Variables and Their Distributions

We first consider univariate random variables. A strict construction of the mathematical definition of a random variable requires a good deal of preliminary development and results. We avoid these details by noting that, essentially, a random variable is a function from a probability space into the real number line. As such, probabilities assigned to events in the probability space are acquired by appropriate subsets of the real line. For statistical purposes, it suffices to focus on these probabilities and describe them via random variables without much consideration of the original probability space.

A.2.1   Univariate Random Variables

Cumulative Distribution Function. The cumulative distribution function (cdf) of a random variable Y is a function F defined by

$$F(y) = P(Y \leq y), \quad -\infty < y < \infty.$$

Although, at first look, this function seems to address only sets of the form $(-\infty, y)$, it is sufficient to determine the probabilities of any reasonable subsets of the real line. As such, the cdf provides one complete description of the probability structure of a random variable.

Properties of the Cumulative Distribution Function. Using standard notation for limits (right-hand and left-hand limits and limits at infinity), the cdf has the following properties.
  (i) $0 \leq F(y) \leq 1$ for all $y \in (-\infty, \infty)$.
 (ii) $F(y)$ is a non-decreasing function of y.
(iii) $F(-\infty) = 0$ and $F(\infty) = 1$.
 (iv) $F(y+) = F(y)$ for all $y \in (-\infty, \infty)$, that is, $F(\cdot)$ is right continuous.

Discrete Random Variables. If the cdf has discontinuities at distinct and well-separated points that are either finite in number or countably infinite, and it is non-increasing between adjacent such points, we will call the random variable with this cdf a discrete random variable.

A discrete random variable takes values only in a finite or countably infinite set of real numbers, say, $\{a_1, a_2, \dots\}$. Its probability structure can be described completely by another function that is often useful in practice.

Probability Mass Function. The probability mass function (pmf) of a discrete random variable Y is a function f defined by

$$f(y) = P(Y = y), \quad y \in (-\infty, \infty).$$

Clearly, $f(y) > 0$ only at a countable number of points, whereas the cdf has discontinuities. We also have $f(y) = F(y) - F(y-).$[2]

Probability Density Function. If the cdf is continuous at all points and has a derivative at all but a countable set of points, it can be reconstructed via another function, f, called a probability density function (pdf), by the relationship

$$F(y) = \int_{-\infty}^{y} f(x)dx.$$

Properties of the Probability Density Function. A probability density function of a random variable Y has the following properties.
  (i) $f(y) \geq 0$ for all $y \in (-\infty, \infty)$.
  (ii) $P(a < Y < b) = \int_{a}^{b} f(y)dy$.
  (iii) $f(y)$ can be taken to equal $\frac{d}{dy}F(y)$ at all points y where F has a derivative and set to any arbitrary finite values elsewhere.

Continuous Random Variables. We will call a random variable continuous if it has a cdf that can be reconstructed from a pdf as defined above. Typically, this means the cdf has a derivative everywhere, except perhaps at a few points.

Convention Regarding Use of the Words "Density" and "Distribution". In this book, as has become common practice in the statistical literature, we use the word "distribution" in a general sense for any description (pdf, pmf, cdf, and possibly other functions) of the complete probability structure of a random variable. Most often, this description is via a pmf or a pdf. In either case we use the word "density," and denote it by the letters p or f, disregarding the distinction between a pmf and a pdf. The context is typically sufficient to clarify whether the random variable is discrete or continuous. (This practice can be shown to be mathematically rigorous by defining an appropriate underlying measure with respect to which the pmf or pdf is defined.) Finally, when referring to a cumulative distribution function, we explicitly call it a cdf and use the upper-case letter F to denote the function.

A.2.2 Bivariate Random Variables

When considering two random variables simultaneously, it is not sufficient to simply describe their separate distributions. The possible set of values for a bivariate *random vector* (we use the word "vector" when more than one variable is considered simultaneously) are points in a coordinate plane. As such, a complete description of the probability structure must include the probability of any reasonable set in the plane, particularly rectangles. To describe the *joint* distribution of two random variables, we need extensions of the cdf, pdf, and pmf.

---

[2] $F(y-)$ denotes the left-hand limit of the cdf $F(\cdot)$ at y.

Bivariate (or Joint) Cumulative Distribution Function. The bivariate cdf of random variables X and Y is a function F defined by

$$F(x, y) = P(X \leq x \cap Y \leq y), \quad -\infty < x < \infty, \ -\infty < y < \infty.$$

Although this function directly addresses only lower left infinite rectangles, it is sufficient to determine the probabilities of any reasonable subsets of the plane. In this sense, the bivariate cdf provides a complete description of the probability structure of two random variables jointly.

Properties of the Bivariate Cumulative Distribution Function. A bivariate cdf has the following properties.

  (i) $0 \leq F(x, y) \leq 1$ for all $x \in (-\infty, \infty)$, $y \in (-\infty, \infty)$.
  (ii) $F(x, \infty)$ and $F(\infty, y)$ are univariate cdfs.
  (iii) $F(b, d) - F(a, d) - F(b, c) + F(a, c) \geq 0$ for all $a \leq b$, $c \leq d$.
  (iv) $F(-\infty, -\infty) = 0$ and $F(\infty, \infty) = 1$,
  (v) $F(x+, y+) = F(x, y)$ for all $x \in (-\infty, \infty)$, $y \in (-\infty, \infty)$, that is, $F(\cdot, \cdot)$ is right continuous.

Bivariate (or Joint) Probability Mass Function. The joint pmf of discrete random variables X and Y is a function f defined by

$$f(x, y) = P(X = x \cap Y = y), \quad x \in (-\infty, \infty), \ y \in (-\infty, \infty).$$

As in the univariate case, $f(x, y) > 0$ only at a countable number of points in the plane where the cdf has discontinuities.

Bivariate (or Joint) Probability Density Function. If the cdf is continuous at all points in the plane and has a mixed partial derivative at all but a countable set of points, it can be related to another function f called a bivariate (or joint) probability density function. The relationship is given by

$$F(x, y) = \int_{-\infty}^{y} \int_{-\infty}^{x} f(s, t) ds dt, \quad f(x, y) = \frac{\partial^2}{\partial x \partial y} F(x, y).$$

A bivariate pdf has properties similar in concept to its univariate counterpart, namely:

  (i) $f(x, y) \geq 0$ for all $-\infty < x < \infty$, $-\infty < y < \infty$;
  (ii) $P(a < X < b, c < Y < d) = \int_{a}^{b} \int_{c}^{d} f(x, y) dy dx$.

Convention Regarding Use of the Words "Density" and "Distribution". We follow the same convention as in the univariate case. See the description given at the end of Section A.2.1.

Marginal Distributions. The joint distribution of two random variables X and Y determines the separate individual distributions of X and of Y. These distributions are called marginal distributions. A marginal distribution fully describes the probability structure of the random variable by itself, without reference to the other. The relevant expressions, with subscripts used on functions to clarify the random variable to which the marginal belongs, are:

$$F_X(x) = F(x, \infty), \qquad F_Y(y) = F(\infty, y);$$
$$f_X(x) = \int_{-\infty}^{\infty} f(x, y)dy, \qquad f_Y(y) = \int_{-\infty}^{\infty} f(x, y)dx;$$
$$f_X(x) = \sum_{all \ y} f(x, y), \qquad f_Y(y) = \sum_{all \ x} f(x, y).$$

Conditional Distributions. These distributions play a crucial role in Bayesian statistics. They describe how the probability structure of one random variable is affected by knowledge of the other. We use the notation $X|Y = y$ to denote the random variable X when Y is known to take the value y. The distribution of this conditional random variable is determined by the joint distribution. The relationships are given by the following expressions:

$$f_{X|Y=y}(x) = \frac{f(x, y)}{f_Y(y)}, \qquad f_{Y|X=x}(y) = \frac{f(x, y)}{f_X(x)}.$$

These relationships hold for pmfs as well as pdfs. Of course, the denominators on the right-hand sides must be positive; otherwise, the conditional density is undefined.

Law of Total Probability. For two random variables,

$$f(y) = \int_{-\infty}^{\infty} f(y|x) f(x) \, dx.$$

This follows from the relationship between the joint distribution and the marginal and conditional distributions stated above.

Bayes' Theorem. For two random variables,

$$f(x|y) = \frac{f(y|x) f(x)}{\int_{-\infty}^{\infty} f(y|x) f(x) \, dx}.$$

A.2.3 Multivariate Random Variables

Extending the development of bivariate random variables to the case of more than two variables is straightforward. We state some of the above results for k joint random variables $X_1, \ldots, X_k$. When convenient, we collect all k random variables as components in a k-dimensional random vector.

Joint Cumulative Distribution Function. The joint cdf is defined as

$$F(x_1, \ldots, x_k) = P(X_1 \leq x_1 \cap \cdots \cap X_k \leq x_k), \quad (x_1, \ldots, x_k) \in \mathbb{R}^k.$$

Here $\mathbb{R}^k$ denotes k-dimensional Euclidean space consisting of all k-tuples of real numbers.

Joint Probability Density Function. If the cdf is continuous at all points in $\mathbb{R}^k$ and has a kth-order mixed partial derivative at all but a countable set of points, it has a probability density function f with the relationships

$$F(x_1, \ldots, x_k) = \int_{-\infty}^{x_k} \cdots \int_{-\infty}^{x_1} f(x_1, \ldots, x_k) dx_1 \cdots dx_k,$$

$$f(x_1, \ldots, x_k) = \frac{\partial^k}{\partial x_1 \cdots \partial x_k} F(x_1, \ldots, x_k).$$

Marginal Distributions. These distributions follow the definitions for bivariate random variables with the single integrals replaced by appropriate multiple integrals:

$$f(x_1) = \int_{-\infty}^{\infty} \cdots \int_{-\infty}^{\infty} f(x_1, x_2, \ldots, x_k) dx_2 \cdots dx_k.$$

This also extends to the joint marginal distribution of a subset of the k random variables. Such a marginal equals the integral of the joint pdf of all k variables over all variables that are not in the subset of interest.

Conditional Distributions. While a large number of conditional distributions are possible, we often focus on one of the k variables conditioned on the rest:

$$f(x_1 | x_2, \ldots, x_k) = \frac{f(x_1, \ldots, x_k)}{f(x_2, \ldots, x_k)}.$$

Again, the general formula is a ratio of the joint density of pooled variables on both sides of the conditioning vertical bar over the joint density of the conditioning variables following the vertical bar.

Exchangeable Random Variables. A set of random variables $X_1, \ldots, X_k$ are exchangeable if and only if the distribution of any permutation of the random variables is the same as the distribution of the random variables in the original order. To make this more precise, suppose $\pi(1), \ldots, \pi(k)$ is any permutation of the integers $1, \ldots, k$. Then exchageability means

$$P(X_{\pi(1)} \leq x_1 \cap \cdots \cap X_{\pi(k)} \leq x_k) = P(X_1 \leq x_1 \cap \cdots \cap X_k \leq x_k).$$

Independence of Random Variables. A set of random variables $X_1, \ldots, X_k$ are independent if and only if their joint distribution equals the product of their marginal distributions. In terms of cdfs, this means

$$F(x_1, \ldots, x_k) = F_{X_1}(x_1) \times \cdots \times F_{X_k}(x_k),$$

where, for example, $F_{X_1}(x_1) = F(x_1, \infty, \ldots, \infty)$. In terms of densities,

$$f(x_1, \ldots, x_k) = f(x_1) \times \cdots \times f(x_k).$$

Under independence, conditional distributions are the same as marginal distributions, that is,

$$f(x_1|x_2) = f(x_1), \ f(x_1, x_2|x_3) = f(x_1, x_2), \ f(x_3|x_1, x_2) = f(x_3), \dots.$$

We use the notation $x_1, \dots, x_n \overset{ind}{\sim}$ to indicate that the random variables $x_1, \dots, x_n$ are independently distributed. Another notational device sometimes used to indicate independence is $x_1 \perp\!\!\!\perp x_2$.

Independent and identically distributed (iid) random variables are useful in specifying models. We use the notation $x_1, \dots, x_n \overset{iid}{\sim}$ to indicate this. While iid random variables are exchangeable, the class of exchangeable random variables is much wider.

One way to describe exchangeable random variables is via a conditionally iid specification. If θ is a random variable and $x_1, \dots, x_n|\theta$ are iid, then the joint distribution of $x_1, \dots, x_n, \theta$ is such that the marginal distribution of $x_1, \dots, x_n$ is exchangeable.

Distribution of a Transformed Random Variable or Vector. Suppose X is a continuous random variable with a pdf $f_X(\cdot)$, and $g(\cdot)$ is an invertible and differentiable function on the space of possible values of X. Then the transformed random variable $Y = g(X)$ has pdf

$$f_Y(y) = \left| \frac{d}{dy} g^{-1}(y) \right| f_X \left(g^{-1}(y) \right).$$

If X is discrete, so is Y with pmf

$$f_Y(y) = f_X \left(g^{-1}(y) \right).$$

Suppose X is a continuous k-dimensional random vector with pdf $f_X(\cdot)$, and $g(\cdot)$ is an invertible function for which all first-order partial derivatives exist and are finite on the space of possible values of X. Then the transformed random vector $Y = g(X)$ has pdf

$$f_Y(y) = \left| \det \left(\frac{\partial}{\partial y} g^{-1}(y) \right) \right| f_X \left(g^{-1}(y) \right),$$

where $\det(M)$ stands for the determinant of a matrix M, and $\frac{\partial}{\partial y} h(y)$ denotes the matrix of first-order partial derivatives of the components of $h(y)$ with respect to the components of y.

A.3 Expectation and Moments

Expectation is a basic notion in considering random variables. It is especially useful for statistical purposes.

Expectation of a Function

Given a random variable X, the expectation of a function $g(\cdot)$ of X is defined as

$$E\left\{g(X)\right\} = \int_{\mathcal{X}} g(x)\, f(x)\, dx,$$

where $\mathcal{X}$ is the space of all possible values of X. This definition works for random variables and random vectors, with $g(\cdot)$ a scalar or vector-valued function. For discrete random variables, the integral is replaced by a sum:

$$E\left\{g(X)\right\} = \sum_{x \in \mathcal{X}} g(x)\, f(x).$$

Expectations do not always exist in that the integral in the definition may not exist. When we refer to an expectation by writing a symbol for it, we make the tacit assumption that the expectation exists and is finite.

Moments

The rth moment of a random variable X is defined as $E(X^r)$. When $r = 1$, we get $E(X)$, which is also called the first moment or the *mean* of X.

Laws of Expectation

Expectation is a linear operation in that

$$E(aX + b) = aE(X) + b,$$

where a and b are scalars and X is a random variable or a random vector. In the random vector case, we also have

$$E(AX + b) = AE(X) + b,$$

where A is a matrix of multiplication-compatible dimensions and b is a vector of the same dimension as X. It is clear from the definition above that the expectation of a constant is the constant itself. The linearity of expectation can also be expressed for a function of X, namely,

$$E\{ag(X) + b\} = aE\{g(X)\} + b, \quad E\{Ag(X) + b\} = AE\{g(X)\} + b,$$

with appropriate dimension compatibility.

Variance

The variance of a random variable X is defined as

$$\mathrm{Var}(X) = E\left(\{X - E(X)\}^2\right).$$

The variance can be expressed in terms of the first two moments of X as

$$\mathrm{Var}(X) = E(X^2) - \{E(X)\}^2.$$

For random vectors X, the notion of variance is more complex. We have the definition

$$\mathrm{Var}(X) = E\left[\{X - E(X)\}\{X - E(X)\}'\right],$$

where M' denotes the matrix transpose of matrix M. In this case, $\mathrm{Var}(X)$ is a square and symmetric matrix with diagonal elements containing the variances of the components of X and off-diagonal elements containing the covariances between two components.

The covariance between two random variables X_1 and X_2 is given by

$$\mathrm{Cov}(X_1, X_2) = E\left[\{X_1 - E(X_1)\}\{X_2 - E(X_2)\}\right].$$

This covariance can be expressed also as

$$\mathrm{Cov}(X_1, X_2) = E(X_1 X_2) - E(X_1)E(X_2).$$

If X_1 and X_2 are independent random variables, $\mathrm{Cov}(X_1, X_2) = 0$, since the expectation of a product of independent random variables equals the product of their expectations. On the other hand, $\mathrm{Cov}(X_1, X_2) = 0$ does not imply independence.

Laws of Variance and Covariance

For a random variable X,

$$\mathrm{Var}(aX + b) = a^2 \mathrm{Var}(X).$$

For a random vector X,

$$\mathrm{Var}(AX + b) = A\,\mathrm{Var}(X)\,A'.$$

Notice that the additive constant does not change the variance, as the variance of a constant is zero. For two random variables X_1 and X_2,

$$\mathrm{Cov}(a_1 X_1 + b_1, a_2 X_2 + b_2) = a_1 a_2 \mathrm{Cov}(X_1, X_2)$$

and

$$\mathrm{Var}(X_1 + X_2) = \mathrm{Var}(X_1) + \mathrm{Var}(X_2) + 2\mathrm{Cov}(X_1, X_2).$$

For independent random variables, the variance of their sum equals the sum of their variances.

Conditional Expectation and Variance

Consider two random variables X and Y. For each possible value y of Y, there is a conditional distribution of X conditioned on $Y = y$. This conditional distribution has a mean (or expectation) denoted by $E(X|Y = y)$. This expectation is a function of y, say $g(y)$. The random variable $g(Y)$ is called the conditional expectation of X given Y and denoted $E(X|Y)$.

If we replace the conditional mean by the conditional variance in the above paragraph, we get the definition of conditional variance. Here $\mathrm{Var}(X|Y = y)$ is a function of y, say $h(y)$. The random variable $h(Y)$ is called the conditional variance of X given Y and denoted $\mathrm{Var}(X|Y)$.

Laws with Conditional Expectations and Variances

The expectation of a random variable X can be expressed as a successive expectation in the following sense:

$$E(X) = E\left\{E(X|Y)\right\}.$$

Notice that the inside expectation on the right-hand side is an integral with respect to the conditional distribution of X, that is, the variable of integration is x. The outside expectation is an integral with respect to the marginal distribution of Y as $E(X|Y)$ is a function of Y.

The variance of a random variable also can be expressed in a similar fashion:

$$\mathrm{Var}(X) = E\left\{\mathrm{Var}(X|Y)\right\} + \mathrm{Var}\left\{E(X|Y)\right\}.$$

Strong Law of Large Numbers

Suppose $X_1, X_2, \ldots$ is a sequence of iid random variables, and $g(\cdot)$ is a function such that $E\left\{g(X_1)\right\}$ and $\mathrm{Var}\left\{g(X_1)\right\}$ are finite. Then, with probability 1,

$$\lim_{n\to\infty} \frac{1}{n} \sum_{i=1}^{n} g(X_i) = E\left[g(X_1)\right].$$

This law also holds under milder conditions on the sequence of random variables, in particular when it is a stationary Markov chain.

Appendix B

Common Distributions

In this appendix we list the various distributions in common use. Table B.1 lists discrete distributions, Table B.2 lists continuous univariate distributions, and Table B.3 continuous multivariate distributions.

TABLE B.1: Discrete univariate and multivariate distributions

Family and variable domain	Notation and parameter domain	Kernel of density	Normalizing constant	Mean	Variance
Bernoulli $x \in \{0,1\}$	$Ber(\pi)$ $\pi \in (0,1)$	$\pi^x(1-\pi)^{1-x}$	1	π	$\pi(1-\pi)$
Binomial $x \in \{0,\dots,n\}$	$Bin(n,\pi)$ $n \in \{0,1,\dots\}, \pi \in (0,1)$	$\frac{n!}{x!(n-x)!}\pi^x(1-\pi)^{n-x}$	1	$n\pi$	$n\pi(1-\pi)$
Multinomial $y_i \in \{0,\dots,n\}$, $\ni \sum_{i=1}^{k} y_i = n$	$Mult_k(n,\boldsymbol{\theta})$ $n \in \{0,1,\dots\}, \boldsymbol{\theta} \in \mathbb{R}^k,$ $\theta_i \in \theta_i > 0 \,\forall i, \sum_{i=1}^{k}\theta_i = 1$	$\prod_{i=1}^{k}\theta_i^{y_i} / \prod_{i=1}^{k} y_i!$	$1/n!$	$E(y_i) = n\theta_i,$ $i=1,\dots,n$	$\mathrm{Var}(y_i) = n\theta_i(1-\theta_i)$ $\mathrm{Cov}(y_i,y_j) = -n\theta_i\theta_j, (i \neq j)$
Poisson $x \in \{0,1,\dots\}$	$Po(\lambda)$ $\lambda \in (0,\infty)$	$\lambda^x/x!$	e^λ	λ	λ

TABLE B.2: Continuous univariate distributions

Family and variable domain	Notation and parameter domain	Kernel of density	Normalizing constant	Mean	Variance
Beta $x \in (0,1)$	$Be(\alpha,\beta)$ $\alpha \in (0,\infty), \beta \in (0,\infty)$	$x^{\alpha-1}(1-x)^{\beta-1}$	$\frac{\Gamma(\alpha)\Gamma(\beta)}{\Gamma(\alpha+\beta)}$	$\frac{\alpha}{\alpha+\beta}$	$\frac{\alpha\beta}{(\alpha+\beta)^2(\alpha+\beta+1)}$
Chi-square $x \in (0,\infty)$	$\chi^2(\nu) \;(= Ga(\nu/2,1/2))$ $\nu \in \{1,2,\dots\}$	$x^{(\nu/2)-1}e^{-x/2}$	$2^{\nu/2}\Gamma(\nu/2)$	ν	2ν
Inverse chi-square $x \in (0,\infty)$	$Inv\chi^2(\nu)$ $\nu \in \{1,2,\dots\}$	$x^{-(\nu/2)-1}e^{-x^{-1}/2}$	$2^{-\nu/2}\Gamma(\nu/2)$	$(\nu-2)^{-1}$, $\nu > 2$	$2(\nu-2)^{-2}\times$ $(\nu-4)^{-1}$, $\nu > 4$
Exponential $x \in (0,\infty)$	$Exp(\lambda)$ $\lambda \in (0,\infty)$	$e^{-\lambda x}$	$1/\lambda$	$1/\lambda$	$1/\lambda^2$
Fisher's F $x \in (0,\infty)$	$F(\nu_1,\nu_2)$ $\nu_1,\nu_2 \in \{1,2,\dots\}$	$x^{(\nu_1/2)-1}\times$ $\left\{1+\frac{\nu_1}{\nu_2}x\right\}^{-(\nu_1+\nu_2)/2}$	$(\nu_2/\nu_1)^{\nu_1/2}\times$ $\frac{\Gamma(\nu_1/2)\Gamma(\nu_2/2)}{\Gamma((\nu_1+\nu_2)/2)}$	$\frac{\nu_2}{\nu-2}$, $\nu > 2$	$\frac{\nu_1+\nu_2-2}{(\nu_2-2)^2(\nu_2-4)}\times$ $\frac{2\nu_2^2}{\nu_1}$, $\nu > 4$
Gamma $x \in (0,\infty)$	$G(\alpha,\beta)$ $\alpha \in (0,\infty), \beta \in (0,\infty)$	$x^{\alpha-1}e^{-x/\beta}$	$\beta^\alpha\Gamma(\alpha)$	$\alpha\beta$	$\alpha\beta^2$
	$Ga(\alpha,\lambda)$ $\alpha \in (0,\infty), \lambda \in (0,\infty)$	$x^{\alpha-1}e^{-\lambda x}$	$\Gamma(\alpha)/\lambda^\alpha$	α/λ	α/λ^2
Inverse gamma $x \in (0,\infty)$	$InvGa(\alpha,\beta)$ $\alpha \in (0,\infty), \beta \in (0,\infty)$	$\left(\frac{1}{x}\right)^{\alpha+1}e^{-\beta/x}$	$\beta^\alpha/\Gamma(\alpha)$	$\frac{\beta}{\alpha-1}$ $\alpha > 1$	$\frac{\beta^2}{(\alpha-1)^2(\alpha-2)}$ $\alpha > 2$
Log-normal $x \in (0,\infty)$	$LN(\mu,\sigma^2)$ $\mu \in (-\infty,\infty), \sigma^2 \in (0,\infty)$	$x^{-1}e^{-\frac{1}{2\sigma^2}(\log(x)-\mu)^2}$	$\sigma\sqrt{2\pi}$	$e^{\mu+\frac{1}{2}\sigma^2}$	$(e^{\sigma^2}-1)e^{2\mu+\sigma^2}$

TABLE B.2: Continuous univariate distributions (continued)

Family and variable domain	Notation and parameter domain	Kernel of density	Normalizing constant	Mean	Variance
Normal $x \in (-\infty,\infty)$	$N(\mu,\sigma^2)$ $\mu \in (-\infty,\infty), \sigma^2 \in (0,\infty)$	$e^{-\frac{1}{2\sigma^2}(x-\mu)^2}$	$\sigma\sqrt{2\pi}$	μ	σ^2
	$No(\mu,\tau)$ $\mu \in (-\infty,\infty), \tau \in (0,\infty)$	$e^{-\frac{\tau}{2}(x-\mu)^2}$	$\tau^{-1/2}\sqrt{2\pi}$	μ	$1/\tau$
		$e^{-\frac{\tau}{2}(x^2-2\mu x)}$	$\tau^{-1/2}\sqrt{2\pi}e^{\tau\mu^2/2}$	μ	$1/\tau$
	$Nor(a,b)$ $a \in (0,\infty), b \in (-\infty,\infty)$	$e^{-\frac{1}{2}(ax^2-2bx)}$	$\frac{\sqrt{2\pi}e^{b^2/(2a)}}{a^{1/2}}$	b/a	$1/a$
Normal-gamma $x \in (-\infty,\infty)$, $y \in (0,\infty)$	$NoGa(\mu,k,\alpha,\beta)$ $\mu \in (-\infty,\infty), k \in (0,\infty),$ $\alpha \in (0,\infty), \beta \in (0,\infty)$	$y^{\alpha-\frac{1}{2}}e^{-\frac{1}{2}ky\{(x-\mu)^2+2\beta/k\}}$	$\frac{\sqrt{2\pi}\Gamma(\alpha)}{k^{1/2}\beta^\alpha}$	$\mu, \alpha/\beta$ $\alpha > 1/2$	$\frac{\beta}{k(\alpha-1)}, \frac{\alpha}{\beta^2}$ $\alpha > 1$
Pareto $x \in (a,\infty)$	$Par(a,b)$ $a \in (0,\infty), b \in (0,\infty)$	$x^{-(b+1)}I_{(a,\infty)}(x)$	$1/(ba^b)$	$\frac{ab}{b-1}, b>1$	$\frac{a^2b}{(b-1)^2(b-2)}, b>2$
Student's t $x \in (-\infty,\infty)$	$t(\nu,\mu,\sigma^2), \quad \nu \in (0,\infty),$ $\mu \in (-\infty,\infty), \sigma \in (0,\infty)$	$\left\{1+\frac{1}{\nu}\left(\frac{x-\mu}{\sigma}\right)^2\right\}^{-(\nu+1)/2}$	$\frac{\sigma\sqrt{\nu\pi}\Gamma(\nu/2)}{\Gamma((\nu+1)/2)}$	$\mu, \nu > 1$	$\frac{\sigma^2\nu}{\nu-2}, \nu > 2$
	$St(\nu,\mu,\tau), \quad \nu \in (0,\infty),$ $\mu \in (-\infty,\infty), \tau \in (0,\infty)$	$\left\{1+\frac{\tau}{\nu}(x-\mu)^2\right\}^{-(\nu+1)/2}$	$\frac{\sqrt{\nu\pi}\Gamma(\nu/2)}{\tau^{1/2}\Gamma((\nu+1)/2)}$	$\mu, \nu > 1$	$\frac{\tau^{-1}\nu}{\nu-2}, \nu > 2$
Uniform $x \in (a,b)$	$U(a,b)$ $a \in (-\infty,\infty), b \in (a,\infty)$	1	$b-a$	$\frac{a+b}{2}$	$\frac{(b-a)^2}{12}$
Weibull $x \in (0,\infty)$	$Weib(\alpha,\lambda)$ $\alpha \in (0,\infty), \lambda \in (0,\infty)$	$x^{\alpha-1}e^{-\lambda x^\alpha}$	$1/(\alpha\lambda)$	$\frac{\Gamma(1/\alpha)}{\alpha\lambda^{1/\alpha}}$	$\frac{2\Gamma(2/\alpha)-\Gamma^2(1/\alpha)}{\alpha\lambda^{2/\alpha}}$

TABLE B.3: Continuous multivariate distributions

Family and variable domain	Notation and parameter domain	Kernel of density	Normalizing constant	Mean	Variance
Dirichlet $\theta \in \mathbb{R}^k, \ni \theta_i > 0$ $\forall i, \sum_{i=1}^k \theta_i = 1$	$D_k(\alpha)$ $\alpha \in \mathbb{R}^k, \ni \alpha_i > 0 \forall i,$ $\sum_{i=1}^k \alpha_i = \alpha_+$	$\prod_{i=1}^k \theta_i^{\alpha_i}$	$\prod_1^k \Gamma(\alpha_i)/\Gamma(\alpha_+)$	α/α_+	
Normal $x \in \mathbb{R}^p$	$N_p(\mu, \Sigma), \ \mu \in \mathbb{R}^p$ $\Sigma \ p \times p$ positive definite	$e^{-\frac{1}{2}(x-\mu)'\Sigma^{-1}(x-\mu)}$	$(2\pi)^{p/2}|\Sigma|^{1/2}$	μ	Σ
	$No_p(\mu, T), \ \mu \in \mathbb{R}^p$ $T \ p \times p$ positive definite	$e^{-\frac{1}{2}(x-\mu)'T(x-\mu)}$	$(2\pi)^{p/2}|T|^{-1/2}$	μ	T^{-1}
	$Nor_p(A,B), \ B \in \mathbb{R}^p$ $A \ p \times p$ positive definite	$e^{-\frac{1}{2}(x'Ax-2B'x)}$	$(2\pi)^{p/2}|A|^{-1/2} \times$ $e^{\frac{1}{2}B'A^{-1}B}$	$A^{-1}B$	A^{-1}
T $x \in \mathbb{R}^p$	$T_p(\nu,\mu,\Sigma), \nu > 0, \mu \in \mathbb{R}^p$ $\Sigma \ p \times p$ positive definite	$\left\{1 + \frac{1}{\nu}(x-\mu)'\Sigma^{-1}(x-\mu)\right\}^{-(\nu+p)/2}$	$c_T|\Sigma|^{1/2}$	μ $\nu > 1$	$\frac{\nu\Sigma}{(\nu-2)}$ $\nu > 2$
	$ST_p(\nu,\mu,T), \nu > 0, \mu \in \mathbb{R}^p$ $T \ p \times p$ positive definite	$\left\{1 + \frac{1}{\nu}(x-\mu)'T(x-\mu)\right\}^{-(\nu+p)/2}$	$c_T|T|^{-1/2}$	μ $\nu > 1$	$\frac{\nu T^{-1}}{(\nu-2)}$ $\nu > 2$
Wishart $X \ p \times p$ matrix, symmetric and positive definite	$W_p(\Omega,\nu), \ \nu \geq p,$ $\Omega \ p \times p$ positive definite	$|X|^{(\nu-p-1)/2}e^{-\frac{1}{2}tr(\Omega^{-1}X)}$	$c_W|\Omega|^{\nu/2}$ [2]	$\nu\Omega$	
	$Wi_p(\Psi,\nu), \ \nu \geq p,$ $\Psi \ p \times p$ positive definite	$|X|^{(\nu-p-1)/2}e^{-\frac{1}{2}tr(\Psi X)}$	$c_W|\Psi|^{-\nu/2}$	$\nu\Psi^{-1}$	
Inverse Wishart $X \ p \times p$ matrix, symmetric and positive definite	$IW_p(\Psi,\nu), \ \nu \geq p,$ $\Omega \ p \times p$ positive definite	$|X|^{-(\nu+p+1)/2}e^{-\frac{1}{2}tr(\Psi X^{-1})}$	$c_W|\Psi|^{\nu/2}$	$\frac{\Psi}{\nu-p-1}$	

[1] $c_T = \frac{(\pi\nu)^{d/2}\Gamma(\nu/2)}{\Gamma((\nu+d)/2)}$

[2] $c_W = 2^{\nu p/2}\pi^{p(p-1)/4}\prod_{i=1}^p \Gamma((\nu+1-i)/2)$

Appendix C

Software for Sampling Posterior Distributions

There are many basic calculations that one can perform in R and the random number generation functions available in it for Bayesian inference, but more complicated probability models will either be too slow or too difficult to program in R. In this Appendix, we provide a brief introduction to software that is available for carrying out Bayesian computation. We focus primarily on WinBUGS, OpenBUGS, JAGS, and Stan. We also touch on the R packages that allow one to interface with these programs, making the analysis more efficient. All of the software and packages we discuss are available free of charge and share some common syntax. They are geared towards simulation from posterior distributions given a model, prior, and data.

The R2WinBUGS and BRugs packages allow one to drive WinBUGS and OpenBUGS from R. This is a major convenience, since this makes it easy to manipulate MCMC output to make pretty pictures of collections of posterior densities, predictive distributions, and so on. Moreover, if one needs to run the same BUGS code many times with slight modifications, it is much simpler to do it from R using one of these packages. Similar functionality is available with Stan and JAGS. Finally, we give brief descriptions of some R packages useful for Bayesian work.

C.1 WinBUGS

The BUGS language can be regarded as a device for communicating models and distributions [232]. This is in contrast to usual scientific computing languages that expect instructions for carrying out calculations. Keeping this distinction in mind is helpful for understanding and writing code.

We describe the basics in three parts: (i) model specification; (ii) input of data and constants; and (iii) iterations and monitoring of variables. We strongly urge the reader to concurrently use the software while reading through the next two examples.

Model specification. This main component of the language asks the user to specify both the sampling model and the priors. For this purpose, two types of statements are available: one declaring the distribution of a variable, the other specifying a variable's mathematical relationship to other variables. For the first purpose, most common distributions are given names with specified parameterizations. A complete table of these distributions is contained in the software manual. We will introduce a few via their use in examples.

Example C.1. In Example 4.6, we generated samples from the posterior distribution of (μ, τ) when the sampling distribution of individual data points is $N(\mu, \tau)$, and independent $N(\mu_0, \tau_0)$ and $Ga(\alpha_0, \lambda_0)$ priors are used for μ and τ, respectively. Here we show how WinBUGS can be used to accomplish the same task.

First, we put into a text file the group of statements on the left in Figure C.1. These model statements can be represented as a directed acyclic graph that specifies relationships between all variables in the model. Such a graph consists of variables as nodes and directed arrows pointing between nodes as determined from the model specification. The graph's visual representation is shown on the right in Figure C.1. Here {mu, tau, y[i], i=1,...,n}, pictured in circles, are stochastic nodes, as these are assigned distributions. The remaining variables, {mu0, tau0, alpha0, lambda0, n} are constants and displayed in rectangles.

```
model{
  for(i in 1:n){
    y[i] ~ dnorm(mu,tau)
  }
  mu ~ dnorm(mu0,tau0)
  tau~dgamma(alpha0,lambda0)
}
```

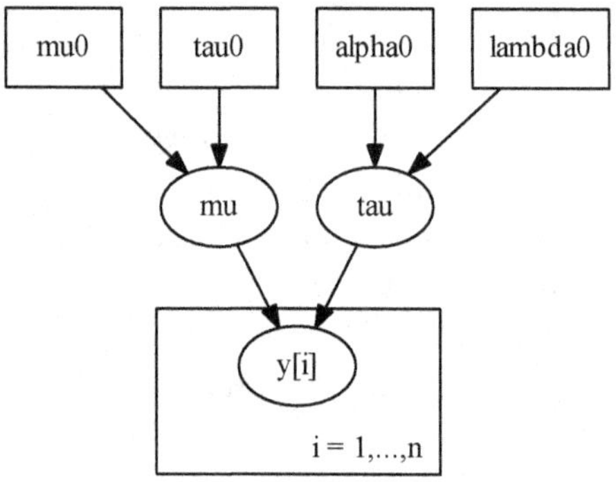

FIGURE C.1: Simple normal-normal model in the BUGS language (left) and the corresponding directed acyclic graph (right).

Notice that WinBUGS automatically infers that the distribution of y[i] is a conditional distribution conditioned on mu and tau, as these are used as parameters in dnorm. We then ask WinBUGS to check this model for proper syntax by clicking the "check model" button on the *Specification Tool* started from the **Model** menu item on the menu bar.

Input of Data and Constants. The next task is to read in the constants and the data. This can be done by highlighting the word "list" from text, such as

```
list(n=403,alpha0=0.1,lambda0=0.1,mu0=150,tau0=0.001)
```

written in an opened text (.txt) or odc (.odc) file, and clicking the "load data" button on the *Specification Tool.* In addition to these constants, we need to input the data. Here we will use the `Weight_00` variable's non-missing response values from the **VetBP** data first introduced in Example 1.1. Using R and some manual editing, this was written into a text file (`dataWeight_00.txt` on the book's website under Chapter 4) as

```
list(y=c(190.4,161.2,...,184.6)),
```

where the ... consist of 400 additional weight values. After all data are read in, we ask WinBUGS to "compile" this model. In this step, WinBUGS performs a good deal of mathematical and coding tasks for us. Knowing which stochastic nodes have been given data values, it prepares to simulate posterior samples for all other nodes conditional on these data. Essentially, it is "deriving" the conditional distributions for the Gibbs sampler for the model, determining what simulation method to use (including the adaptive rejection sampler for log-concave distributions), and putting all this code together for iterative simulation of samples from the posterior.

If we want to monitor multiple chains, we need to input the number of chains using the "num of chains" button on the *Specification Tool*, after the data are loaded and before compiling.

MCMC Iterations and Monitoring of Variables. To start the simulations, WinBUGS needs initial values for all stochastic nodes that are not given data values. On the *Specification Tool*, the "load inits" button can be used in a manner similar to the "load data" button. An alternative is to let WinBUGS generate initial values ("gen inits"), which it does using the priors for these nodes. It is also possible to load initial values for some variables and generate them for the rest. We note, however, that there will be instances when it is necessary to specify initial values. This is often indicated by certain error messages when attempting to have BUGS generate initial values. If multiple chains are specified, then the same number of sets of distinct initial values are required. BUGS will keep requesting them until all have been specified.

At this point, WinBUGS is ready to start the Markov chain. We now click "samples" from the **Inference** menu, which brings up the *Sample Monitor Tool*. Here we type in the node names (`mu, tau`) one at a time and click the highlighted "set" button. When done, we need to type *, which informs BUGS that we have set all of the stochastic variables that we want to monitor. The other input items on this tool are relevant only after the samples are generated.

Next, we go back to the **Model** menu and click on the *Update Tool*. Here, we must indicate how many iterates are to be simulated. A thinning value can be specified here also, but this is not recommended when first running your program. The "refresh" button gives an indication of how much time is needed for the number of iterates specified there. For example, if it is set to 100, one can see how long each set of 100 iterates takes to simulate. Clicking the "update" button starts the sampling. This tool can be used repeatedly to add iterations if we wish.

To see the results, we return to the *Sample Monitor Tool*. The "history" button shows a plot of the chain, starting at the specified iteration. Looking at the chain from the very beginning, we see that convergence occurs rapidly; a burn-in of 100 iterations is quite sufficient. Now starting at iteration 101, we click the "density" button to see the posterior densities of mu and tau. The "stats" button puts out some summaries for each variable, and the "auto corr" button generates autocorrelation plots. Finally, the "coda" button generates two files, one containing the posterior samples sequentially, and another containing indexing information for extraction of the MCMC generated samples for each of the variables. As we see below, it is much more convenient to use R to convey input to WinBUGS and to extract samples from it to analyze in R.

C.1.1 OpenBUGS

OpenBUGS developed as an open-source version of WinBUGS and is very similar to it. It is also free of charge and readily available for downloading from the internet. There are some differences from WinBUGS, mainly enhancements, that are explained on the website openbugs.info. All of the above description of how WinBUGS works, including the code and the graphics interface, applies identically to OpenBUGS.

C.1.2 Censored Data in BUGS

BUGS handles censored data (see Chapters 11 and 12) in a special way. One sets the censored times to missing and uses a built-in function for censoring, I(L,U). The I(L,U) function follows a distributional statement for a stochastic node and means that the value lies between the values L and U.

For survival analysis with accelerated failure-time (AFT) regression models, the construct works as follows. If the ith individual's time is not censored, the value of t[i] is the actual time of the event (i.e., t[i]$=t_i$). If the ith individual's time is censored, the value of t[i] is missing and entered as NA. If an observation is right censored at c_i, we set L[i] $= c_i$. That is, the lower bound is the censored observation time. For the upper bound, we leave it blank to indicate that there is no upper limit. In our program, we write I(c[i],). If the observation is left censored at c_i, set U[i] to c_i and set L[i] equal to 0, since the actual time cannot be negative. If we have interval censored data, we use L[i] equal to the lower bound of the interval and U[i] equal to the upper bound. For uncensored observations, t[i] $= t_i$, the observed time to the event. If the observation is not missing (i.e., t[i] is not set to NA), the constraints given in I(L,U) are ignored.

Below are some BUGS programming statements that specify a log-normal AFT model for Example 12.1 (see Chapter 12). The log-normal regression model uses reference priors, and the BUGS program includes a subset of the data listed at the end. In the code, the distribution of the times is specified in the statement

```
t[i] ~ dlnorm(mu[i], tau) I(c[i],)
```

The statement tells BUGS that the outcome times have a log-normal distribution with mean mu[i] and precision tau. Furthermore, the statement constrains the times that are missing (i.e., =NA) to be larger than c[i]. Again, if the time t[i] has a value and does not equal NA, the constraint is ignored. In the program below, c[i] equals 0 for all uncensored times.

```
model{
 for(i in 1:106){
   sAge[i] <- (age[i]-mean(age[ ]))/sd(age[ ])
   sYr[i] <- (Yr[i]-mean(Yr[ ]))/sd(Yr[ ])
   t[i] ~ dlnorm(mu[i], tau) I(c[i],)
   mu[i] <- beta[1] + beta[2]*equals(stage[i],2)
                    + beta[3]*equals(stage[i],3)
                    + beta[4]*equals(stage[i],4)
            + beta[5]*sAge[i] + beta[6]*sYr[i]
# 5 month survival probabilities using covariates in the data
   S[i] <- 1- phi((log(5)-mu[i])*sqrt(tau))
# Medians corresponding to the covariates in the data
   med[i] <- exp(mu[i])
 }
 for(i in 1:6){
   beta[i] ~ dnorm(0,0.000001)
   rm[i] <- exp(beta[i])  # RMs for each variable
   prob[i] <- step(beta[i])
 }
 tau ~ dgamma(0.001,0.001)
 sigma <- sqrt(1/tau)
}
list(beta=c(0,0,0,0,0,0),tau=1)  # Initial values
stage[ ] t[ ] age[ ] Yr[ ] c[ ]
1 0.6 77 76 0
1 1.3 53 71 0
1 2.4 45 71 0
1 NA  57 78 2.5
1 3.2 58 74 0
1 NA 51 77 3.2
The last 84 data lines have been removed to save space
END
```

We note that one does not have to use the above approach for handling censored data if one is fitting a proportional hazards regression model as given in Section 12.2.2. An example program is in the folder for Chapter 12 on the book's website. The file has PHRegression in the name.

C.1.3   Interface with R: **R2WinBUGS** and **BRugs**

R2WinBUGS and BRugs are R packages that enable one to interact with WinBUGS or OpenBUGS. These R packages allow data manipulation and preparation, convenient input of constants and data, and extraction of posterior samples for further processing and graphing in R. Here are some highlights of the packages, including R code to illustrate their use.

R2WinBUGS. With R2WinBUGS, we need several things to interact with one of the BUGS programs. We need (i) the BUGS program (the program statements either in a named text file or a character object in R), (ii) data lists for input, (iii) a vector with the names of model parameters whose posterior samples we want to save, and (iv) a function to initialize the chains. The following example illustrates the use of R2WinBUGS. The approach involves reading data into R and then writing R commands to drive WinBUGS or OpenBUGS in R.

Example C.2. We continue with Example C.1, where the variable `Weight_00` was taken from the **VetBP** data set. The data set is contained in the file `VetBP.csv` on the book's website under Chapter 3. The model specification (BUGS) code is also there in `wtmodel.txt`. Both files should be placed in the R working directory.

The BUGS code fits a simple model with a Gaussian likelihood, Gaussian prior for the mean, and a gamma prior for the precision, the reciprocal of the variance. Note that one specifies a normal or Gaussian distribution in the BUGS language in terms of the mean and the precision, not the mean and the standard deviation (as in R) or variance.

```
model{ # Likelihood
  for(i in 1:n){
     y[i] ~ dnorm(mu, tau) }
#  Prior
   mu ~ dnorm(mu0, tau0)
   tau ~ dgamma(alpha0, lambda0)
# Parameter of interest
   sigma <- 1/sqrt(tau)
   cv <- sigma/mu    }
```

The following R code uses WinBUGS to generate posterior samples and subsequently summarize inferences and graphs. The R function bugs() instructs R to run WinBUGS to generate posterior iterates. Inferences for the standard deviation $\sigma = 1/\sqrt{\tau}$ and coefficient of variation $cv = \sigma/\mu$ are illustrated.

We run the program in R using the R package R2WinBUGS, which can call OpenBUGS or WinBUGS (the default). The R commands below specify the data, the values of parameters of the prior distributions, and the names of the parameters to monitor. There is also a function that will generate initial values in R for the parameters `mu` and `tau`. The last command instructs R to call WinBUGS and save the results in the R object called `VetBP.sim`.

```
library("R2WinBUGS")
VetBPdata <- read.csv("VetBP.csv", header=T)
# indices of non-missing observations
ok <- !is.na(VetBPdata$Weight_00)
```

```
# vector of non-missing observations
y <- VetBPdata$Weight_00[ok]
n <- length(y)
alpha0 <- 0.1; lambda0 <- 0.1;
mu0 <- 150; tau0 <- 0.001
data <- list("n", "y", "mu0", "tau0", "alpha0", "lambda0")
inits <- function() {
  list(mu = rnorm(1, mean=120, sd=5),
       tau = runif(1, min=0.1, max=10))
}
parameters <- c("mu", "tau", "sigma", "cv")


# Run using the default, WinBUGS
VetBP.sim <- bugs(data, inits, parameters, "wtmodel.txt",
                  n.chains=3, n.iter=10000, debug=F, useWINE=F)
```

The R2WinBUGS package includes versions of the print( ) and plot( ) commands specifically for the MCMC samples that are returned via the bugs command. Here is the default output of the print( ) command.

```
> print(VetBP.sim)
Inference for Bugs model at "VetBP_BUGS.txt", fit using WinBUGS,
 3 chains, each with 10000 iterations (first 5000 discarded), n.thin = 15
 n.sims = 1002 iterations saved
            mean  sd   2.5%    25%   50%    75%  97.5% Rhat n.eff
mu         210.0 2.1  205.8  208.5  210  211.4  214.1    1  1000
sigma       44.1 1.6   41.0   42.9   44   45.1   47.4    1  1000
deviance  4195.5 2.1 4194.0 4194.0 4195 4196.0 4200.0    1   800

For each parameter, n.eff is a crude measure of effective sample size,
and Rhat is the potential scale reduction factor (at convergence, Rhat=1).

# Deviance Information Criterion
DIC info (using the rule, pD = Dbar-Dhat) #We discuss DIC in Chapter 10
pD = 2.0 and DIC = 4197.5
DIC is an estimate of expected predictive error (lower deviance is better).
```

One can also use the R package R2WinBUGS with OpenBUGS. One simply specifies the name of the program in the program= argument of the bugs( ) command as in the following statement.

```
# Run with OpenBUGS
VetBP.sim <- bugs(data, inits, parameters, "wtmodel.txt",
                  n.chains=3, n.iter=10000, program="openbugs")
```

We next use the features of the R package coda to check some characteristics of the MCMC output (with result in Figure C.2).

```
 # Coerce to mcmc object for use with coda then plot
MCMCout <- as.mcmc(VetBP.sim$sims.matrix)
```

```
str(MCMCout)
plot(MCMCout[,c(1,3)])  #  Plot mu and sigma
```

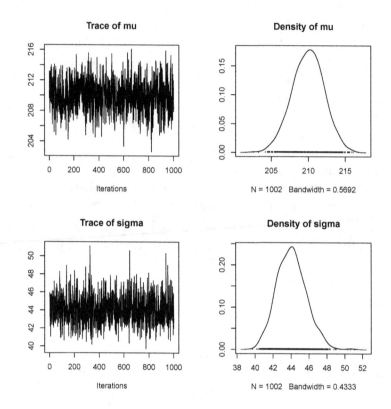

FIGURE C.2: Output of plot() function on object generated by R package coda.

We check autocorrelations with the coda function autocorr.

```
> autocorr(MCMCout[,c(1,3)])
, , mu


                  mu          sigma
Lag 0    1.00000000   0.093958603
Lag 1    0.03522100  -0.010263788
Lag 5   -0.05131544   0.024386797
Lag 10   0.06082433   0.002685143
Lag 50   0.03939281   0.004553790


, , sigma


                  mu          sigma
Lag 0    0.093958603  1.0000000000
Lag 1    0.008429359 -0.0358526279
```

```
Lag 5    0.040119814  -0.0174528540
Lag 10   0.019199481  -0.0008152195
Lag 50  -0.037513675   0.0243738396
```

Note that the autocorrelations for μ appear in the first column in the first set, and those for σ in the second column in the second set. The other columns contain cross-correlations. The autocorrelations can be plotted with **autocorr.plot(MCMCout[,1:2])**; the resulting graphs are shown in Figure C.3.

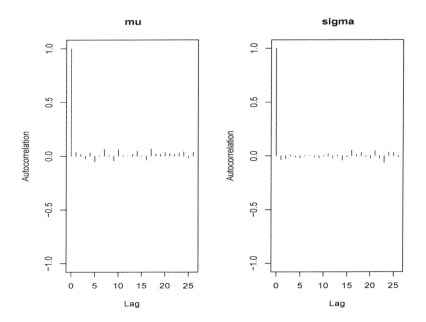

FIGURE C.3: Autocorrelation plots from coda.

Additionally, we can create a new parameter as a function of model parameters and use the saved posterior samples to infer its posterior distribution and characteristics related to it. For example, the following statements in R compute the coefficient of variation and plot its posterior distribution (see Figure C.4).

```
# Posterior for coefficient of variation.
cvs <- MCMCout[,4]
summary(cvs)
pdf("VetBP_CV_plots.pdf")
hist(cvs,probability=TRUE)
lines(density(cvs))
dev.off()
```

BRugs. This is an alternative interface with OpenBUGS. It is more direct and less automated than R2WinBUGS.

- BRugs supplies several functions that are equivalent to clicking various buttons

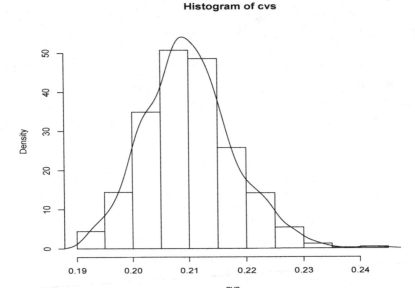

FIGURE C.4: Posterior density of the coefficient of variation of the `Weight_00` variable.

on the three pop-up tools (*Specification*, *Update*, and *Sample Monitor*) in OpenBUGS.

- The `modelData` function provides two forms of data input. One form loads data directly from a text file containing data in OpenBUGS format. The other form takes a list of names of R objects matching variables in the syntax-checked model and passes the list to OpenBUGS in the appropriate format. This second form allows data reading and preparation to be performed in R. Data can be loaded in steps by using this function multiple times.

- The `samplesSample` function is somewhat like the *coda* button in WinBUGS. It extracts samples for a monitored variable. Again, this is very useful, as it makes posterior samples available in R for all post-MCMC manipulations and graphing.

For Example C.2, we replace the `bugs()` function call when using the R package R2WinBUGS with BRugs commands as follows.

```
library("BRugs")

modelCheck("wtmodel.txt")
modelData(bugsData(
    list("y", "n","mu0", "tau0", "alpha0", "lambda0"))
    )
modelCompile(numChains=3)
```

```
# initial values for three chains
mu <- rnorm(1, mean=120, sd=5)
tau <- runif(1, min=0.1, max=10)
modelInits(bugsData(list("mu","tau")))
mu <- rnorm(1, mean=120, sd=5)
tau <- runif(1, min=0.1, max=10)
modelInits(bugsData(list("mu","tau")))
mu <- rnorm(1, mean=120, sd=5)
tau <- runif(1, min=0.1, max=10)
modelInits(bugsData(list("mu","tau")))

modelUpdate(500) # burn-in 500 iterations

samplesSet(c("mu","tau")) # specify nodes to monitor
modelUpdate(1000)

samplesStats("*")
samplesHistory("*")
samplesDensity("*")
samplesBgr("*")
samplesAutoC("*", 1)

# extract samples
musamples <- samplesSample("mu")
tausamples <- samplesSample("tau")
```

The R objects **musamples** and **tausamples** can be used in subsequent post-processing to accomplish inference for functions of these.

C.2 JAGS

JAGS [261], which humbly derives its name from Just Another Gibbs Sampler, is available for download at http://mcmc-jags.sourceforge.net/ and runs on multiple operating systems. In fact, the motivation for the development of JAGS was to have a BUGS-like program that will run in the Unix environment. JAGS is open-source, and there is an active users' group. The program shares many features with the original BUGS program, and the syntax is similar to that of WinBUGS, although there are some differences. Of particular interest for biostatisticians are the differences in the way the programs handle censored observations.

We discuss the way to work with censoring when fitting an AFT regression model (see Section 12.1) in JAGS in the next section. We note that one does not have to use the same approach for handling censored data if one is fitting a proportional hazards regression model as given in Section 12.2.2. An example program is in the folder for Chapter 12 on the book's website. The file has PHRegression in the name.

Another difference between JAGS and WinBUGS or OpenBUGS is the ability to transform data within JAGS but separately from the programming carried out within the *model* block. One specifies these transformations in a set of programming statements enclosed in braces preceded by the keyword *data*. That is, the JAGS program would start with

```
data{
   ...
   programming statements for data transformation
   ...
}
```

followed by statements specifying the sampling distribution and prior distributions

```
model{
   ...
   programming statements
   ...
}
```

The programming statements could include things like standardizing covariates, computing logarithms, and similar one-time manipulations of the data. The advantage of having a separate *data* block is that the transformations will only occur once at the start of the program and not repeatedly at every iteration. Of course, one could also pass the transformed data to JAGS from R.

One can easily call JAGS from within the R programming environment, making it easy to use the graphical and analytical tools available there. There is the rjags package and a so-called wrapper package called R2jags that provides functionality similar to R2WinBUGS. The jagsUI package is another wrapper for rjags that tries to look and feel like R2WinBUGS, so one can easily move from JAGS to either WinBUGS or OpenBUGS.

C.2.1   Censored Data in JAGS

JAGS handles censored data (see Chapters 11 and 12) differently than BUGS. Censoring is different from truncation, and unlike BUGS, JAGS can handle both. Censoring simply means that we know that the observation could be larger than some value, although there was also a chance it could have been smaller. Truncation, on the other hand, means that the random variable cannot take values outside of the constrained range. An example of a truncated distribution is the half-normal distribution, which corresponds to the part of a normal density with mode at 0 but only allowing non-negative values. For example, one might specify a half-normal distribution for a standard deviation.

For censored data, JAGS uses the built-in function dinterval(,). For survival analysis with JAGS, dinterval(,) is used as a distribution. The function takes two arguments. If we write y[i] ~ dinterval(t[i], c[i]), then y[i] equals 0 if $t[i] \le c[i]$ and 1 if $t[i] > c[i]$.

In our survival analysis setting, we specify pairs (t_i, c_i) for each individual's event time and (potential) censoring time. Each individual has to have a potential censoring time, so we set c_i to a very large number (call it tMax) if t_i is an uncensored observation. The large number might be the largest possible follow-up time in the study under analysis.

We pass to JAGS an observation for each individual to indicate if the time is censored or not. For example, we can create a variable named is.censored[i] for each individual that we pass to JAGS with the data. This variable will equal 1 if the observation is a censored time and 0 if it is the time the patient experienced the event. We write in our JAGS program that this indicator variable has a distribution with the syntax is.censored[i] ~ dinterval(t[i], c[i]). In the statement, t[i] is either an actual time or missing (=NA), depending on whether the observation was the time of the actual event or a censoring time, respectively. The variable c[i] equals tMax if t[i] is an uncensored observation or a number a tiny bit larger than the follow-up time if t[i] is a censored observation. We wrote that c[i] should be a little larger than the censored follow-up time, because the function will expect 0 if t[i] equals c[i]. As a result of is.censored[i] equaling 1 when the observation is censored and t[i] is missing, JAGS will impute a value for the censored time that is larger than c[i], thanks to the program statement is.censored[i] ~ dinterval(t[i], c[i]).

We give the JAGS statements for the larynx cancer example in Chapter 12 (see Example 12.1). We fit a log-normal AFT regression to the data. In the program, the statements that specify the AFT model are the following.

```
is.censored[i] ~ dinterval(t[i], c[i])
t[i] ~ dlnorm(mu[i], tau)
```

We see that the variable is.censored[i] will be 0 or 1, depending on whether t[i] is less than or equal to c[i] or not. We specify t[i] as missing in the data we pass to JAGS, so only imputed values that are greater than c[i] will be *allowed*. Uncensored observations are treated as log-normally distributed observations in the program.

```
model {
  ### Create standardized covariates & means
  for (i in 1:(oldn + predn)) {
    sAge[i] <- (age[i]-mean(age[1:oldn]))/sd(age[1:oldn])
    sYr[i] <- (yr[i]-mean(yr[1:oldn]))/sd(yr[1:oldn])
    mu[i] <- beta[1] + beta[2]*equals(stage[i],2)
            + beta[3]*equals(stage[i],3)
            + beta[4]*equals(stage[i],4)
            + beta[5]*sAge[i] + beta[6]*sYr[i]
    # 5 month survival probabilities using covariates in the data
    S[i] <- 1- phi((log(5)-mu[i])*sqrt(tau))
```

```
   # Medians corresponding to the covariates in the data
     med[i] <- exp(mu[i])
   }
### Model observed subjects
for (i in 1:oldn) {
     is.censored[i] ~ dinterval(t[i], c[i])
     t[i] ~ dlnorm(mu[i], tau)
   }
   # Make predictions for combinations of covariates
   for(i in 1:predn) {
       predt[i] ~ dlnorm(mu[i + oldn], tau)
   }

   for (i in 1:6) {
      beta[i] ~ dnorm(0,0.000001)
      rm[i] <- exp(beta[i])   # RMs for each variable
   }
   tau ~ dgamma(0.001,0.001)
   sigma <- sqrt(1/tau)
}
```

C.3   Stan and rstan

Stan [64] is another program that one can use for fitting complex Bayesian models to analyze data. Like the BUGS-based programs (WinBUGS, OpenBUGS, and JAGS), Stan uses simulation to generate posterior samples. After the Markov chain has converged, one can treat the sample the program generated like random samples from the posterior distribution of interest. Stan has a very active users' group that contributes many example programs for fitting complex models.

A key difference between Stan and the BUGS-based programs is how Stan forms the Markov chain. Stan uses Hamiltonian Monte Carlo, whereas BUGS and related programs use methods based on the Metropolis–Hastings algorithm which includes Gibbs sampling (cf. Sections 4.4.1 and 4.4.2). We provide an overview of Hamiltonian Monte Carlo in Section 4.4.4.

There are a few other differences between Stan and WinBUGS that are worth pointing out. One difference is that one can compile a Stan program into a dynamic shared object that one can execute multiple times to generate samples. With the resulting object, one can carry out inference with this model and the same or similar data multiple times without the need to recompile the program. WinBUGS, Open-BUGS, and JAGS require that one use an interpreter that is part of the respective package each time one wishes to run a program to analyze data. Thus, while it may take longer initially to compile a **Stan** program than it takes to interpret a comparable program in **WinBUGS**, one will save time later if one wishes to reuse the same **Stan** program with the same or different data.

An idiosyncrasy of **Stan**, or really of the Hamiltonian Monte Carlo algorithm's reliance on gradients for directing proposals, is that one cannot have model parameters or latent variables that have discrete probability distributions. While this restriction to continuous parameters may seem highly limiting, one can sometimes find ways to work around it for many models. We show one such method in Chapter 9 where we discuss zero-inflated Poisson models (Section 9.2.2). The **Stan** code for that model is available on the book's website for Chapter 9.

Structure of a **Stan** Program

Programs for characterizing models in **Stan** are built around specifying a likelihood and a prior distribution. In this respect, **Stan** is similar to the **BUGS**-like programs. The actual structure of a **Stan** program is different, however. Also, all programming statements have to end with a semicolon (;).

Stan programs consist of blocks. Some blocks are required, and some are optional. The six main blocks that make up a Stan program are, in order, a *data* block, a *transformed data* block, a *parameters* block, a *transformed parameters* block, a *model* block, and a *generated quantities* block. At a minimum, one will probably want to use three of the blocks, namely, the *data*, *parameters*, and *model* blocks. In addition to the general program blocks, one can also write one's own functions for use in a Stan program. User-written function blocks are contained in separate *function* blocks that appear at the start of the Stan program, before the *data* block.

Each block starts with the name of the block as a keyword, followed by the block's statements enclosed in curly braces. Here is a brief description of each block. We note that none of the blocks are required, although a blank file will generate a warning. Furthermore, declarations of variables must precede program statements within a block. Finally, included blocks must be in the order in which we present them here.

The *data* block. This block tells **Stan** which variables in the program are fixed quantities that one inputs to **Stan**. These quantities do not change while the **Stan** program is executing. The primary quantities that appear in the data block are the observations and any fixed quantities that one uses in the program, such as the parameters in prior distributions. Within the data block, one specifies the data type of each quantity. There are many data types in **Stan**. The ones that we use most often are integer, real, vector, and matrix or array.

The *transformed data* block. This block allows one to create new fixed quantities or carry out mathematical calculations on entities defined in the data block. **Stan** includes many built-in functions that one can use to carry out transformations of the data, such as taking logarithms, square roots, standardizing, and so on. Within this block, one first defines the new derived variables' names, along with their respective data types. The declarations precede the program statements that involve the quantities.

The *parameters* block. After introducing the data and any other fixed quantities or transformations of each, one tells Stan about the random unobserved quantities in the probability model one is fitting to the data. The *parameters* block tells Stan about the model parameters and any other unobserved variables one may have in the model. Again, we first declare the data types before we use any variables. Examples of unobservables that one might define in a *parameters* block are the rate parameter in a Poisson distribution or the mean and standard deviation in a normal model.

The *transformed parameters* block. Just as one could carry out calculations and transformations with the fixed quantities defined in the data block, one can carry out transformations of parameters using Stan's built-in functions. The transformed parameters block will contain statements that create new parameters from parameters given in the parameters block and, possibly, the data. An example of a simple transformed parameter is the standard deviation, defined as the square root of the variance, with the variance defined in the parameters block. When fitting a regression, the expected value of an observation will be declared as a transformed parameter and then defined as some function of regression coefficients (given in the parameters block) and covariates in the data block or transformed data block. Another example is a vector of missing values that one wishes to impute as functions of covariates.

The *model* block. This block comes next in the Stan program. It describes the prior distribution of the parameters (parameters block) and the likelihood. The syntax in the model block is similar to the syntax in the BUGS language. In particular, one uses the tilde ("~") to characterize a variable's distribution, whether parameters or the likelihood. Again, all statements in Stan must end with a semicolon. No variables may be introduced in the model block, with a few exceptions such as indexing variables in loops. In several complex problems, one may wish to compute the likelihood explicitly instead of declaring the distribution of the data outcomes.

The *generated quantities* block. This last block consists of statements that operate on the Markov chain iterates at each iteration of the sampler. One would generate predicted values in this block. In a regression model, for example, one may wish to consider different sets of covariates. In this block, one would write the statements to compute predicted means or predicted observations for observations with a new set of covariates. One could also generate any other functions of the data and parameters that one does not need to define in the sampling model (prior and likelihood).

Stan includes a host of built-in functions for distributions and specialized data types, such as a correlation matrix data type. As noted above, one can also write one's own functions and put these in a function block at the beginning of the program (i.e., before the data block).

There is a package rstan that makes it easy to run Stan programs from within R. The package contains R functions for running Stan, retrieving output from Stan once the program is done, and evaluating the generated samples for convergence, etc.

Example C.3. We illustrate Stan by returning to Example C.2 but use Stan for posterior inference instead of OpenBUGS. In that example, we fit a simple normal model to make inference about the average weights of the veterans in the **VetBP** data set. The targets of inference were the mean, standard deviation, and the coefficient of variation of the men's weights. The model in Example C.2 consists of a Gaussian likelihood, a Gaussian prior for the mean, and a Gamma prior for the precision (i.e., the reciprocal of the variance). The probability model is

$$y \mid \mu, \sigma^2 \sim N(\mu, \sigma^2)$$
$$\mu \sim N(\mu_0, \sigma_\mu^2) \quad \text{indep.} \quad \sigma^2 \sim \text{Inv-gamma}(\alpha_0, \lambda_0)$$
$$\text{or } \mu \sim N(\mu_0, \sigma_\mu^2) \quad \text{indep.} \quad \tau \sim gamma(\alpha_0, \lambda_0).$$

The Stan program, available on the book's website in a file named `wtmodel.stan` fits the same model.

One thing we wish to emphasize is the difference between Stan and the BUGS-like languages for characterizing normal or Gaussian distributions. The BUGS language programs specify the normal distribution in terms of the mean and the precision. In Stan, we specify the normal distribution in terms of the mean and the standard deviation. We will often, therefore, specify a prior distribution for the standard deviation when we use Stan. We could instead put a prior distribution on the variance or precision in Stan, but we would have to be careful about transformation of variables in any computation involving the densities. We refer the reader to the web for a discussion of transforming variables in Stan.

```
data {
  int N;          // Number of observations
  vector[N] y;    // Dependent variable
  real alpha0;
  real lambda0;
  real mu0;
  real tau0;
}

parameters {
  real mu;
  real<lower=0> precision;
}

transformed parameters{
// Stan uses the standard deviation,
// not the variance or precision.
real sigma;
sigma = 1/sqrt(precision);
}
```

```
model {
  mu ~ normal(mu0, sqrt(1/tau0));
  precision ~ gamma(alpha0, lambda0);
  for (i in 1:N) {
    y[i] ~ normal(mu, sigma);
  }
}
```

There are a few things to notice about this Stan program. First of all, there are more statements than we had in the BUGS-language program in Example C.2 to accomplish the same thing. Many of the extra programming statements concern declarations of variables in the program. With a few exceptions, all variables that appear in a Stan program have to be declared at the start of the appropriate block. There are also more statements in the Stan program, because we wanted to use the precisions for the normal distributions to match the WinBUGS analysis in Example C.2. We could manage to save a few lines of code in the *model* block by specifying the likelihood without a `for` statement. We could instead write

```
model {
  mu ~ normal(mu0, sqrt(1/tau0));
  precision ~ gamma(alpha0, lambda0)
  y ~ normal(mu, sigma);
}
```

Stan knows that y is a vector, because we declared it to be so in the *data* block. Since the observations are conditionally independent (given μ and σ) and y is a vector, Stan will substitute the appropriate statements when compiling the code. We wrote the likelihood specification as a loop to match the earlier WinBUGS example. Note that one of the advantages of declaring variables in Stan, especially vectors and matrices, is the ability to exploit the built-in vectorization capabilities of Stan.

We now review some of the features of the R package rstan for interacting with Stan from within the R environment. We first create the necessary objects in R to pass to the Stan program. Then we run Stan and generate posterior samples that we store in a `stanfit` object. We then carry out some inferences based on the MCMC output. The inferences are the same as the ones we include in Example C.2. One can either have the Stan code in a text file or make the Stan program a character object in R.

The R function `stan()` instructs Stan to generate posterior iterates. The R statements that follow provide inferences for the standard deviation $\sigma = 1/\tau$ and coefficient of variation $cv = \sigma/\mu$.

With the rstan package, one can pass data to Stan and retrieve the results of the MCMC in a similar manner as for WinBUGS, OpenBUGS, or JAGS. The statements below input the data, the names of the model parameters, and randomly generate (in R) initial values for random quantities. The call to the function `stan()` first converts the Stan program statements to C++, compiles the resulting C++ program, and then runs it to generate posterior samples.

There is another way to run **Stan** from R. While the function `stan()` actually accomplishes three steps, one can call the corresponding three specific functions in the **rstan** library in sequence if one wants more control over the process, perhaps for debugging. The three steps are as follows.

- `stanc()` This function translates the model statements in the **Stan** language to code in C++.

- `stan_model()` This function compiles the C++ code into a binary shared object. The function also loads this executable shared object into the current R session.

- `sampling` This function actually runs the executable program to draw samples. The output is "wrapped" into an object of class **stanfit**.

Here is an example of statements in R that will prepare the files that **rstan** will send to **Stan** when we run it from R. The data are in the file VetBP.csv.

```
library(rstan)
library(coda)
# Read the data into object VetBPdata
VetBPdata = read.csv("VetBP.csv", header=T)
# Remove missing values
#   Get indices of non-missing observations
ok <- !is.na(VetBPdata$Weight_00)
#   Create vector of non-missing observations
y <- VetBPdata$Weight_00[ok]
n <- length(y) # Variable with the sample size.
# Set the hyperparameters.
alpha0 <- 0.1; lambda0 <- 0.1;
mu0 <- 150; tau0 <- 0.001
# Create a list object with elements for
# the data block.
data <- list("n", "y", "mu0", "tau0", "alpha0", "lambda0")
# Create a function that will generate
# random initial values for the MCMC chains.
inits <- function() {
  list(mu = rnorm(1, mean=120, sd=5),
      tau = runif(1, min=0.1, max=10))
}
# Create a character vector with the names
# of the parameters in the Stan model.
parameters <- c("mu", "sigma")
```

Now, run **Stan** from R.

```
VetBP.sim = stan("wtmodel.stan", data=data,
   pars=parameters, init=inits, chains=3, iter=10000))
```

After Stan has finished running and performed the requested number of iterations, it returns control to the user's R session. At this point, one can examine the MCMC output that Stan returned. Summary statistics and plots are available via some functions in the rstan package or other R packages (e.g., the coda and bayesplot packages) that are available for carrying out Bayesian inference with MCMC output.

Summary statistics via the statement `print(VetBP.sim)` are as follows.

```
Inference for Stan model: wtmodel.
3 chains, each with iter=10000; warmup=5000; thin=1;
post-warmup draws per chain=5000, total post-warmup draws=15000.

          mean se_mean   sd     2.5%      25%      50%      75%    97.5% n_eff Rhat
mu      209.91   0.02 2.20   205.63   208.43   209.92   211.39   214.20 12279    1
sigma    44.10   0.01 1.54    41.23    43.04    44.06    45.11    47.31 12838    1
lp__  -1729.95   0.01 1.00 -1732.67 -1730.33 -1729.64 -1729.24 -1728.98  6846    1

Samples were drawn using NUTS(diag_e) at Wed Jul  1 16:13:04 2020.
For each parameter, n_eff is a crude measure of effective sample size,
and Rhat is the potential scale reduction factor on split chains (at
convergence, Rhat=1).
```

We next use the features of the R package coda to check some characteristics of the MCMC output. We first extract the output from Stan into an object that is appropriate for coda. In this example, we create a list mcmc object with the R function `As.mcmc.list` that keeps the three Markov chains separate. (Note that the capital "A" in the function's name is important for use with a stanfit object.)

```
MCMCout <- As.mcmc.list(VetBP.sim)
summary(MCMCout)


Iterations = 5001:10000
Thinning interval = 1
Number of chains = 3
Sample size per chain = 5000

1. Empirical mean and standard deviation for each variable,
   plus standard error of the mean:

          Mean    SD Naive SE Time-series SE
mu       209.9 2.197 0.017935        0.01928
sigma     44.1 1.545 0.012611        0.01346
lp__   -1729.9 1.003 0.008189        0.01226


2. Quantiles for each variable:

            2.5%       25%       50%       75%     97.5%
mu        205.63    208.43    209.92    211.39    214.20
sigma      41.23     43.04     44.06     45.11     47.31
lp__   -1732.67  -1730.33  -1729.64  -1729.24  -1728.98
```

The `coda` plot function generates the graph shown in Figure C.5.

```
plot(MCMCout)
```

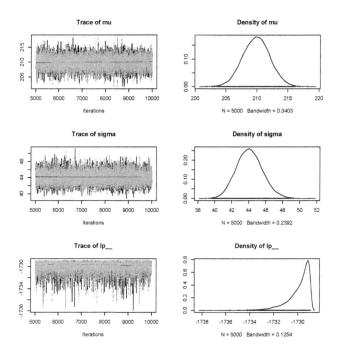

FIGURE C.5: Plots of Stan's MCMC output with R package `coda`.

We can check autocorrelations with the **rstan** function `stan_ac()`, which produces a plot (Figure C.6). Note that the autocorrelations for μ appear on the left-hand side of the figure and those for σ on the right-hand side.

We can create a new parameter as a function of model parameters and use the saved posterior samples to infer its posterior distribution and characteristics related to it. For example, the following statements in R compute the coefficient of variation and plot its posterior distribution (see Figure C.7). We extract the MCMC samples from the **stanfit** object **VetBP.sim** using the **rstan** package function `extract()`. Recall that **Stan** returned the standard deviation, not the variance or precision. We note that we could also have generated posterior samples of the coefficient of variation in our **Stan** program.

```
Stan.out = extract(VetBP.sim, permute=FALSE)\\
CV = Stan.out[,,2]/Stan.out[,,1]\\
summary(CV)
```

```
    chain:1            chain:2            chain:3
Min.   :0.1841    Min.   :0.1845    Min.   :0.1836
```

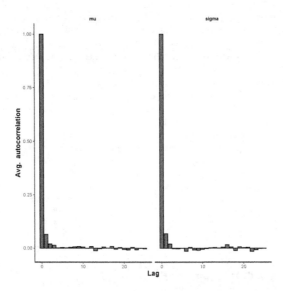

FIGURE C.6: Plots of Stan's MCMC output with function `stan_ac`.

```
1st Qu.:0.2049     1st Qu.:0.2049     1st Qu.:0.2048
Median :0.2098     Median :0.2100     Median :0.2099
Mean    :0.2101    Mean    :0.2103    Mean    :0.2102
3rd Qu.:0.2151     3rd Qu.:0.2155     3rd Qu.:0.2153
Max.    :0.2397    Max.    :0.2432    Max.    :0.2401
```

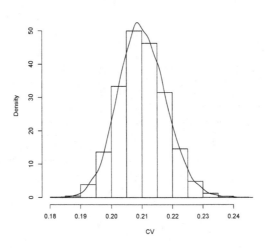

FIGURE C.7: Posterior distribution based on Stan's MCMC output.

Overall, the inference with Stan is similar to results in Example C.2.

C.3.1   Censored Data in **Stan**

Stan does not have the same capability as BUGS or JAGS for handling censored data in a model for AFT regression. Instead, we take advantage of **Stan**'s method for computing the log-likelihood and built-in functions for evaluating log densities and survival functions.

As with BUGS and JAGS, we use the larynx cancer data to illustrate a **Stan** program for fitting an AFT regression model. We create two vectors of observations: one vector consists of uncensored observations, and the other has all of the censored observations. We then compute the regressions for each individual in each of the two sets that we use as the individual's mean. We let **Stan** evaluate the density of each uncensored observation by indicating the sampling distribution using the appropriate density function. We cannot do the same thing for the censored observations, but we can add the log of the sampling distribution's survival function to the overall log-likelihood via the **Stan** keyword **target**. That is, we increment the log-likelihood using built-in **Stan** functions. The calculation of the log-likelihood in the laryngeal cancer example is contained in the *model* block and appears as follows for a log-normal AFT regression analysis.

```
for(i in 1:Nobs) {
    tobs[i] ~ lognormal(muobs[i], sigma);
}
for(i in 1:Ncens) {
    target += lognormal_lccdf(tcens[i]| mucens[i], sigma);
}
```

The observed failure times are in the data vector **tobs[]**, and the censored times are in the vector **tcens[]**. We tell **Stan** to model the observed failure times as **lognormal(,)** with mean equal to the regression that we compute in the transformed parameters block. For the censored observations, we increment the log-likelihood via the keyword **target**, evaluating the log of the log-normal survival function (**lognormal_lccdf(t, mean, sigma)**) at the censored time. The survival function has the AFT regression function as the mean for the observation and the standard deviation **sigma**. (The **_lccdf** in the **Stan** function **lognormal_lccdf(t, mean, sigma)** stands for "log complementary cumulative distribution function," i.e., the log of 1 minus the cdf.)

The following **Stan** program fits a log-normal AFT regression to the larynx cancer data in Example 12.1. The program uses the same priors for β and the precision τ as the examples in BUGS and JAGS earlier in this appendix.

```
data {
    int<lower=0> Nobs;
    int<lower=0> Ncens;
    vector<lower=0>[Nobs] tobs;
    vector<lower=0>[Ncens] tcens;
    vector[90] age;
    vector[90] yr;
```

```
    int stageobs[Nobs];
    vector[Nobs] ageobs;
    vector[Nobs] yrobs;
    int stagecens[Ncens];
    vector[Ncens] agecens;
    vector[Ncens] yrcens;
}
transformed data{
    vector[Nobs] sAgeobs;
    vector[Nobs] sYrobs;
    vector[Ncens] sAgecens;
    vector[Ncens] sYrcens;
    sAgeobs = (ageobs-mean(age))/sd(age);
    sYrobs = (yrobs-mean(yr))/sd(yr);
    sAgecens = (agecens-mean(age))/sd(age);
    sYrcens = (yrcens-mean(yr))/sd(yr);
}
parameters {
    vector[6] beta;
    real<lower=0> tau;
}
transformed parameters {
    real sigma;
    vector[Nobs] muobs;
    vector[Ncens] mucens;
    sigma = sqrt(1/tau);
    for(i in 1:Nobs) {
        muobs[i] = beta[1] + beta[2] * (stageobs[i] == 2) +
            beta[3]*(stageobs[i] == 3) + beta[4]*(stageobs[i] == 4) +
            beta[5]*sAgeobs[i] + beta[6]*sYrobs[i];
    }
    for(i in 1:Ncens) {
        mucens[i] = beta[1] + beta[2] * (stagecens[i] == 2) +
            beta[3]*(stagecens[i] == 3) + beta[4]*(stagecens[i] == 4) +
            beta[5]*sAgecens[i] + beta[6]*sYrcens[i];
    }
}
model {
    for(i in 1:Nobs) {
        tobs[i] ~ lognormal(muobs[i], sigma);
    }
    for(i in 1:Ncens) {
        target += lognormal_lccdf(tcens[i]| mucens[i], sigma);
    }
    for(i in 1:6) {
```

```
      beta[i] ~ normal(0, 1 / sqrt(0.000001));
    }
  tau ~ gamma(0.001,0.001);
}
```

We note that one does not have to use the same approach we just presented for censored data if one is fitting a proportional hazards regression model as given in Section 12.2.2. An example program is in the folder for Chapter 12 on the book's website. The file has PHRegression in the name. The basic idea is the same as given in Section 12.2.2 and is conceptually the same as in the programs for WinBUGS, OpenBUGS, and JAGS.

C.4   R Packages

WinBUGS has made it easier for researchers to implement the Bayesian inferential paradigm in their work. It began as a Microsoft® Windows® implementation of BUGS. In the above subsections we have seen enhancements and alternatives to WinBUGS that adapt to various operating systems. It is also possible to run Windows programs on computers that are using other operating systems. One example is WINE, which allows one to run Windows programs on various Unix-based platforms, such as Solaris, BSD, Linux, and Mac OSX. Although WINE does not emulate Windows (in fact, the original acronym WINE stands for "Wine Is Not an Emulator"), it does allow one to run many Windows programs. The R function R2WinBUGS discussed in the previous section can also be used in WINE by specifying via an argument in the function that the code is running in WINE, and making sure that WinBUGS is set up to run via WINE.

Despite the large array of models one can implement in WinBUGS, sometimes there may be difficulties actually running the models or, in some situations, the specific Bayesian model is outside the scope of WinBUGS. Several R packages have targeted such situations, providing functionality to fit such models via R functions. Such packages are, of course, evolving continually, with new ones appearing with regularity. We briefly list some examples her:

- MCMCPack is a package written for R that fits many different Bayesian regression models using MCMC. The built-in regression models carry out posterior simulation and return objects that one can evaluate directly with the R package coda. The package includes models that are used commonly in the social and behavioral sciences, such as linear regression; logistic regression; probit regression, including probit models for ordinal outcomes; Poisson regression; and hierarchical extensions of some of these. It also includes change-point models and some functions that are useful in general, such as functions for the Wishart and Dirichlet distributions. MCMCPack carries out posterior sampling via routines written mostly in programming languages, such as C^{++}, that can carry out the calculations much more quickly than R can.

- LearnBayes [5] is a sizable collection of R functions that help in learning and using the basic ingredients of Bayesian analysis. Functions are available to carry out analysis of many commonly used models introduced in this book.

- DPpackage [176, 175] contains a set of R functions for fitting Bayesian nonparametric and semiparametric models. While we do not address such models in a distinct chapter in this book, references are made to these, especially for survival modeling, in Chapters 11 and 12. The package includes functions for semiparametric density estimation, ROC curve analysis, fitting models for interval censored data, binary regression models, generalized linear mixed models, among others. The Bayesian nonparametric models are based on the Dirichlet process (Section 3.3.2) or Pólya tree models.

- DPWeibull [295, 294] contains functions to analyze time-to-event or survival data via a semiparametric model based on Dirichlet process mixtures of Weibull distributions. Analysis of data with and without covariates is available, including some graphical displays of results. The package also provides for analysis of competing-risks data and handles most commonly seen censored data as well as time-varying covariates.

- spBayesSurv [364, 365] addresses semiparametric survival analysis models, including for spatially correlated data. Several different types and approaches to models are implemented and various types of censoring are allowed. The package also provides calculations of three different model choice criteria.

- BART [74, 240, 301, 302] provides nonparametric regression analyses for various types of outcomes (continuous, binary, multinomial, survival) using ensembles of Bayesian additive regression trees. It also includes corresponding models that allow a Dirichlet prior on probabilities for choosing covariates at tree nodes (DART [230]). Some post-processing functions are provided, as are the posterior tree ensembles themselves (for possible later processing by the user).

Bibliography

[1] C. J. Adcock. A Bayesian approach to calculating sample sizes. *The Statistician*, 37(4/5):433–439, 1988.

[2] C. J. Adcock. Sample size determination: A review. *The Statistician*, 46(2):261–283, 1997.

[3] J. Aitchison and I. R. Dunsmore. *Statistical Prediction Analysis*. Cambridge University Press, Cambridge, 1st edition, 1975.

[4] H. Akaike. A new look at the statistical model identification. *IEEE Transactions on Automatic Control*, 19(6):716–723, 1974.

[5] J. Albert. LearnBayes: Functions for learning Bayesian inference. *R-package Version 2.15.1*, 2018. https://CRAN.R-project.org/package=LearnBayes.

[6] P. K. Andersen and R. D. Gill. Cox's regression model for counting processes: A large sample study. *Annals of Statistics*, 10(4):1100–1120, 12 1982.

[7] F. J. Anscombe. Sequential medical trials. *Journal of the American Statistical Association*, 58(302):365–383, 1963.

[8] S. G. Arbuck. Workshop on phase I study design. Ninth NCI/EORTC New Drug Development Symposium, Amsterdam, March 12, 1996. *Annals of Oncology*, 7(6):567–73, 1996.

[9] P. Armitage. *Sequential Medical Trials*. Thomas, Springfield, IL, 1960.

[10] P. Armitage. Reply to discussion 'On the allocation of treatments in sequential medical trials' by J.A. Bather and 'The search for optimality in clinical trials' by P. Armitage. *International Statistical Review / Revue Internationale de Statistique*, 53(1):36, 1985.

[11] P. Armitage. The search for optimality in clinical trials. *International Statistical Review / Revue Internationale de Statistique*, 53(1):15–24, 1985.

[12] B. C. Arnold and S. J. Press. Compatible conditional distributions. *Journal of the American Statistical Association*, 84(405):152–156, 1989.

[13] H. Aslanidou, D. K. Dey, and D. Sinha. Bayesian analysis of multivariate survival data using Monte Carlo methods. *Canadian Journal of Statistics / Revue Canadienne de Statistique*, 26(1):33–48, 1998.

[14] J. Babb, A. Rogatko, and S. Zacks. Cancer phase I clinical trials: Efficient dose escalation with overdose control. *Statistics in Medicine*, 17(10):1103–20, 1998.

[15] S. Banerjee, B. Carlin, and A. Gelfand. *Hierarchical Modeling and Analysis for Spatial Data*. Chapman and Hall/CRC, Boca Raton, FL, 2nd edition, 2015.

[16] C. M. Barker, W. O. Johnson, B. F. Eldridge, B. K. Park, F. Melton, and W. K. Reisen. Temporal connections between *culex tarsalis* abundance and transmission of western equine encephalomyelitis virus in California. *American Journal of Tropical Medicine and Hygiene*, 82(6):1185–1193, 2010.

[17] M. S. Bartlett. A comment on D. V. Lindley's statistical paradox. *Biometrika*, 44(3/4):533–534, 1957.

[18] R. H. Bartlett, D. W. Roloff, R. G. Cornell, A. F. Andrews, P. W. Dillon, and J. B. Zwischenberger. Extracorporeal circulation in neonatal respiratory failure: A prospective randomized study. *Pediatrics*, 76(4):479–87, 1985.

[19] J. A. Bather. On the allocation of treatments in sequential medical trials. *International Statistical Review / Revue Internationale de Statistique*, 53(1):1–13, 1985.

[20] J. A. Bather. Reply to discussion 'On the allocation of treatments in sequential medical trials' by J.A. Bather and 'The search for optimality in clinical trials' by P. Armitage. *International Statistical Review / Revue Internationale de Statistique*, 53(1):35–36, 1985.

[21] M. J. Bayarri and J. O. Berger. P values for composite null models. *Journal of the American Statistical Association*, 95:1127–1142, 2000.

[22] M. J. Bayarri and J. O. Berger. The interplay of Bayesian and frequentist analysis. *Statistical Science*, 19(1):58–80, 2004.

[23] E. J. Bedrick, R. Christensen, and W. Johnson. A new perspective on priors for generalized linear models. *Journal of the American Statistical Association*, 91:1450–1460, 1996.

[24] E. J. Bedrick, R. Christensen, and W. Johnson. Bayesian binomial regression: Predicting survival at a trauma center. *The American Statistician*, 51(3):211–218, 1997.

[25] E. J. Bedrick, R. Christensen, and W. O. Johnson. Bayesian accelerated failure time analysis with application to veterinary epidemiology. *Statistics in Medicine*, 19(2):221–237, 2000.

[26] R. E. Bellman. *Dynamic Programming*. Princeton University Press, Princeton, NJ, 1957.

[27] D. A. Belsley, E. Kuh, and R. E. Welsch. *Regression Diagnostics: Identifying Influential Data and Sources of Collinearity*. John Wiley & Sons, New York, 1980.

[28] D. J. Bem, J. Utts, and W. O. Johnson. Must psychologists change the way they analyze their data? *Journal of Personality and Social Psychology*, 101(4):716–719, 2011.

[29] J. O. Berger. *Statistical Decision Theory and Bayesian Analysis*. Springer-Verlag, New York, 1993.

[30] J. O. Berger. The case for objective Bayesian analysis. *Bayesian Analysis*, 1(3):385–402, 2006.

[31] J. O. Berger and M. Delampady. Testing precise hypotheses. *Statistical Science*, 2(3):317–335, 1987.

[32] J. O Berger and T. Sellke. Testing a point null hypothesis: The irreconcilability of p values and evidence. *Journal of the American Statistical Association*, 82(397):112–122, 1987.

[33] J. O. Berger and R. L. Wolpert. *The Likelihood Principle*. Institute of Mathematical Statistics, Hayward, CA, 2nd edition, 1988.

[34] J. M. Bernardo. Reference posterior distributions for Bayesian inference. *Journal of the Royal Society, Series B*, 41(2):113–147, 1979.

[35] J. M. Bernardo and A. F. M. Smith. *Bayesian Theory*. John Wiley & Sons, Chichester, 1994.

[36] D. A. Berry. *Statistics: A Bayesian Perspective*. Duxbury Press, Belmont, CA, 1996.

[37] D. A. Berry, C. Cirrincione, I. C. Henderson, M. L. Citron, D. R. Budman, L. J. Goldstein, S. Martino, E. A. Perez, H. B. Muss, L. Norton, C. Hudis, and E. P. Winer. Estrogen-receptor status and outcomes of modern chemotherapy for patients with node-positive breast cancer. *Journal of the American Medical Association*, 295(14):1658–67, 2006.

[38] D. A. Berry and B. Fristedt. *Bandit Problems: Sequential Allocation of Experiments*. Chapman & Hall, London, 1985.

[39] D. A. Berry and C. H. Ho. One-sided sequential stopping boundaries for clinical-trials: A decision-theoretic approach. *Biometrics*, 44(1):219–227, 1988.

[40] D. A. Berry, P. Mueller, A. P. Grieve, M. K. Smith, T. Parke, and M. Krams. Bayesian designs for dose-ranging drug trials. In C. Gatsonis, R. E. Kass, B. Carlin, A. Carriquiry, and A. Gelman, editors, *Case Studies in Bayesian Statistics, Vol. 5*, pages 99–181. Springer-Verlag, New York, 2002.

[41] S. M. Berry, B. P. Carlin, J. J. Lee, and P. Müller. *Bayesian Adaptive Methods for Clinical Trials*. CRC Press, Boca Raton, FL, 2011.

[42] M. Betancourt. A conceptual introduction to Hamiltonian Monte Carlo. Preprint, arXiv:1701.02434, 2017.

[43] J. Blum and V. Susarla. On the posterior distribution of a Dirichlet process given randomly right censored observations. *Stochastic Processes and their Applications*, 5(3):207–211, 1977.

[44] G. E. P. Box. Science and statistics. *Journal of the American Statistical Association*, 71(356):791–799, 1976.

[45] G. E. P. Box. Sampling and Bayes' inference in scientific modelling and robustness. *Journal of the Royal Statistical Society, Series A*, 143(4):383–404, 1980.

[46] G. E. P. Box and D. R. Cox. An analysis of transformations. *Journal of the Royal Statistical Society, Series B*, 26(2):211–252, 1964.

[47] A. J. Branscum, I. A. Gardner, and W. O. Johnson. Bayesian modeling of animal- and herd-level prevalences. *Preventive Veterinary Medicine*, 66(1–4):101–112, 2004.

[48] A. J. Branscum, I. A. Gardner, and W. O. Johnson. Estimation of diagnostic test sensitivity and specificity through Bayesian modeling. *Preventive Veterinary Medicine*, 68:145–163, 2005.

[49] A. J. Branscum, W. O. Johnson, T. E. Hanson, and A. T. Baron. Flexible regression models for ROC and risk analysis, with or without a gold standard. *Statistics in Medicine*, 34(30):3997–4015, 2015.

[50] A. J. Branscum, W. O. Johnson, T. E. Hanson, and I. A Gardner. Bayesian semiparametric ROC curve estimation and disease diagnosis. *Statistics in Medicine*, 27(13):2474–2496, 2008.

[51] A. J. Branscum, A. M. Perez, W. O. Johnson, and M. C. Thurmond. Bayesian spatiotemporal analysis of foot-and-mouth disease data from the Republic of Turkey. *Epidemiology and Infection*, 136(6):833–842, 2008.

[52] N. E. Breslow and D. G. Clayton. Approximate inference in generalized linear mixed models. *Journal of the American Statistical Association*, 88(421):9–25, 1993.

[53] A. E. Brockwell and J. B. Kadane. A gridding method for Bayesian sequential decision problems. *Journal of Computational and Graphical Statistics*, 12(3):566–584, 2003.

[54] L. D. Broemeling. *Bayesian Analysis of Linear Models*. Marcel Dekker, New York, 1985.

[55] L. D. Broemeling. *Bayesian Biostatistics and Diagnostic Medicine*. Chapman and Hall/CRC, Boca Raton, FL, 2007.

[56] S. P. Brooks and A. Gelman. General methods for monitoring convergence of iterative simulations. *Journal of Computational and Graphical Statistics*, 7(4):434–455, 1998.

[57] J. Brophy and L. Joseph. A Bayesian meta-analysis of randomized megatrials for the choice of thrombolytic agents in acute myocardial infarction. In D. K. Stangl and D. A. Berry, editors, *Meta-Analysis in Medicine and Health Policy*, pages 83–104. Marcel Dekker, New York, 2000.

[58] J. M. Brophy and L. Joseph. Placing trials in context using Bayesian-analysis. GUSTO revisited by Reverend Bayes. *Journal of the American Medical Association*, 273(11):871–875, 1995.

[59] D. R. Budman, D. A. Berry, C. T. Cirrincione, I. C. Henderson, W. C. Wood, R. B. Weiss, C. R. Ferree, H. B. Muss, M. R. Green, L. Norton, and E. Frei. Dose and dose intensity as determinants of outcome in the adjuvant treatment of breast cancer. The Cancer and Leukemia Group B. *Journal of the National Cancer Institute*, 90(16):1205–11, 1998.

[60] J. Cao, J. J. Lee, and S. Alber. Comparison of Bayesian sample size criteria: ACC, ALC, and WOC. *Journal of Statistical Planning and Inference*, 139(12):4111–4122, 2009.

[61] B. P. Carlin and A. E. Gelfand. An iterative Monte Carlo method for nonconjugate Bayesian analysis. *Statistics and Computing*, 1:119–128, 1991.

[62] B. P. Carlin, J. B. Kadane, and A. E. Gelfand. Approaches for optimal sequential decision analysis in clinical trials. *Biometrics*, 54(3):964–975, 1998.

[63] B. P. Carlin and T. A. Louis. *Bayesian Methods for Data Analysis*. Chapman and Hall/CRC, Boca Raton, FL, 2009.

[64] B. Carpenter, A. Gelman, M. Hoffman, D. Lee, B. Goodrich, M. Betancourt, M. Brubaker, J. Guo, P. Li, and A. Riddell. Stan: A probabilistic programming language. *Journal of Statistical Software*, 76(1):1–32, 2017.

[65] G. Casella and R. Berger. *Statistical Inference*. Thomson Learning, Pacific Grove, CA, 2nd edition, 2002.

[66] G. Casella and E. I. George. Explaining the Gibbs sampler. *The American Statistician*, 46:167–174, 1992.

[67] J. E. Cavanaugh and A. A. Neath. Generalizing the derivation of the Schwarz information criterion. *Communications in Statistics: Theory and Methods*, 28(1):49–66, 1999.

[68] C. Celeux, F. Forbes, C. P. Robert, and D. M. Titterington. Deviance information criteria for missing data models. *Bayesian Analysis*, 1:651–673, 2006.

[69] M.-H. Chen, M. de Castro, M. Ge, and Y. Zhang. Bayesian regression models for competing risks. In J. P. Klein, H. C. VanHouwelingen, J. G. Ibrahim, and T. H. Scheike, editors, *Handbook of Survival Analysis*, pages 179–198. Chapman and Hall/CRC, Boca Raton, FL, 2014.

[70] M.-H. Chen, D. K. Dey, P. Müller, D. Sun, and K. Ye. *Frontiers of Statistical Decision Making and Bayesian Analysis: In Honor of James O. Berger.* Springer-Verlag, New York, 2010.

[71] Y. K. Cheung. *Dose Finding by the Continual Reassessment Method.* CRC Press, Boca Raton, FL, 2011.

[72] Y. K. Cheung and R. Chappell. Sequential designs for phase I clinical trials with late-onset toxicities. *Biometrics*, 56(4):1177–1182, 2000.

[73] S. Chib and E. Greenberg. Understanding the Metropolis-Hastings algorithm. *The American Statistician*, 49(4):327–335, 1995.

[74] H. A. Chipman, E. I. George, and R. E. McCulloch. BART: Bayesian additive regression trees. *Annals of Applied Statistics*, 4(1):266–298, 2010.

[75] Y.-K. Choi, W. O. Johnson, and M. C. Thurmond. Diagnosis using predictive probabilities without cut-offs. *Statistics in Medicine*, 25(4):699–717, 2006.

[76] R. Christensen. *Log-Linear Models and Logistic Regression.* Springer-Verlag, New York, 2nd edition, 1997.

[77] R. Christensen. *Plane Answers to Complex Questions: The Theory of Linear Models.* Springer, New York, 4th edition, 2011.

[78] R. Christensen and W. Johnson. A conversation with Seymour Geisser. *Statistical Science*, 22(4):621–636, 2007.

[79] R. Christensen, W. Johnson, A. Branscum, and T. Hanson. *Bayesian Ideas and Data Analysis: An Introduction for Scientists and Statisticians.* Chapman and Hall/CRC, Boca Raton, FL, 2010.

[80] D. Clayton. Some approaches to the analysis of recurrent event data. *Statistical Methods in Medical Research*, 3(3):244–262, 1994.

[81] D. G. Clayton. A model for association in bivariate life tables and its application in epidemiological studies of familial tendency in chronic disease incidence. *Biometrika*, 65(1):141–151, 1978.

[82] W. S. Cleveland. LOWESS: A program for smoothing scatterplots by robust locally weighted regression. *The American Statistician*, 35(1):54, 1981.

[83] G. A. Colditz, M. J. Stampfer, W. C. Willett, C. H. Hennekens, B. Rosner, and F. E. Speizer. Prospective study of estrogen replacement therapy and risk of breast cancer in postmenopausal women. *Journal of the American Medical Association*, 264(20):2648–2653, 1990.

[84] D. Collett. *Modelling Survival Data in Medical Research*. CRC Press, Boca Raton, FL, 2015.

[85] R. D. Cook. Detection of influential observation in linear regression. *Technometrics*, 19(1):15–18, 1977.

[86] R. D. Cook and S. Weisberg. *Residuals and Influence in Regression*. Chapman & Hall, New York, 1982.

[87] R. D. Cook and S. Weisberg. *Applied Regression Including Computing and Graphics*. John Wiley & Sons, 2009.

[88] D. R. Cox. Regression models and life-tables (with discussion). *Journal of the Royal Statistical Society, Series B*, 34(2):187–220, 1972.

[89] M. De Backer, P. De Keyser, C. De Vroey, and E. Lesaffre. A 12-week treatment for dermatophyte toe onychomycosis terbinafine 250mg/day vs. itraconazole 200mg/day—a double-blind comparative trial. *British Journal of Dermatology*, 134(s46):16–17, 1996.

[90] M. De Iorio, W. O. Johnson, P. Müller, and G. L. Rosner. Bayesian nonparametric nonproportional hazards survival modeling. *Biometrics*, 65(3):762–771, 2009.

[91] M. H. DeGroot. *Optimal Statistical Decisions*. John Wiley & Sons, Hoboken, NJ, 2004.

[92] M. Delampady and J. O. Berger. Lower bounds on Bayes factors for multinomial distributions, with application to chi-squared tests of fit. *Annals of Statistics*, 18(3):1295–1316, 1990.

[93] P. Dellaportas and A. F. M. Smith. Bayesian inference for generalized linear and proportional hazards models via Gibbs sampling. *Applied Statistics*, 42(3):443–459, 1993.

[94] N. Dendukuri and L. Joseph. Bayesian approaches to modeling the conditional dependence between multiple diagnostic tests. *Biometrics*, 57(1):158–167, 2001.

[95] L. Devroye. *Non-Uniform Random Variate Generation*. Springer-Verlag, New York, 1986.

[96] D. K. Dey, S. K. Ghosh, and B. K. Mallick. *Generalized Linear Models: A Bayesian Perspective*. CRC Press, Boca Raton, FL, 2000.

[97] M. Ding, G. Rosner, and P. Müller. Bayesian optimal design for phase II screening trials. *Biometrics*, 64(3):886–894, 2008.

[98] N. R. Draper and H. Smith. *Applied Regression Analysis*. John Wiley & Sons, New York, 1998.

[99] S. Duane, A. D. Kennedy, B. J. Pendleton, and D. Roweth. Hybrid Monte Carlo. *Physics Letters B*, 195(2):216–222, 1987.

[100] R. L. Dykstra and P. Laud. A Bayesian nonparametric approach to reliability. *Annals of Statistics*, 9(2):356–367, 1981.

[101] J. H. Edmonson, T. R. Fleming, D. G. Decker, G. D. Malkasian, E. O. Jorgensen, J. A. Jefferies, M. J. Webb, and L. K. Kvols. Different chemotherapeutic sensitivities and host factors affecting prognosis in advanced ovarian carcinoma versus minimal residual disease. *Cancer Treatment Reports*, 63(2):241–247, 1979.

[102] R. M. Elashoff, G. Li, and N. Li. *Joint Modeling of Longitudinal and Time-to-Event Data*. CRC Press, Boca Raton, FL, 2017.

[103] C. Enøe, M. P. Georgiadis, and W. O. Johnson. Estimation of sensitivity and specificity of diagnostic tests and disease prevalence when the true disease state is unknown. *Preventive Veterinary Medicine*, 45(1-2):61–81, 2000.

[104] X. Fan. *Bayesian Nonparametric Inference for Competing Risks Data*. Ph.D. Dissertation, Medical College of Wisconsin, 2008.

[105] FDA. *Guidance for Industry Estimating the Maximum Safe Starting Dose in Initial Clinical Trials for Therapeutics in Adult Healthy Volunteers*, 2005.

[106] FDA. *Guidance for the Use of Bayesian Statistics in Medical Device Clinical Trials*. U.S. Department of Health and Human Services, Food and Drug Administration, Center for Devices and Radiological Health, Silver Spring, Maryland, February 2010.

[107] P. Feigl and M. Zelen. Estimation of exponential survival probabilities with concomitant information. *Biometrics*, 21(4):826–838, 1965.

[108] T. S. Ferguson. Bayesian analysis of some nonparametric problems. *Annals of Statistics*, 1(2):209–230, 1973.

[109] T. S. Ferguson and E. G. Phadia. Bayesian nonparametric estimation based on censored data. *Annals of Statistics*, 7(1):163–186, 1979.

[110] D. Field, C. Davis, D. Elbourne, A. Grant, A. Johnson, and D. Macrae. UK collaborative randomised trial of neonatal extracorporeal membrane oxygenation. *Lancet*, 348(9020):75–82, 1996.

[111] L. S. Freedman, D. Lowe, D. J. Spiegelhalter, and P. Macaskill. Stopping rules that incorporate clinical opinion. *Controlled Clinical Trials*, 4(2):152–152, 1983.

[112] L. S. Freedman and D. J. Spiegelhalter. The assessment of subjective opinion and its use in relation to stopping rules for clinical trials. *The Statistician*, 32(1-2):153–160, 1983.

[113] L. S. Freedman and D. J. Spiegelhalter. Using clinical opinion in the design of fixed-sized trials. *Controlled Clinical Trials*, 5(3):302–302, 1984.

[114] L. S. Freedman and D. J. Spiegelhalter. Comparison of Bayesian with group sequential methods for monitoring clinical trials. *Controlled Clinical Trials*, 10(4):357–367, 1989.

[115] L. S. Freedman and D. J. Spiegelhalter. Application of Bayesian statistics to decision-making during a clinical trial. *Statistics in Medicine*, 11(1):23–35, 1992.

[116] L. S. Freedman, D. J. Spiegelhalter, and M. K. B. Parmar. The what, why and how of Bayesian clinical trials monitoring. *Statistics in Medicine*, 13(13–14):1371–1383; discussion 1385–1389, 1994.

[117] E. J. Freireich, E. A. Gehan, D. P. Rall, L. H. Schmidt, and H. E. Skipper. Quantitative comparison of toxicity of anticancer agents in mouse, rat, hamster, dog, monkey, and man. *Cancer Chemotherapy Reports*, 50(4):219–244, 1966.

[118] L. M. Friedman, C. Furberg, and D. L. DeMets. *Fundamentals of Clinical Trials*. Springer, New York, 4th edition, 2010.

[119] D. Gamerman. Sampling from the posterior distribution in generalized linear mixed models. *Statistics and Computing*, 7:57–68, 1997.

[120] P. H. Garthwaite and J. M. Dickey. Quantifying expert opinion in linear-regression problems. *Journal of the Royal Statistical Society, Series B*, 50(3):462–474, 1988.

[121] P. H. Garthwaite, J. B. Kadane, and A. O'Hagan. Statistical methods for eliciting probability distributions. *Journal of the American Statistical Association*, 100(470):680–701, 2005.

[122] J. L. Gastwirth, W. O. Johnson, and D. M. Reneau. Bayesian analysis of screening data: Application to AIDS in blood donors. *Canadian Journal of Statistics*, 19(2):135–150, 1991.

[123] S. Geisser. The inferential use of predictive distributions. In V. P. Godambe and D. A. Sprott, editors, *Foundations of Statistical Inference*, pages 456–469. Holt, Reinhart, and Winston, Toronto, 1971.

[124] S. Geisser. *A Predictivistic Primer.* North-Holland, New York, 1980.

[125] S. Geisser. On prior distributions for binary trials. *The American Statistician*, 38(4):244–247, 1984.

[126] S. Geisser. Influential observations, diagnostics and discovery tests. *Journal of Applied Statistics*, 14(2):133–142, 1987.

[127] S. Geisser. *Predictive Inference: An Introduction.* Chapman & Hall, New York, 1993.

[128] S. Geisser and W. F. Eddy. Predictive approach to model selection. *Journal of the American Statistical Association*, 74(365):153–160, 1979.

[129] A. E. Gelfand and D. K. Dey. Bayesian model choice: Asymptotics and exact calculations. *Journal of the Royal Statistical Society, Series B*, 56(3):501–514, 1994.

[130] A. E. Gelfand, S. E. Hills, A Racine-Poon, and A. F. M. Smith. Illustration of Bayesian inference in normal data models using Gibbs sampling. *Journal of the American Statistical Association*, 85(412):972–985, 1990.

[131] A. E. Gelfand, S. K. Sahu, and B. P. Carlin. Efficient parametrizations for normal linear mixed models. *Biometrika*, 82(3):479–488, 1995.

[132] A. E. Gelfand and A. F. M. Smith. Sampling-based approaches to calculating marginal densities. *Journal of the American Statistical Association*, 85:398–409, 1990.

[133] A. Gelman, J. B. Carlin, H. S. Stern, D. B. Dunson, A. Vehtari, and D. B. Rubin. *Bayesian Data Analysis.* Chapman & Hall/CRC, Boca Raton, FL, 3rd edition, 2014.

[134] A. Gelman, J. B. Carlin, H. S. Stern, and D. B. Rubin. *Bayesian Data Analysis.* Chapman & Hall, London, 1995.

[135] A. Gelman, J. Hwang, and A. Vehtari. Understanding predictive information criteria for Bayesian models. *Statistics and Computing*, 24(6):997–1016, 2014.

[136] A. Gelman, A. Jakulin, M. G. Pittau, Y.-S. Su, et al. A weakly informative default prior distribution for logistic and other regression models. *Annals of Applied Statistics*, 2(4):1360–1383, 2008.

[137] A. Gelman, X.-L. Meng, and H. S. Stern. Posterior predictive assessment of model fitness via realized discrepancies (with discussion). *Statistica Sinica*, 6(4):733–760, 1996.

[138] A. Gelman and D. B. Rubin. Inference from iterative simulation using multiple sequences. *Statistical Science*, 7(4):457–472, 1992.

[139] E. I. George and R. E. McCulloch. Variable selection via Gibbs sampling. *Journal of the American Statistical Association*, 88(423):881–889, 1993.

[140] E. I. George and R. E. McCulloch. Approaches for Bayesian variable selection. *Statistica Sinica*, 7(2):339–373, 1997.

[141] M. P. Georgiadis, W. O. Johnson, I. A. Gardner, and R. Singh. Correlation-adjusted estimation of sensitivity and specificity of two diagnostic tests. *Applied Statistics*, 52(1):63–76, 2003.

[142] J. Geweke. Evaluating the accuracy of sampling-based approaches to the calculation of posterior moments. In J. M. Bernardo, J. O. Berger, A. P. Dawid, and A. F. M. Smith, editors, *Bayesian Statistics 4*, Oxford, 1992. Oxford University Press.

[143] W. R. Gilks and P. Wild. Adaptive rejection sampling for Gibbs sampling. *Applied Statistics*, 41:337–348, 1992.

[144] J. Gill and L. D. Walker. Elicited priors for Bayesian model specifications in political science research. *Journal of Politics*, 67(3):841–872, 2005.

[145] J. Gittins, K. Glazebrook, and R. Weber. *Multi-Armed Bandit Allocation Indices*. John Wiley & Sons, Chichester, 2nd edition, 2011.

[146] M. Goldstein. Subjective Bayesian analysis: Principles and practice. *Bayesian Analysis*, 1(3):403, 2006.

[147] M. Gönen, W. O. Johnson, Y. Lu, and P. H. Westfall. Comparing objective and subjective Bayes factors for the two-sample comparison: The classification theorem in action. *The American Statistician*, 73(1):22–31, 2018.

[148] S. N. Goodman. Toward evidence-based medical statistics. 1: The p-value fallacy. *Annals of Internal Medicine*, 130(12):995–1004, 1999.

[149] S. N. Goodman. Towards evidence-based medical statistics. 2: The Bayes factor. *Annals of Internal Medicine*, 130(12):1005–1013, 1999.

[150] S. N. Goodman, M. L. Zahurak, and S. Piantadosi. Some practical improvements in the continual reassessment method for phase I studies. *Statistics in Medicine*, 14(11):1149–1161, 1995.

[151] C. K. Grieshaber and S. Marsoni. Relation of preclinical toxicology to findings in early clinical trials. *Cancer Treatment Reports*, 70(1):65–72, 1986.

[152] M. Gruber. *Improving Efficiency by Shrinkage: The James–Stein and Ridge Regression Estimators*. Marcel Dekker, New York, 1998.

[153] C. E. Guse, D. J. Peterson, A. L. Christiansen, J. Mahoney, P. Laud, and P. M. Layde. Translating a fall prevention intervention into practice: A randomized community trial. *American Journal of Public Health*, 105(7):1475–1481, 2015.

[154] K. M. Guskiewicz and J. P. Mihalik. Biomechanics of sport concussion: Quest for the elusive injury threshold. *Exercise and Sport Sciences Reviews*, 39(1):4–11, 2011.

[155] P. Gustafson. Large hierarchical Bayesian analysis of multivariate survival data. *Biometrics*, 53(1):230–42, 1997.

[156] P. Gustafson. Bayesian analysis of frailty models. In Klein, JP and Van-Houwelingen, HC and Ibrahim, JG and Scheike, TH, editor, *Handbook of Survival Analysis*, pages 475–488. Chapman & Hall/CRC, Boca Raton, FL, 2014.

[157] P. Gustafson, A. E. Gelfand, S. K. Sahu, W. O. Johnson, T. E. Hanson, L. Joseph, and J. Lee. On model expansion, model contraction, identifiability and prior information: Two illustrative scenarios involving mismeasured variables [with comments and rejoinder]. *Statistical Science*, 20(2):111–140, 2005.

[158] T. Hanson, E. Bedrick, W. Johnson, and M. Thurmond. A mixture model for bovine abortion and foetal survival. *Statistics in Medicine*, 22:1725–1739, 2003.

[159] T. Hanson, W. Johnson, and P. Laud. Semiparametric inference for survival models with step process covariates. *Canadian Journal of Statistics*, 37(1):60–79, 2009.

[160] W. K. Hastings. Monte Carlo sampling methods using Markov chains and their applications. *Biometrika*, 57(1):97–109, 1970.

[161] I. C. Henderson, D. A. Berry, G. D. Demetri, C. T. Cirrincione, L. J. Goldstein, S. Martino, J. N. Ingle, M. R. Cooper, D. F. Hayes, K. H. Tkaczuk, G. Fleming, J. F. Holland, D. B. Duggan, J. T Carpenter, E. Frei, R. L. Schilsky, W. C. Wood, H. B. Muss, and L. Norton. Improved outcomes from adding sequential paclitaxel but not from escalating doxorubicin dose in an adjuvant chemotherapy regimen for patients with node-positive primary breast cancer. *Journal of Clinical Oncology*, 21(6):976–983, 2003.

[162] J. Herson. Predictive probability early termination plans for phase II clinical trials. *Biometrics*, 35(4):775–83, 1979.

[163] S. P. Hey and J. Kimmelman. Are outcome-adaptive allocation trials ethical? *Clinical Trials*, 12(2):102–106, 2015.

[164] J. P. Hobert and G. Casella. The effect of improper priors on Gibbs sampling in hierarchical linear mixed models. *Journal of the American Statistical Association*, 91(436):1461–1473, 1996.

[165] J. A. Hoeting, D. Madigan, A. E. Raftery, and C. T. Volinsky. Bayesian model averaging: A tutorial (with comments). *Statistical Science*, 14(4):382–417, 1999.

[166] P. Hoff. *A First Course in Bayesian Statistical Methods*. Springer, New York, 2009.

[167] M. D. Hoffman and A. Gelman. The No-U-Turn sampler: Adaptively setting path lengths in Hamiltonian Monte Carlo. *Journal of Machine Learning Research*, 15(1):1593–1623, 2014.

[168] T. R. Holford. The analysis of rates and of survivorship using log-linear models. *Biometrics*, 36(2):299–305, 1980.

[169] S. L. Hui and S. D. Walter. Estimating the error rates of diagnostic tests. *Biometrics*, 36(1):167–171, 1980.

[170] J. G. Ibrahim and M.-H. Chen. Prior elicitation and variable selection for generalized linear mixed models. In D. K. Dey, S. K. Ghosh, and B. K. Mallick, editors, *Generalized Linear Models: A Bayesian Perspective*, pages 41–53. Marcel Dekker, New York, 2000.

[171] J. G. Ibrahim, M.-H. Chen, and D. Sinha. *Bayesian Survival Analysis*. Springer Series in Statistics. Springer, New York, 2001.

[172] J. G. Ibrahim and P. W. Laud. On Bayesian analysis of generalized linear models using Jeffreys's prior. *Journal of the American Statistical Association*, 86(416):981–986, 1991.

[173] J. P. A. Ioannidis. Why most published research findings are false. *PLoS Medicine*, 2(8):e124, 2005.

[174] H. Ishwaran and M. Zarepour. Exact and approximate sum representations for the Dirichlet process. *Canadian Journal of Statistics*, 4:269–283, 1994.

[175] A. Jara. DPpackage (version 1.1-4): Bayesian nonparametric modeling in R, 2012. http://cran.r-project.org.

[176] A. Jara, T. E. Hanson, F. A. Quintana, P. Mueller, and G. L. Rosner. DPpackage: Bayesian non- and semi-parametric modelling in R. *Journal of Statistical Software*, 40(5):1–30, 2011.

[177] H. Jeffreys. An invariant form for the prior probability in estimation problems. *Proceedings of the Royal Society of London, Series A*, 186(1007):453–461, 1946.

[178] R. A. Johnson and D. W. Wichern. *Applied Multivariate Statistical Analysis*. Prentice Hall, Englewood Cliffs, NJ, 5th edition, 2002.

[179] V. E. Johnson. A Bayesian χ^2 test for goodness-of-fit. *Annals of Statistics*, 32(6):2361–2384, 2004.

[180] V. E. Johnson and J. D. Cook. Bayesian design of single-arm phase II clinical trials with continuous monitoring. *Clinical Trials*, 6(3):217–226, 2009.

[181] V. E. Johnson and D. Rossell. On the use of non-local prior densities in Bayesian hypothesis tests. *Journal of the Royal Statistical Society, Series B*, 72(2):143–170, 2010.

[182] W. Johnson. Influence measures for logistic regression: Another point of view. *Biometrika*, 72(1):59–65, 1985.

[183] W. Johnson and S. Geisser. A predictive view of the detection and characterization of influential observations in regression analysis. *Journal of the American Statistical Association*, 78(381):137–144, 1983.

[184] W. Johnson and S. Geisser. Estimative influence measures for the multivariate general linear model. *Journal of Statistical Planning and Inference*, 11(1):33–56, 1985.

[185] W. Johnson, J. Utts, and L. Pearson. Bayesian robust estimation of the mean. *Applied Statistics*, 35(1):63–72, 1986.

[186] W. O. Johnson. Predictive influence in the log normal survival model. In J. C. Lee, W. O. Johnson, and A. Zellner, editors, *Prediction and Modelling in Statistics and Econometrics: Essays in Honor of Seymour Geisser*, pages 104–121, Amsterdam, 1996. Elsevier.

[187] W. O. Johnson and J. L. Gastwirth. Bayesian inference for medical screening tests: Approximations useful for the analysis of acquired immune deficiency syndrome. *Journal of the Royal Statistical Society, Series B*, 53(2):427–439, 1991.

[188] W. O. Johnson, J. L. Gastwirth, and L. M. Pearson. Screening without a "gold standard": The Hui-Walter paradigm revisited. *American Journal of Epidemiology*, 153(9):921–924, 2001.

[189] W. O. Johnson, G. Jones, and I. A. Gardner. Gold standards are out and Bayes is in: Implementing the cure for imperfect reference tests in diagnostic accuracy studies. *Preventive Veterinary Medicine*, 167:113–127, 2019.

[190] W. O. Johnson, E. Ward, and D. L. Gillen. Bayesian methods in public health. *Handbook on Statistics: Disease Modeling and Public Health*, 36:407–442, 2017.

[191] G. Jones and W. O. Johnson. Prior elicitation: Interactive spreadsheet graphics with sliders can be fun, and informative. *The American Statistician*, 68(1):42–51, 2014.

[192] G. Jones, W. O. Johnson, T. E. Hanson, and R. Christensen. Identifiability of models for multiple diagnostic testing in the absence of a gold standard. *Biometrics*, 66(3):855–863, 2010.

[193] L. Joseph and P. Belisle. Bayesian sample size determination for normal means and differences between normal means. *The Statistician*, 46(2):209–226, 1997.

[194] L. Joseph, T. W. Gyorkos, and L. Coupal. Bayesian estimation of disease prevalence and the parameters of diagnostic tests in the absence of a gold standard. *American Journal of Epidemiology*, 141(3):263–272, 1995.

[195] L. Joseph and D. B. Wolfson. Interval-based versus decision theoretic criteria for the choice of sample size. *The Statistician*, 46(2):145–149, 1997.

[196] J. B. Kadane. *Principles of Uncertainty*. Chapman & Hall/CRC, Boca Raton, FL, 2011.

[197] J. B. Kadane, J. M. Dickey, R. L. Winkler, W. S. Smith, and S. C. Peters. Interactive elicitation of opinion for a normal linear model. *Journal of the American Statistical Association*, 75(372):845–854, 1980.

[198] J. B. Kadane and N. A. Lazar. Methods and criteria for model selection. *Journal of the American Statistical Association*, 99(465):279–290, 2004.

[199] J. B. Kadane and L. J. Wolfson. Experiences in elicitation. *The Statistician*, 47(1):3–19, 1998.

[200] D. Kahneman and A. Tversky. Subjective probability: A judgement of representativeness. In D. Kahneman, P. Slovic, and A. Tversky, editors, *Judgment under Uncertainty: Heuristics and Biases*, pages 43–47. Cambridge University Press, Cambridge, 1982.

[201] J. D. Kalbfleisch. Non-parametric Bayesian analysis of survival time data. *Journal of the Royal Statistical Society, Series B*, 40(2):214–221, 1978.

[202] E. L. Kaplan and P. Meier. Nonparametric estimation from incomplete observations. *Journal of the American statistical association*, 53(282):457–481, 1958.

[203] O. Kardaun. Statistical survival analysis of male larynx-cancer patients—A case study. *Statistica Neerlandica*, 37(3):103–125, 1983.

[204] J. P. Klein and M. L. Moeschberger. *Survival Analysis: Techniques for Censored and Truncated Data*. Springer, New York, 2nd edition, 2003.

[205] K. P. Kleinman and J. G. Ibrahim. A semi-parametric Bayesian approach to generalized linear mixed models. *Statistics in Medicine*, 17(22):2579–2596, 1998.

[206] K. P. Kleinman and J. G. Ibrahim. A semiparametric Bayesian approach to the random effects model. *Biometrics*, 54(3):921–938, 1998.

[207] A. Kottas. Nonparametric Bayesian survival analysis using mixtures of Weibull distributions. *Journal of Statistical Planning and Inference*, 136(3):578–596, 2006.

[208] M. Krams, K. R. Lees, W. Hacke, A. P. Grieve, J.-M. Orgogozo, G. A. Ford, and Investigators for the ASTIN Study. Acute stroke therapy by inhibition of neutrophils (ASTIN). *Stroke*, 34(11):2543–2548, 2003.

[209] L. Kuo, A. F. M. Smith, S. MacEachern, and M. West. Bayesian computations in survival models via the Gibbs sampler. In J. P. Klein and P. K. Goel, editors, *Survival Analysis: State of the Art*, pages 11–24. Kluwer Academic Publishers, Dordrecht, The Netherlands, 1992.

[210] N. Laird. Nonparametric maximum likelihood estimation of a mixing distribution. *Journal of the American Statistical Association*, 73(364):805–811, 1978.

[211] N. Laird and D. Olivier. Covariance analysis of censored survival data using log-linear analysis techniques. *Journal of the American Statistical Association*, 76(374):231–240, 1981.

[212] N. M. Laird and J. H. Ware. Random-effects models for longitudinal data. *Biometrics*, 38(4):963–974, 1982.

[213] K. K. G. Lan and D. L. DeMets. Discrete sequential boundaries for clinical trials. *Biometrika*, 70:659–663, 1983.

[214] P. Laud, P. Damien, and T. Shively. Sampling truncated distributions via rejection algorithms. *Communications in Statistics: Simulation and Computation*, 39(6):1111–1121, 2010.

[215] P. W. Laud. *Bayesian nonparametric inference in reliability*. Ph.D. Dissertation, University of Missouri, Columbia, MO, 1977.

[216] P. W. Laud, P. Damien, and S. G. Walker. Computations via auxiliary random functions for survival models. *Scandinavian Journal of Statistics*, 33(2):219–226, 2006.

[217] P. W. Laud and J. G. Ibrahim. Predictive model selection. *Journal of the Royal Statistical Society, Series B*, 57(1):247–262, 1995.

[218] J. J. Lee and D. D. Liu. A predictive probability design for phase II cancer clinical trials. *Clinical Trials*, 5(2):93–106, 2008.

[219] E. Lesaffre and B. Spiessens. On the effect of the number of quadrature points in a logistic random-effects model: An example. *Aplied Statistics*, 50:325–335, 2001.

[220] R. J. Lewis and D. A. Berry. Group sequential clinical-trials – A classical evaluation of Bayesian decision-theoretic designs. *Journal of the American Statistical Association*, 89(428):1528–1534, 1994.

[221] R. J. Lewis, A. M. Lipsky, and D. A. Berry. Bayesian decision-theoretic group sequential clinical trial design based on a quadratic loss function: A frequentist evaluation. *Clinical Trials*, 4(1):5–14, 2007.

[222] C.-S. Li. Identifiability of zero-inflated Poisson models. *Brazilian Journal of Probability and Statistics*, 26(3):306–312, 2012.

[223] D. V. Lindley. On a measure of the information provided by an experiment. *Annals of Mathematical Statistics*, 27(4):986–1005, 1956.

[224] D. V. Lindley. A statistical paradox. *Biometrika*, 44(1–2):187–192, 1957.

[225] D. V. Lindley. *Bayesian Statistics; A Review*. Society for Industrial and Applied Mathematics, Philadelphia, 1972.

[226] D. V. Lindley. The choice of sample size. *The Statistician*, 46(2):129–138, 1997.

[227] D. V. Lindley. The choice of sample size—Reply. *The Statistician*, 46(2):163–166, 1997.

[228] D. V. Lindley and A. F. M. Smith. Bayes estimates for the linear model. *Journal of the Royal Statistical Society, Series B*, 34(1):1–41, 1972.

[229] J. K. Lindsey. Exact sample size calculations for exponential family models. *The Statistician*, 46(2):231–237, 1997.

[230] A. R. Linero. Bayesian regression trees for high-dimensional prediction and variable selection. *Journal of the American Statistical Association*, 113(522):626–636, 2018.

[231] R. J. Little. Calibrated Bayes: A Bayes/frequentist roadmap. *The American Statistician*, 60(3):213–223, 2006.

[232] D. Lunn, C. Jackson, N. Best, A. Thomas, and D. Spiegelhalter. *The BUGS Book: A Practical Introduction to Bayesian Analysis*. CRC Press, Boca Raton, FL, 2012.

[233] D. Lunn, D. Spiegelhalter, A. Thomas, and N. Best. The BUGS project: Evolution, critique and future directions. *Statistics in Medicine*, 28(25):3049–3067, 2009.

[234] S. N. MacEachern. Dependent Dirichlet processes. Unpublished manuscript, Department of Statistics, The Ohio State University, 2000.

[235] I. Mahmood and J. D. Balian. The pharmacokinetic principles behind scaling from preclinical results to phase I protocols. *Clinical Pharmacokinetics*, 36(1):1–11, 1999.

[236] S. S Mahmood, D. Levy, R. S. Vasan, and T. J. Wang. The Framingham Heart Study and the epidemiology of cardiovascular disease: A historical perspective. *The Lancet*, 383(9921):999–1008, 2014.

[237] M. McCrea. *Mild Traumatic Brain Injury and Postconcussion Syndrome: The New Evidence Base for Diagnosis and Treatment*. Oxford University Press, Oxford, 2008.

[238] P. McCullagh. Regression models for ordinal data. *Journal of the Royal Statistical Society, Series B*, 42(2):109–142, 1980.

[239] P. McCullagh and J. A. Nelder. *Generalized Linear Models*. Chapman and Hall, London, 2nd edition, 1989.

[240] R. McCulloch, R. Sparapani, R. Gramacy, C. Spanbauer, and M. Pratola. BART: Bayesian additive regresssion trees. *R-package Version 2.7*, 2019. https://CRAN.R-project.org/package=BART.

[241] R. McElreath. *Statistical Rethinking: A Bayesian Course with Examples in R and Stan*. Chapman and Hall/CRC, Boca Raton, FL, 2nd edition, 2020.

[242] N. Metropolis, A. W. Rosenbluth, M. N. Rosenbluth, A. H. Teller, and E. Teller. Equation of state calculations by fast computing machines. *Journal of Chemical Physics*, 21(6):1087–1092, 1953.

[243] T. J. Mitchell and J. J. Beauchamp. Bayesian variable selection in linear regression. *Journal of the American Statistical Association*, 83(404):1023–1032, 1988.

[244] J. Mullahy. Specification and testing of some modified count data models. *Journal of Econometrics*, 33(3):341–365, 1986.

[245] P. Müller, D. A. Berry, A. P. Grieve, M. Smith, and M. Krams. Simulation-based sequential Bayesian design. *Journal of Statistical Planning and Inference*, 137(10):3140–3150, 2007.

[246] A. B. Nattinger, P. W. Laud, R. Bajorunaite, R. A. Sparapani, and J. L. Freeman. An algorithm for the use of Medicare claims data to identify women with incident breast cancer. *Health Services Research*, 39(6p1):1733–50, 2004.

[247] A. B. Nattinger, L. E. Pezzin, R. A. Sparapani, J. M. Neuner, T. K. King, and P. W. Laud. Heightened attention to medical privacy: Challenges for unbiased sample recruitment and a possible solution. *American Journal of Epidemiology*, 172(6):637–44, 2010.

[248] R. M Neal. MCMC using Hamiltonian dynamics. In S. Brooks, A. Gelman, G. Jones, and X. L. Meng, editors, *Handbook of Markov Chain Monte Carlo*. Chapman and Hall/CRC, Boca Raton, FL, 2011.

[249] J. A. Nelder and R. W. M. Wedderburn. Generalized linear models. *Journal of the Royal Statistical Society, Series A*, 135(3):370–384, 1972.

[250] A. Nishimura and D. Dunson. Recycling intermediate steps to improve Hamiltonian Monte Carlo. *Bayesian Analysis*, 2020.

[251] M. Norris, W. O. Johnson, and I. A. Gardner. Modeling bivariate longitudinal diagnostic outcome data in the absence of a gold standard. *Statistics and its Interface*, 2(2):171–185, 2009.

[252] P. C. O'Brien and T. R. Fleming. A multiple testing procedure for clinical trials. *Biometrics*, 35(3):549–556, 1979.

[253] A. O'Hagan, C. E. Buck, A. Daneshkhah, J. R. Eiser, P. H. Garthwaite, D. J. Jenkinson, J. E. Oakley, and T. Rakow. *Uncertain Judgements: Eliciting Experts' Probabilities*. Wiley, London, 2006.

[254] J. O'Quigley, M. Pepe, and L. Fisher. Continual reassessment method: A practical design for phase I clinical trials in cancer. *Biometrics*, 46:33–48, 1990.

[255] P. P. O'Rourke, R. K. Crone, J. P. Vacanti, J. H. Ware, C. W. Lillehei, R. B. Parad, and M. F. Epstein. Extracorporeal membrane oxygenation and conventional medical therapy in neonates with persistent pulmonary hypertension of the newborn: A prospective randomized study. *Pediatrics*, 84(6):957–963, 1989.

[256] G. Parmigiani and L. Inoue. *Decision Theory: Principles and Approaches*. John Wiley & Sons, Chichester, 2009.

[257] G. Parveen, M. F. Khan, H. Ali, T. Ibrahim, and R. Shah. Determination of lethal dose (LD_{50}) of venom of four different poisonous snakes found in Pakistan. *Biochemistry & Molecular Biology Journal*, 3(3):18, 2017.

[258] M. S. Pepe. *The Statistical Evaluation of Medical Tests for Classification and Prediction*. Oxford University Press, Oxford, 2004.

[259] L. B. Perry, R. A. Van Dyke, and R. A. Theye. Sympathoadrenal and hemodynamic effects of isoflurane, halothane, and cyclopropane in dogs. *Anesthesiology*, 40(5):465–470, 1974.

[260] S. Piantadosi. Translational clinical trials: An entropy-based approach to sample size. *Clinical Trials*, 2(2):182–192, 2005.

[261] M. Plummer. JAGS: A program for analysis of Bayesian graphical models using Gibbs sampling, 2003. https://sourceforge.net/projects/mcmc-jags/files/Manuals/4.x/jags_user_manual.pdf/download.

[262] S. J. Pocock. Group sequential methods in the design and analysis of clinical trials. *Biometrika*, 64:191–199, 1977.

[263] R. F. Potthoff and S. N. Roy. A generalized multivariate analysis of variance model useful especially for growth curve problems. *Biometrika*, 51(3-4):313–326, 1964.

[264] J. W. Pratt, H. Raiffa, and R. Schlaifer. The foundations of decision under uncertainty: An elementary exposition. *Journal of the American statistical association*, 59(306):353–375, 1964.

[265] F. A. Quintana, W. O. Johnson, L. E. Waetjen, and E. B. Gold. Bayesian nonparametric longitudinal data analysis. *Journal of the American Statistical Association*, 111(515):1168–1181, 2016.

[266] A. E. Raftery and S. M Lewis. One long run with diagnostics: Implementation strategies for Markov chain Monte Carlo, Comment on Practical Markov Chain Monte Carlo by Chares Geyer. *Statistical Science*, 7(4):493–497, 1992.

[267] H Raiffa and R Schlaifer. *Applied Statistical Decision Theory*. Division of Research, Graduate School of Business Adminitration, Harvard University, Boston, 1961.

[268] D. Ratkowsky. *Nonlinear Regression Modeling*. Marcel Dekker, New York, 1983.

[269] J. A. Rice. *Mathematical Statistics and Data Analysis*. Wadsworth, Belmont CA, 1995.

[270] D. Rizopoulos. *Joint Models for Longitudinal and Time-To-Event Data: With Applications in R*. CRC Press, Boca Raton, FL, 2012.

[271] C. P. Robert. *The Bayesian Choice: From Decision-Theoretic Foundations to Computational Implementation*. Springer-Verlag, New York, 2001.

[272] B. Rosner. *Fundamentals of Biostatistics*. Duxbury Press, Belmont, CA, 2006.

[273] G. L. Rosner. Bayesian monitoring of clinical trials with failure-time endpoints. *Biometrics*, 61(1):239–45, 2005.

[274] G. L. Rosner, J. C. Panetta, F. Innocenti, and M. J. Ratain. Pharmacogenetic pathway analysis of irinotecan. *Clinical Pharmacology & Therapeutics*, 84(3):393–402, 2008.

[275] S. Ross. *A First Course in Probability*. Pearson, Harlow, 9th edition, 2014.

[276] D. Rossell, P. Müller, and G. L. Rosner. Screening designs for drug development. *Biostatistics*, 8(3):595–608, 2007.

[277] R. M. Royall. Ethics and statistics in randomized clinical trials. *Statistical Science*, 6(1):52–62, 1991.

[278] V. Sambucini. A Bayesian predictive two-stage design for phase II clinical trials. *Statistics in Medicine*, 27(8):1199–224, 2008.

[279] L. J. Savage. *The Foundations of Statistics*. Dover Publications, New York, 1972.

[280] H. Scheffé. *The Analysis of Variance*. Wiley, 1999.

[281] H. Schmidli, S. Gsteiger, S. Roychoudhury, A. O'Hagan, D. Spiegelhalter, and B. Neuenschwander. Robust meta-analytic-predictive priors in clinical trials with historical control information. *Biometrics*, 70(4):1023–1032, 2014.

[282] D. Schwartz and J. Lellouch. Explanatory and pragmatic attitudes in therapeutical trials. *Journal of Clinical Epidemiology*, 62(5):499–505, 2009.

[283] G. Schwarz. Estimating the dimension of a model. *Annals of Statistics*, 6(2):461–464, 1978.

[284] J. W. Seaman III, J. W. Seaman Jr., and J. D. Stamey. Hidden dangers of specifying noninformative priors. *The American Statistician*, 66(2):77–84, 2012.

[285] S. R. Searle. *Linear Models*. Wiley, New York, 1971.

[286] S. R. Searle, G. Casella, and C. E. McCulloch. *Variance Components*. Wiley, New York, 2009.

[287] P. Sebastiani and H. P. Wynn. Maximum entropy sampling and optimal Bayesian experimental design. *Journal of the Royal Statistical Society, Series B*, 62(1):145–157, 2000.

[288] SEER. Surveillance, Epidemiology and End Results program at seer.cancer.gov, 2011.

[289] SEER-Medicare. SEER-Medicare Linked Database at healthcaredelivery.cancer.gov/seermedicare, 2011.

[290] T. Sellke, M. J. Bayarri, and J. O. Berger. Calibration of p values for testing precise null hypotheses. *The American Statistician*, 55(1):62–71, 2001.

[291] J. Sethuraman. A constructive definition of Dirichlet priors. *Statistica Sinica*, 4(2):639–650, 1994.

[292] B. Shahbaba, S. Lan, W. O. Johnson, and R. M. Neal. Split Hamiltonian Monte Carlo. *Statistics and Computing*, 24(3):339–349, 2014.

[293] Y. Shi. *Weibull Mixture Models for Regression in the Context of Time-to-event Data.* Ph.D. Dissertation, Medical College of Wisconsin, Milwaukee, WI, 2017.

[294] Y. Shi. DPWeibull: Dirichlet process Weibull mixture model for survival data. *R-package Version 1.5*, 2020. https://CRAN.R-project.org/package=DPWeibull.

[295] Y. Shi, P. Laud, and J. Neuner. A dependent Dirichlet process model for survival data with competing risks. *Lifetime Data Analysis*, 2020.

[296] Y. Shi, M. Martens, A. Banerjee, and P. Laud. Low information omnibus (LIO) priors for Dirichlet process mixture models. *Bayesian Analysis*, 14(3):677–702, 2019.

[297] D. Sinha, J. G. Ibrahim, and M.-H. Chen. A Bayesian justification of Cox's partial likelihood. *Biometrika*, 90(3):629–641, 2003.

[298] P. J. Smith and T. J. Thompson. Correcting for confounding in analyzing receiver operating characteristic curves. *Biometrical Journal*, 38(7):857–863, 1996.

[299] G. W. Snedecor and W. G. Cochran. *Statistical Methods.* Iowa State University Press, Ames, 6th edition, 1967.

[300] R. Sparapani, B. R. Logan, R. E. McCulloch, and P. W. Laud. Nonparametric competing risks analysis using Bayesian additive regression trees. *Statistical Methods in Medical Research*, 29(1):57–77, 2020.

[301] R. Sparapani, C. Spanbauer, and R. McCulloch. Nonparametric machine learning and efficient computation with Bayesian additive regression trees: The BART R package. *Journal of Statistical Software*, 2019.

[302] R. A. Sparapani, B. R. Logan, R. E. McCulloch, and P. W. Laud. Nonparametric survival analysis using Bayesian additive regression trees (BART). *Statistics in Medicine*, 35(16):2741–2753, 2016.

[303] R. A. Sparapani, L. E. Rein, S. S. Tarima, T. A. Jackson, and J. R. Meurer. Non-parametric recurrent events analysis with BART and an application to the hospital admissions of patients with diabetes. *Biostatistics*, 21(1):69–85, 2020.

[304] D. J. Spiegelhalter, N. G. Best, B. R. Carlin, and A. van der Linde. Bayesian measures of model complexity and fit. *Journal of the Royal Statistical Society, Series B*, 64(4):583–616, 2002.

[305] D. J. Spiegelhalter and L. S. Freedman. A predictive approach to selecting the size of a clinical trial, based on subjective clinical opinion. *Statistics in Medicine*, 5(1):1–13, 1986.

[306] D. J. Spiegelhalter, L. S. Freedman, and P. R. Blackburn. Monitoring clinical trials: Conditional or predictive power? *Controlled Clinical Trials*, 7(1):8–17, 1986.

[307] D. J. Spiegelhalter, L. S. Freedman, and M. K. Parmar. Applying Bayesian ideas in drug development and clinical trials. *Statistics in Medicine*, 12(15–16):1501–1511; discussion 1513–1517, 1993.

[308] D. J. Spiegelhalter, L. S. Freedman, and M. K. B. Parmar. Bayesian approaches to randomized trials. *Journal of the Royal Statistical Society, Series A*, 157:357–387, 1994.

[309] N. Stallard, P. F. Thall, and J. Whitehead. Decision theoretic designs for phase II clinical trials with multiple outcomes. *Biometrics*, 55(3):971–977, 1999.

[310] P. Strazzullo, S. M. Kerry, A. Barbato, M. Versiero, L. D'Elia, and F. P. Cappuccio. Do statins reduce blood pressure? *Hypertension*, 49(4):792–798, 2007.

[311] J. R. Stroud, P. Müller, and G. L. Rosner. Optimal sampling times in population pharmacokinetic studies. *Applied Statistics*, 50(3):345–359, 2001.

[312] W. W. Stroup. *Generalized Linear Mixed Models: Modern Concepts, Methods and Applications*. CRC Press, Boca Raton, FL, 2012.

[313] V. Susarla and J. Van Ryzin. Nonparametric Bayesian estimation of survival curves from incomplete observations. *Journal of the American Statistical Association*, 71(356):897–902, 1976.

[314] S. B. Tan and D. Machin. Bayesian two-stage designs for phase II clinical trials. *Statistics in Medicine*, 21(14):1991–2012, 2002.

[315] P. Thall, P. Fox, and J. Wathen. Statistical controversies in clinical research: Scientific and ethical problems with adaptive randomization in comparative clinical trials. *Annals of Oncology*, 26(8):1621–1628, 2015.

[316] P. F. Thall and J. D. Cook. Dose-finding based on efficacy-toxicity trade-offs. *Biometrics*, 60(3):684–693, 2004.

[317] P. F. Thall, R. E. Millikan, P. Mueller, and S. J. Lee. Dose-finding with two agents in phase I oncology trials. *Biometrics*, 59(3):487–496, 2003.

[318] P. F. Thall and K. E. Russell. A strategy for dose-finding and safety monitoring based on efficacy and adverse outcomes in phase I/II clinical trials. *Biometrics*, 54(1):251–64, 1998.

[319] P. F. Thall and R. Simon. A Bayesian approach to establishing sample-size and monitoring criteria for phase II clinical trials. *Controlled Clinical Trials*, 15(6):463–481, 1994.

[320] P. F. Thall and R. Simon. Practical Bayesian guidelines for phase IIB clinical-trials. *Biometrics*, 50(2):337–349, 1994.

[321] P. F. Thall and S. C. Vail. Some covariance-models for longitudinal count data with overdispersion. *Biometrics*, 46(3):657–671, 1990.

[322] P. F. Thall and J. K. Wathen. Practical Bayesian adaptive randomisation in clinical trials. *European Journal of Cancer*, 43(5):859–866, 2007.

[323] The GUSTO Investigators. An international randomized trial comparing four thrombolytic strategies for acute myocardial infarction. *New England Journal of Medicine*, 329(10):673–682, 1993.

[324] P. Therasse, S. G. Arbuck, E. A. Eisenhauer, J. Wanders, R. S. Kaplan, L. Rubinstein, J. Verweij, M. Van Glabbeke, A. T. van Oosterom, M. C. Christian, and S. G. Gwyther. New guidelines to evaluate the response to treatment in solid tumors. *JNCI: Journal of the National Cancer Institute*, 92(3):205–216, 2000.

[325] M. V. Thomas, A. Branscum, C. S. Miller, J. Ebersole, M. Al-Sabbagh, and J. L. Schuster. Within-subject variability in repeated measures of salivary analytes in healthy adults. *Journal of Periodontology*, 80(7):1146–1153, 2009.

[326] M. C. Thurmond, W. O. Johnson, C. A. Muñoz-Zanzi, C.-L. Su, and S. K. Hietala. A method of probability diagnostic assignment that applies Bayes theorem for use in serologic diagnostics, using an example of *Neospora caninum* infection in cattle. *American Journal of Veterinary Research*, 63(3):318–325, 2002.

[327] L. Tierney. Markov chains for exploring posterior distributions. *Annals of Statistics*, 22:1701–1728 (discussion 1728–1762), 1994.

[328] L. Tierney and J. B. Kadane. Accurate approximations for posterior moments and marginal densities. *Journal of the American Statistical Association*, 81(393):82–86, 1986.

[329] L. Tierney, R. E. Kass, and J. B. Kadane. Approximate marginal densities of nonlinear functions. *Biometrika*, 76(3):425–433, 1989.

[330] M. Tighiouart, A. Rogatko, and J. S. Babb. Flexible Bayesian methods for cancer phase I clinical trials. Dose escalation with overdose control. *Statistics in Medicine*, 24(14):2183–96, 2005.

[331] L. Trippa, G. L. Rosner, and P. Mueller. Bayesian enrichment strategies for randomized discontinuation trials. *Biometrics*, 68(1):203–211, 2012.

[332] A. Tsiatis. A nonidentifiability aspect of the problem of competing risks. *Proceedings of the National Academy of Sciences of the United States of America*, 72(1):20–22, 1975.

[333] A. A. Tsiatis. The asymptotic joint distribution of the efficient scores test for the proportional hazards model calculated over time. *Biometrika*, 68(1):311–315, 1981.

[334] B. W. Turnbull and L. Weiss. A likelihood ratio statistic for testing goodness of fit with randomly censored data. *Biometrics*, 34(3):367–375, 1978.

[335] F. Tuyl, R. Gerlach, and K. Mengersen. A comparison of Bayes-Laplace, Jeffreys, and other priors: The case of zero events. *The American Statistician*, 62(1):40–44, 2008.

[336] F. Tuyl, R. Gerlach, and K. Mengersen. Posterior predictive arguments in favor of the Bayes-Laplace prior as the consensus prior for binomial and multinomial parameters. *Bayesian Analysis*, 4(1):151–158, 2009.

[337] J. Utts. Replication and meta-analysis in parapsychology (with discussion). *Statistical Science*, 6:363–403, 1991.

[338] J. Utts and R. Heckard. *Mind on Statistics, 5th Edition*. Brooks-Cole/ Cengage Learning, Boston, 2015.

[339] J. Utts, M. Norris, E. Suess, and W. Johnson. The strength of evidence versus the power of belief: Are we all Bayesians? In C. Reading, editor, *Data and Context in Statistics Education: Towards an Evidence-Based Society. Proceedings of the Eighth International Conference on Teaching Statistics*, Voorburg, 2010. International Statistical Institute.

[340] S. Ventz, M. Cellamare, S. Bacallado, and L. Trippa. Bayesian uncertainty directed trial designs. *Journal of the American Statistical Association*, 114(527):962–974, 2018.

[341] S. Ventz and L. Trippa. Bayesian designs and the control of frequentist characteristics: A practical solution. *Biometrics*, 71(1):218–226, 2015.

[342] S. G. Walker, P. Damien, P. W. Laud, and A. F. M. Smith. Bayesian nonparametric inference for random distributions and related functions. *Journal of the Royal Statistical Society, Series B*, 61(3):485–527, 1999.

[343] F. Wang and A. E. Gelfand. A simulation-based approach to Bayesian sample size determination for performance under a given model and for separating models. *Statistical Science*, 17(2):193–208, 2002.

[344] J. H. Ware. Investigating therapies of potentially great benefit: ECMO. *Statistical Science*, 4(4):298–306, 1989.

[345] R. L. Wasserstein and N. A. Lazar. The ASA statement on p-values: Context, process, and purpose. *The American Statistician*, 70(10):129–133, 2016.

[346] S. Watanabe. Asymptotic equivalence of Bayes cross validation and widely applicable information criterion in singular learning theory. *Journal of Machine Learning Research*, 11:3571–3594, 2010.

[347] J. K. Wathen and P. F. Thall. A simulation study of outcome adaptive randomization in multi-arm clinical trials. *Clinical Trials*, 14(5):432–440, 2017.

[348] L. J. Wei. An application of an urn model to the design of sequential controlled clinical trials. *Journal of the American Statistical Association*, 73(363):559–563, 1978.

[349] L. J. Wei. The generalized Polya's urn design for sequential medical trials. *Annals of Statistics*, 7(2):291–296, 1979.

[350] D. A. Weiner, T. J. Ryan, C. H. McCabe, J. W. Kennedy, M. Schloss, F. Tristani, B. R. Chaitman, and L. D. Fisher. Exercise stress testing: Correlations among history of angina, st-segment response and prevalence of coronary-artery disease in the Coronary Artery Surgery Study (CASS). *New England Journal of Medicine*, 301(5):230–235, 1979.

[351] S. Weisberg. *Applied Linear Regression*. John Wiley & Sons, Hoboken, NJ, 2005.

[352] R. Wetzels, R. P. P. P. Grasman, and E.-J. Wagenmakers. A default Bayesian hypothesis test for ANOVA designs. *The American Statistician*, 66(2):104–111, 2012.

[353] J. Whittle, M. M. Schapira, K. E. Fletcher, A. Hayes, J. Morzinski, P. Laud, D. Eastwood, K. Ertl, L. Patterson, and K. E. Mosack. A randomized trial of peer-delivered self-management support for hypertension. *American Journal of Hypertension*, 27(11):1416–1423, 2014.

[354] P. Wild and W. R. Gilks. Algorithm AS 287: Adaptive rejection sampling from log-concave density functions. *Applied Statistics*, 42:701–708, 1993.

[355] J. D. Wright, J. P. Hughes, Y. Ostchega, S. S. Yoon, and T. Nwankwo. Mean systolic and diastolic blood pressure in adults aged 18 and over in the united states, 2001–2008. Technical report, National Center for Health Statistics, Hyattsville, MD: National Center for Health Statistics., 2011.

[356] T. W. Yen, X. Fan, R. Sparapani, P. W. Laud, A. P. Walker, and A. B. Nattinger. A contemporary, population-based study of lymphedema risk factors in older women with breast cancer. *Annals of Surgical Oncology*, 16(4):979–988, 2009.

[357] Y. Yuan, H. Q. Nguyen, and P. F. Thall. *Bayesian Designs for Phase I-II Clinical Trials*. CRC Press, Boca Raton, FL, 2016.

[358] Y. Yuan and G. Yin. Bayesian phase I/II adaptively randomized oncology trials with combined drugs. *Annals of Applied Statistics*, 5:924–942, 2011.

[359] S. L. Zeger and M. R. Karim. Generalized linear models with random effects: A Gibbs sampling approach. *Journal of the American Statistical Association*, 86(413):79–86, 1991.

[360] M. Zelen. Play the winner rule and the controlled clinical trial. *Journal of the American Statistical Association*, 64(325):131–146, 1969.

[361] A. Zellner. On assessing prior distributions and Bayesian regression analysis with g-prior distributions. In P. K. Goel and A. Zellner, editors, *Bayesian Inference and Decision Techniques: Essays in Honor of Bruno de Finetti*, pages 233–243. North-Holland, Amsterdam, 1986.

[362] J. Zhang, N. Yoganandan, F. A. Pintar, Y. Guan, B. Shender, G. Paskoff, and P. Laud. Effects of tissue preservation temperature on high strain-rate material properties of brain. *Journal of Biomechanics*, 44(3):391–396, 2011.

[363] L. Zhang, K. H. Yang, and A. I. King. A proposed injury threshold for mild traumatic brain injury. *Journal of Biomechanical Engineering*, 126:226–236, 2004.

[364] H. Zhou and T. Hanson. A unified framework for fitting Bayesian semiparametric models to arbitrarily censored survival data, including spatially referenced data. *Journal of the American Statistical Association*, 113(522):571–581, 2018.

[365] H. Zhou and T. Hanson. spBayesSurv: Bayesian modeling and analysis of spatially correlated survival data. *R-package Version 1.1.4*, 2020. https://CRAN.R-project.org/package=spBayesSurv.

Index

Printed in the United States
By Bookmasters